Pharmacodynamic Models of Selected Toxic Chemicals in Man

Volume 1: Review of Metabolic Data

Pharmacodynamic Models of Selected Toxic Chemicals in Man

Volume 1: Review of Metabolic Data

Prepared for the
Directorate-General of Employment,
Social Affairs and Education
of the Commission of the European Communities

by
M. C. Thorne, D. Jackson
and A. D. Smith

Associated Nuclear Services
60 East Street, Epsom, Surrey, England

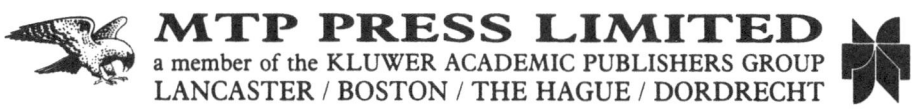

MTP PRESS LIMITED
a member of the KLUWER ACADEMIC PUBLISHERS GROUP
LANCASTER / BOSTON / THE HAGUE / DORDRECHT

for the Commission of the European Communities

Published in the UK and Europe by
MTP Press Limited
Falcon House
Lancaster, England

British Library Cataloguing in Publication Data
Thorne, M. C.
  Pharmacodynamic models of selected toxic
  chemicals in man.
  1. Toxicology—Methodology
  2. Chemicals—Physiological effect
  3. Pharmacokinetics
  I. Title   II. Jackson, D.   III. Smith,A. D.
  615.9'07   RA1199

ISBN-13: 978-94-010-8348-5

Published in the USA by
MTP Press
A division of Kluwer Boston Inc.
101 Philip Drive
Norwell, MA 02061, USA

Library of Congress Cataloging-in-Publication Data
Thorne, M. C.
  Pharmacodynamic models of selected toxic
  chemicals in man.

  (ANS report; no. 512-2)
  Includes bibliographies and index.
  Contents: v. 1. Review of metabolic data—
  v. 2. Routes of intake and implementation of
  pharmacodynamic models/A. D. Smith and M. C. Thorne.
  1. Carcinogens—Metabolism.   2. Pharmacokinetics.
  3. Carcinogens—Metabolism—Mathematical models.
  I. Jackson, D.   II. Smith, A. D. (Anthony David)
  III. Title.   IV. Series. [DNLM: 1. Models, Chemical.
  2. Poisons—pharmacodynamics.   QV 600 T511p]
  RC268.6.S65   1986   616.99'4071   86-124

ISBN 978-94-010-8348-5   ISBN 978-94-009-4163-2 (eBook)
DOI 10.1007/978-94-009-4163-2

EUR 10409

Publication arranged by
Commission of the European Communities
Directorate-General Telecommunications,
Information Industries and Innovation,
Luxembourg

Contents

Preface

These volumes present the results of two studies undertaken for the Directorate General of Employment, Social Affairs and Education of the Commission of the European Communities. The aim was to review available data concerning the metabolism of a selection of toxic chemicals in man and to develop mathematical models representing this metabolism. Volume 1 is the report from the first study and presents reviews of the data for each of the substances and proposes models for their metabolic behaviour. Volume 2 is the report of the second study and contains a review of new data relevant to the development of metabolic models for each substance. The modelling of uptake and retention by the two major routes of uptake (the respiratory system and the gastrointestinal tract) is also reviewed. The implementation of the models in a computer code is described and results are presented illustrating organ concentrations and rates of excretion for typical regimes of exposure.

1
Foreword

This report contains the results of a study undertaken by Associated Nuclear Services (ANS) for the Directorate General of Employment, Social Affairs and Education of the Commission of the European Communities (CEC). This study was entitled "Models for the Metabolism of Chemical Carcinogens in Man".

2
Summary

This report includes results of a review of the metabolism of selected actual and potential human carcinogens and proposals for pharmacokinetic models to represent that metabolism. It is thought that these models, and the reviews upon which they are based, will provide information relevant to the development of monitoring programmes for these various substances and in the interpretation of dose-response data obtained under different exposure regimes and as a result of different routes of administration.

The substances included in this review comprise arsenic, beryllium, cadmium, lead, nickel, chromium, asbestos, benzene, vinyl chloride monomer, benzidine and its congeners, carbon tetrachloride and methyl iodide. For all of these, except benzidine and carbon tetrachloride, it has proved possible to develop pharmacokinetic models relevant to some aspects of their metabolism.

In the main report, these various models are described together with comments on the limits of their applicability. The detailed reviews upon which these models are based and which contain collateral information of interest are presented as a series of appendices.

3
Introduction

There are numerous naturally occurring and man-made substances which can be toxic to man, including elements, small organic molecules and fibrous materials such as asbestos. In recent years, particular attention has been directed to those substances which can elicit a carcinogenic response in animals or man and this has led to comprehensive reviews of the evidence for such a carcinogenic response in a wide range of materials (International Agency for Research on Cancer, 1982).

Once a material has been identified as toxic, and, in particular, potentially carcinogenic, to man, there is a requirement to limit exposure to the substance such that the risks attendant upon exposure are eliminated, or reduced to an acceptable level. In some cases, this can be done by eliminating utilisation of the material, but this is not always possible, for one of several reasons.

-   The material may be ubiquitous in the environment and may be an essential trace element for human metabolism, e.g. arsenic or nickel.
-   The material may be of major economic significance for an industrial economy and not be replacable with an acceptable alternative, e.g. vinyl chloride monomer.

-   The substance may be used in structural materials and demolition may constitute a substantial hazard, e.g. asbestos.

In these circumstances, it is necessary to set levels limiting exposure to the substance and to monitor that these levels are being achieved. Such levels may be set in terms of limiting air concentrations of the substance; limiting concentrations of the substance or its derivatives in monitorable materials such as urine, faeces, blood or exhaled air; or limiting physiological effects of the substance, such as changes in serum enzyme levels.

In formulating such standards, recourse has to be made to toxicity data derived from case reports, epidemiological studies and animal experiments.   However, these data may be only related indirectly to the types of exposure conditions which are currently occurring, or are projected as likely to occur in the future.   In these circumstances, it is necessary to develop models to relate currently available information to the quantities of interest. Broadly, two types of model need to be considered.

-   Toxicological models which relate exposure to effect, at the whole body, tissue, cellular or molecular level.

-   Pharmacokinetic models which relate exposure to a substance to levels of that substance, its derivatives, or other induced substances, in tissues, tissue components and excreta.

The present report deals only with pharmacokinetic models.   It is emphasised that while such models form a component of toxicological models they are, in general, not sufficient for the development of such models, which also require a detailed knowledge of the processes which control the toxic response. Also, the present report is primarily concerned with pharmacokinetic models for human metabolism, though a considerable number of data are also included on pharmacokinetics in animals. It is emphasised that the development of toxicological models on the basis of animal experimentation requires a sound knowledge of differences in the pharmacokinetics of the substance in different animal species, at different dose levels and by different routes of exposure or administration.

The models developed are directed to three applications.

-   Relation of intakes of a substance to time-dependent concentrations of that substance, its derivatives, or other induced substances, in various target organs and tissues of the body.

-   Relation of intakes of a substance to time-dependent concentrations or amounts of that substance, its derivatives, or other induced substances, in potentially monitorable materials such as urine, faeces, blood and expired air.

-   Relation of concentrations, or amounts, of the substance, its derivatives, or other induced materials, in potentially monitorable materials, to concentrations of the substance, or its derivatives, in target organs or tissues.

Because of limitations in the data, it has not proved possible to develop models that satisfy all these applications for all the substances considered.

The report consists of two main sections and a series of appendices.   Section 4 is concerned with general information relevant to several of the models.   Thus, it includes information on generalised models appropriate to the lung and gastrointestinal tract.   Section 5 contains a brief summary of the various models which have been developed in the course of the study.

There are twelve appendices to the report.   Each consists of a review of a particular substance.   The appendices are as follows.

Appendix	Substance
1	Arsenic
2	Beryllium
3	Cadmium
4	Lead
5	Nickel
6	Chromium
7	Asbestos
8	Benzene
9	Vinyl chloride
10	Benzidine
11	Carbon tetrachloride
12	Methyl iodide

Each appendix contains information on the physical and chemical properties of the substance, its production and uses, its effects and its metabolism. As appropriate, the appendices also contain pharmacokinetic models and illustrative calculations made using those models. As far as possible, the reviews, and the models based on them, have been directed towards the problem of assessing, and quantifying the importance of, factors such as:

- different routes of exposure;

- effects of age, state of health, quantity of chemical administered and dietary status;

- possible effects of medical intervention at high levels of exposure.

Whilst it has generally been possible to make qualitative comments on these matters, it has not been possible, in all cases, to incorporate them in the models.

4
General Considerations

There are two aspects of the models which are general to several of the substances considered. These are:

- the gastrointestinal tract model for the metals and metalloids;
- the lung model for the metals.

In addition, it is noted that four of the organic substances considered, viz. benzene, vinyl chloride monomer, benzidine and its congeners, and carbon tetrachloride, are metabolised by the mixed function oxidase system. Thus, a brief note on this system is also included as background information.

4.1   The gastrointestinal tract model

A specific gastrointestinal tract model has not been developed for the purpose of this study. Instead, it is recommended that the model set out by the International Commission on Radiological Protection (1979) in its recommendations on limiting exposure of workers to radioactive materials be used. This model, which is a compartmental model with constant rate coefficients, is set out in Fig. 1.

4.2   The lung model

A generalised lung model is recommended for compounds of beryllium, cadmium, lead, nickel and chromium. This model is that recommended by the International Commission on Radiological Protection (1979) and is illustrated in Fig. 2. The lung is divided into four main regions:

- the nasal passages (NP);

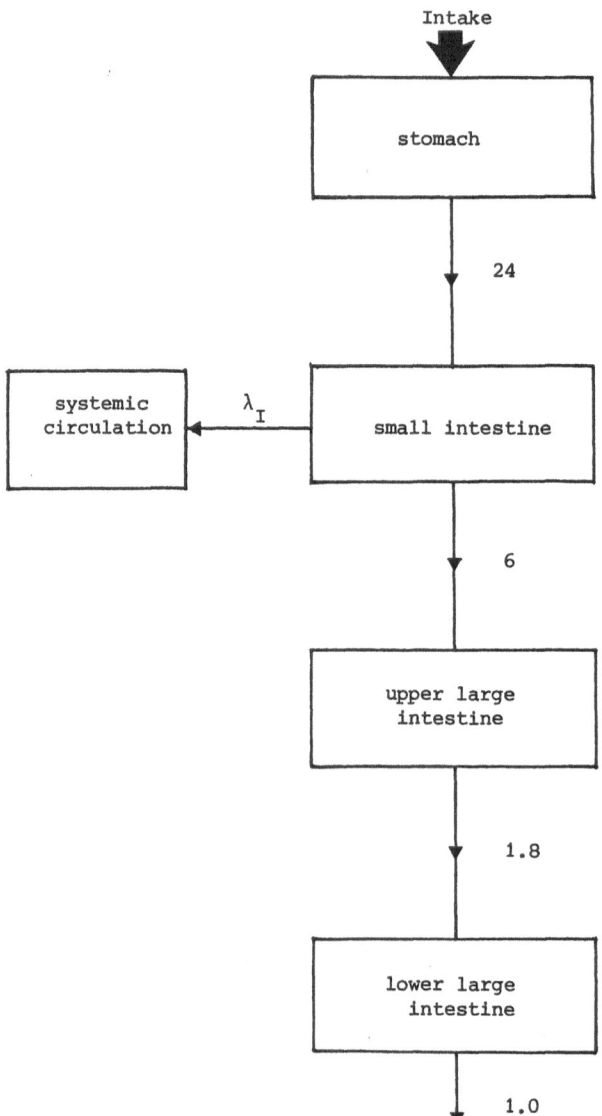

Notes: Rate contants given in units of d^{-1} .
        The value of λ_I can be calculated using

$$\lambda_I = 6f_1/(1-f_1)$$

where f_1 is the fractional absorption of the substance
from the gastrointestinal tract. If f_1 is unity, the
substance can be considered to go directly from the
stomach to the systemic circulation with a rate coefficient
of 24 d^{-1} .
From International Commission on Radiological Protection (1979).

FIGURE 1. THE GENERAL GASTROINTESTINAL TRACT MODEL FOR THE METALS AND
           METALLOIDS.

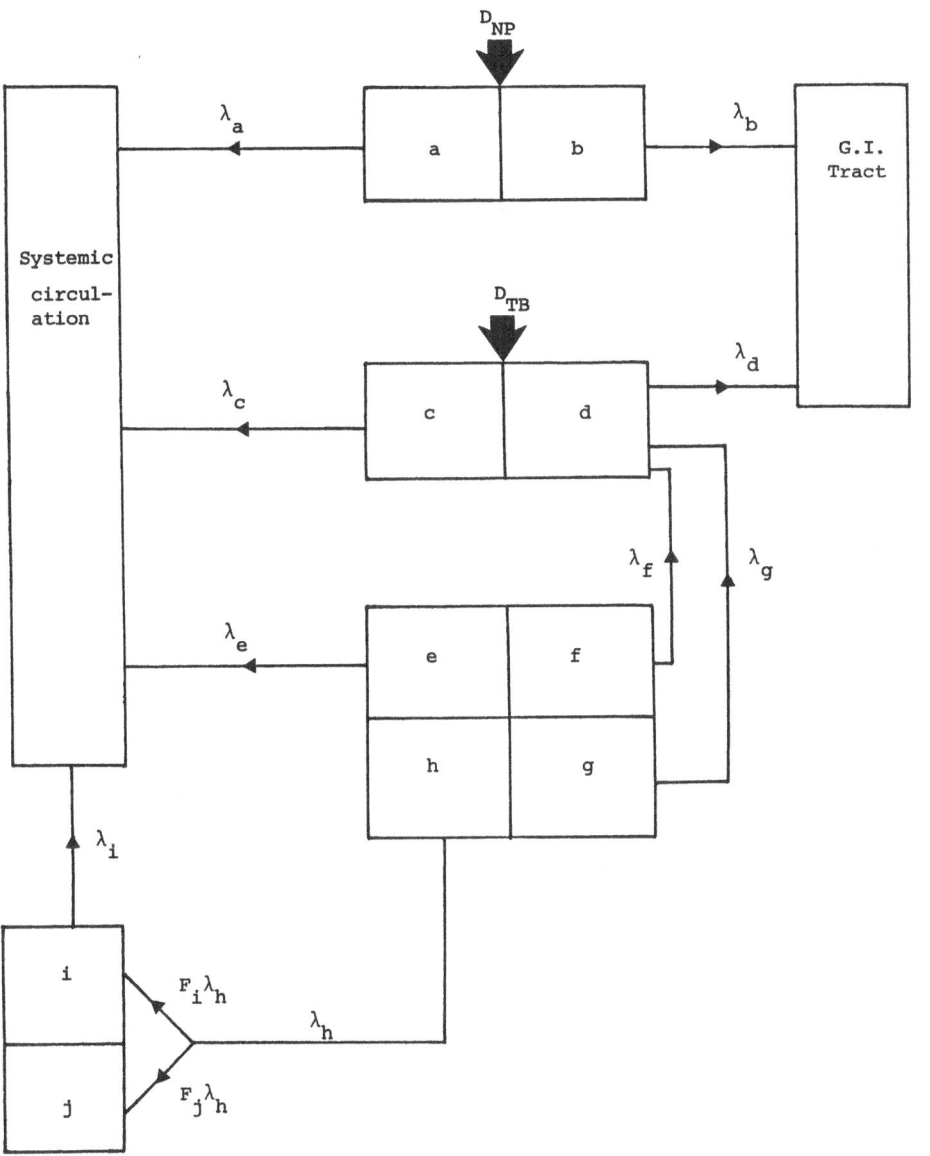

Note: Adapted from the International Commission on Radiological Protection (1979

FIGURE 2.   MATHEMATICAL MODEL TO DESCRIBE CLEARANCE FROM THE RESPIRATORY
SYSTEM.

-   the trachea and bronchii (TB);
-   the pulmonary region (P); and
-   the pulmonary lymph nodes (LN).

Deposition is to the NP, TB and P regions, with the fractional deposition of inhaled material in each being determined by the mass median aerodynamic diameter (MMAD) of the aerosol inhaled (see Fig. 3).   Partition of this deposition between the individual compartments within a particular region and the rates of clearance from those compartments are determined by the chemical characteristics of the inhaled aerosol.   Thus, overall, the model is characterised by the following set of first-order differential equations.

$$\frac{d}{dt}\, q_a(t) = I(t).D_{NP}.F_a - \lambda_a q_a(t)$$

$$\frac{d}{dt}\, q_b(t) = I(t).D_{NP}.F_b - \lambda_b q_b(t)$$

$$\frac{d}{dt}\, q_c(t) = I(t).D_{TB}.F_c - \lambda_c q_c(t)$$

$$\frac{d}{dt}\, q_d(t) = I(t).D_{TB}.F_d + \lambda_f q_f(t) + \lambda_g q_g(t) - \lambda_d q_d(t)$$

$$\frac{d}{dt}\, q_e(t) = I(t).D_P.F_e - \lambda_e q_e(t)$$

$$\frac{d}{dt}\, q_f(t) = I(t).D_P.F_f - \lambda_f q_f(t)$$

$$\frac{d}{dt}\, q_g(t) = I(t).D_P.F_g - \lambda_g q_g(t)$$

$$\frac{d}{dt}\, q_h(t) = I(t).D_P.F_h - \lambda_h q_h(t)$$

$$\frac{d}{dt}\, q_i(t) = F_i \lambda_h q_h(t) - \lambda_i q_i(t)$$

$$\frac{d}{dt}\, q_j(t) = F_j \lambda_h q_h(t)$$

where $I(t)$ is the rate of intake of material;

D_{NP}, D_{TB} and D_P are the fractional depositions in the regions of the lung, as shown in Fig. 3;

F_a to F_j are the partition fractions between the various compartments; and

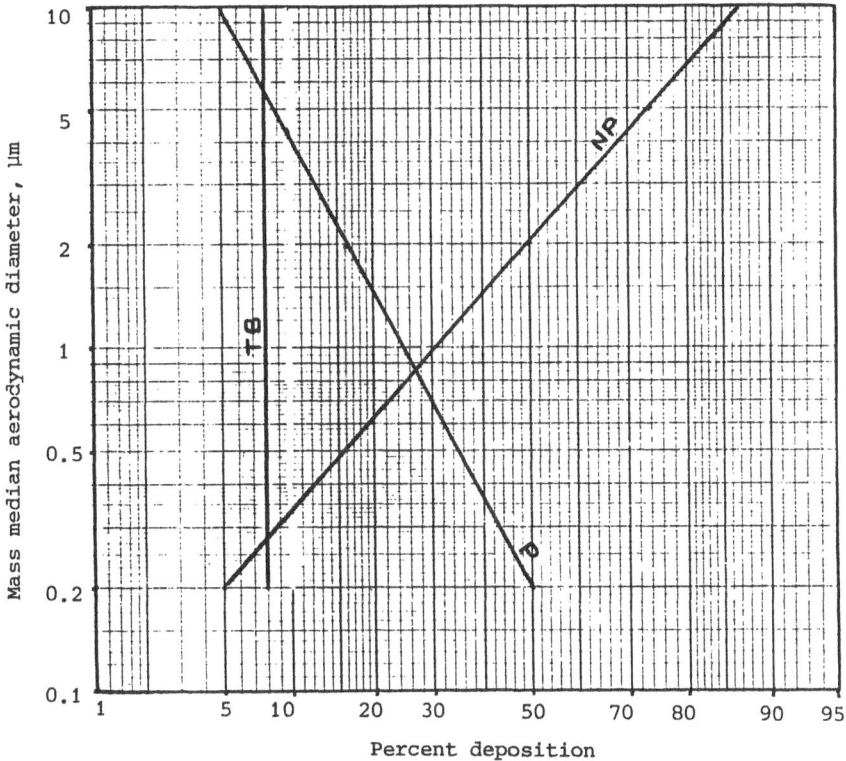

Percent deposition

Notes: The percentage of activity or mass of an aerosol which
         is deposited in the N-P, T-B and P regions is given in
         relation to the mass median aerodynamic diameter (MMAD)
         of the aerosol distribution. The model is intended for
         use with aerosol distributions with MMADs between 0.2
         and 10μm and with geometric standard deviation of less
         than 4.5.
         Adapted from the International Commission on Radiological
         Protection (1979).

FIGURE 3.   DEPOSITION OF DUST IN THE RESPIRATORY SYSTEM.

TABLE 1

PARAMETERS VALUES FOR THE LUNG MODEL

Compartment	Class					
	D		W		Y	
	F	λ (d^{-1})	F	λ (d^{-1})	F	λ (d^{-1})
a	0.5	69.3	0.1	69.3	0.01	69.3
b	0.5	69.3	0.9	1.73	0.99	1.73
c	0.95	69.3	0.5	69.3	0.01	69.3
d	0.05	3.47	0.5	3.47	0.99	3.47
e	0.8	1.39	0.15	0.0139	0.05	0.00139
f	-	-	0.4	0.693	0.4	0.693
g	-	-	0.4	0.0139	0.4	0.00139
h	0.2	1.39	0.05	0.0139	0.15	0.00139
i	1.0	1.39	1.0	0.0139	0.9	0.000693
j	-	-	-	-	0.1	0.000693

Note:

Based on values given by the International Commission on Radiological Protection (1979).

λ_a to λ_i are the rate coefficients, as shown in Fig. 2.

Values of F_a to F_i and λ_a to λ_i are defined according to the chemical form of the substance. Three classes of materials are used; D, W and Y. These correspond to clearance from the lung in periods of the order days, weeks and years respectively. Values of F_a to F_i and λ_a to λ_i for these three classes of materials are given in Table 1.

4.3   The mixed function oxidase system

The mixed function oxidase system is an enzyme system resident on the endoplasmic reticulum, particularly in cells of the liver. It is a general purpose system for the detoxification of a wide variety of substances by means of oxidation reactions. There are a large number of reviews covering the operation of this system and the reader is referred to those of Snyder and Remmer (1979), Powis and Jansson (1979), Mansuy (1981), and Philpot and Wolf (1981) for recent accounts.

A general scheme for the mechanism of the mixed function oxidase system is presented in Fig. 4. The system is driven by single electron transfers from the reduced form of nicotinamide adenine dinucleotide phosphate (NADP) which is designated NADPH, or the reduced form of nicotinamide adenine dinucleotide (NADH). The key points to note about the system are that it requires the presence of NADPH to operate, hence the need for a NADPH generating system in in vitro studies; that the enzyme system can be induced by a wide range of drugs (see Snyder and Remmer, 1979); and that the system can oxidise a wide range of substrates, including benzene, vinyl chloride monomer, benzidine and its congeners, and carbon tetrachloride. Thus, many of the experimental studies reported concerning these substances are really experiments on the mixed function oxidase system.

In general, as previously noted, this system serves as a detoxification process. However, in the cases of all four substances noted above, the substrate is thought to be biologically inert and it is the mixed function oxidase system which produces the active metabolite, in the form of an epoxide, a CCl_3 radical, or a derivative of one of these. In such cases, the active metabolite is produced local to the mixed function oxidase system and may react with it, suppressing or destroying its activity. It seems that this mechanism is probably responsible for the dose-dependent kinetics recorded for several of the substances reviewed in this study.

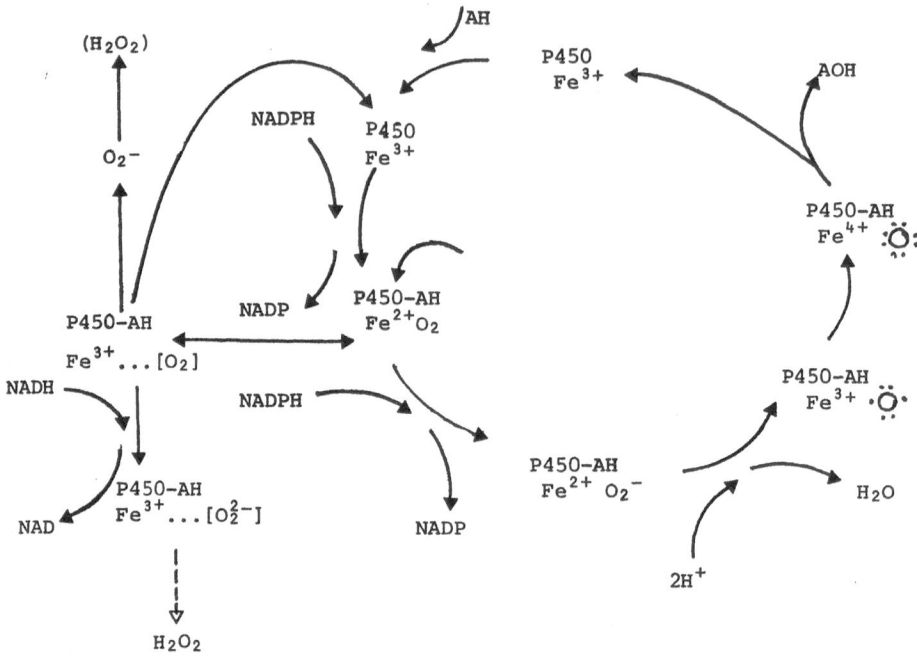

Notes: Derived from Powis and Jannson (1979).
          AH is the substrate and AOH the oxidised form:
          P450 represents cytochrome P450 in its various oxidation
          states.
          NAD represents nicotinamide adenine dinucleotide.
          NADP represents nicotinamide adenine dinucleotide phosphate.
          The NADPH-NADP reaction involves NADPH-cytochrome P450
          reductase, while the NADH-NAD reaction involves NADH-
          cytochrome b_5 reductase and cytochrome b_5 as an electron
          carrier.

FIGURE 4. MECHANISM OF THE MIXED FUNCTION OXIDASE SYSTEM.

5
Metabolic Models

The metabolic models developed in this study are summarised below. For a detailed justification, and illustrative calculations, the reader is referred to the appropriate appendix.

5.1   Arsenic

5.1.1   Fractional gastrointestinal absorption

A value of 0.5 to 1.0 can be used for most compounds of the element. Exceptions are arsenilic acid and arsenic trioxide in solid form. For arsenilic acid a best estimate value is 0.3. For solid arsenic trioxide no value can be recommended, since the degree of absorption will be strongly dependent on particle size and the pH of the gastric juice.

5.1.2   Retention in, and translocation from, the lung

The following define a model for arsenic retention in, and translocation from, the lungs.

-   The deposition of arsenic containing aerosols in the lungs is similar to that of other aerosols.

-   In deeply inhaling smokers, ∿10% of arsenic incorporated in cigarettes will be deposited in the lungs.

-   All compounds of arsenic which have been studied have been found to be cleared from the lungs with a half-life of a few days; a biphasic model in which 75% of deposited material is cleared with a half-life of 4 days and 25% is cleared with a half-life of 10 days is recommended as appropriate to man.

-   Virtually all arsenic translocated from the lungs enters the blood either directly or via the gastrointestinal tract.

-   A fraction of 0.6 of inhaled arsine can be assumed to be virtually instantaneously absorbed from the lungs, with the residual fraction being exhaled.

5.1.3   Retention in the body

Most compounds of arsenic exhibit an early phase of rapid excretion and considerable methylation of arsenic occurs within the body. Data on distribution and retention in man are relatively limited, but the following functions appear to give a reasonable model for the retention of arsenic following entry of a unit quantity of the element into the systemic circulation:

$$R_{LIVER}(t) = 0.16 \ e^{-1.54t} + 0.025 \ e^{-0.014t} + 0.013 \ e^{-0.0005t}$$

$$R_{KIDNEY}(t) = 0.03 \ e^{-1.54t} + 0.005 \ e^{-0.014t} + 0.002 \ e^{-0.0005t}$$

$$R_{OTHER}(t) = 0.06 \ e^{-1.54t} + 0.47 \ e^{-0.014t} + 0.235 \ e^{-0.0005t}$$

where t is in hours.

Summing these retention functions gives:

$$R_{WHOLE \ BODY}(t) = 0.25 \ e^{-1.54t} + 0.5 \ e^{-0.014t} + 0.25 \ e^{-0.0005t}$$

and differentiating gives the total rate of excretion;

$$E = 38.5 \ e^{-1.54t} + 0.7 \ e^{-0.014t} + 0.0125 \ e^{-0.0005t} \ \% \ h^{-1}$$

for activity injected directly into the systemic circulation. This excretion can be assumed to be entirely in urine. For man, the dynamics of arsenic excretion in urine are better defined than those for loss in blood or hair, and urinary monitoring is the preferred method of assay with respect to occupational exposure. Post-mortem hair samples may be useful in retrospective analysis of arsenic exposure, but more work is required before these can be unambiguously interpreted in terms of the time course of such exposure. Data quantifying transfer of arsenic to, and across, the human placenta are not available, though this process is known to occur.

5.2   Beryllium

5.2.1   Fractional gastrointestinal absorption

For the purpose of modelling, the fractional gastrointestinal absorption of all compounds of beryllium can be taken as 0.005.

5.2.2   <u>Retention in, and translocation from, the lung</u>

For retention in, and translocation from, the lung it is appropriate to use the ICRP lung model, but changing the long-term component of class W retention from a 50 to a 100 day half-life. With this modification, beryllium sulphate can be assigned to inhalation class W, whereas compounds of beryllium which are present in colloidal or particulate form, such as the phosphate and oxide, as well as ores such as beryl and bertrandite, should be assigned to inhalation class Y. Beryllium citrate should probably be assigned to class D, but exposure to this compound is unlikely to be a significant practical problem.

5.2.3   <u>Systemic metabolism</u>

Following instantaneous entry of a unit quanitity of beryllium into the systemic circulation, the following retention functions can be taken to apply:

$$R_{WHOLE\ BODY}(t) = 0.4\ e^{-2.0t} + 0.16\ e^{-0.046t} + 0.44\ e^{-0.00046t}$$

$$R_{BONE}(t) = 0.03\ e^{-2.0t} + 0.35\ e^{-0.00046t}$$

$$R_{LIVER}(t) = 0.01\ e^{-2.0t} + 0.03\ e^{-0.046t} + 0.01\ e^{-0.00046t}$$

$$R_{KIDNEY}(t) = 0.002\ e^{-2.0t} + 0.03\ e^{-0.046t} + 0.01\ e^{-0.00046t}$$

$$R_{MUSCLE}(t) = 0.16\ e^{-2.0t} + 0.02\ e^{-0.046t} + 0.03\ e^{-0.00046t}$$

$$R_{OTHER}(t) = 0.198\ e^{-2.0t} + 0.08\ e^{-0.046t} + 0.04\ e^{-0.00046t}$$

where t is time in days.

5.2.4   <u>Excretion</u>

Following the instantaneous entry of a quantity of beryllium into the systemic circulation, the time dependence of urinary and faecal excretion can be taken to be described by:

$$E_u(t) = 64\ e^{-2.0t} + 0.41\ e^{-0.046t} + 0.011\ e^{-0.00046t}$$

$$E_f(t) = 16\ e^{-2.0t} + 0.33\ e^{-0.046t} + 0.009\ e^{-0.00046t}$$

where

$E_u(t)$ is the urinary excretion rate (% introduced beryllium d^{-1});

$E_f(t)$ is the faecal excretion rate (% introduced beryllium d^{-1}); and

    t is time in days.

5.2.5   Skin absorption

Absorption of beryllium through the intact skin does not need to be included in a metabolic model, though skin reactions from contact exposure can occur.

5.2.6   Placental transfer and transfer via milk

No data have been found concerning transfer of beryllium to the placenta or developing foetus, or for transfer to human milk. Data from studies on dairy cows indicate that ingestion of beryllium contaminated milk will not be a major route of exposure, even for the offspring of occupationally exposed individuals.

5.3   Cadmium

5.3.1   Fractional gastrointestinal absorption

Reported values for the fractional gastrointestinal absorption of cadmium in man are normally <0.1 and fall in the range 0.004 to 0.1.   An appropriate value for all compounds and complexes of cadmium, over recorded ranges of dietary intake, is taken to be 0.05.

5.3.2   Retention in, and translocation from, the lung

Of cadmium deposited in the human lung, between 0.1 and 0.5 is absorbed, with values for absorption typically around 0.25. Oxides, halides, sulphides and nitrates of cadmium are assigned to ICRP inhalation class W and all other compounds, apart from hydroxides, are assigned to class D.   The position on cadmium hydroxide is unclear, due to insufficient data, and it may be properly assigned to class W or class Y.

5.3.3   Retention in the body

Of cadmium entering the systemic circulation, a fraction of about 0.1 is apparently available for early excretion with a biological half-life of 1.5 days.   The remainder of the cadmium is apparently retained in all organs and tissues with a biological half-life of about 25 years, though a range of 20 to 30 years can be expected. On this basis, a reasonable representation of the whole-body retention of cadmium, following entry of a unit quantity of the element into the systemic circulation, is:

$$R(t) = 0.1e^{-0.693t/1.5} + 0.9e^{-0.693t/9125}$$

where t is in days.

Data for the distribution of cadmium in man suggest that fractions of 0.2, 0.3, 0.1 and 0.01 of cadmium deposited in the body be assigned to the liver, kidneys, bone and blood respectively.

5.3.4   Excretion

Cadmium is generally excreted primarily in the faeces, although urinary excretion has been reported to be the main route of loss in some cases.   In the absence of clinical mahifestations of cadmium poisoning, associated with renal and/or hepatic dysfunction, the daily excretion of cadmium typically represents some 0.005 to 0.01% of the total body burden.   Loss of cadmium in hair, sweat or saliva is detectable, but not significant compared with urinary or faecal excretion.   In general, for man, several reviews suggest that urinary levels of cadmium can be taken to reflect the total body burden, and blood levels of cadmium to reflect the average daily intake for the preceeding few months.   However, more data are required before such values can be interpreted unambiguously.

5.3.5   Skin absorption

No data have been found concerning the skin absorption of cadmium, and this does not appear to require inclusion in the metabolic model.

5.3.6   Cross-placental transfer and transfer in milk

At cadmium levels likely to be encountered in the environment, the placenta apparently forms an effective barrier to the transport of cadmium to the foetus and it is unlikely that pregnancy will substantially modify the metabolic model proposed.   At higher levels of exposure, the placenta itself may be affected and some data suggest that, following high level exposure of the mother, the new born have a lower birth weight than those derived from non-exposed mothers.   Data concerning the loss of cadmium in milk are very variable.   In view of the degree of uncertainty with respect to loss in milk, no recommendations are made concerning the effect of lactation on the metabolism of cadmium, or on transfer of the element via this route.

5.4   Lead

5.4.1   Gastrointestinal absorption

A best estimate of the fractional absorption of lead from the gastrointestinal tract of adults is 0.3, but values ranging between 0.05 and 0.65 have been reported. Absorption can be modified by a number of factors including the chemical and physical form of lead ingested, associated dietary intakes, periods of fasting or undernourishment, and the status of the individual with regard to iron and calcium stores. Drugs which alter the rate of gastric emptying are expected to modify the fractional absorption. For children, a fractional absorption value of 0.5 is taken to be appropriate.

5.4.2   Retention in the respiratory system

Lead deposited in the lungs is almost completely absorbed, and very little muco-ciliary clearance of the respiratory tract has been reported. Translocation of lead to the systemic circulation occurs rapidly, and it is probable that 90% of deposited lead is cleared with a biological half-life of 7 to 14 hours, although a small fraction of this (up to 10%) may be cleared with a half-life of 1 hour. The remaining lead deposited in the lung is cleared with a biological half-life of approximately 70 hours.

5.4.3   Systemic metabolism

Following entry of a unit quantity of lead into the systemic circulation, the whole-body retention [R(t)] is well represented by:

$$R(t) = 0.69e^{-0.693t/12} + 0.191e^{-0.693t/180} + 0.119e^{-0.693t/10000}$$

where t is in days.

The long-term component of retention is associated predominantly with slow clearance from bone. Retention of lead in bone and other tissues is well described by the following functions.

$$R_{BONE}(t) = 0.55[0.6e^{-0.693t/12} + 0.2e^{-0.693t/180} + 0.2e^{-0.693t/10000}]$$

$$R_{LIVER}(t) = 0.25[0.8e^{-0.693t/12} + 0.18e^{-0.693t/180} + 0.02e^{-0.693t/10000}]$$

$$R_{KIDNEY}(t) = 0.02[0.8e^{-0.693t/12} + 0.18e^{-0.693t/180} + 0.02e^{-0.693t/10000}]$$

$$R_{OTHER}(t) = 0.18[0.8e^{-0.693t/12} + 0.18e^{-0.693t/180} + 0.02e^{-0.693t/10000}]$$

where t is in days.

No specific modifications to the retention functions are recommended for high levels of lead intake, or for different physiological states of the individual. However, the following general comments are of relevance.

- Lead may be released from bone into the bloodstream as a result of physiological stress including pregnancy, trauma and infection.

- Disease can modify distribution and retention functions, e.g. elevated aortic lead concentrations are associated with atherosclerosis.

- Calcification, fatty change and fibrosis associated with ageing can modify retention.

- Nutritional status, such as calcium and iron body stores, can influence retention.

5.4.4   Other metabolic information

Essentially no absorption of metallic lead occurs through intact skin, though uptake can occur where skin lesions or abrasions are present. No estimates can be made of the rate or amount of such intake, as it will be highly dependent on the individual case. Cross-placental transfer of lead is linearly related to umbilical flow-rate and foeto-toxic levels of lead can be transferred. Lead is detectable in human milk; the concentration is related to blood lead content and probably never exceeds 1.0 µg ml^{-1}.

5.4.5   Excretion of lead

Urine, faeces and sweat can all form significant pathways for the excretion of lead. Of lead absorbed, it is likely that urinary and sweat losses will be very similar. Loss in faeces primarily reflects recent dietary intake, but some absorbed lead is excreted in the bile and from the intestinal mucosa. It is probable that there is a loss of approximately 1 µg lead per day due to translocation to hair, but reported estimates have varied up to 30 µg per day.

5.5   Nickel

5.5.1   Gastrointestinal absorption

A best estimate of fractional absorption from the gastrointestinal tract is 0.05, but a range of 0.01 to 0.20 is not unusual, depending on chemical form administered, nature of the diet, nickel status and state of health. Absorption does not seem to be modified substantially by the amount of nickel present in the diet.

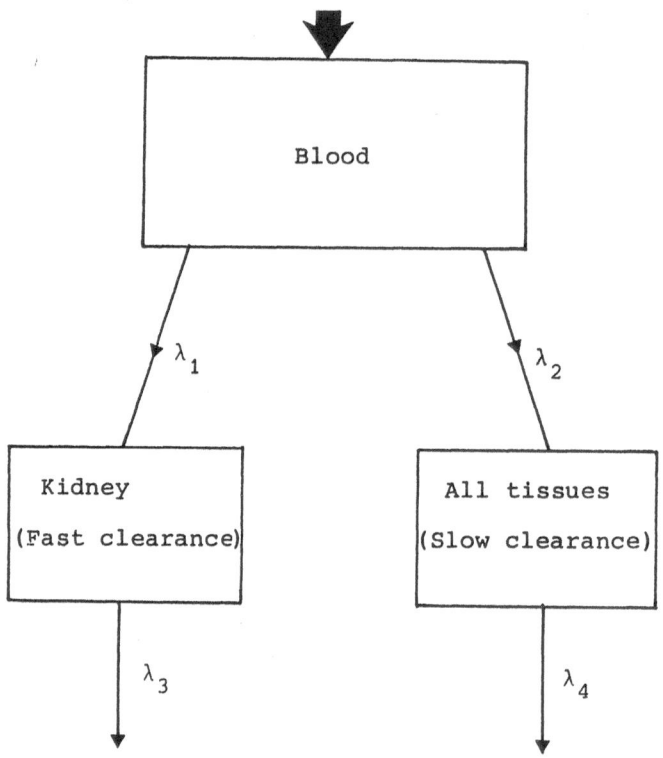

Note:
 (1) Kidney content = [Kidney(Fast clearance)]

              + 0.005 [All tissues(slow clearance)]

   Blood content = [Blood] + 0.002 [All tissues(slow clearance)]

   Other tissues = 0.993 [All tissues(slow clearance)]

FIGURE 5. SIMPLE MODEL FOR THE METABOLISM OF NICKEL IN MAN AFTER ENTRY
OF THE ELEMENT INTO THE SYSTEMIC CIRCULATION.

5.5.2   Retention in the respiratory system

'It is assumed that all nickel entering the respiratory system as nickel carbonyl is deposited there and that it is then translocated to the systemic circulation with a biological half-life of 0.1 d. After entry into the systemic circulation, the metabolic model for other inorganic compounds of nickel is assumed to apply. However, it is emphasised that further work on nickel carbonyl metabolism is required before a detailed model can be developed.
For other compounds of nickel, the ICRP lung model is taken to apply, using the following classification:

Inhalation class	Compounds
W	oxides, hydroxides, carbides, Ni_3S_2 (amorphous and crystalline)
	NiS (amorphous and crystalline)
D	all other commonly occuring compounds

This classification is likely to over-estimate, rather than under-estimate, the mobility of the nickel sulphides.

5.5   Systemic metabolism

The model illustrated in Fig. 5 should be used, in conjunction with the following rate coefficients:

$\lambda_1 = 1.05$ d^{-1}.

$\lambda_2 = 0.45$ d^{-1}.

$\lambda_3 = 6.0$ d^{-1}.

$\lambda_4 = 5.78 \times 10^{-4}$ d^{-1}.

In estimating urinary and faecal excretion it can be assumed that 90% of material leaving the 'all tissues (slow clearance)' compartment goes to urinary excretion and that the remainder goes to faecal excretion.
The model does not apply to nickel entering the body by intramuscular injection or implantation. Clearance from the site of intramuscular injection will be very dependent upon the type of material injected and the location of the site.
The same model can be used when chelation therapy is employed. However, at the time of injection of the chelate, nickel in blood should be partitioned into two fractions. One fraction can be assumed to be Ni^{2+} and will continue to behave in the same fashion as before. The second fraction will be the nickel-chelate complex and will behave metabolically as the chelate.

5.5.4   Transfer to the foetus

In the absence of specific data for man, nickel concentrations in the foetus can be assumed to be similar to those in the mother at any time.

5.5.5   Transcutaneous absorption

The data available are not sufficient to define a quantitative model, but it may be prudent to assume that, when a nickel salt in solution is applied to the skin, a total of about 1% of the nickel is absorbed and enters the systemic circulation in the first 24 hours post-application.

5.5.6   Effects of state of health

Renal dysfunction is likely to have a profound modifying effect on the retention of nickel in the body, but has not been studied and cannot currently be quantified.

5.5.7   Administration of toxic levels

The data available are not sufficient to justify any modifications to the models for different levels of exposure.

5.6   Chromium

5.6.1   Fractional gastrointestinal absorption

An f_1 value of 0.05 is recommended for all inorganic salts of chromium. No distinction is made between intakes of trivalent or hexavalent chromium.   Dietary, or biologically incorporated chromium, is absorbed more efficiently and an f_1 value of 0.25 is assigned to all dietary intakes of chromium.

5.6.2   Retention in, and translocation from, the lung

Chromium is assigned to the following inhalation classes, in accordance with ICRP recommendations:

Chemical Group	Inhalation class
oxides and hydroxides	Y
halides and nitrates	W
all other compounds	D

Chromium entering the gastrointestinal tract following clearance from the lungs is assumed to be present in inorganic form, probably trivalent, and an f_1 value of 0.05 is taken to be applicable.

5.6.3   Retention in the body

Following entry of a unit quantity of chromium into the systemic circulation retention in the bone of man is adequately represented by:

$$R_{BONE}(t) = 0.05e^{-0.693t/10000}$$

where t is in days

Retention of chromium in tissues other than bone is taken to be represented by:

$$R_{OTHER}(t) = 0.95\ a[0.35e^{-0.693t/0.5} + 0.26e^{-0.693t/13} + 0.39e^{-0.693t/200}]$$

where t is in days and

a   takes values of 0.2, 0.02, 0.04, 0.02 and 0.72 for lung, liver, kidneys, spleen and all other tissues respectively.

No modification to the retention function is recommended for high levels of dietary chromium intake.   However, the following assumptions are recommended for patients with haemochromatosis:

- retention in bone is unaffected;

- biological half-lives of retention in soft-tissues are not significantly modified, although data indicate that a long-term component of retention of 160 d may be more appropriate;

- fractions of 0.58, 0.2 and 0.22 are assigned to short, medium and long-term components of retention respectively;

- clearance of chromium from the blood is more rapid, due to a reduction in the long-term retained fraction.

5.6.4   Excretion of chromium

In view of the wide variability in reported concentrations of chromium in both urine and faeces, no model is proposed relating body burden to urinary excretion.   However, it is noted that in excess of 80% of chromium absorbed to the systemic circulation is excreted in the urine.   Glomerular filtration and tubular reabsorption are both of significance in the renal excretion of chromium. Nearly all chromium in urine is incorporated in low molecular weight complexes, protein-bound chromium is excreted only to a very small degree.

5.6.5   Skin absorption of chromium

Up to 23% of chromium in a solution of sodium chromate administered to the intact skin may be absorbed over one hour, depending on the molarity of the solution. A fractional absorption of 0.1 is taken to be appropriate for all forms of hexavalent chromium in contact with skin for appreciable periods. Absorption of trivalent chromium is assumed to be negligible.

5.6.6   Cross placental transfer and transfer in milk

Insufficient data are available to modify the proposed retention function in respect of physiological changes associated with pregnancy and lactation. However, it is clear that substantial depletion of maternal chromium stores may occur during both pregnancy and subsequent lactation.   Plasma chromium levels in pregnant women are almost half those in healthy non-pregnant women of similar age. In cows, it has been estimated that over 40% of maternal chromium may be lost in milk, but this conclusion is very tentative and its relevance to the case of lactating women is not readily determined.

5.7   Abestos

5.7.1   Ingestion

No recommendations are made concerning a metabolic model for ingested asbestos.   The reasons for this are discussed in Section 7.6 of Appendix 7.

5.7.2   Inhalation

For inhaled asbestos the following recommendations are made.

- Of inhaled asbestos, 50% can be assumed to be deposited in the lung, including both upper and lower components of the respiratory tract.
- Of inhaled amphibole asbestos, 10% can be assumed to be retained in the lung with a half-life of 200 d and the rest rapidly excreted.
- Of inhaled chrysotile asbestos, 2.5% can be assumed to be retained in the lung with a half-life of 200 d and the rest rapidly excreted.
- For the purpose of monitoring, all asbestos leaving the lungs may be assumed to be lost from the body via faecal excretion, though some transfer to other tissues undoubtedly occurs.
- For assessment of intakes of asbestos by inhalation the following retention functions are recommended.

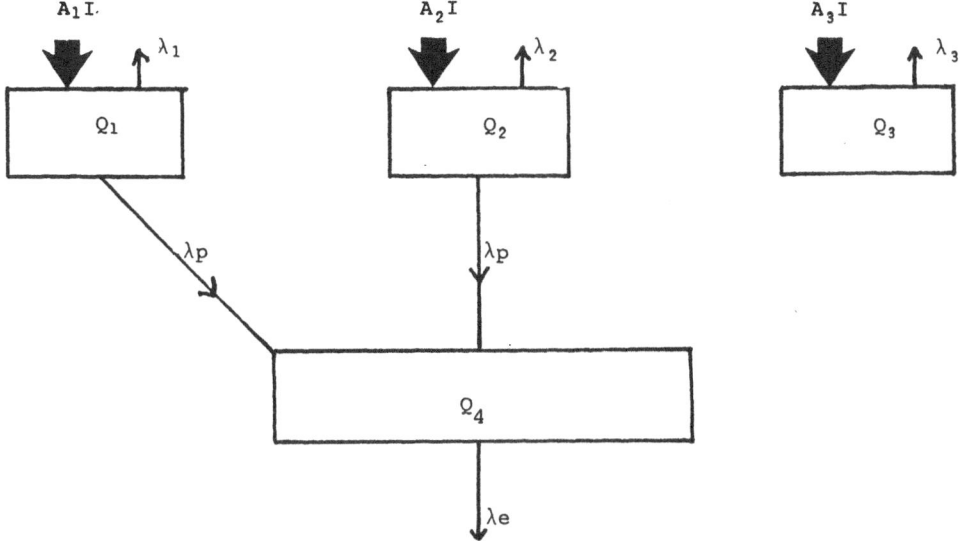

NOTES: A_1 to A_3 are the fractions of inhaled benzene deposited in the various retention compartments;

I is the rate of inhalation of benzene;

λ_1 to λ_3 are the rates of loss to exhalation;

λp is the rate of conversion to phenol and other metabolites of benzene;

λe is the rate of excretion of benzene metabolites;

Q_1 to Q_3 are the amounts of benzene retained in the body;

Q_4 is the amount of benzene metabolites retained in the body.

FIGURE 6   A SIMPLE MODEL FOR SIMULATING THE RETENTION OF INHALED BENZENE AND THE EXCRETION OF BENZENE METABOLITES IN URINE.

Chrysotiles:

$$R(t) = 0.925e^{-0.693t/1} + 0.05e^{-0.693t/10} + 0.025e^{-0.693t/200}$$

Amphiboles:

$$R(t)\ 0.85e^{-0.693t/1} + 0.05e^{-0\ 693t/10} + 0.1e^{-0.693t/200}$$

The corresponding faecal excretion functions are as follows.

Chrysotiles:

$$E_f(t) = 64e^{-0.693t/1} + 0.35e^{-0.693t/10} + 0.0087e^{-0.693t/200}$$

Amphiboles:

$$E_f(t) = 59e^{-0.693t/1} + 0.35e^{-0.693t/10} + 0.035e^{-0.693t/200}$$

where $E_f(t)$ is the percentage excretion per day; and
t is in days.

It is noted that there is undoubtedly a small fraction of asbestos
which is retained in the lung with a biological half-life of much
more than 200 d.   This asbestos is probably long-fibred and it is
emphasised that neither the period of its retention, nor the processes of its transfer from the lung, can currently be quantified.

5.8   Benzene

        A model is given only for inhalation exposure to benzene,
since   other   routes   are   of   little   significance   in   comparison.
Furthermore, the model relates specifically to monitoring for benzene
exposure, since the distribution of benzene and its metabolites in
man, or any other species, has not been characterised adequately and
the   particular   metabolites   responsible   for   the   toxic   effects   of
benzene have not been identified clearly.   The model is illustrated
in Fig. 6.
        About   50%   of   inhaled   benzene   is   retained   in   the   body
following inhalation, though some of this is rapidly re-excreted in
the   exhaled   air,   such   that,   in   a   3 h   exposure,   concentrations   of
benzene   in   exhaled   air   are   70%   of   concentrations   in   inhaled   air.
Further, following cessation of exposure three components of loss are
identified with rate constants ~5 h^{-1}, 1 h^{-1} and 0.02 h^{-1}.   Benzene
retained in the body will be available for excretion into the exhaled
air, or conversion into phenol and other derivatives for excretion in
the urine.   It is not clear whether the transformation to phenol
operates on benzene associated with all components of retention, but
as a first approach to modelling it is assumed that transformation to
phenol occurs only in the two most rapidly turning-over compartments.
Phenol and other metabolites produced from benzene are assumed to be
excreted   entirely   in   the   urine.   The   reason   for   exclusion   of   the
component with slow turnover is that it is probably associated with
fat and is, therefore, not available for cellular oxidation.   Values

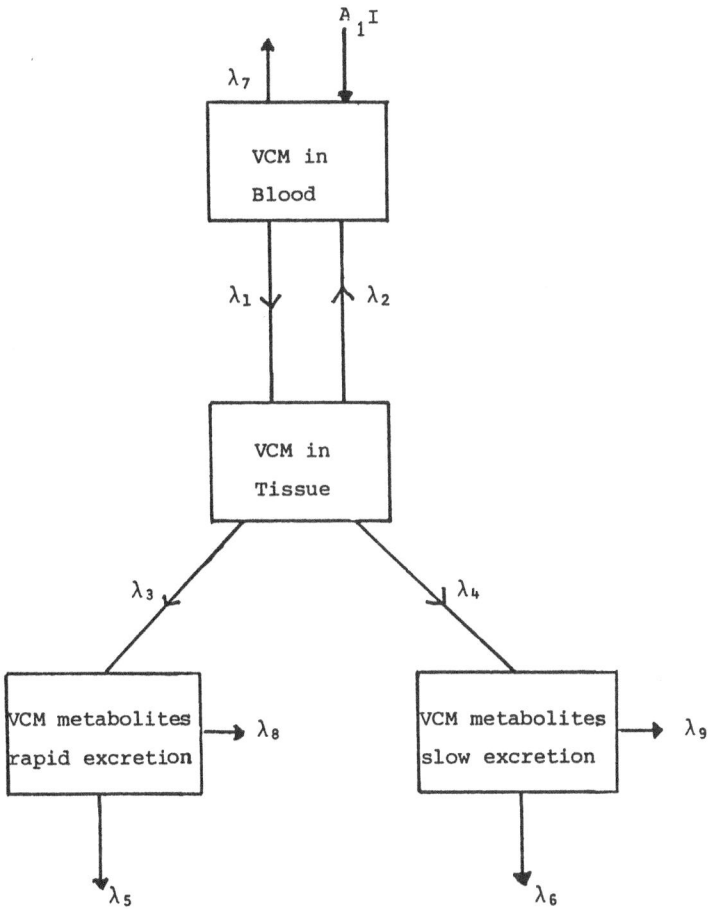

NOTES: I = Intake rate

A_1 = Fraction of inhaled VCM entering blood
λ_1, λ_2 = Blood: Tissue exchange rates
λ_3, λ_4 = Metabolic rates
λ_5, λ_6 = Excretion rates for identifiable metabolites
λ_7 = Unchanged VCM exhalation rate
λ_8, λ_9 = Rates of breakdown to non-specific metabolites

FIGURE 7   MODEL FOR VINYL CHLORIDE MONOMER (VCM)
                METABOLISM IN MAN

of the model parameters have been calculated from the data available and are listed below.

$$\lambda_1 = 4.72 \ h^{-1} \qquad A_1 = 0.3$$
$$\lambda_2 = 0.72 \ h^{-1} \qquad A_2 = 0.6$$
$$\lambda_3 = 0.02 \ h^{-1} \qquad A_3 = 0.02$$
$$\lambda_p = 0.5 \ h^{-1}$$
$$\lambda_e = 0.09 \ h^{-1}$$

At high levels of exposure, phenolic inhibition of cytochrome P450 will cause reduction in λ_p, but the data available are not sufficient to quantify this. If this effect were to be modelled, the use of a Michaelis-Menten type of saturable expression would probably be appropriate.

5.9   Vinyl chloride monomer

A model for the metabolism of vinyl chloride monomer is shown in Fig. 7. This model is for the interpretation of exhaled air and urinary metabolite measurements and is not a complete representation of vinyl chloride metabolism. Taking the only well-defined specific urinary metabolite of vinyl chloride monomer to be thiodiglycolic acid, and assuming that rat and human metabolism are closely similar, the following model parameter values are recommended.

Parameter	Value (h^{-1})
λ_1	18
λ_2	6
λ_3	3
λ_4	0.3
λ_5	0.03
λ_6	0.0038
λ_7	50
λ_8	0.13
λ_9	0.0162

The fraction of inhaled vinyl chloride monomer reaching blood, A_1, is taken to be unity.

5.10   Benzidine

The major potential route of exposure to benzidine and its congeners has been identified as transcutaneous. Unfortunately, the degree of systemic uptake by this route cannot be quantified, except that it can be in excess of 1% of the material applied to the skin. Furthermore, the time course of such uptake has not been studied.

While there are two papers available concerning the metabolism of benzidine and its congeners at early times after exposure, i.e. in the first few days, the evidence suggests that metabolites of benzidine and its congeners are bound in tissues for many weeks.

On the basis of the data available, it is not currently possible to propose a metabolic model for benzidine that would be useful either in monitoring exposure or in interpreting dose response data.

5.11   Carbon tetrachloride

Data on the metabolism of CCl_4 are very limited. Significant transcutaneous absorption can occur, but human studies appear to be limited to immersion of one thumb for a thirty minute period. In respect of ingestion, investigations on man are limited to a single individual exposed to a very large volume of CCl_4 in combination with methanol, while experiments on rats were conducted for purposes other than the understanding of CCl_4 pharmacokinetics.

Inhalation, potentially the most significant route of exposure has been little better investigated and data on monkeys and man are insufficient to generate a pharmacokinetic model applicable to exposure regimes other than those studied.

In terms of monitoring for exposure to CCl_4, analysis of the expired air seems a potentially useful method, particularly since components of loss of unchanged CCl_4 with half lives ~50 h may occur. If such a method were to be used, detailed experiments would have to be undertaken to characterise the uptake and loss of CCl_4 by humans at different levels.

5.12   Methyl iodide

On the basis of data currently available, it is not possible to construct a detailed pharmacokinetic model for methyl iodide. If an individual is exposed to the vapour, ~75% of that inhaled will typically enter the circulation and be metabolised. Metabolism, which may occur in blood, liver and in other organs or tissues, involves the release of the iodide ion and further metabolism of the methyl group. In the liver, this further metabolism typically involves conjugation with glutathione. Conjugation and subsequent excretion of the conjugated products have not been quantified in any detail. Furthermore, the products formed and excreted are unlikely to be specific to methyl iodide exposure.

With respect to the iodide released, an individual exposed to an atmosphere containing 5 ppm of methyl iodide would inhale ~2.7×10^5 µg of methyl iodide, corresponding to an uptake of 1.8×10^5 µg of iodine into the systemic circulation. This is very much more than the typical daily intake of iodine of 200 µg (International Commission on Radiological Protection, 1979) and suggests that exposure to methyl iodide could, in some circumstances, be monitored using a metabolic model for iodine. Such a model, which takes account of the effect of different levels of iodine intake on iodide metabolism, has been developed by Coughtrey et al. (1983). This model in illustrated in Fig. 8. For adult man, values of the various rate coefficients are as listed below.

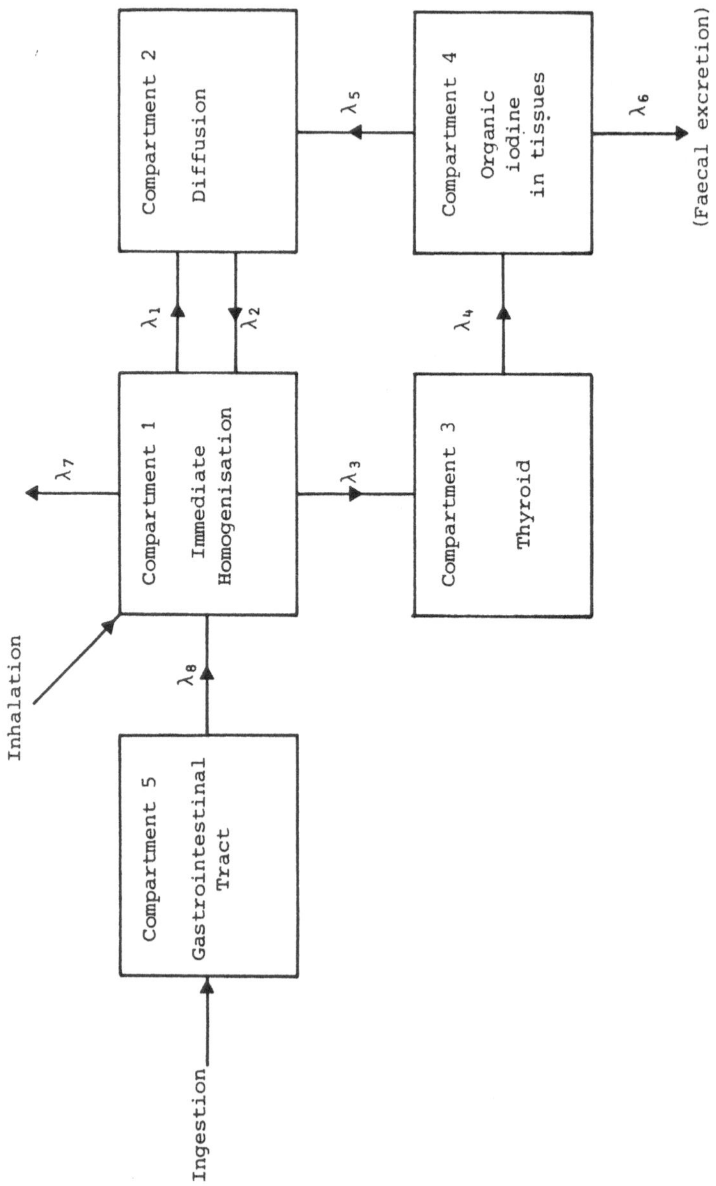

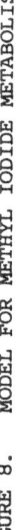

FIGURE 8.   MODEL FOR METHYL IODIDE METABOLISM

Coefficient	Value (d^{-1})
λ_1	48
λ_2	18.7
λ_4	8.75×10^{-3}
λ_5	5.25×10^{-2}
λ_6	5.83×10^{-3}
λ_7	6.9

A value for λ_3 is estimated by consideration of the requirement to maintain homeostatic equilibrium. Thus,

$$\lambda_3 = \lambda_7(\lambda_5+\lambda_6)q_4/(I_{ING}+U_{INH}-\lambda_6 q_4)$$

where I_{ING} (mg d^{-1}) is the daily intake of iodine by ingestion;

U_{INH} (mg d^{-1}) is the daily uptake of iodine by inhalation; and

q_4 (mg) is the mass of organic iodine in tissues, which may be taken as 1.2 mg.

Thus, in this model, the thyroid effectively regulates its uptake of iodide and any excess is excreted in the urine.

It is noted that dietary iodine intakes can be very variable, depending on both locality and diet, and that this may need to be taken into account when using the above model for workplace monitoring.

6
Acknowledgements

We would like to thank A. Martin and W.J. Hunter for helpful discussions during the course of this study and P.J. Coughtrey for helpful comments on several sections of the text. Particular thanks must go to A. Keadell, L.J. Charlwood, and I. Harrington for preparation of the figures and especially to our typists J. Darby, G. Tiplady and M. Razzell for coping with a large manuscript so rapidly and accurately.

7
References

Coughtrey, P.J., Jackson, D. and Thorne, M.C. 1983. Radio-nuclide Distribution and Transport in Terrestrial and Aquatic Ecosystems. Vol.3, A.A., Balkema, Rotterdam, 1983.

International Agency for Research on Cancer, 1982. Chemicals, Industrial Processes and Industries Associated with Cancer in Humans, IARC Monographs Supplement 4.

International Commission on Radiological Protection, 1979. Limits for Intakes of Radionuclides by Workers. Part 1, Annals of the ICRP, Vol.2, Nos. 3/4.

Mansuy, D., 1981. Use of model systems in biochemical toxicology. Heme models. In: Hodgson E., Bend J.R. and Philpot R.M. (Eds.) Reviews in Biochemical Technology 3. Elsevier/North-Holland, New York, pp.283-320.

Philpot, R.M. and Wolf, C.R., 1981. The properties and distribution of the enzymes of pulmonary cytochrome P-450-dependent monooxygenase systems. In: Hogson E., Bend J.R. and Philpot R.M. (Eds.). Reviews in Biochemical Technology 3, Elsevier/North-Holland, New York, pp.51-76.

Powis, G., and Jansson, I., 1979. Stoichiometry of the mixed function oxidase. Pharmac. Ther., 7, 297-311.

Snyder, R. and Remmer, H. 1979. Classes of hepatic microsomal mixed function oxidase inducers. Pharmac. Ther., 7, 203-244, 1979.

Appendix 1
Arsenic

CONTENTS

1.1   INTRODUCTION

Arsenic is defined as a metalloid and exhibits valence states -3, 0, +3 and +5. From a biological and toxicological point of view, three main groups of compounds of the element may be defined. These are:

- inorganic compounds;
- organic compounds;
- arsine gas.

Over the last 50 years, a large number of reviews have been published concerning the distribution, metabolism and toxicology of arsenic and much of the information in this chapter is drawn from some of the more recent of these reviews (Fowler et al., 1979; NAS, 1977; IARC, 1980; Pershagen and Vahter, 1979; Nordberg et al., 1979; Leonard and Lauwerys, 1980; Axelson, 1980; Pershagen, 1980; Fowler, 1977; ICRP, 1981; Underwood, 1977).

The production of a wide variety of arsenic compounds has been reviewed by the IARC (1980). Compounds produced to a significant extent include arsenilic acid, elemental arsenic, arsenic pentoxide, arsenic sulphide, arsenic trioxide, arsine, calcium arsenate, dimethylarsinic acid, lead arsenate, the disodium salt of methanearsonic acid, the monosodium salt of methanearsonic acid, potassium arsenate, potassium arsenite, sodium arsenate, sodium arsenite and sodium cacodylate. In the context of environmental levels of arsenic and in the development of metabolic models, it is appropriate to note distinctions between As^{3+} compounds, As^{5+} compounds, monomethylarsonic acid, dimethylarsinic (cacodylic) acid and arsine gas.

The acute and chronic toxicity of specific arsenic compounds has long been recognized (Fowler, 1977; Tsuchiya, 1977; Tseng, 1977; Ishinishi et al., 1977; Kyle and Pearse, 1965; Levvy, 1947; Nordberg et al., 1979; Pershagen and Vahter, 1979; Done and Peart, 1971; Dinman, 1969; NAS, 1977; IARC, 1980) and the reader is referred to Pershagen and Vahter (1979) for a brief review. With respect to carcinogenesis, the IARC (1980) have summarised relevant human and animal data. Other recent reviews on the subject include those by Axelson (1980), Pershagen (1981) and Leonard and Lauwerys (1980). On the basis of the available data, the IARC (1980) concluded that "there is inadequate evidence for the carcinogenicity of arsenic compounds in animals". However, they also stated that "there is sufficient evidence that inorganic arsenic compounds are skin and lung carcinogens in humans [but] the data suggesting an increased risk for cancer at other sites are inadequate for evaluation".

1.2   INTAKE RATES

1.2.1   Typical dietary intakes

Arsenic is ubiquitous in the environment with concentrations in rocks and soils ranging from <1 ppm to >10^2 ppm (Fowler, 1977). Bowen (1979) listed the following concentrations (μg g^{-1} d.w.):

TABLE 1

ARSENIC CONCENTRATION IN FOODSTUFFS AND
OTHER BIOLOGICAL MATERIALS [1]

Material	Concentration ($\mu g\ g^{-1}$)	Notes
Cereals		
Wheat	0.007-0.3	2,4
	0.09-0.16	2,4
	0.09-0.16	2,4
Wheat flour	0.01-0.09	2,4
Corn (grain)	<0.01-0.4	2,4
	<0.01-0.05	2,4
	0.05-0.07	2,4
	<0.05-0.1	2,4
Corn (stalk and leaves)	0.04	3
	0.6-2.5	2
	1.83-1.9	2
	0.1-1.94	2
	0.71	2
Corn (seedling)	3.0	2
Corn (pop)	0.1	2,4
Barley	<0.1-0.55	2
Rye	<0.1	2
Oats	<0.1-2.28	2
	0.09-0.13	2
Straw	0.28	
Millett	<0.1	2
Rice (grain)	<0.07-3.53	2,4
Rice	0.4	2,4
Rice (whole plant)	0.8-5.0	2
Bread	0.016-0.03	2,4
Bread (whole wheat)	0.008-0.02	2,4
Bread (ginger)	0.05-0.07	2,4
Vegetables		
Soybean	0.08	2,4
	0.05-1.22	2,4
	0.05-1.22	2,4
Soybean (fodder)	0.07-2.12	2
	0.07-2.12	2
Soybean (oil)	0.09	2,4
Beans (green)	∿0.04	2,4
	0.01-0.08	2,4
	trace	2
	trace	2

TABLE 1 (Contd.)

Material	Concentration ($\mu g\ g^{-1}$)	Notes
Vegetables (contd.)		
Beans (pod)	0.27	2,4
(leaves)	0.21	2
Beans	0.05-0.40	2,4
	0.07	2,4
Beans (vines)	0.18	2
Beans (roots)	0.29	2
Beans (kidney)	0.33	2,4
Beans (lima)	0.4	2,4
Beans (yellow eye, leaf)	0.08-1.14	2
Beans (black wax, leaf)	1.57	2
Beans (black wax)	0.08	2,4
Pea	<0.01-0.49	2,4
	0.01-0.4	2,4
Pea (pod)	0.05	2,4
Pea (vine)	0.12-2.82	2
Pea (root)	22.70	2,5
Peanut	0.01-0.3	2
Carrot	0.03-0.8	2,4
	<0.01-0.08	2,4
Carrot (tops)	0.0-0.57	2
(roots)	0.32	2,4
Potato	0.0076-1.25	2,4
	0.01-0.5	2,4
	0.2	2,4
	trace - 0.1	2,4
Potato (peelings)	0.4-2.4	2
Potato (sweet)	0.00	2,4
Onion	0.015-1.54	2,4
	0.08-0.36	2,4
Onion (tops)	3.19	2
Turnip	0.036-0.83	2,4
	<0.01	2,4
Turnip (greens)	0.03	2
Parsnips	0.2	2,4
Beet (tops)	0.07-3.48	2
(roots)	0.1-1.3	2,4
	0.34	2,4
Beets	1.27	2,4
Radish	0.01-1.22	2,4
Tomato	0.01-2.95	2,4
	0.08-0.09	2,4
	<0.2	2,4
	trace	2
	trace	2
Tomato (stalk and leaves)	<0.2	2
	6.75	2
Tomato (root)	<0.2	2
	0.26-0.49	2

TABLE 1 (Contd.)

Material	Concentration ($\mu g\ g^{-1}$)	Notes
Vegetables (contd.)		
Eggplant	0.18-0.77	2,4
	0-6.14	2,4
Eggplant (roots)	0.98	2
Cucumber	0.02-2.4	2,4
Pickle (sweet)	0.14	2,4
Lettuce	0.01-3.78	2,4
	0.12	2,4
Lettuce (roots)	0.47	2
Parsley	0.1-8.0	2,4
Watercress	1.84-2.1	2,6
Spinach	0.04-2.25	2,4
Kale	0.11-0.22	2,4
	0.01-0.99	2,4
Kale (roots)	0.39	2
Swiss chard	~0.05-0.08	2,4
Cabbage	0.0-2.01	2,4
Chicory	0.62	2,4
	0.1	3
Lentil	0.70	2,4
	0.1	2,4
Celery	0.2-0.75	2,4
Celery (whole plant)	2.32	2
Celery (stalks)	0.60	2,4
Celery (root)	1.00	2,4
Salsify	0.11	3
Asparagus	0.1	2,4
Mushroom (canned)	0.45-0.79	2
Cauliflower	0.86	2,4
Endive	0.21	2,4
Pepper	0.39	2,4
	0.00	2,4
Pepper (roots)	1.57	2
Squash	0.023-0.034	2,4
Apple	0.04-1.72	2,4
	0.03-1.91	2,4
	0.07-1.35	2,4
Apple butter	0.43-2.41	2,4
Apple juice/cider	0.065-0.165	7
Orange	~0.4	2,4
Orange juice	0.008-0.12	7
Pear	~0.5	2,4
Pear (skin)	0.4-0.6	2,4
Peach	0.07-1.5	2,4
Apricot	0.15-1.5	2,4
Lemon	0.5	2,4
Lemon (leaves)	0.35	2

TABLE 1 (Contd.)

Material	Concentration (μg g^{-1})	Notes
Pineapple	0.08	2,4
Banana	0.06	2,4
Pumpkin	0.09	2,4
Blueberry (leaves)	0.78	2
(stems)	0.27	2
(roots)	2.40	2
Grapes	0.75-1.20	2,4
	0.05	2,4
Grapes (leaves)	2.3	2
Grapefruit (leaves)	2.0-3.0	2
Mandarin	0.85	2,4
Beverages		
Wine	0.005-0.15	3,4
	0.01-0.02	3,4
	<0.1	3,4
Wine (white)	0.06-0.56	3,4
(red)	0.03-1.38	3,4
(fruit)	0.06-0.11	3,4
(port)	0.02-0.07	3,4
Grape juice	not detected	3
Lemonade	0.0-0.005	3,4
Whiskey	0.02-0.07	3,4
Beer	0.01-2.0	3,4
Ale	<0.02	3,4
Malt	0.26-0.35	7
Hops (sun-dried)	0.08-0.15	2
Hops (sulphured)	0.03-0.82	2
Liquid fruit products	0.09-0.21	3,4
Tree fruits		
Walnuts	0.07	2,4
Walnuts (black)	0.13	3
Hazelnuts	0.78	2,4
Dates	0.12	3,4
Filberts	0.11	2,4
Almonds	0.3	2,4
Forage crops		
Grass	0.1-0.7	2
	0.5-0.94	2
	0.5	2
Clover	<0.1-0.17	2
	0.46	2
Clover (red)	0.37	2
	0.11-0.39	2
Clover (white)	3.64	2

TABLE 1 (Contd.)

Material	Concentration ($\mu g \ g^{-1}$)	Notes
Forage crops (contd.)		
Hay	0.52	2
Alfalfa	0.05-3.38	2
	1.97	2
Alfalfa (roots)	3.15	2
Sudangrass	0.70	2
	trace	2
	trace	2
Vetch	1.22	2
Vetch (roots)	7.15	2
Sunflower	<1.0-2.0	2
Miscellaneous		
Baking powder	1.0	
Cottonseed	0.05	
Cottonseed products	0.58	4
Sugar	0.15	4
Glucose	0.2	4
Honey	0.14	4
Pectin	1.0-3.55	
Organic food colour	3.0	
Gelatin	1.0	
Chocolate	0.07-1.53	
Jam	0.0-0.1	4
Jam and marmalades	0.04-0.08	4
Mustard (paste)	0.28	
Rhubarb	<0.1	
Tobacco	trace - 42.8	
Seaweeds		
Various [8]	4.0-60.0	2
	3.8-18.0	2
	107-109	2
	47.0-93.8	2
	45.0-52.5	2
	26.0-30.0	2
	45.0	2
	11.2	2
	39.0	2
	24-65	2
	28-67.5	2
	7.5	2
	6.0	2
	4.5-17.2	2
	15-34	2
	15-22	2

TABLE 1 (Contd.)

Material	Concentration ($\mu g\ g^{-1}$)	Notes
Domestic animals		
Beef	0.008	3,4
Calf muscle	0.52	3,4
Calf liver	0.15	3,4
Liver	0.063	3,4
Veal	0.005-0.01	3,4
Pork (muscle)	0.22-0.32	3,4
	<0.02	3,4
Salami	0.14-0.20	3,4
Chicken (meat)	0.02	3,4
(kidney)	0.05	3,4
	0.02	3,4
(liver)	<2.2	3,4
	0.02	3,4
	0.08	3,4
(bone marrow)	0.0-0.4	3
Egg yolk	0.005	3,4
Meat (canned)	0.01-0.18	3,4
	0.2-4.13	2
Fat	0.13-0.54	2
Milk and milk products		
Milk	0.0005-0.07	3,4
Milk (dried)	<0.5	2,4
Milk (sterilised)	0.03-0.04	3,4
Milk (condensed)	0.01-0.014	3,4
Butter	0.07	3,4
Marine invertebrates [9]		
Shrimp	1.27-41.6	3,4
Shrimp (Eng.potted)	8.2-18.8	3,4
(edible portion)	0.95-31.2	3,4
(canned)	0.08	3,4
Palamon serratus (cooked)	1.0-2.7	3,4
Crab (dressed)	18.8-62.6	3,4
(canned)	0.71	3,4
(muscle)	6.1	3,4
Carcinus maenas (cooked)	2.5-7.0	3,4
Cancer paguris (cooked)	2.1-33.4	3,4
Clam (minced)	0.85	3,4
	1.42-2.56	3,4
(canned)	0.36	3,4

TABLE 1 (Contd.)

Material	Concentration ($\mu g\ g^{-1}$)	Notes
Marine invertebrates (Contd.)		
Prawn	34.1	3,4
Prawn (Dublin Bay)	27.0–130.5	3,4
(American tinned)	10.5–30.0	3,4
(Japanese tinned)	15.0–63.8	3,4
Oyster	0.3–3.7	3
Oyster (English)	2.2–7.5	3
(Portugese)	24.8–52.5	3
(American tinned)	0.4–0.8	3,4
(canned)	0.22	3,4
(smoked)	1.0	3,4
Lobster	2.27–54.5	3
Lobster (canned)	0.94	3,4
(fillet)	5.3	3,4
(fillet)	14.0	3.4
(cooked)	10.8–17.2	3,4
(muscle)	0.022	3,4
(whole)	0.453	3
(Norwegian, cooked)	7.2–19.4	3,4
Scallop	27.0–63.8	3
Mussel	2.58–89.2	3
Cockle	5.1–8.4	3
	1.3–2.4	3
	3.7–6.6	3
Whelk	9.0–30.0	3
Periwinkle (cooked)	3.6–6.3	3,4
Crayfish (cooked)	12–54.6	3,4
Crayfish	15–33.8	3
	0.8–1.5	3
Squid	6.5	3,4
Squid (raw)	0.8–7.5	3
(cooked)	0.4–3.3	3,4
Cuttlefish (cooked)	0.8–6.8	3,4
Anchovy	7.1–10.7	3,4
Octopus (tentacles)	0.12	3,4
(raw)	2.6–40.3	3,4
(cooked)	3.0–31.0	3,4
Fish		
Cod	~4	3,4
Cod (fillet)	2.2	3,4
(muscle)	0.4–0.8	3,4
Cod (liver oil)	1.4–10.0	3
Black marlin (muscle)	0.1–1.65	3,4
Tuna	0.71–4.6	3,4
Tunny	9.6	2

<u>TABLE 1</u> (Contd.)

Material	Concentration ($\mu g \ g^{-1}$)	Notes
<u>Fish</u> (Contd.)		
Haddock	5.54-10.8	2
Mullet (red)	1.54	3,4
Dogfish	0.53	3,4
Plaice	4.5-7.5	3,4
Sole	5.2	3,4
Dab	2.2-3.0	3,4
Caviar (Russian)	3.8	3
Freshwater fish	0-0.4	3
Bass (large mouthed)	0.01-1.86	3,4
Bass (white)	0.08-1.20	3,4
	0.28-0.48	3,4
Catfish	0.07-0.3	3,4
Herring (fillet)	3.8	3,4
(muscle)	2.0	3,4
Mackerel (fillet)	2.2-3.5	2
North Atlantic finfish	<1.0-6.4	3
Salmon	0.09	3,4
Fish muscle	3.06-6.8	3,4

Notes: 1. Data from NAS(1977), Appendices A and B, untreated values only.
2. Dry weight basis.
3. Wet weight basis.
4. Used in estimates of food concentrations.
5. Anomalous result - much higher concentration than in plants treated with arsenic.
6. Excluded because of method of cultivation.
7. Difficult to interpret, since specified as dry weight.
8. Data for whole seaweeds only, seaweed oils usually exhibit higher concentrations of arsenic.
9. Edible species and edible fractions identified as far as possible, some whole animal data listed for comparison.

Geosphere

granite and basalt	1.5
limestone and sandstone	1
shale	13
soil	6
seawater	0.0037
freshwater	0.0005

Biosphere

land plants	0.02-7
edible vegetables	0.01-1.5
mammalian muscle	0.007-0.09
marine fish	0.2-10

In terms of human diet, marine and freshwater fish and invertebrates appear to be the richest source of the element with oysters containing 3 μg g^{-1} and prawns up to 174 μg g^{-1} (ICRP, 1975). On the basis of a detailed study of arsenic in foods Jelinek and Corneliussen (1977) have given estimates of the average daily intake of arsenic in US diets. Their results, converted from μg As$_2$O$_3$ to μg As, are given below.

Federal year	Arsenic intake (μg d^{-1})	Percentage from meat, fish and poultry
1967	52	43
1968	104	33
1969	57	45
1970	43	84
1971	13	88
1972	9	100
1973	8	60
1974	16	76

Much of the drop in the early 1970s is attributed to decreased use of arsenic containing pesticides on food crops. This also explains the higher percentage contribution of meat, fish and poultry to the total dietary intake.

It is noted that the dietary intakes quoted above are rather lower than those given by some other authors. Thus, the ICRP (1975, 1981) estimated 1000 μg d^{-1}, while Nordberg et al. (1979) quoted the following values from a variety of studies:

Dietary intake (μg d^{-1})	Comments
410	Institutional diet containing no seafood
70-170	Japanese diet
500-4200	Canadian, French, UK and US diets
40-1400	Hospital diets

Food product	Assumed concentration at consumption (μg g^{-1})	Far East		Near East		Africa		Latin America		Europe		North America		Oceania	
		(2)	(3)	(2)	(3)	(2)	(3)	(2)	(3)	(2)	(3)	(2)	(3)	(2)	(3)
Cereals	0.006	404	2.4	446	2.7	330	2.0	281	1.7	375	2.3	185	1.1	243	1.5
Starchy roots	0.1	156	15.6	44	4.4	473	47.3	247	24.7	377	37.7	136	13.6	144	14.4
Sugar	0.1	22	2.2	37	3.7	29	2.9	85	8.5	79	7.9	113	11.3	135	13.5
Pulses and nuts	0.3	56	16.8	47	14.1	37	11.1	46	13.8	15	4.5	19	5.7	11	3.3
Vegetables and fruits	0.1	128	12.8	398	39.8	215	21.5	313	31.3	316	31.6	516	51.6	386	38.6
Meat	0.04	24	1.0	35	1.4	40	1.6	102	4.1	111	4.4	248	9.9	312	12.5
Eggs	0.04	3	0.1	5	0.2	4	0.2	11	0.4	23	0.9	55	2.2	31	1.2
Fish	1.3(4)	27	35.1	12	15.6	16	20.8	18	23.4	38	49.4	26	33.8	22	28.6
Milk	0.05	51	2.6	214	10.7	96	4.8	240	12.0	494	24.7	850	42.5	574	28.7
Fats and oils	0.3	9	2.7	20	6.0	19	5.7	24	7.2	44	13.2	56	16.8	45	13.5
Total			91.2		98.6		117.8		127.1		176.6		188.5		155.8

REGION

Notes: 1. Data on food consumption rates are taken from Reference Man (ICRP,1975)
2. Consumption (g d^{-1})
3. Arsenic intake (μg d^{-1})
4. Assuming 90% fish and 10% shellfish consumption.

TABLE 2

ESTIMATED DAILY DIETARY INTAKES OF ARSENIC IN VARIOUS REGIONS[1]

Fowler et al. (1979) quoted values for a US institutional diet of 40 µg d^{-1} and for a normal US diet of 190 µg d^{-1}. Reference to the paper of Schroeder et al. (1966), on which these figures were based, shows that the correct values are 410 µg d^{-1} and 900 µg d^{-1} respectively. Fowler et al. (1979) also quote Japanese intakes of 70-370 µg d^{-1}. In comparison, Lisella et al. (1972) estimated average dietary intakes of 900 µg d^{-1}. In order to obtain a new estimate of dietary intakes, use has been made of the detailed information on arsenic concentrations in biological materials given in Appendices A and B of the National Academy of Sciences report on arsenic (NAS, 1977). Relevant data are listed in Table 1 and the following arsenic concentrations are estimated from a selection of the data presented there:

Foodstuff	Arsenic concentration (µg g^{-1} w.w.)
	Best estimate
Cereals and cereal products	0.006
Vegetables	0.1
Beverages including milk and wine	0.05
Tree fruits (nuts and dates)	0.3
Meat and meat products	0.04
Marine invertebrates	4
Marine fish	1
Sugar, honey, jam and marmalade	0.1
Butter and oils	0.3

The best estimates listed above can be used, in conjunction with the dietary information summarised by the ICRP (ICRP, 1975, p. 349), to give estimated dietary intakes of between 90 and 190 µg d^{-1} (see also Table 2). Finally, it is useful to note that Table 2 implies that the percentage contributions to arsenic intake in the North American diet are as follows:

Meat, eggs and fish	24%
Milk	23%
Vegetables, fruits, nuts, pulses and starchy roots	38%
Other	15%

In comparison, the data of Jelinek and Corneliussen (1977) for the period 1967 to 1974 yield values of 52%, 9%, 12% and 27% respectively.

In conclusion, while it is noted that arsenic levels in the US diet have declined markedly in recent years, for comparison with data on tissue levels of arsenic measured in various countries over several decades it is appropriate to assume a normal level of dietary intake of about 150 µg d^{-1}, though individuals may have intake rates an order of magnitude higher or lower than this. The data on arsenic concentrations in foodstuffs (Table 1) indicate that dietary intakes in excess of 1000 µg d^{-1} are very unlikely, unless specific local contamination is present.

1.2.2   Arsenic in drinking water

Concentrations of arsenic in drinking water are usually low. McCabe et al. (1970) reported that less than 1% of more than 18000 community water supplies in the USA exhibited arsenic concentrations exceeding 0.01 mg l^{-1}. However, higher concentrations have been recorded (IARC, 1980). For example, Fowler et al. (1979) cited a variety of papers to illustrate that river and lake waters may contain up to 1 mg l^{-1}, while high carbonate spring waters in California, Rumania, Kamchatka (USSR) and New Zealand are reported to contain 0.4-1.3 mg l^{-1} (Schroeder and Balassa, 1966). In Antofagasta (Chile), dermatologic lesions in a high percentage of inhabitants are associated with levels of arsenic in water-based drinks of 0.6 to 0.8 mg l^{-1} and levels in carbonated drinks of 0.3 to 0.7 mg l^{-1} (Borgono et al., 1977). In Japan, symptoms of poisoning were associated with drinking well waters contaminated with arsenic at a level of 1 to 3 mg l^{-1} (Tsuchiya, 1977), while in Taiwan artesian well water containing 0.01 to 1.82 mg l^{-1} of arsenic has been associated with increased incidence of Blackfoot disease (a peripheral vascular disorder resulting in gangrene of the extremities) and skin cancer (Tseng, 1977). In Lane County, Oregon, some chronic arsenic toxicity is reported at arsenic in water levels of about 0.4 mg l^{-1} (Whanger et al., 1977).

There seems to be agreement that the content of arsenic in surface waters in non-polluted areas does not exceed 0.01 mg l^{-1} (Pershagen and Vahter, 1979; Nordberg et al., 1979). Assuming water intake rates of 1.65 l d^{-1} for men and 1.2 l d^{-1} for women (ICRP, 1975), the normal daily intake of arsenic in drinking water will not exceed 17 µg. This is in agreement with the values 8 to 18 µg d^{-1} for all beverages which can be obtained from data presented by Jelinek and Corneliussen (1977). However, significant toxicity symptoms are unlikely to be observed until water concentrations reach ~0.4 mg l^{-1}, corresponding to intakes ~600 µg d^{-1}. Thus, in specific areas, arsenic in drinking water could be the main source of human exposure and relatively high chronic intakes could occur without the appearance of a detectable excess of symptoms of acute or chronic intoxication among the exposed population. Extremely high levels of arsenic (>100 mg l^{-1}) have been reported for waters from areas of thermal activity (Pershagen and Vahter, 1979), but such waters are clearly not fit for human consumption.

The relationship between the different forms of arsenic in surface waters from various parts of the world remains largely unknown (Pershagen and Vahter, 1979). However, both organic and inorganic species are reported to be present (Braman and Foreback, 1973; Crecelius, 1974). The main organic species are generally present in lower amounts than the inorganic forms arsenite and arsenate (Pershagen and Vahter, 1979) and are possibly produced from them by bacterial and fungal metabolism (IARC, 1980).

1.2.3   Inhalation of arsenic

Burning of coal and smelting of metals are major sources of arsenic air pollution (Nordberg et al., 1979). In their review, Nordberg et al. (1979) quote concentrations of 0.04 to 0.14 µg m^{-3}, as a yearly average in suspended matter in British town air; 0.56 and 0.07 µg m^{-3}, as winter and summer means in Prague and <0.01 to 0.36 μg m^{-3} in urban areas of the United States. They also note air concentrations $\sim$1-4 μg m^{-3} have been measured in the vicinity of smelter operations. This fact was also noted by Pershagen and Vahter (1979), who pointed out that, in 1974, only 73 of the 280 US National Air Surveillance Network sites had quarterly average concentrations in excess of 10^{-3} μg m^{-3} and only 13 sites, mainly highly urbanised areas and smelter locations showed levels of above 0.02 μg m^{-3} The IARC (1980) quoted the following data concerning arsenic levels in air:

	Level (μg m^{-3})
US stations 1950, 1953, 1961 and 1964	N.D.-0.75($\bar{x}$=0.03)
US urban areas 1968-69 (average)	0.02
US rural areas 1968-69 (maximum)	0.02
UK (7 sites)	<0.0015-0.037
Industrial area, Osaka, Japan	0.025-0.090
Non-ferrous smelters	0-0.854
Pesticide plants	0.003-0.8

They also noted concentrations of 0.6-141 μg m^{-3} at 46 to 91 m from one US cotton gin, while, at 300 m from several cotton gins producing 5 bales of cotton per day, they quoted arsenic in air concentrations of 0.25 μg m^{-3} (gins with uncontrolled emissions) and 0.037 μg m^{-3} (gins with well controlled emissions). At 50 m from the gins, air concentrations were about a factor of 20 to 50 higher.

To interpret these concentrations, it is useful to note that Reference Man (ICRP, 1975) inhales 23 m^3 of air per day. Thus, even if the average arsenic concentration in air is as high as 0.2 μg m^{-3}, the daily intake by this route will be less than 5 μg. In the vicinity of smelters and cotton gins air concentrations of about 1 μg m^{-3} are likely to occur, leading to intakes by inhalation of $\sim$20 μg d^{-1}.

In this context, it is relevant to note that Gabor and Coldea (1977) have observed enhanced hair levels of arsenic in residents living in an ore smelting area where the average arsenic content in air was 3.6 μg m^{-3}. This corresponds to daily intakes by inhalation of $\sim$80 μg d^{-1}, but these are undoubtedly supplemented by enhanced dietary intakes.

The smoking of tobacco can provide a significant supplementary source of inhaled arsenic. While tobacco grown on soils not treated with arsenicals usually has a content of arsenic below 3 μg g^{-1}, the use of insecticides containing arsenic has resulted in enhanced levels in tobacco products, particularly in the US (Nordberg et al., 1979). Levels of up to 40 μg g^{-1} were recorded, but, during the last 20 years, reduced use of arsenical insecticides has caused levels to decrease to less than 8 μg g^{-1} (Nordberg et al., 1979). It is estimated that only 10 to 20% of this arsenic is volatilised in the smoke (Arnold et al., 1970; Holland et al., 1959), indicating that smokers consuming 20 cigarettes d^{-1} (or $\sim$20 g tobacco) will inhale no more than $\sim$30 μg of arsenic.

Organ, tissue or fluid	Concentration in μg g⁻¹ (number of samples)	Weighted mean (μg g⁻¹) (2)	Unweighted mean (μg g⁻¹) (2)	Number of samples (2)
Adrenal	0.0129(22),0.0261(22)	0.0195	0.0195	44
Aorta	0.0105(29),0.0189(29)	0.0147	0.0147	58
Blood (total)	0.19(103),0.0042(8),0.0025(7), 0.063(?),0.06(?),0.084(3), 0.092(15),0.011(?),0.042(5)	0.152 (3)	0.061	141
Blood (erythrocytes)	0.0027(7)	0.0027	0.0027	7
Blood (plasma)	<0.01(1),0.0024(16)	0.0024	0.0012 —	16
Blood (serum)	0.043(3),0.02(39)	0.022	0.0315	42
Bone	2.21(341),0.08(20)	2.09 (4)	1.15	361
Brain	0.0026(19),0.10(8)	0.031	0.053	27
Breast	0.027(3)	0.027	0.027	3
Hair	0.18(2),0.705(1000),0.65(650), 1.75(776),0.71(121),2.1(66), 0.26(16),1.07(10),0.9(42), 0.13(24),0.32(16),3.7(120), 0.51(43),0.29(200),0.23(11), 0.52(?)	1.06	0.88	3,100
Heart	0.0057(23),0.0074(23),0.0044(21)	0.0059	0.0058	67
Kidney	0.3(8),0.0059(25),0.0113(25), 0.0016(7),0.35(8)	0.077	0.133	73
Liver	0.46(6),0.0095(27),0.0167(27), 0.011(7),0.0065(5),0.097(17), 0.019(20)	0.051	0.089	109
Lung	0.0026(2),0.064(45),0.02(4), 0.01(7),0.08(56),0.113(56), 0.023(56),0.016(2)	0.067	0.041	228
Lymph node	0.2(6),0.074(18),0.024(3)	0.096	0.099	27
Milk	0.036(?)	-	0.036	-
Muscle (skeletal)	0.139(8),0.025(24),0.004(6),0.002(6)	0.040	0.043	44

TABLE 3

THE DISTRIBUTION OF STABLE ARSENIC IN HUMAN TISSUES   (1)

Organ, tissue or fluid	Concentration in μg g^{-1} (number of samples)	Weighted mean (μg g^{-1}) (2)	Unweighted mean (μg g^{-1}) (2)	Number of samples (2)
Nails	1.05(16),0.362(124),1.97(20), 1.0(42),3.3(?),0.225(10),0.2(1)	0.683	1.16	213
Ovary	0.2(5),0.016(13)	0.067	0.108	18
Pancreas	0.021(30),0.005(7)	0.018	0.013	37
Placenta	0.0055(6),0.0052(?)	0.0055	0.0054	6
Prostate	0.0084(10)	0.0084	0.0084	10
Skin	0.088(5),0.035(2),0.048(76),0.038(56), 0.092(2),0.072(1),0.06(1)	0.046	0.062	143
Stomach	0.0059(21),0.0099(21)	0.0079	0.0079	42
Spleen	0.003(7),0.0038(23),0.0071(23)	0.0051	0.0046	53
Thymus	0.0094(11)	0.0094	0.0094	11
Thyroid	0.0105(22),0.0198(22),0.009(3)	0.015	0.013	47
Tongue	0.0154(9),0.009(9)	0.012	0.012	18
Tooth (dentine)	0.1(?),0.022(4)	0.022	0.061	4
Tooth (enamel)	0.07(75), <0.02(28)	0.05–0.06	0.035–0.045	103
Trachea	0.008(9)	0.008	0.008	9
Urine	0.036(4),0.084(50),0.023(20), 0.120(2),0.015(2),0.041(13)	0.061	0.053	91
Urine (24h collection) (5)	0.129(16),0.077(2),0.016(2), 0.017(1),0.0046(1),0.139(?),0.034(5)	0.090	0.060	27
Uterus	0.019(23)	0.019	0.019	23

Notes: 1. Data are from Iyengar et al. (1978), but are all converted to fresh weight using the dry and ash weight fractions given. In the cases of breast, lymph node and placenta, the fresh to dry weight conversion factor for muscle is used.

2. Weighted means are based on all studies where the number of subjects is specified, unweighted means are based on all studies, giving equal weight to each. Number of samples is the sum over all studies used in the weighted mean calculation.

3. Heavily biased to one study of 103 samples analysed by mass spectrometry.

4. Two studies with substantially different results.

5. Based on an assumed urine volume of 1.4 l.

TABLE 3   (Contd.)

1.2.4   Summary

Based on the information presented in this section, normal intake rates for arsenic can be estimated as follows:

Route of intake	Typical intake rate ($\mu g\ d^{-1}$)	Comments
Diet	150	Specific individuals and groups may have daily intake rates an order of magnitude higher or lower than this.
Drinking water	<17	Up to ~600 $\mu g\ d^{-1}$ in some areas. Above this level, toxicity symptoms become apparent in relatively small populations.
Air	<5	~20 $\mu g\ d^{-1}$ or higher near non-ferrous smelters and cotton gins.
Smoking	<30	Based on a daily consumpti of 20 g of tobacco.

It is noted that these intakes do not include the component due to the use of arsenic containing pharmaceuticals. This will only affect a small number of relatively readily identifiable individuals.

1.3   DISTRIBUTION OF ARSENIC IN HUMAN TISSUES

Iyengar et al. (1978) reviewed the elemental composition of a wide range of human tissues and body fluids. Table 3 is derived from their review and shows the concentrations of arsenic in various human organs, tissues and tissue fluids. For convenience of comparison, all concentrations have been converted to μg arsenic per gram of fresh tissue, using the dry and ash weight fractions listed by Iyengar et al. (1978). These data are also displayed in graphical form in Fig. 1. On the basis of the information presented there, and in Table 3, the following conclusions may be drawn.

- Arsenic is concentrated in hair and nails where it is typically found at a level of 1 $\mu g\ g^{-1}$.
- Arsenic may concentrate in bone, but the relatively low concentrations found in dentine tend to contradict this hypothesis.
- Dietary arsenic is not accumulated in human erythrocytes.
- Excluding hair and nails, arsenic is relatively uniformly distributed throughout all organs and tissues of the human body, though it may be concentrated to some extent in kidneys, liver and ovaries.

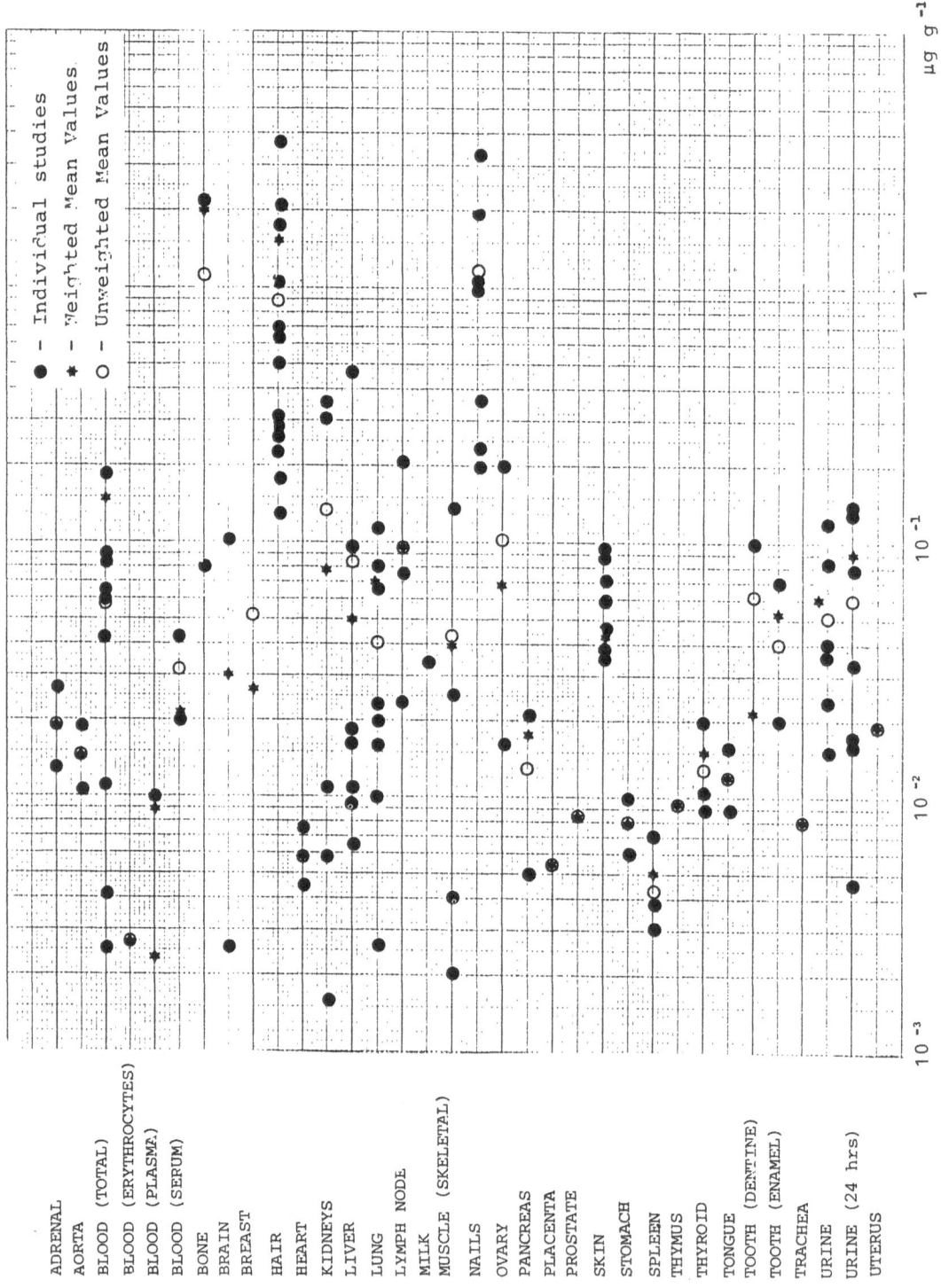

FIGURE 1.   THE DISTRIBUTION OF STABLE ARSENIC IN HUMAN TISSUES

- A typical concentration of arsenic in soft tissues is 0.04 $\mu g\,g^{-1}$, except for liver, kidneys and ovaries where a value of 0.1 $\mu g\,g^{-1}$ is more usual.
- Concentrations of arsenic in urine are similar to concentrations of arsenic in total blood and are typically 0.07 $\mu g\,g^{-1}$.

Arsenic concentrations in tissues are also discussed by Fowler et al. (1979) and by the IARC (1980). Fowler et al. (1979) quoted the following tissue concentrations (dry weight basis) for healthy persons from Scotland who died in accidents.

Tissue or fluid	Concentration ($\mu g\,g^{-1}$)
Whole blood	0.036
Bone	0.053
Hair	0.460
Nail	0.283
Lung	0.078
Skin	0.080
Other tissues	0.012-0.062

Concentrations in organs from Japanese who generally had consumed relatively high quantities of seafood were also given. These are summarised below (wet weight basis).

Tissue or fluid	Concentration ($\mu g\,g^{-1}$)
Bone (femur)	0.118
(rib)	0.074
Hair	0.174
Nail	0.892
Other tissues	0.020-0.078

More detailed autopsy data on a variety of previously healthy subjects who had died as a result of violence are given by Smith (1967). These subjects were all residents of Glasgow and Smith noted that they may not be representative of other areas. The data given by Smith are summarised below.

		Concentration (μg g^{-1} d.w.)			
Tissue	No. of samples	Minimum	Maximum	Median	Mean
Adrenal	22	0.002	0.293	0.029	0.061
Aorta	29	0.003	0.570	0.031	0.063
Blood (whole)*	12	0.001	0.920	0.038	0.147
Bone	20	0.010	0.240	0.057	0.080
Brain	19	0.001	0.036	0.013	0.016
Breast	3	0.030	0.221	-	0.095
Hair*	1250	0.030	8.17	0.510	0.650
Heart	23	0.002	0.078	0.024	0.027
Kidney	25	0.002	0.363	0.033	0.050
Liver	27	0.005	0.246	0.028	0.057
Lung	56	0.006	0.514	0.082	0.113
Muscle (pectoral)	24	0.012	0.431	0.063	0.091
Nail*	124	0.020	2.90	0.300	0.362
Ovary	13	0.013	0.260	0.037	0.071
Pancreas	30	0.005	0.410	0.045	0.088
Prostate	10	0.010	0.090	0.046	0.045
Skin	76	0.009	0.590	0.090	0.124
Spleen	23	0.001	0.132	0.020	0.032
Stomach	21	0.003	0.104	0.037	0.037
Teeth	75	0.003	0.635	0.050	0.070
Thymus	11	0.003	0.332	0.015	0.047
Thyroid	22	0.001	0.314	0.042	0.079
Uterus	23	0.010	0.188	0.031	0.058

Note: * Indicates data from live subjects.

All the above data are compatible with the conclusions derived from examination of the heterogeneous mass of data summarised by Iyengar et al. (1978).

1.4   METABOLISM

1.4.1   Gastrointestinal absorption

Several reviews have discussed the gastrointestinal absorption of compounds of arsenic (Pershagen and Vahter, 1979; Nordberg et al., 1979; Fowler et al., 1979; IARC, 1980; ICRP, 1981). On the basis of the available data, Fowler et al. (1979) made the following comments:

Species	Compound	Fractional absorption	Reference	Comments
Man	Arsenic in drinking water	~0.5	Valentine et al., 1979.	Estimated from drinking water and urine concentrations using a daily water intake of 1.5 l.
Rat	Arsenic in pig flesh Arsenic trioxide	0.24 (0.21-0.26) 0.50 (0.20-0.76)	Overby and Frost, 1962.	Estimated from urinary and faecal excretions.
Rat	Arsenic in shrimps Arsenic trioxide Stock diet	>0.96 >0.87 >0.78	Coulson et al., 1935.	Estimated from urinary and faecal excretion.
Man	Arsenic in shrimps Arsenic trioxide Dietary	>0.98 1 >0.67	Coulson et al., 1935.	Estimated from urinary and faecal excretion.
Man	Liquid arsenicalis	>0.96	Bettley and O'Shea, 1975.	Estimated from faecal excretion.
Pig	Arsenilic acid	0.15-0.46	Overby and Frost, 1960.	Estimated from urinary and faecal excretion over the last two days of a 12 day arsenilic acid feeding period.

TABLE 4

THE GASTROINTESTINAL ABSORPTION OF COMPOUNDS OF ARSENIC

Species	Compound	Fractional absorption	Reference	Comments
Man	Arsenic in fish	0.77 (0.64-0.90)	Freeman et al., 1979.	Estimated from urinary excretion over 9 days. Takes no account of residual tissue retention and biliary excretion.
Rat Rabbit Guinea pig	10-10' oxybisphenoxarsine oxybisphenoxarsine oxybisphenoxarsine	~0.2 ~0.4 ~0.4	Kronenberg and Hartung 1981.	Based on faecal excretion over 7 days, using C-14 label for assay and thus neglecting metabolic transformation.
Rabbit	Monosodium acid methanearsenate	0.52 (0.42-0.61)	Exon et al., 1974.	Based on urinary and faecal excretion: biliary excretion neglected thus underestimating absorption.
Man	As^{3+} and As^{5+} in wine As^{5+} rich well water	>0.8 <0.5	Crecelius, 1977	Based on urinary excretion to 61h. Value based on mass balance to 70h post-ingestion and does not take account of arsenic retained in the body or excreted in the faeces.
Cynomologus monkey	Fish arsenic Arsenic trioxide	0.90 (0.84-0.99) 0.98 (0.96-0.99)	Charbonneau et al., 1978.	Estimated from faecal excretion to 14 days.
Mouse	As^{3+} As^{3+}	0.98 0.96	Vahter and Norin, 1980	Based on faecal excretion to 48h, corrected for biliary contribution using results from sub-cutaneous administration (correction <5%)

TABLE 4   (Contd.)

Species	Compound	Fractional absorption	Reference	Comments
Rat	Sodium arsenate	~0.75	Dutkiewicz, 1977.	Comparison of faecal excretion over 10 days following intravenous and oral administration.
Rat	Dimethylarsinic acid	~1	Stevens et al., 1977.	Comparison of blood concentrations 0.2 to 100 days after intravenous and oral administration.
Hamster	Arsenic acid	0.36	Charbonneau et al., 1980.	Author's estimate.
Mouse	As^{5+} As^{3+}	0.96	Vahter, 1981.	Based on urinary excretion and residual body content 48h after administration.
Rat	As^{5+} As^{3+}	0.82 0.86	Vahter, 1981.	Based on urinary excretion and residual body content 48h after administration.
Man	Arsenic acid	0.94 (0.89-0.96)	Pomroy et al., 1980.	Based on faecal excretion during 7 days after administration.
Mouse	Arsenic acid	>0.8	Gerber et al., 1982.	Based on gastrointestinal tract content after 3,5 and 7 days of feeding an arsenic contaminated diet.
Man	?	>0.90	Arnold et al., 1970.	Based on whole-body retention.

TABLE 4 (Contd.)

- Both human and animal data indicate that over 80% of an ingested dose of dissolved inorganic trivalent arsenic is absorbed from the gastrointestinal tract.

- A few animal studies indicate that absorption following ingestion of pentavalent inorganic arsenic will be about the same as for inorganic trivalent forms.

- Organic arsenic compounds in seafoods are more than 80% absorbed from the gastrointestinal tract in both animals and humans.

- Feed promoters, such as arsinilic acid, are absorbed to only 15 to 40%.

- In the case of arsenic trioxide, which is only slightly soluble in water, the gastrointestinal absorption will be dependent on factors such as particle size and pH of the gastric juice.

A variety of data (Table 4) support these conclusions.

With respect to the speed and location of arsenic absorption, Tsutsumi et al. (1975) studied the uptake of arsenic from a ligated ileocaecal portion of rabbit intestine. In control animals, ~30% of infused As_2O_3 was absorbed into the blood within 60 minutes. When dimercaprol (BAL) or thioctic acid were administered, either parenterally, or directly into the loop, absorption decreased.

Comparison of blood concentrations in rats following oral and intravenous administration of sodium arsenate (Dutkiewicz, 1977) demonstrated that gastrointestinal absorption is essentially complete by 15 h post-administration. In comparison, Stevens et al. (1977) estimated a half-life of 248 minutes for transfers of dimethylarsenic acid from the gastrointestinal tract of rats to their blood. However, examination of their data suggests that the true half-time could be rather lower, since gastrointestinal absorption appeared to be essentially complete by 3 h after administration.

In man, the rapid transfer of arsenic from blood to urine (see Section 4.3) can be used, in conjunction with the data of Crecelius (1977), to argue for an absorption half-time of a few hours.

In conclusion, it seems likely that arsenic is absorbed rapidly from the small intestine. For model calculations, the fractional absorption may be taken as 0.5 to 1.0 for most compounds of the element, exceptions to this are feed promoters, such as arsinilic acid, and arsenic trioxide in solid form. For arsinilic acid, a best estimate of fractional absorption is 0.3. For solid arsenic trioxide no firm recommendation can be given, since gastrointestinal absorption will be strongly dependent on particle size and pH of the gastric juice. For dietary arsenic, a best estimate of fractional absorption is 0.9.

1.4.2   Retention in the respiratory system

The metabolism of arsenic following inhalation or intratracheal instillation has been much less investigated than has the metabolism of the element subsequent to oral administration. The ICRP (1966) assigned all commonly occurring compounds of arsenic to inhalation class W, representing a biological half-life in the deep lung of weeks, rather than days or years. Other reviewers appear to have given little attention to the dynamics of arsenic retention in the lungs and its transfer from there to the gut or blood.

Two studies have investigated the metabolism of arsenic inhaled in cigarette smoke (Holland et al., 1959; Arnold et al., 1970). In the work of Holland et al. (1959), eleven volunteers who had terminal lung cancer were studied. Eight inhaled the smoke, in their usual manner, from a cigarette impregnated in its distal half with [As-74] sodium arsenate. The other three inhaled [As-74] sodium arsenate in aerosol form. Arsenic distribution and retention was studied using external gamma counting together with urinary and faecal assay.

Uptakes of activity following smoking represented 4.8 to 8.8% of that injected into the cigarettes (i.e.~40% of inhaled activity when account is taken of the volatilised fraction as discussed in Section 1.2.3), whereas uptake following inhalation of the aerosol represented 32 to 62% of the amount nebulised. These uptakes are consistent with those expected for aerosols with an activity median aerodynamic diameter of about 1 μm (ICRP, 1966). Both cigarette and aerosol arsenic appeared to be similarly spatially distributed in the lungs and their retention was also reported to be similar.

Of the initial arsenic uptake by the lungs, ~75% was retained in that tissue with a half-life of just over one day, while ~25% was retained with a half-life ~10 days. Excretion was almost entirely in the urine with ~30% of uptake being excreted on the first day and ~45% in total over the first 10 days after inhalation.

Arnold et al. (1970) reported that 15 to 20% of arsenic contained in each cigarette was released in the smoke and that uptake was strongly dependent on smoking habits, i.e. 0.23%, 2% and 5-10% of the arsenic contained in each cigarette for individuals not inhaling, slightly inhaling and deeply inhaling respectively. The figure of 5-10% for deeply inhaling subjects represents a fractional uptake of 0.3 to 0.6 of inhaled arsenic, which is consistent with the result reported by Holland et al. (1959). Of absorbed arsenic, 50% was eliminated in the first 4.5 d and 75% in the first 11 d after inhalation. For comparison, after ingestion, 50% elimination occurred in 3 d and 80% in 10 d. These data suggest that inhaled arsenic is relatively rapidly cleared from the lungs of man.

Arnold et al. (1970) also undertook studies on the distribution of As-74 in guinea pigs and rats following inhalation. In the guinea pig the arsenic was almost completely cleared from the lung in a period of six days and only in the skeleton was there evidence for a substantial component of long-term retention. In the rat, the lung and most other tissues exhibited long-term retention of arsenic, but this was almost undoubtedly due to arsenic contained in blood (Section 1.4.3).

Other relevant data on the metabolism of inhaled arsenic in man are given by Smith et al. (1977), who compared arsenic levels in urine with airborne arsenic exposure. The relative proportions of the various arsenic species in urine was independent of the level of exposure, viz. 9% As(III), 6% As(V), 20% methylarsonic acid and 65% dimethylarsinic acid. Urinary excretion of As(III), methylarsonic and dimethylarsinic acids was more closely related to "irrespirable" particulate exposure than to "respirable" particulate exposure. This was presumably because "irrespirable" particles comprised much of the exposure and are more effectively trapped in the lung plus upper airways than are respirable particles which are mainly trapped in the deep lung or exhaled.

TABLE 5

RATIO OF BLOOD TO MUSCLE CONCENTRATIONS OF ARSENIC IN RATS AND RABBITS (1)

Time (h)	Ratio of blood to muscle concentration	
	Rat	Rabbit
6	37.6	0.64
24	67.5	0.33
48	140.0	0.30
96	99.4	

Note: 1. From Ducoff et al. (1948)

TABLE 6

DISTRIBUTION OF CARRIER – FREE RADIO – ARSENIC IN VARIOUS SPECIES 48 HOURS AFTER INTRAMUSCULAR INJECTION (1)

Tissue	Total organ content (% injected activity)						
	Rat	Cat	Dog	Rabbit	Guinea pig	Chick	Mouse
Blood	44.5	5.62	0.10	0.27	0.25	0.19	0.07
Liver	1.46	0.65	–	1.01	1.21	0.15	0.09
Kidney	0.47	0.10	–	0.37	0.06	0.06	0.12
Spleen	0.50	0.30	–	0.008	0.01	0.01	0.05
Bone	1.91	0.98	–	0.98	1.10	0.80	0.24
Muscle	2.46	1.85	–	2.13	2.95	1.40	0.70

Note: 1. From Lanz et al. (1950)

The study of Smith et al. (1977) demonstrates that, in common with arsenic administered via other routes, inhaled arsenic is methylated in the human body and that both monomethyl and dimethyl forms are significant metabolites.

Other data on inhaled arsenic are available for rabbits (Bencko et al., 1968), but these do not add significantly to the information presented above. Following intratracheal instillation of dimethylarsinic acid (Stevens et al., 1977) or sodium arsenate (Dutkiewicz, 1977) into rats, the arsenic enters blood virtually as quickly as if it had been intravenously injected.

On the basis of the data presented above, the following conclusions may be drawn.

- The deposition of arsenic containing aerosols in the lungs is similar to that of other aerosols and, in deeply inhaling smokers, ∿10% of arsenic in cigarettes will be deposited in the lungs.

- All compounds of arsenic which have been studied have been found to be cleared from the lungs with a half-life of a few days; a biphasic model in which 75% of deposited material is cleared with a half-life of 4 days and 25% is cleared with a half-life of 10 days is probably the most reasonable to use for man.

- Virtually all arsenic translocated from the lungs enters the blood either directly or via the gastrointestinal tract.

Finally, it is important to note that the above remarks do not apply to the toxic, arsenic containing, gas arsine. As with other gases, a large fraction of inhaled arsine is very rapidly absorbed from the lungs. Experiments on mice (Levvy, 1947) indicated that this fraction is ∿0.64 over a wide range of levels of exposure. These experiments also demonstrated that arsenic inhaled as arsine is much more avidly retained in the tissues of mice than is arsenic injected as arsenite. This is probably because of the high concentration of arsine arsenic in blood relative to other tissues (Levvy, 1947).

1.4.3   Systemic metabolism

A wide variety of studies have demonstrated that arsenic is accumulated in the blood of rats (e.g. Hunter et al., 1942; Ducoff et al., 1948; Lanz et al., 1959; Klaasen, 1974; Cikrt and Bencko, 1974; Dutkiewicz, 1977; Kronenberg and Hartung, 1981) and from such experiments it can be estimated that up to 80% of absorbed arsenic can be accumulated in the blood (Pershagen and Vahter, 1979). This is in distinct contrast to the situation in other species, as is illustrated by the inter-species comparisons set out in Tables 5 to 8, and can be attributed to the binding ˙ of arsenic to globin in rat erythrocytes (Pershagen and Vahter, 1979).

The affinity of rat erythrocytes for arsenic, and the consequent long-term retention in blood, makes the rat an inappropriate species for investigation of the metabolism and excretion of arsenic. Data from experiments on rats are not, therefore, considered further.

TABLE 7

TISSUE DISTRIBUTION OF RADIOACTIVITY AFTER
ADMINISTRATION OF (C-14) 10-10' OXYBISPHENOXARSINE
TO RATS, GUINEA PIGS AND RABBITS   (1)

| Tissue | Percent dose/100 g wet tissue (3) | | |
	Rat	Guinea Pig	Rabbit
Liver	9.52 (100)	11.98 (100)	0.26 (100)
Kidney	7.10 (75)	3.10 (26)	0.27 (128)
Spleen	5.02 (52)	0.53 (4)	0.05 (21)
Heart	2.52 (25)	0.60 (5)	0.08 (36)
Lung	4.58 (47)	1.20 (10)	0.14 (59)
Brain	4.65 (48)	1.30 (11)	0.26 (115)
Stomach	1.26 (13)	0.85 (7)	0.10 (43)
Intestines	2.53 (26)	0.85 (7)	0.09 (46)
Bladder	1.35 (14)	0.65 (5)	0.12 (48)
Adrenal	2.55 (26)	2.08 (17)	- -
Testes	1.66 (18)	0.30 (3)	0.12 (38)
Skin	1.85 (19)	0.85 (7)	0.16 (75)
Fat	0.63 (7)	0.48 (4)	0.04 (18)
Gall bladder	- -	4.82 (40)	0.28 (128)
Muscle	1.10 (11)	0.68 (6)	0.05 (19)
Blood (2)	12.90 (133)	0.50 (4)	0.04 (23)
Plasma (2)	0.15 (2)	0.40 (3)	0.01 (4)
Bile (2)	- -	0.48 (4)	0.26 (90)

Notes: 1. From Kronenberg and Hartung (1981)
        2. Per 100 ml.
        3. Values in parenthesis are normalised to
            liver as 100.

TABLE 8

CONCENTRATION OF As-74 IN VARIOUS
TISSUES OF THE RAT 2h and 7d AFTER
INTRAVENOUS INJECTION   (1)

Tissue	Concentration (% I.A. g^{-1})	
	2 hour	7 day
Blood	0.65	1.0
Plasma	0.0018	0.0014
Liver	0.025	0.06
Spleen	0.03	0.25
Kidney	0.06	0.06
Heart	0.03	0.13
Lung	0.035	0.14
Testes	0.005	0.0013
Brain	0.003	0.0015

Note: 1. From Klaassen (1974)

TABLE 9

EARLY EXCRETION OF ARSENIC IN VARIOUS SPECIES

Species	Reference	Comments
Rabbit	Marafante et al. 1980.	After intraperitoneal injection of sodium arsenite, urinary and faecal excretion in the first 24h were 55.5 ± 18.5 and 6.2 ± 4.3% of the injected activity respectively. Chemical species in urine were 37% inorganic arsenic, 2.6% monomethylarsenic and 60.4% dimethylarsinic acid.
Man	Holland et al. 1959.	∿30% of inhaled arsenic is excreted in the urine in the first day after intake.
Man	Arnold et al. 1970.	After inhalation in cigarette smoke, 50% of absorbed arsenic is eliminated in 4½ days and 7.5% in 11 days. After ingestion, 50% is eliminated in three days and 80% in ten days.
Man	Coulson et al. 1935.	Rapid arsenic excretion following ingestion of shrimp arsenic and arsenic trioxide (see Figure 2).
Man	Bettley and O'Shea 1975.	Rapid urinary arsenic excretion after oral dosing of normal and carcinoma patients with liquid arsenicalis (see Figure 3).
Man	Freeman et al. 1979.	Rapid urinary excretion after ingestion of arsenic in fish. (see Figure 4).
Rabbit and guinea pig	Kronenberg and Hartung, 1981.	Excretion of 10-10' oxybisphenoxarsine (OBPA) by rabbits and guinea pigs (see Figure 5).
Man	Hunter et al. 1942.	Excretion after single and multiple injections of arsenite (see Figures 6,7,8).

TABLE 9   (Contd.)

Species	Reference	Comments
Man	Mealey et al. 1959.	Urinary excretion parallels plasma concentration in subject intra-venously injected with arsenic primarily ·in the As^{3+} state. Renal clearance corresponds to 3.54 l of plasma h^{-1} and the initial dilution volume is 14.1 l.
Man	Crecelius, 1977	Urinary excretion of various chemical species of arsenic after oral administration of arsenite-rich wine, arsenate rich drinking water and crab meat containing organo-arsenic compounds. (see Figures 9,10 and 11).
Dog and cow	Lasko and Peoples 1975.	Urinary excretion of methylated and inorganic arsenic after feeding with sodium arsenate and potassium arsenite. Half-time of loss after feeding ∿1 day.
Monkey	Charbonneau et al. 1978.	Excretion of inorganic and fish arsenic by monkeys after ingestion (see Figure 12).
Rabbit	Bertolero et al. 1981.	Excretion over the first four days after intraperitoneal injection becomes dominated by demethylarsinic acid by day 2. (see Figure 13).
Mouse	Vahter, 1981.	20% of As^{3+} and 35% of As^{5+} lost from the body in the first 48 hours after oral dosing.
Man	Pomroy et al. 1980.	Urinary and faecal excretion after administration of a single dose of (^{74}As) arsenic acid to six volunteers (see Figure 14)

1.4.3.1   Whole-body retention

A variety of studies on animals have demonstrated the rapid early excretion of various compounds of arsenic in several species, almost exclusively in the urine (Pershagen and Vahter, 1979). This information is summarised in Table 9 and the associated figures. The most comprehensive set of human data are those of Mealey et al.(1975) who administered arsenic, predominantly as As^{3+} into five subjects. The plasma concentration curve in these subjects was well described by:

$$C_p(t) = 7.0 \exp(-1.54t) + 0.070 \exp(-0.025t) + 0.015 \exp(-0.003t)$$

where $C_p(t)$ (% injected activity l^{-1}) is the plasma concentration; and

t is the time in hours after injection.

The urinary excretion curve was similar to the plasma clearance curve and, at early times, represented a renal clearance rate of 3.54 l of plasma h^{-1}. Assuming this renal clearance rate to apply at all times, the urinary excretion could be represented by

$$U(t) = 24.78 \exp(-1.54t) + 0.2478 \exp(-0.025t) + 0.0531 \exp(-0.003t)$$

where $U(t)$ (% injected activity h^{-1}) is the urinary excretion rate.

Integrating this function over all time implies that ~44% of injected arsenic is excreted in urine, whereas, in practice, 18 to 39% was recovered at the end of one hour, 36 to 56% at the end of four hours and 57 to 90% recovered at the end of nine days. In one patient, who was followed for 18 days, 96.6% of the total injected dose was detected in the urine.

Examination of the urinary excretion curve presented by Mealey et al. (1959), suggests that a more adequate representation may be

$$U(t) = 40.7 \exp(-1.54t) + 1.0 \exp(-0.02t) + 0.03 \exp(-0.0012t)$$

This expression gives 21%, 30%, 81% and 86% of administered arsenic excreted in urine at 1h, 4h, 9d and 18d post-injection respectively. It is useful to note that the half-lives and relative proportions of the two longer-term components of retention are consistent with results from other human and animal studies on a variety of arsenical compounds (Fig. 2 to 8), but that, in these other studies, integration of urinary excretion over the first day post-administration has obscured the component of very rapid excretion. The distinction between the plasma clearance curve and the urinary excretion curve probably reflect the processes of arsenic methylation which have been identified in man and other mammalian species (Marafante et al., 1980; Buchet et al., 1980; Tam et al., 1978; Tam et al., 1979; Smith et al., 1977; Crecelius, 1977; Lasko and Peoples, 1975; Charbonneau et al., 1980; Bertolero et al., 1981; Vahter, 1981; Mahieu et al., 1981) and the processes of arsenite-arsenate transformation (Bencko et al., 1976; Ginsburg, 1965).

Mainly on the basis of data from the studies of Mealey et al. (1959), the ICRP (1981) commented that the whole-body retention in man

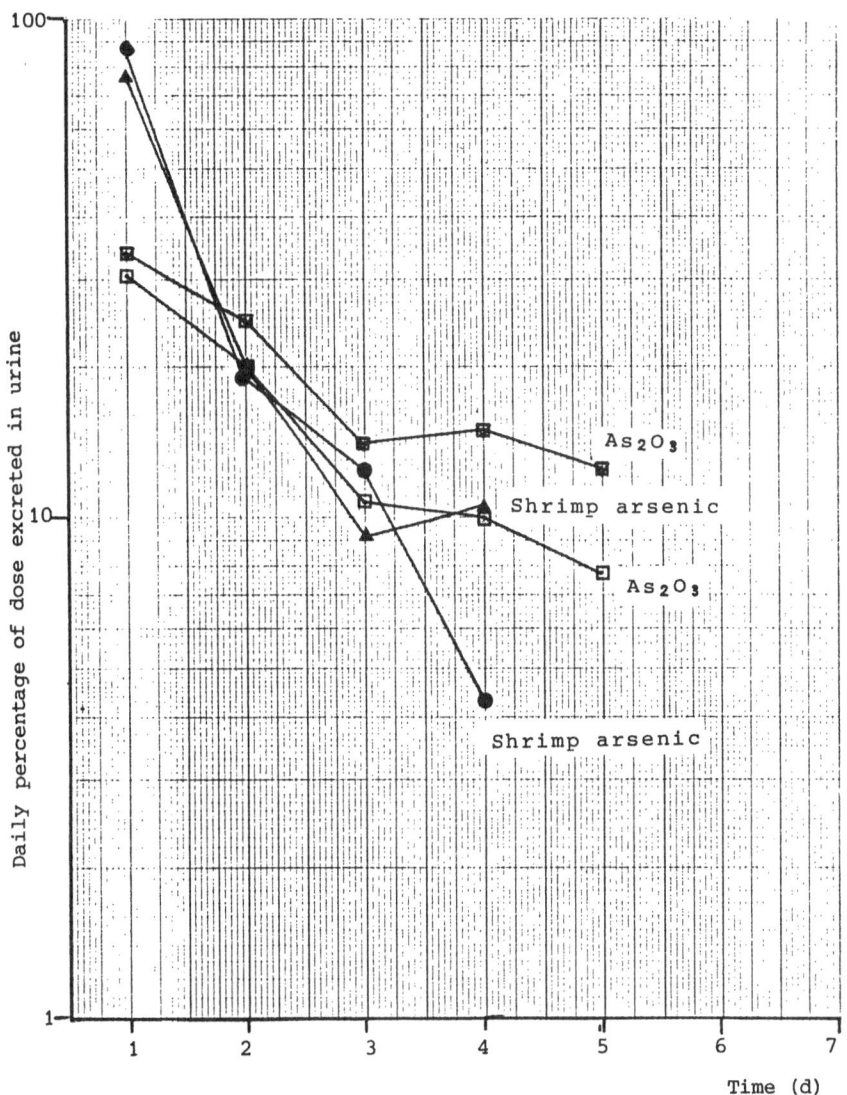

FIGURE 2.   EXCRETION OF ARSENIC BY MAN SUBSEQUENT
TO INGESTION (FROM COULSON ET AL.   (1935),
UNCORRECTED FOR NORMAL EXCRETION).

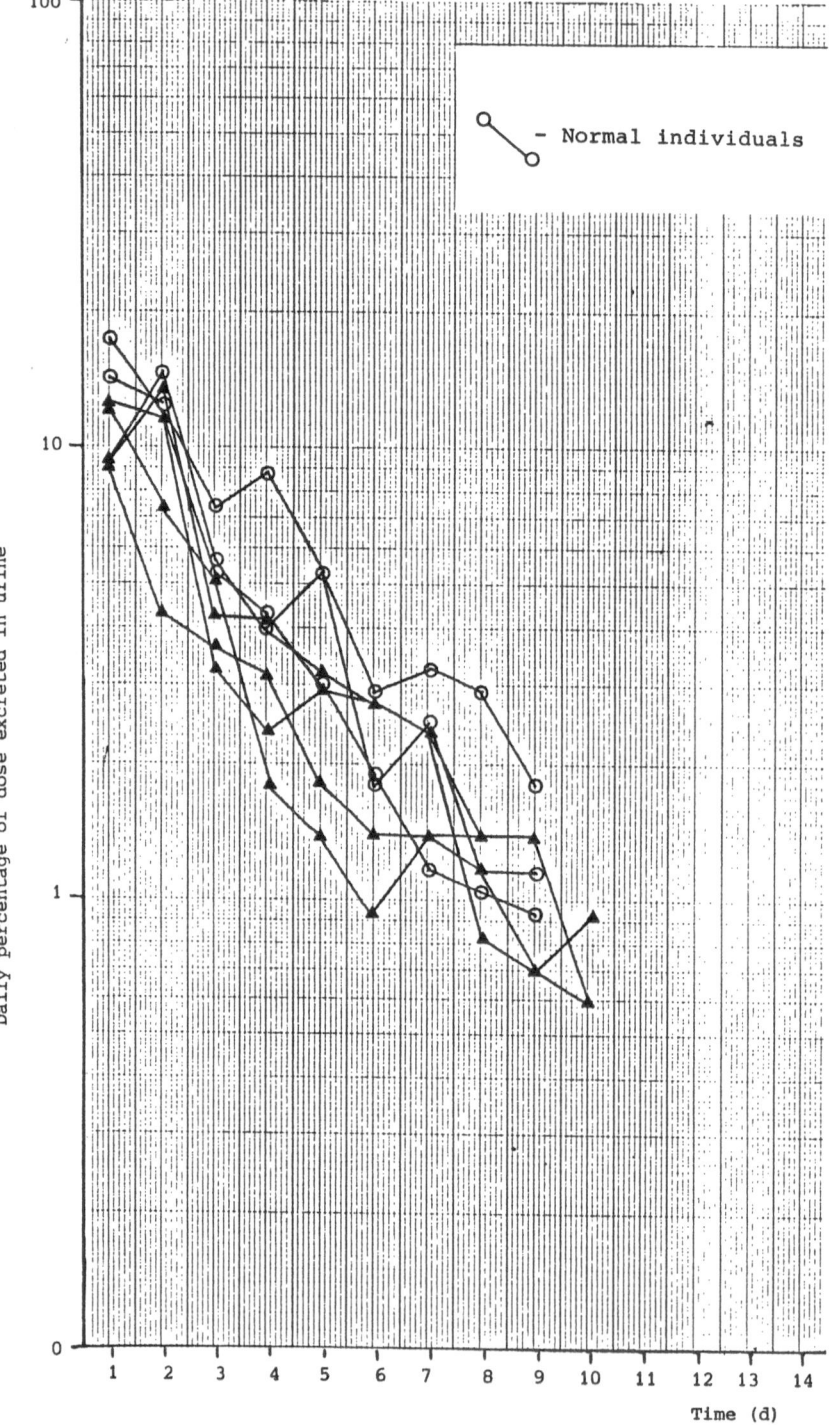

FIGURE 3. URINARY EXCRETION OF ARSENIC IN NORMAL AND
CARCINOMA PATIENTS (FROM BETTLEY AND O'SHEA 1975)

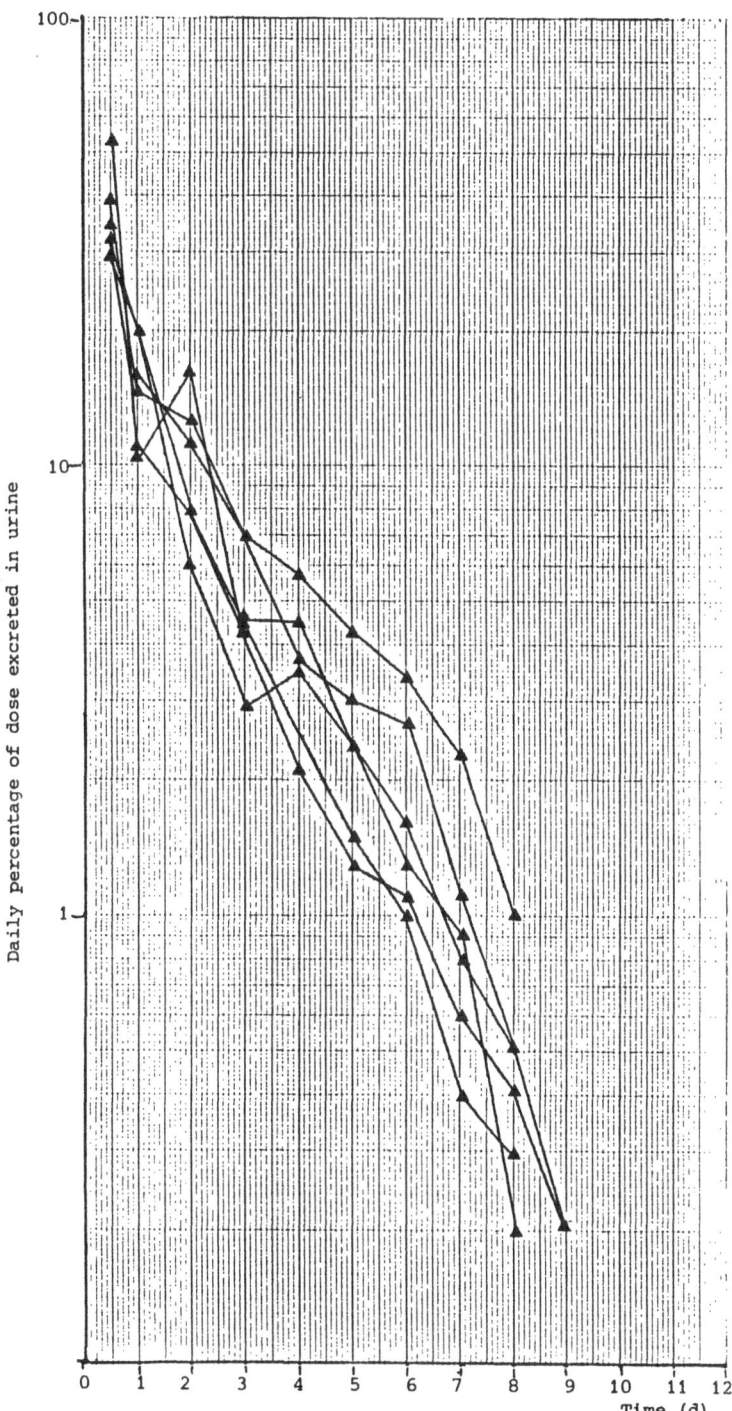

FIGURE 4. URINARY EXCRETION OF ARSENIC IN NORMAL
SUBJECTS FOLLOWING CONSUMPTION OF ARSENIC
CONTAINING FISH (FROM FREEMAN ET AL. 1979).

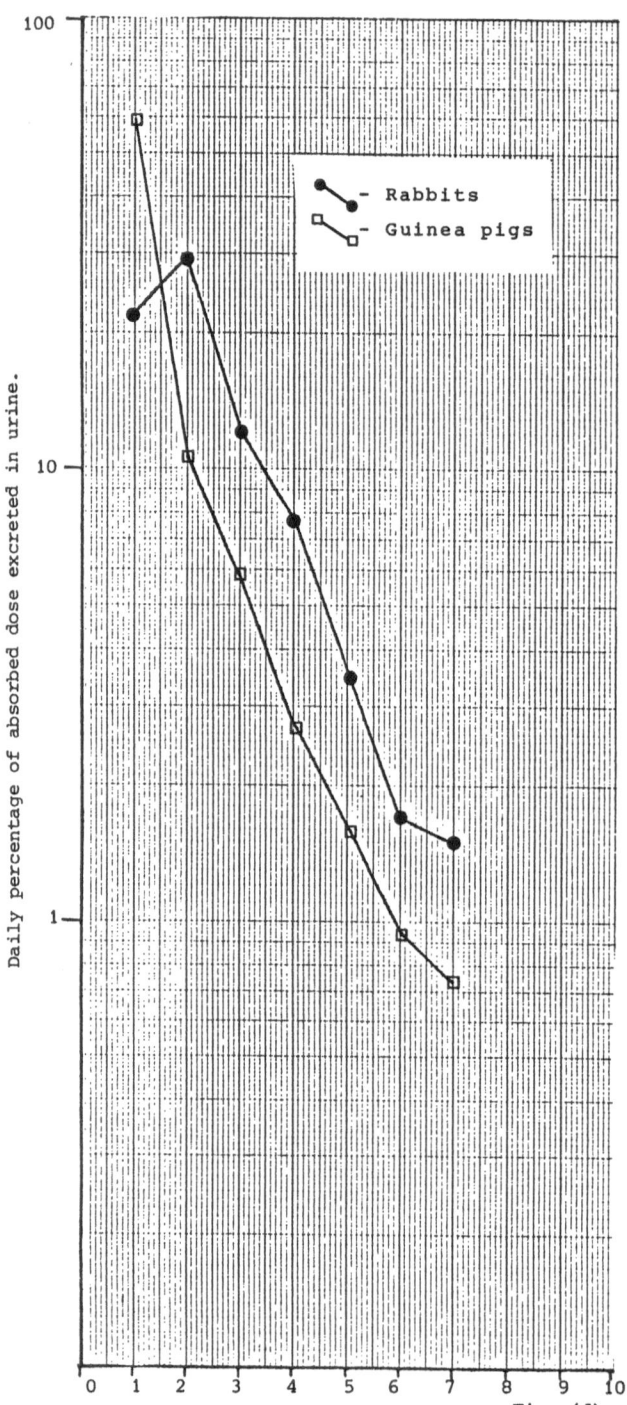

FIGURE 5.   URINARY EXCRETION OF 10-10 OXYBIOPHENOXARSINE
             BY GUINEA PIGS AND RABBITS (FROM KRONENBERG AND
             HARTUNG 1981).
Note: Corrected to absorbed dose during faecal excretion.

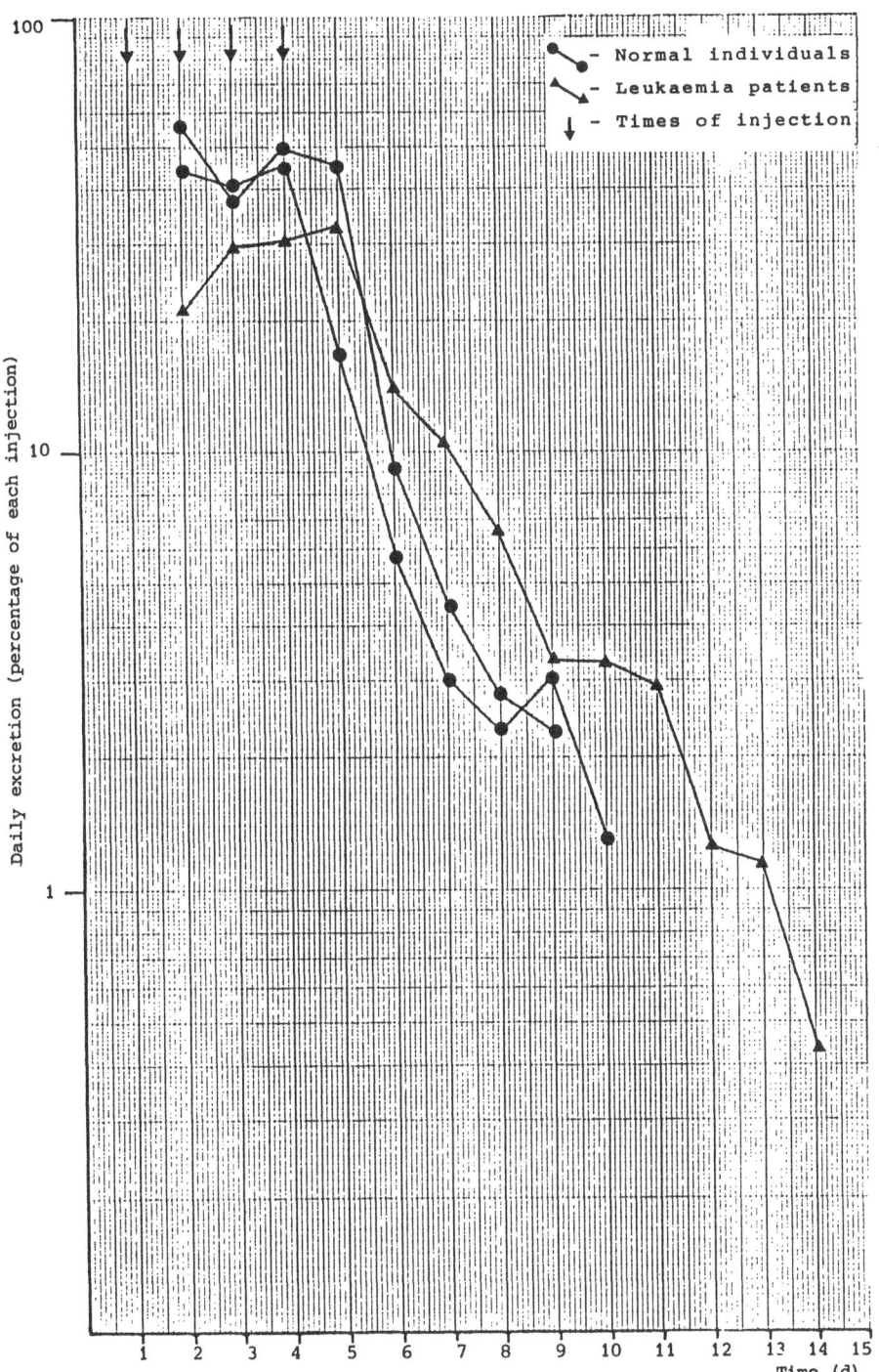

FIGURE 6. URINARY EXCRETION OF ARSENIC BY MAN AFTER
SUBCUTANEOUS INJECTION OF ARSENITE (FROM
HUNTER ET AL. 1942).

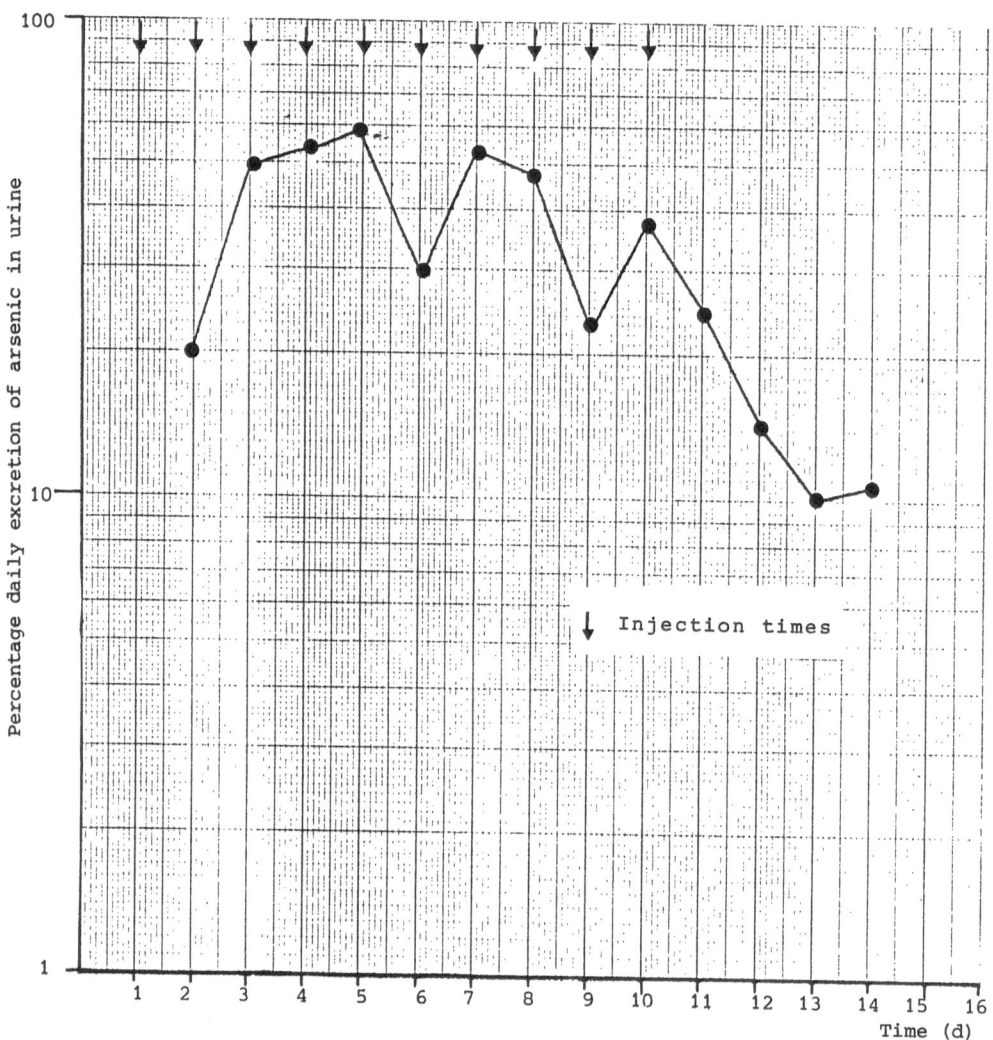

FIGURE 7.   URINARY EXCRETION OF ARSENIC BY A LEUKAEMIC
MAN DURING AND AFTER REPEATED SUBCUTANEOUS
INJECTIONS OF ARSENITE(FROM HUNTER ET AL. 1942).

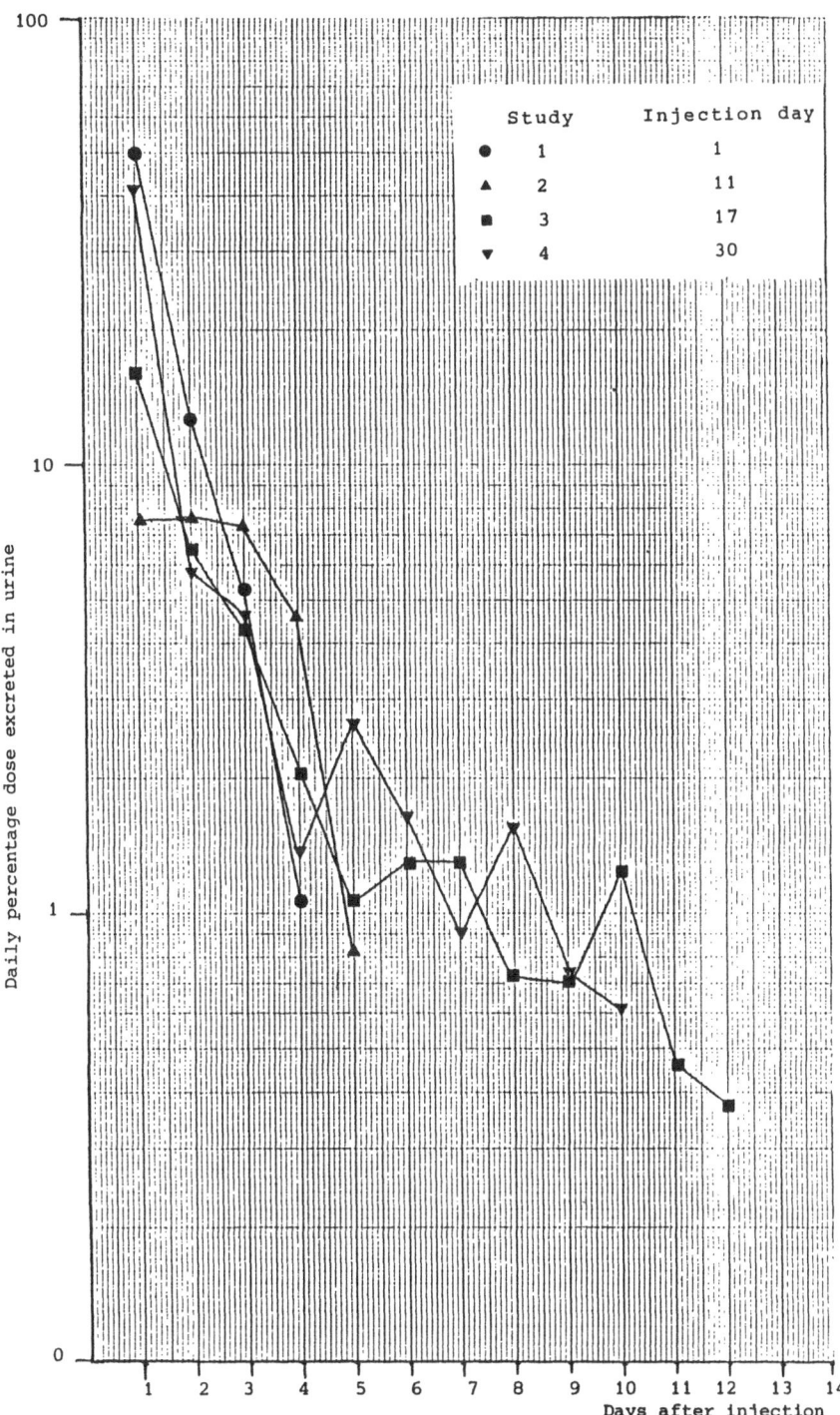

FIGURE 8.   URINARY EXCRETION OF ARSENIC AFTER A SINGLE
            SUBCUTANEOUS INJECTION OF ARSENITE TO A
            LEUKAEMIC HUMAN (FROM HUNTER ET AL.   1942).

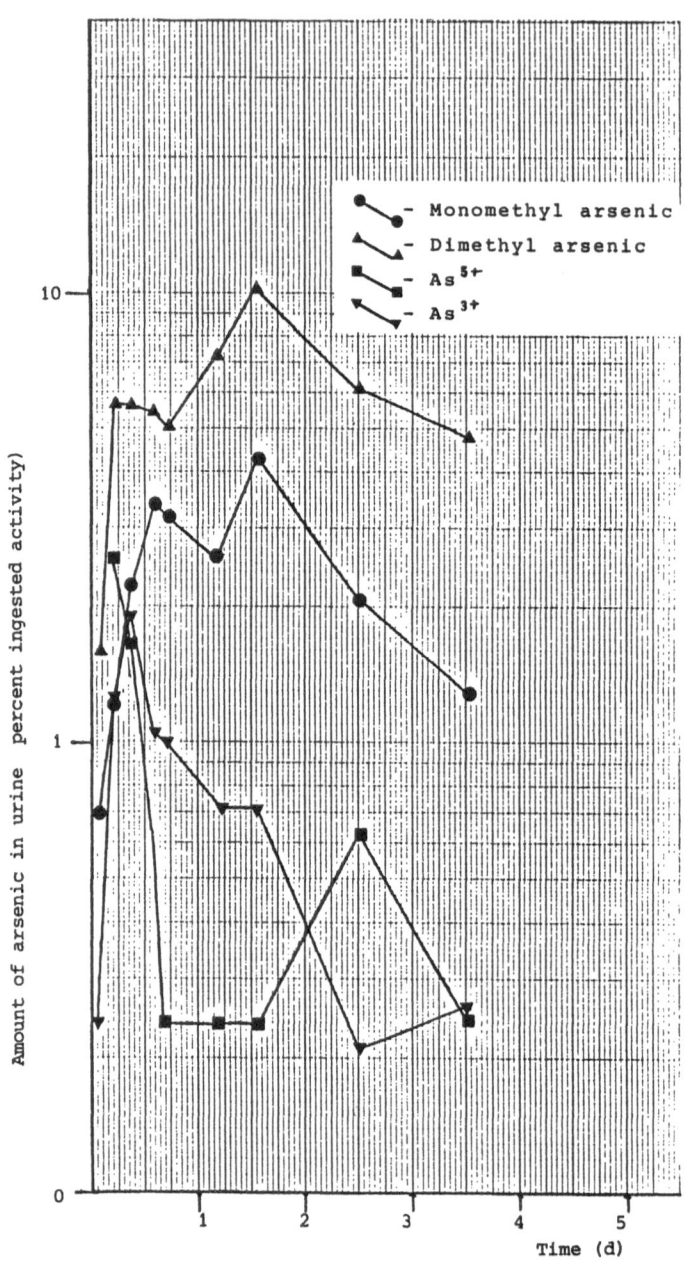

FIGURE 9.   URINARY EXCRETION OF ARSENIC AFTER
            INGESTION OF CONTAMINATED WINE (FROM
            CRECELIUS   1977).

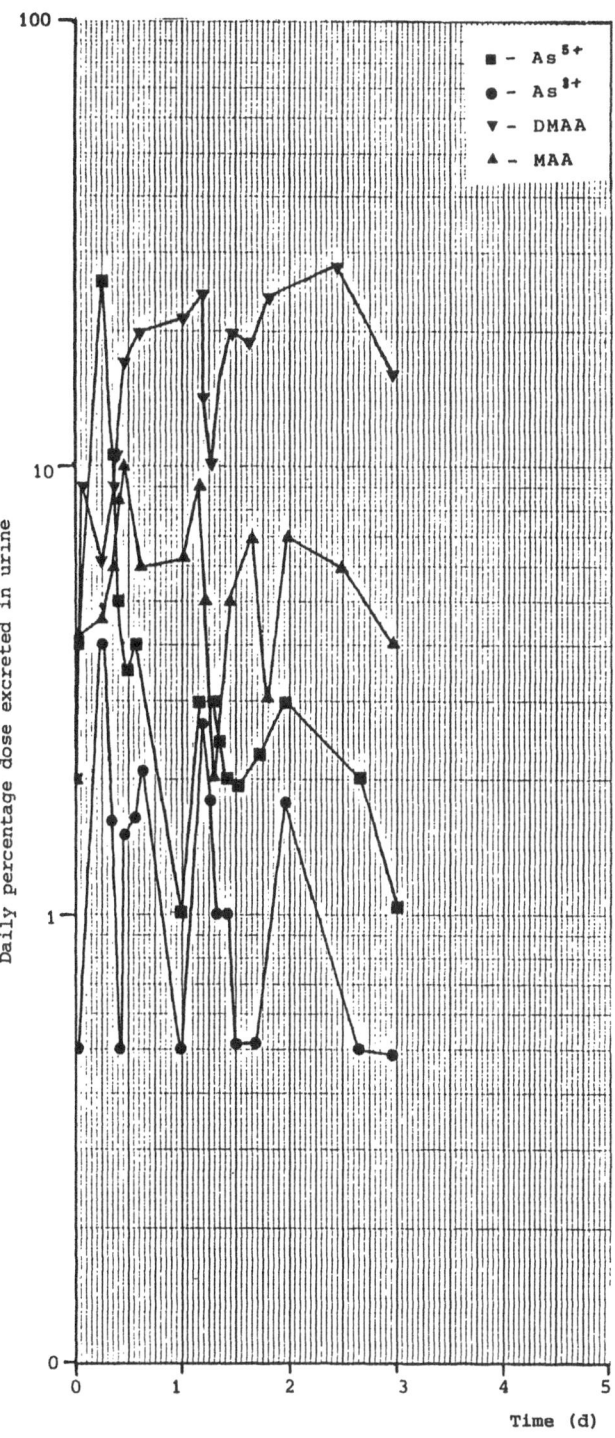

FIGURE 10.   URINARY EXCRETION OF ARSENIC AFTER
             INGESTION OF WELL WATER CONTAINING
             250µg As^{5+} (FROM CRECELIUS 1977).

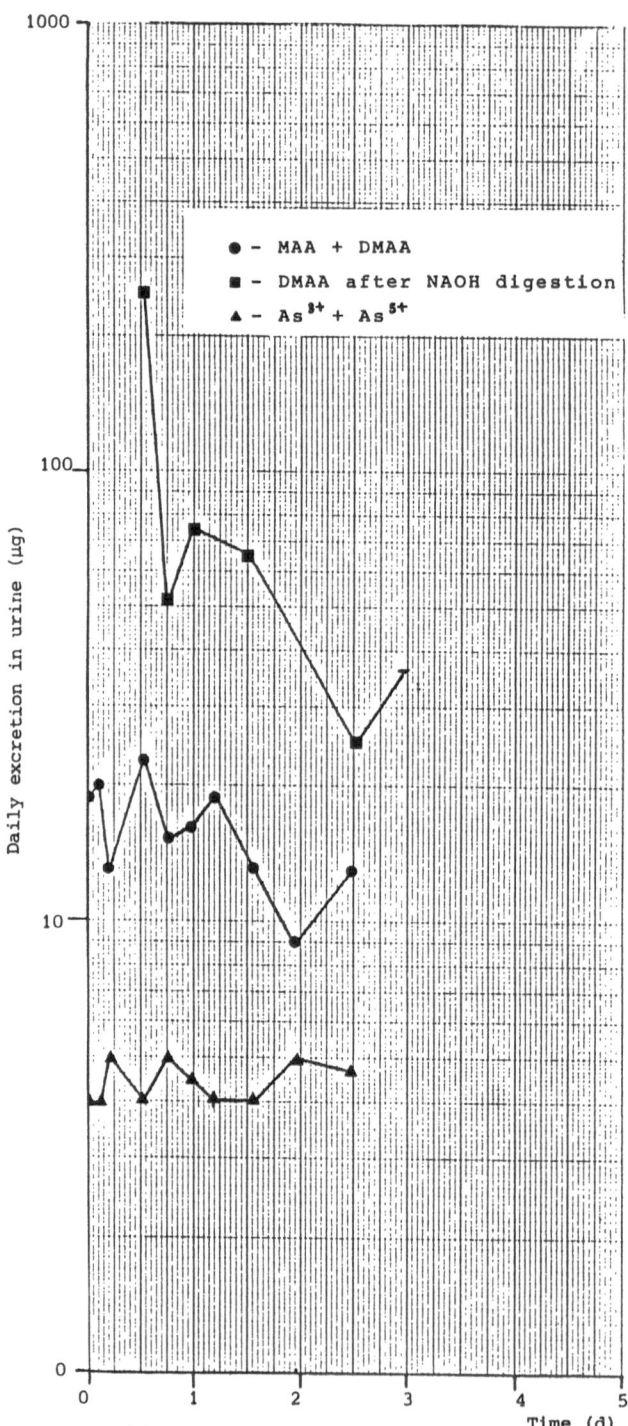

FIGURE 11.   URINARY EXCRETION OF ARSENIC AFTER
INGESTION OF CRAB MEAT CONTAINING 2000µg
OF AN ORGANO-ARSENIC COMPOUND (FROM
CRECELIUS   1977).

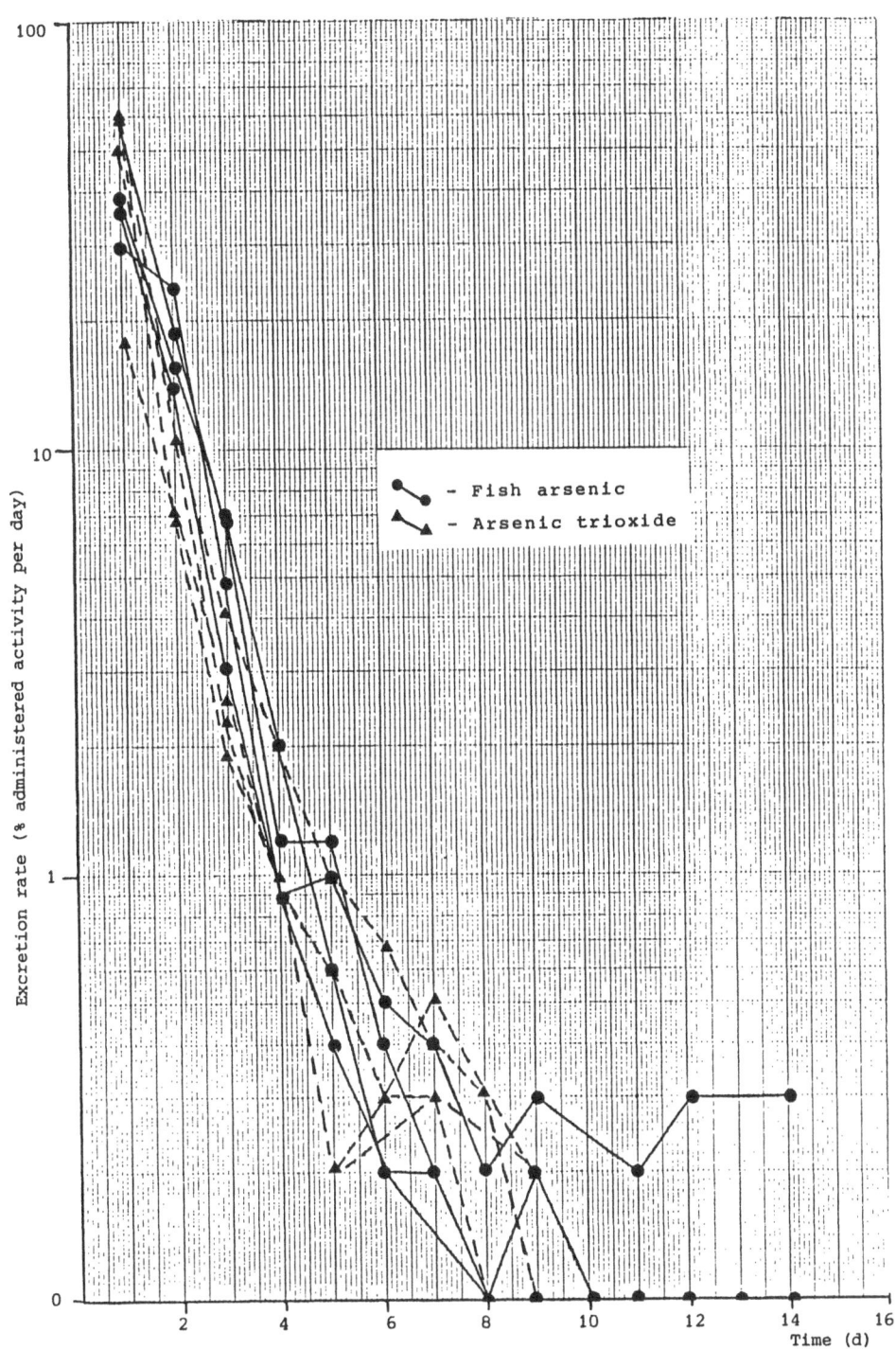

FIGURE 12.   URINARY EXCRETION OF ARSENIC BY MONKEYS AFTER
             ORAL DOSING (FROM CHARBONNEAU ET AL.   1978).

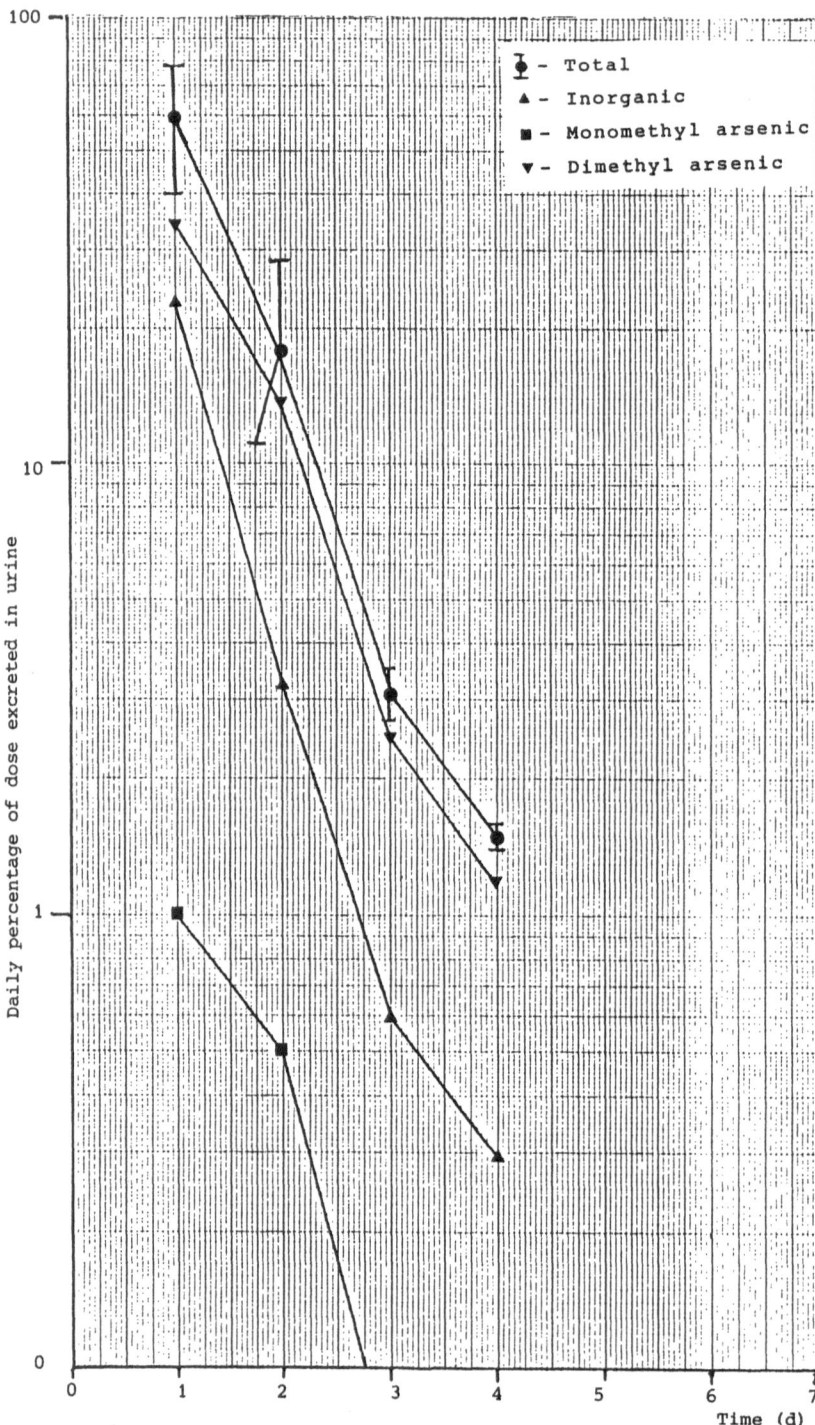

FIGURE 13.   URINARY EXCRETION OF ARSENIC IN RABBITS AFTER
INTRA-PERITONEAL INJECTION OF SODIUM ARSENITE
(FROM BERTOLERO ET AL. 1981).

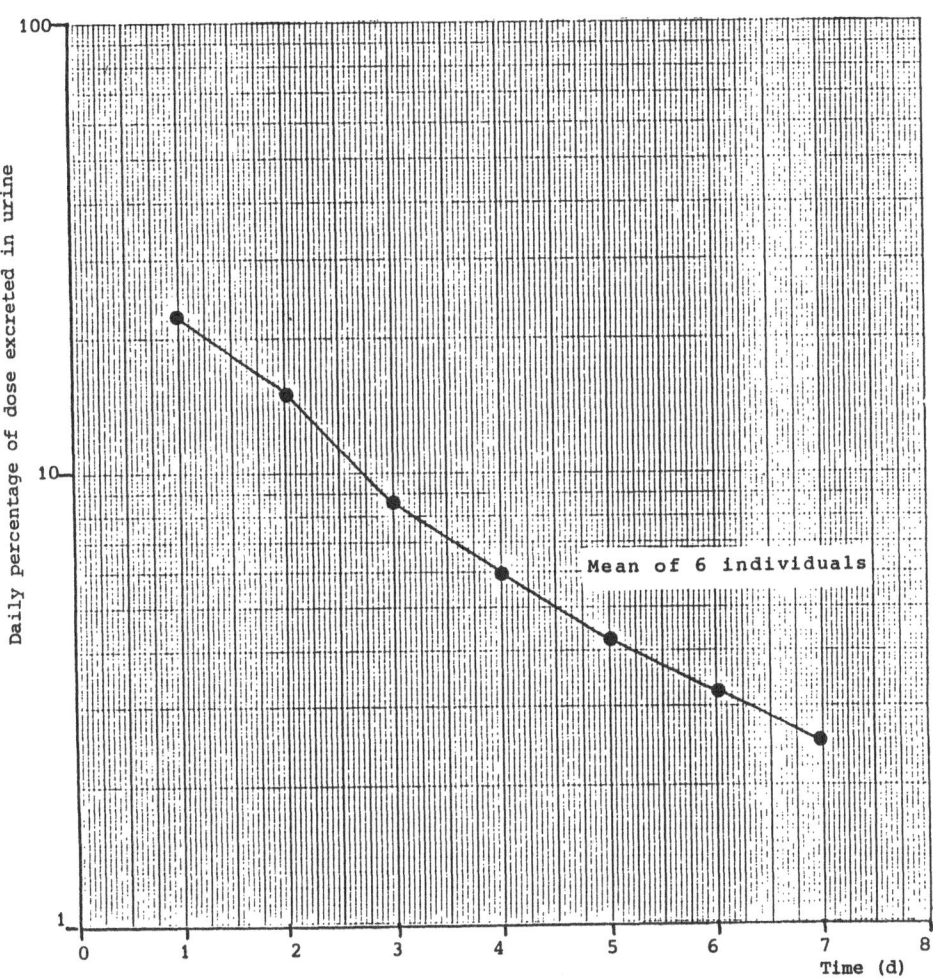

FIGURE 14.   URINARY EXCRETION OF ARSENIC BY MAN AFTER A SINGLE
ORAL DOSE OF ARSENIC ACID (FROM POMROY ET AL.   1980).

of a unit quantity of arsenic, intravenously injected as arsenite, is likely to be well represented by:

$$R(t) = 0.35 \exp(-1.444t) + 0.28 \exp(-0.0263t) + 0.37 \exp(-0.003t).$$

Alternatively, $R(t)$ can be derived by neglecting faecal excretion, integrating $U(t)$ and normalising to unity at time zero. This yields:

$$R(t) = 0.25 \exp(-1.54t) + 0.50 \exp(-0.02t) + 0.25 \exp(-0.0012)$$

This latter function for whole-body retention can be used to estimate the relationship between the daily dietary intake of arsenic and the average concentration in tissues, using the relationship:

$$C = A \; f_1 \int_0^\infty R(t) \; dt/24M$$

where C ($\mu g \; g^{-1}$) is the concentration in tissues;
  A ($\mu g \; d^{-1}$) is the daily intake;
  f_1 is the fractional gastrointestinal absorption;
  M (g) is the mass of the whole-body; and
  24 is the conversion from days to hours.

Taking f_1 to be 0.9 for dietary arsenic (see Section 4.1) and using 70 kg as the mass of the body (ICRP, 1975), the above expression reduces to:

$$C = 1.25 \times 10^{-4} A$$

If the daily intake of arsenic in food and drinking water is taken to be ~170 $\mu g \; d^{-1}$ (Section 1.2.4), the average tissue concentration of the element is estimated to be 0.002 $\mu g \; g^{-1}$. This is about a factor of two lower than the average tissue concentration listed in Section 1.3. A possible reason for this inconsistency is that the urinary excretion function givey by Mealey et al. (1959) over-estimates the rate of urinary excretion at times long after entry of arsenic into the systemic circulation. In this context, it is relevant to note that the data of Mealey et al. extended to only 280h post-injection and that urinary excretion rates exhibited considerable variability in the period 40 to 280h post-injection. In view of these considerations, the data of Mealey et al. can reasonably be interpreted to yield a whole-body retention function for trivalent arsenic as:

$$R(t) = 0.25 \exp(-1.54t) + 0.50 \exp(-0.02t) + 0.25 \exp(-0.0005t)$$

where t is in hours.

This expression yields:

$$C = 2.81 \times 10^{-4} A \; \mu g \; g^{-1}$$

which, for a daily intake of 170 μg, corresponds to an equilibrium tissue concentration of 0.048 $\mu g \; g^{-1}$.

This result may be compared with the results of Pomroy et al. (1980) who administered carrier free [As-74] arsenic acid to six volunteers and studied retention over 100 days. This administration was via the oral

Material	0.5h		2h		6h		24h	
	As(V)	As(III)	As(V)	As(III)	As(V)	As(III)	As(V)	As(III)
Kidney	1.17±0.22	0.74±0.06	0.97±0.11	1.01±0.07	0.72±0.05	0.61±0.07	0.03±0.00	0.05±0.02
Liver	0.93±0.17	2.02±0.07	0.57±0.04	0.92±0.05	0.26±0.02	0.31±0.02	0.02±0.00	0.04±0.01
Bile	1.86±0.08	3.31±0.57	0.51±0.11	5.30±0.95	0.34±0.06	0.94±0.19	-	-
Brain	0.01±0.00	0.01±0.00	0.03±0.00	0.04±0.00	0.05±0.00	0.06±0.00	<0.01	<0.01
Skeleton	0.08±0.01	0.07±0.00	0.12±0.02	0.16±0.02	0.18±0.04	0.18±0.03	0.02±0.01	0.01±0.01
Skin	0.07±0.01	0.06±0.01	0.10±0.01	0.15±0.01	0.11±0.01	0.13±0.01	0.02±0.01	0.06±0.01

Notes: 1. Standard errors given.
2. Data from Vahter and Norin (1980).

TABLE 10

ARSENIC CONCENTRATIONS (μg As g^{-1}) IN ORGANS AND TISSUES OF MICE
0.5 - 24h FOLLOWING A SINGLE ORAL ADMINISTRATION OF As(V) or As(III)

TABLE 11

ARSENIC CONCENTRATIONS (% I.A. g^{-1}) IN TISSUES OF PREGNANT MICE AFTER INTRAPERITONEAL INJECTION OF (As-73) ARSENIC ACID ON DAY 12 OF PREGNANCY

Organ or tissue	3h	6h	12h	24h	2d	3d	4d	7d
Blood	30	15	1.7	0.17	0.25	0.07	0.06	–
Skin	14	25	6.6	3	2	0.8	1.3	1
Bone	–	15	12	3	3.5	3	3	0.7
Brain	6	7	2	0.25	0.17	0.12	0.07	0.04
Muscle	20	13	4	1	0.6	0.4	0.3	0.17
Uterus	4	1.7	1.5	0.4	0.15	0.25	0.35	0.04
Ovary	2	1.7	0.4	0.06	0.05	0.05	0.04	0.035
Placenta	0.17	0.04	–	0.01	0.01	0.008	0.008	0.005
Foetus	0.07	0.05	–	0.007	0.005	0.004	0.003	–

Note: Data obtained from graphs presented by Gerber at al. (1982)

TABLE 12

DISTRIBUTION OF ARSENIC IN GUINEA PIGS
($ I.A. g^{-1} tissue) AFTER ORAL ADMINISTRATION

Organ or tissue	3h	16h	3d	6d	7d	8d	9d
Liver	33.2	29.30	24.40	13.35	15.10	15.96	8.82
Spleen	5.90	6.15	6.99	6.30	6.25	6.05	8.04
Blood	1.56	8.88	5.88	4.85	4.17	4.40	3.45
Lung	3.12	5.17	5.93	4.91	3.05	2.96	3.36
Heart	4.23	4.69	5.90	5.05	3.65	3.72	4.81
Kidney	11.45	27.50	20.00	17.87	13.55	14.89	16.05
Adrenal	4.40	4.06	3.26	6.07	-	-	-
Stomach	28.50	6.58	6.99	8.40	5.21	4.08	3.36
Muscle	2.25	3.78	13.95	22.70	24.50	24.00	24.08
Bone	2.35	2.93	3.40	-	13.12	12.06	12.85
Brain	3.04	0.96	3.30	10.50	11.40	11.88	15.18

Note: from Arnold et al. (1970)

TABLE 13

ARSENIC RESIDUES IN PIGS ($\mu g\ g^{-1}$) FED 250 g ARSENILIC
ACID PER TON AND KILLED AT INTERVALS AFTER WITHDRAWAL
OF ARSENIC FROM THE DIET

Days after withdrawal	As_2O_3 ($\mu g\ g^{-1}$ wet tissue)					
		Kidney		Muscle		
	Liver	Cortex	Medulla	Back	Leg	Diaphragm
0	6.25	5.5	1.0	0.5	-	0.5
1	3.1	2.0	1.0	<0.5	<0.5	<0.5
2	3.5	2.0	1.0	<0.5	<0.5	<0.5
3	2.1	1.0	0.5	<0.5	<0.5	<0.5
4	1.0	0.5	0.5	<0.5	<0.5	<0.5
5	2.0	1.0	1.0	1.0	0.5	1.0
6	1.0	1.0	0.5	0.5	0.5	0.5

Note: from Gitter and Lewis (1969)

Animal No.	1	2	6	3	4	5	9	10	11	12	13	14	15	20
Total As (mg kg^{-1})	4.95	3.5	0.97	1.0	1.0	0.94	3.3	3.2	3.1	3.1	3.3	1.56	1.3	1.05
Time from last dose to killing (d)	2	2	1	2	4	6	1	2	4	6	8	1	1	0.63
Whole blood	0.05	0	0.11	0.04	0	0	0.05	0.05	*	*	*	0.076	0.06	0.029
Liver	0.61	1.8	2.0	0.63	0.075	0.02	0.85	0.3	0.36	0.06	0.1	0.71	0.52	0.31
Spleen	0.19	1.2	0.58	0.20	0.04	0.01	0.26	0.12	0.38	0.06	0.02	0.16	0.16	0.067
Kidney	0.57	0.5	3.22	0.32	0.13	0.04	0.63	0.45	0.35	0.13	0.10	0.65	0.58	0.29
Brain	0.23	0.5	0.14	0.29	0.06	0.04	0.20	0.15	0.17	0.08	0.17	0.09	0.13	0.062
Bone marrow	0.19	–	0.45	0.12	0.02	0	0.36	0.10	0.15	0	0.016	0.24	0.16	0.065
Lung	–	–	0.72	0.19	0.03	0	0.27	0.13	0.10	0.026	0.025	0.29	0.17	0.12
Muscles	–	–	0.33	0.19	0.04	0.015	0.25	0.15	0.16	0.05	0.10	0.17	0.14	0.087
Thyroid	–	–	–	–	–	–	–	0.09	0.10	0	0	0.08	0.10	0.085
Testes	–	–	–	–	–	–	–	–	–	–	–	0.09	0.05	0.038
Epididymis	–	–	–	–	–	–	–	–	–	–	–	0.75	0.47	0.71
Urine	–	–	–	–	–	–	–	–	–	–	–	0.8	0.25	0.79
Bile	–	–	–	–	–	–	–	–	–	–	–	–	–	0.13

Notes: 1. From Hunter et al. (1942)
        2. Values for blood, urine and bile are per cc and not per g.
        *   Undetectable.

TABLE 14

DISTRIBUTION OF ARSENIC IN GUINEA PIGS (μmol g^{-1}) FOLLOWING SUB-CUTANEOUS
INJECTION OF POTASSIUM ARSENITE

Sex	Male					Virgin female			Pregnant female	
Total As (mg kg^{-1})	0.62	1.2	3.2	3.4	0.91	0.96 (3)	0.99	3.91	1.1	3.3
Time from last dose to killing (d)	1	2	1	4	1	1	1	1	1	1
Whole blood	0	0.17	0.05	0.05	0.04	0	0.084	0.069	0.13	0.05
Liver	0.10	0.12	0.73	0.40	0.24	0.034	0.39	0.63	0.14	0.66
Spleen	0.07	0.13	0.29	0.17	0.09	0.009	0.13	0.22	0.09	0.18
Kidney	0.11	0.40	0.88	0.82	0.30	0.01	0.49	0.83	0.25	0.89
Brain	0.02	0.04	0.13	0.072	0.034	0.005	0.057	0.10	0.044	0.10
Bone marrow	–	–	0.23	0.10	0.054	0.005	0.15	0.11	0.095	0.10
Lung	–	–	0.59	0.20	0.26	0.05	0.62	0.78	0.28	0.75
Muscle	–	–	0.33	0.32	0.074	0	0.25	0.20	0.12	0.19
Thyroid	–	–	0.18	0.10	0.11	0.02	0.15	0.23	0.10	0.19
Testes	–	–	0.16	0.12	0.052	0	0.08	0.14	0.10	0.15
Epididymis	–	–	0.38	0.87	0.13	0.01	0.12	0.11	0.17	0.18
Bile	–	–	0.32	–	0.15	0	0.34	0.64	0.54	0.06
Urine	–	–	–	–	2.0	0.25	2.75	8.3	5.1	None

Notes: 1. From Hunter et al (1942)
2. Values for blood, bile and urine are per cc and not per g.
3. Absorption from injection very low.

TABLE 15

DISTRIBUTION OF ARSENIC IN RABBITS (μmol g^{-1}) FOLLOWING
SUB-CUTANEOUS INJECTION OF POTASSIUM ARSENITE

TABLE 16

DISTRIBUTION OF ARSENIC IN A SINGLE
HUMAN AT DEATH FOUR DAYS AFTER
SUB-CUTANEOUS INJECTION OF ARSENIC

Organ or tissue	Concentration	
	umol g^{-1}	Normalised to pect. muscle
Liver	0.4	1.9
Spleen	0.2	0.95
Kidney	0.54	2.6
Cerebrum	0.15	0.71
Cerebellum	0.14	0.67
Lung	0.06	0.29
Pect. muscle	0.21	1.0
Heart muscle	0.10	0.48
Heart thrombus	0.13	0.62
Pancreas	0.17	0.81
Adrenals	0.10	0.48
Lymph node	0.10	0.48
Testes	0.14	0.62
Vert. marrow	0.12	0.57
Fem. marrow	0	0

Note: data from Hunter et al. (1942)

Tissue	Time to death (d)										
	0.042	0.71	1.38	1.79	4	7	9	9.5	18	21	71
Heart	4.92	–	1.37	0.62	0.32	0.31	0.25	0.05	0.18	–	0.043
Aorta	–	–	0.50	–	–	–	0.18	0.03	–	–	–
Spleen	3.35	2.67	5.14	0.76	0.58	0.34	0.35	0.09	–	–	–
Liver	12.10	6.18	7.35	2.96	1.39	1.13	0.75	0.30	0.83	0.42	0.81
Kidney	36.88	16.71	5.60	2.81	2.10	1.15	1.19	0.23	0.27	–	0.347
Pancreas	3.76	2.23	1.75	0.61	–	0.36	0.22	0.082	0.13	–	0.006
Muscle	0.63	0.79	0.90	0.59	–	–	0.484	0.16	–	0.15	0.071
Bone	–	1.05	0.77	–	–	–	0.24	0.02	0.14	0.10	–
Lung	–	–	2.12	0.70	0.31	0.21	0.21	0.10	–	–	0.10
Brain	0.155	0.77	0.28	0.195	0.13	0.15	0.15	0.05	0.06	0.06	0.011
Scalp	–	0.32	0.56	0.71	–	1.77	0.03	0.33	0.34	0.20	–
Adrenal	3.78	–	–	0.59	0.24	0.39	0.10	–	0.15	–	–
Testis	–	–	1.19	1.14	–	–	0.23	0.094	–	–	–
Intestine	–	–	–	–	–	–	0.42	0.104	–	–	–
Thyroid	–	–	2.31	0.42	0.64	1.01	0.87	–	–	0.29	–

Note: 1. Data from Mealey et al. (1959), expressed as % I.A. kg^{-1} and normalised to 70 kg body weight.

TABLE 17

CONCENTRATION OF As-74 IN VARIOUS AUTOPSY SAMPLES
FOLLOWING INTRAVENOUS INJECTION OF As^{3+} (1)

TABLE 18

CONCENTRATION OF ARSENIC (ppm) IN TISSUES
AND EXCREMENTS OF RABBITS EXPOSED TO 50 ppm
MONOSODIUM ACID METHANEARSENATE IN FEED

Tissue	Weeks of exposure				
	2	4	7	12	17
Liver	0.57	0.37	0.44	0.37	0.78
Kidney	0.56	0.47	0.56	0.49	1.40
Muscle	<0.1	0.27	0.26	0.54	0.36
Bone	<0.1	<0.15	<0.1	<0.1	3.52
Hair	<0.25	1.30	2.42	3.58	2.29
Faeces	11.30	8.10	8.50	8.80	8.40
Urine	15.10	9.10	13.30	8.40	6.20

Note: from Exon et al. (1974)

TABLE 19

DISTRIBUTION OF ARSENIC IN RABBITS AT
VARIOUS TIMES AFTER INTRAVENOUS
INJECTION OF SODIUM ARSENITE   (1)

| Time to death (d) | 0.25 | 1 | 2 | 4 |
Sex	♀	♂	♂	♀
Tissue:				
Blood	0.64	0.33	0.30	–
Spleen	1.75	0.81	1.90	–
Heart	1.28	0.48	0.30	0.60
Lung	2.89	2.67	–	–
Kidney	4.67	1.70	1.50	–
Liver	11.53	2.30	–	4.80
Muscle	1.00	1.00	1.00	1.00
Femoral marrow	–	6.89	3.90	7.00
Brain	0.33	0.37	0.20	–

Note: Data from Ducoff et al. (1948)
         normalised to muscle.

TABLE 20

DISTRIBUTION OF ARSENIC IN MICE AT
VARIOUS TIMES AFTER INJECTION
OF SODIUM   ARSENITE   (1)

| Tissue | Time to death   (d) | | | |
	0.25	0.50	1.0	2.0
Kidney	0.84	0.27	0.088	0.078
Liver	0.67	0.29	0.103	0.054
Spleen	0.49	0.26	0.077	0.107
Muscle	0.50	0.21	0.077	–

Note: Data from Ducoff et al. (1948) averaged
         over normal and tumour bearing mice and
         normalised to % I.A. g^{-1}.

TABLE 21

DISTRIBUTION OF ARSENIC IN A MORIBUND
FEMALE INTRAVENOUSLY   INJECTED WITH
SODIUM ARSENITE

Tissue	Distribution (1)
Liver	4.07
Kidney	2.59
Spleen	1.41
Parotid tumour	1.37
Heart	1.28
Jejunum	1.25
Vertebral marrow	1.25
Mesenteric lymph node	1.12
Stomach	1.03
Pancreas	1.02
Muscle (quadriceps)	1.00
Ileum	0.97
Lung	0.95
Femoral marrow	0.95
Adrenal	0.75
Ovary	0.73
Thyroid	0.67
Skin	0.59
Brain	0.22
Femoral cortical bone	0.21

Note: data from Ducoff et al. (1948)
           normalised to muscle.

Tissue	Rat						Average	Standard error
	1	2	3	4	5	6		
Kidney	1.044	1.29	1.53	1.18	1.566	1.791	1.400	0.113
Liver	1.022	2.62	1.59	0.841	0.775	0.978	1.304	0.288
Adult filarids	1.310	1.83	1.65	1.738	0.874	0.214	1.269	0.282
Epidermis	0.549	1.93	0.956	1.16	0.654	1.016	1.044	0.200
Spleen	0.753	1.51	0.667	0.466	0.879	1.484	0.960	0.179
Lung	0.918	1.34	0.833	0.695	0.593	0.478	0.810	0.124
Muscle	0.475	0.866	0.791	0.352	0.285	0.440	0.535	0.097
Heart	0.422	0.842	0.411	0.340	0.332	0.345	0.449	0.080
Blood	0.207	0.989	0.196	0.180	0.169	0.264	0.334	0.132
Dermis	0.320	0.401	0.196	0.131	0.266	0.267	0.264	0.038
Thyroid	0.267	0.585	0.199	0.000	0.586	0.000	0.273	0.108
Brain	0.172	0.299	0.196	0.123	0.201	0.176	0.195	0.024

Note: from Lawton et al. (1945); units are $\mu g\ g^{-1}$ wet weight for an administration of 1.6 $\mu g\ g^{-1}$.

TABLE 22

ARSENIC CONCENTRATION IN ADULT COTTON RATS INFECTED WITH
LITOMOSOIDES CARINII AT 24 HOURS AFTER INTRAPERITONEAL
INJECTION OF SODIUM ARSENITE (1)

Organ or tissue	Concentration (% I.A. kg^{-1})									Average tissue weight (g)
	0.083h	0.5h	1h	3h	12h	24h	48h	96h	168h	
Heart	36	5	30	45	5	6	13	3	1	8.99
Lungs	33	160	70	110	30	10	42	5	6	17.10
Liver	64	20	80	160	30	8	10	2	3	109.98
Kidney	163	136	292	177	42	13	40	10	2	21.16
Blood serum	550	23	33	29	10	16	2	n.d.	n.d.	233.40 (cm³)
Spleen	270	60	30	40	10	5	10	3	4	1.92
Stomach	11	27	22	30	6	4		4	1	32.73
Large intestine	54	10	13	20	16	2	36	4	2	n.r. (4)
Small intestine	81	38	65	60	10	3	20	2	2	n.r.
Muscle	20	10	10	16	6	4	9	3	n.d.	1575.00
Bone	20	32	33	50	7	13	19	13	4	283.00
Skin – fur	51	23	30	17	10	10	10	10	4	13.70
Testes	4	18		14	6	4	8	10	n.d.	7.60
Salivary gland	148	27	40	25	18	3	11	3	5	1.40
Thyroid	42	6	50	43	12	18	23	3	57	0.40
Adrenal	22	5	32	24	18	23	15		1	0.46
Teeth	46	15		54	138	8	24	12	2	7.50
Toe nails		23	17	45	38	3	24	15	5	3.90
Eyes	37	3		6	n.d. (3)	3	7		2	6.00
Ear cartilage	46	41			7	4	5	18	8	8.76 (5)
Brain	4	6	5	11	3	6	8	n.d.	n.d.	10.30
Bladder urine	75	1320	1060	257	1110	445	760	23	7	n.r.
Bile	4	2	10	13	4	6	7	1	n.d.	n.r.
Tumour (2)	9	38	24	43	12	29	8	n.d.	4	n.r.
Peritoneal fluid		32	14		15				n.d.	n.r.
Fat		9	5	6	n.d.	n.d.	5	4	2	n.r.
Marrow	19	101	29	28	3	n.d.	11	2	n.d.	n.r.

Notes: 1. From Dupont et al. (1942)
        2. Testicular Brown-Pearce rabbit epithelioma.
        3. n.d. = not detectable or <50% above background.
        4. n.r. = not recorded.
        5. One ear total.

TABLE 23

DISTRIBUTION OF ARSENIC IN RABBITS AFTER ADMINISTRATION OF SODIUM ARSENATE   (1)

Organ or tissue	Concentration (% I.A. g^{-1} s.e.)				
	5h	16h	48h	96h	144h
Liver	0.197±0.031	0.041±0.008	0.023±0.005	0.018±0.003	0.015±0.002
Lung	0.211±0.038	0.036±0.006	0.014±0.003	0.012±0.003	0.008±0.002
Kidney	0.183±0.029	0.087±0.017	0.027±0.007	0.020±0.005	0.016±0.004
Spleen	0.054±0.015	0.011±0.003	0.009±0.004	0.008±0.003	0.005±0.001
Heart	0.036±0.009	0.008±0.002	0.006±0.002	0.005±0.002	0.003±0.001
Testes	0.025±0.007	0.007±0.002	0.006±0.001	0.005±0.002	0.002±0.002
Brain	0.012±0.002	0.005±0.003	0.003±0.002	0.001±0.001	0.001±0.001
Skel. muscle	0.019±0.006	0.017±0.004	0.014±0.002	0.010±0.003	0.007±0.002

Note: data from Bertolero et al. (1981)

TABLE 24

ARSENIC DISTRIBUTION IN RABBITS FOLLOWING INTRAPERITONEAL INJECTION OF (As-74)O_2^- (1)

route and the mean whole-body retention function for the six individuals was:

$$R(t) = 0.659 \exp(-0.0138t) + 0.304 \exp(-0.0030t)$$
$$+ 0.037 \exp(-0.00075t)$$

This expression yields:

$$C = 1.8 \times 10^{-4}A$$

which, for a daily intake of 170 µg, corresponds to an equilibrium tissue concentration of 0.031 µg g^{-1}.

Taking the results of Mealey et al. (1959) and Pomroy et al. (1980), together with other results on the rapid early excretion of arsenic, it is probably appropriate to use the following function for whole-body retention of arsenic acid, following its entry into the systemic circulation:

$$R(t) = 0.25 \exp(-1.54t) + 0.5 \exp(-0.014t) + 0.25 \exp(-0.0005t)$$

Taken together with an f_1 of 0.9, this expression yields:

$$C = 2.87 \times 10^{-4}A$$

which, for A=170 µg d^{-1}, yields an equilibrium tissue concentration of 0.048 µg g^{-1}.

1.4.3.2   Distribution of arsenic

The distribution of stable arsenic in body tissues was discussed in Section 1.3, where it was concluded that, excluding hair and nails, arsenic is relatively uniformly distributed throughout all organs and tissues of the human body. Data on the tissue distribution of arsenic in various species following various modes of administration are summarised in Tables 6 and 10 to 24. In general, liver and kidney exhibit particularly high concentrations at early times, but at longer times after administration this enhancement generally becomes less marked. Data for man, normalised to muscle as unity, are shown in Fig. 15 and corresponding data for rabbits are shown in Fig. 16.

The data presented in these tables and figures suggest that the concentration of arsenic in the kidneys and liver is about ten times the concentration in other tissues in the first few hours after administration, but that at times long after administration the average concentration in these tissues is likely to be only about twice the average for other tissues. On this basis, and using the whole-body retention function derived in Section 1.4.3.1, the following tissue retention functions are obtained:

$$R_{LIVER}(t) = 0.16 \exp(-1.54t) + 0.025 \exp(-0.014t) + 0.013 \exp(-0.0005t)$$

$$R_{KIDNEY}(t) = 0.03 \exp(-1.54t) + 0.005 \exp(-0.014t) + 0.002 \exp(-0.0005t)$$

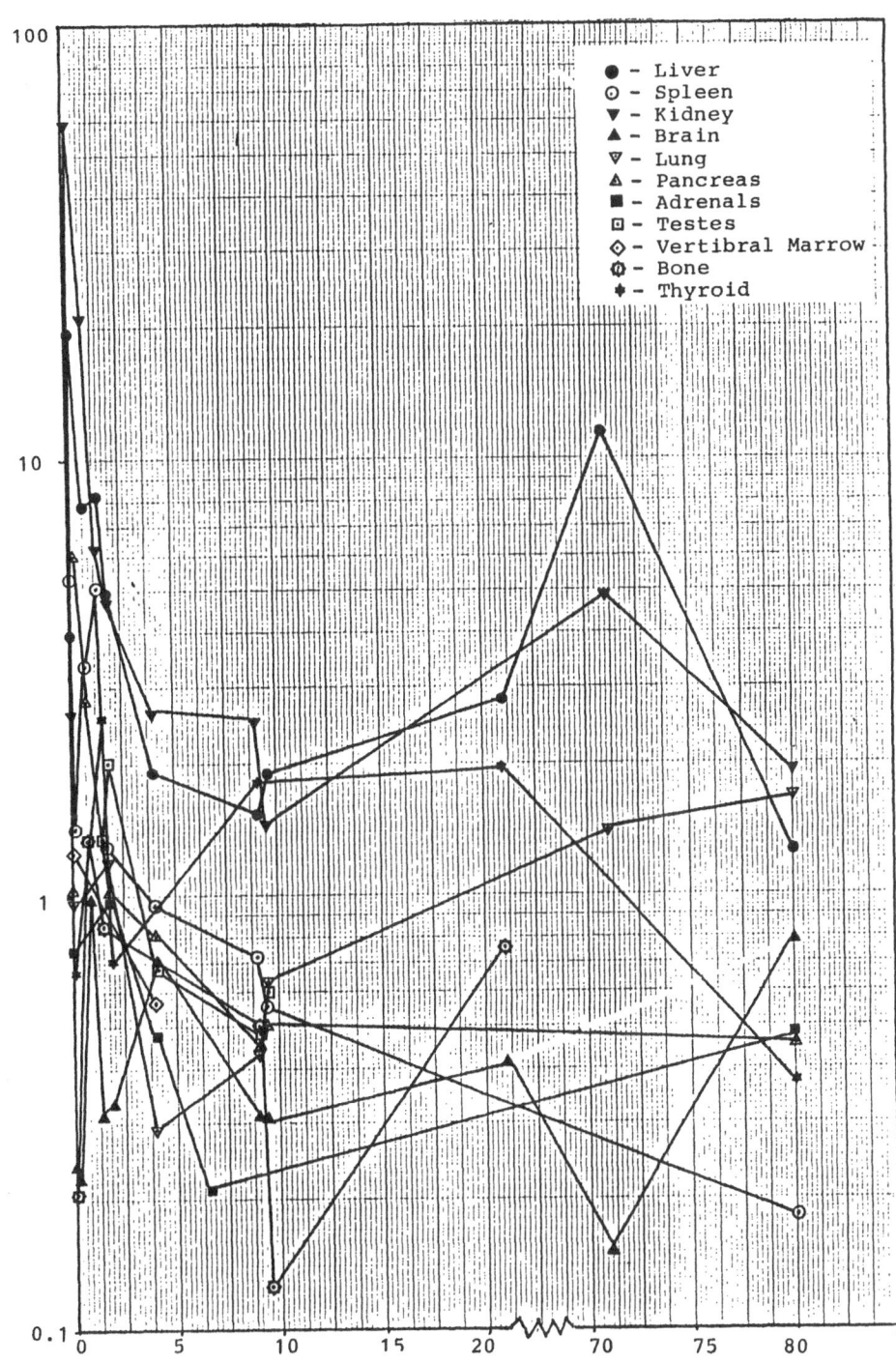

FIGURE 15.   DISTRIBUTION OF ARSENIC IN MAN AS DETERMINED
FROM AUTOPSY SPECIMENS.

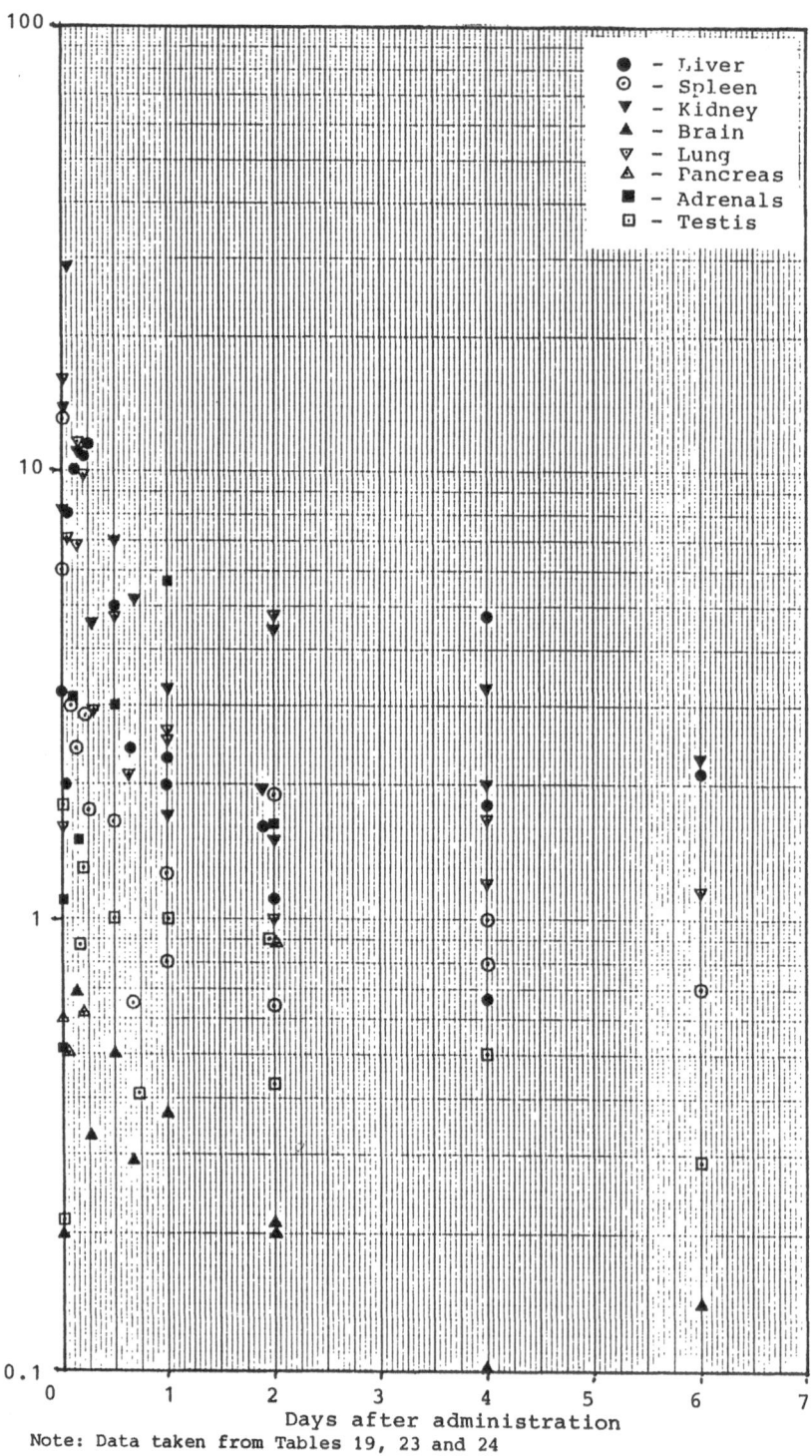

Note: Data taken from Tables 19, 23 and 24

FIGURE 16.   DISTRIBUTION OF ARSENIC IN RABBITS

$$R_{OTHER}(t) = 0.06 \exp(-1.54t) + 0.47 \exp(-0.014t) + 0.235 \exp(-0.0005t)$$

where t is in hours.

Using these retention functions, together with an f_1 of 0.9 and an arsenic intake rate of 170 µg d⁻, it is possible to calculate equilibrium levels of arsenic in tissues and compare these with the values given in Table 3. This is done below.

Tissue	Concentration ($\mu g \ g^{-1}$)	
	Calculated	Measured †
Liver	0.099	0.051
Kidney	0.090	0.077
Other	0.047	0.040*

Note: † Weighted mean from Table 3.
        * Value for muscle.

Arsenic in hair has often been considered as a useful indicator of exposure to arsenic, but the dynamics of uptake do not appear to have been studied extensively. Smith (1964) has commented that values quoted for the time taken for arsenic to appear in hair after ingestion vary from 12 hours to a week, while the time taken to return to normal levels after chronic exposure is given values between 3 months and a year. His own data indicate that root values are in relatively close equilibrium with the blood stream, at least at early times (0-4h) after ingestion, and that the return to normal levels is much more rapid than had been suggested by earlier workers.

1.4.3.3   Transfer to the foetus

The placenta is permeable to arsenic during the early critical stages of embryogenesis and the element has been shown to be teratogenic in the mouse, rat and hamster (Ferm, 1977). The placenta appears to be permeable only to arsenic in its ionic form, organic arsenicals apparently do not cross the placenta with any great ease, but are stored in it in fairly high concentrations (Leonard and Lauwerys, 1980). There do not appear to be sufficient data available to develop a model for arsenic retention in, and transfer across, the human placenta.

1.5   MODEL SUMMARY

The following model is recommended for arsenic on the basis of data discussed in previous sections of this review.

1.5.1   Fractional gastrointestinal absorption

A value of 0.5 to 1.0 can be used for most compounds of the element. Exceptions are arsenilic acid and arsenic trioxide in solid form. For arsenilic acid a best estimate value is 0.3. For solid arsenic trioxide no value can be recommended, since the degree of absorption will be strongly dependent on particle size and the pH of the gastric juice.

1.5.2   Retention in, and translocation from, the lungs

The following conclusions define a model for arsenic retention in, and translocation from, the lungs.

- The deposition of arsenic containing aerosols in the lungs is similar to that of other aerosols.

- In deeply inhaling smokers, ~10% of arsenic incorporated in cigarettes will be deposited in the lungs.

- All compounds of arsenic which have been studied have been found to be cleared from the lungs with a half-life of a few days; a biphasic model in which 75% of deposited material is cleared with a half-life of 4 days and 25% is cleared with a half-life of 10 days is recommended as appropriate to man.

- Virtually all arsenic translocated from the lungs enters the blood either directly or via the gastrointestinal tract.

- A fraction of 0.6 of inhaled arsine can be assumed to be virtually instantaneously absorbed from the lungs, with the residual fraction being exhaled.

1.5.3   Retention in the body

Most compounds of arsenic exhibit an early phase of rapid excretion and considerable methylation of arsenic occurs within the body. Data on distribution and retention in man are relatively limited, but the following functions appear to give a reasonable model for the retention of arsenic following entry of a unit quantity of the element into the systemic circulation:

$$R_{LIVER}(t) = 0.16 \exp(-1.54t) + 0.025 \exp(-0.014t) + 0.013 \exp(-0.0005t)$$

$$R_{KIDNEY}(t) = 0.03 \exp(-1.54t) + 0.005 \exp(-0.014t) + 0.002 \exp(-0.0005t)$$

$$R_{OTHER}(t) = 0.06 \exp(-1.54t) + 0.47 \exp(-0.014t) + 0.235 \exp(-0.0005t)$$

where t is in hours.

Summing these retention functions gives:

$$R_{WHOLE\ BODY}(t) = 0.25 \exp(-1.54t) + 0.5 \exp(-0.014t) + 0.25 \exp(-0.0005t)$$

and differentiating gives the total rate of excretion;

$$E = 38.5 \exp(-1.54t) + 0.7 \exp(-0.014t) + 0.0125 \exp(-0.0005t) \%I.A.\ h^{-1}$$

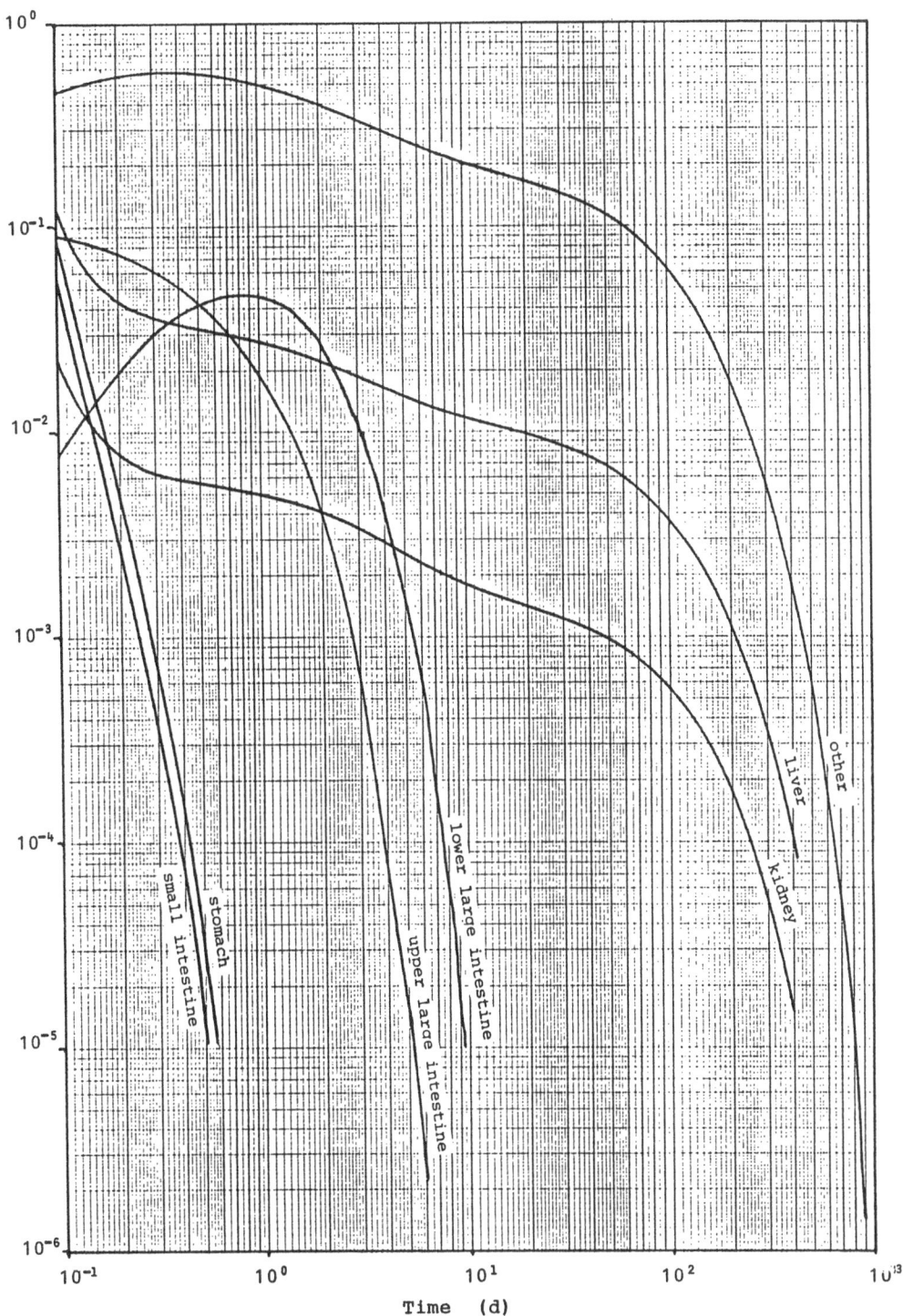

FIGURE 17   ARSENIC RETENTION FOLLOWING INGESTION   OF A UNIT
              QUANTITY OF THE ELEMENT.

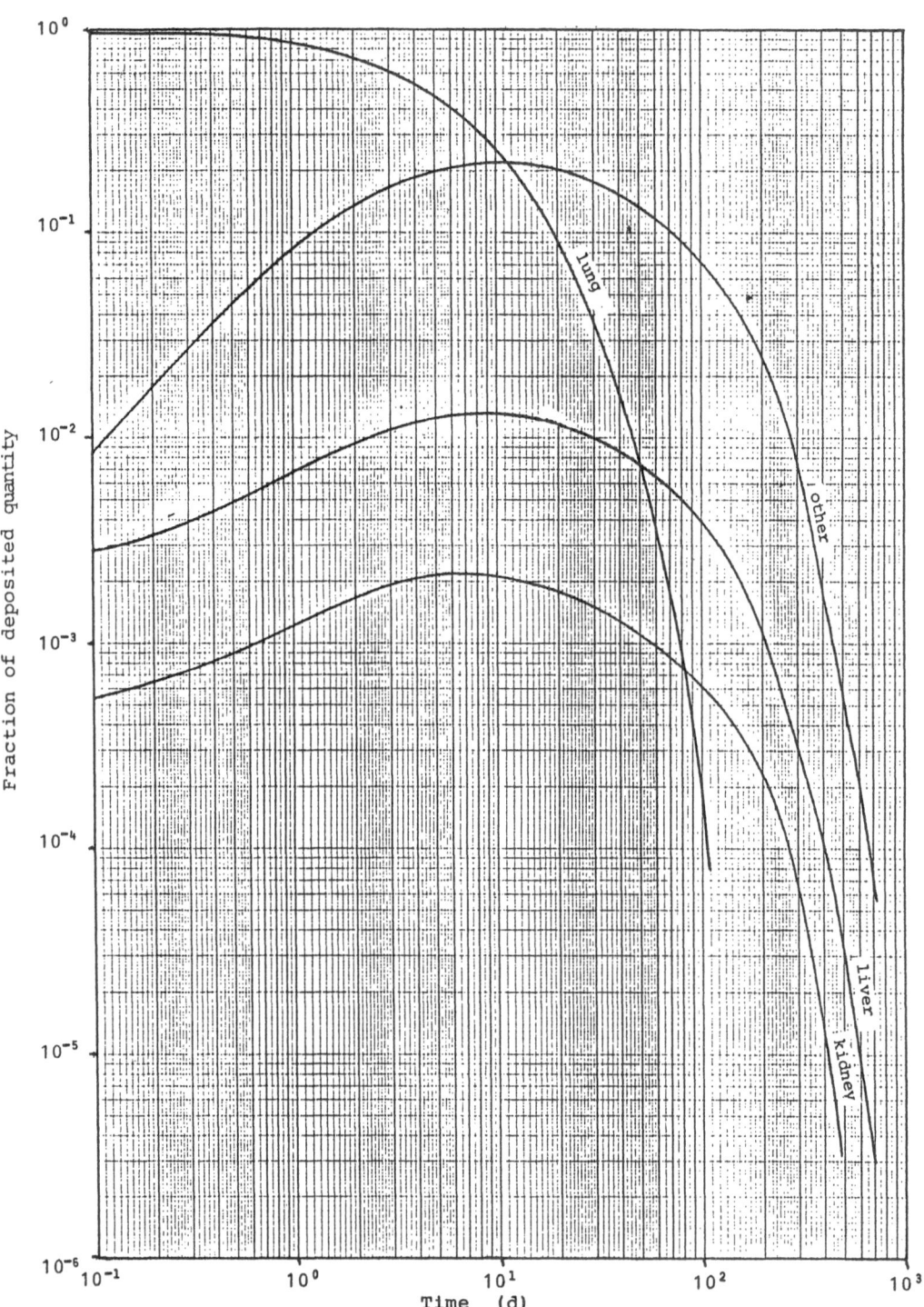

FIGURE 18   ARSENIC RETENTION FOLLOWING INHALATION OF A UNIT
QUANTITY OF THE ELEMENT.

for activity injected directly into the systemic circulation. This excretion can be assumed to be entirely in urine. For man, the dynamics of arsenic excretion in urine are better defined than those for loss in blood or hair, and urinary monitoring is the preferred method of assay with respect to occupational exposure. Post-mortem hair samples may be useful in retrospective analysis of arsenic exposure, but more work is required before these can be unambiguously interpreted in terms of the time course of such exposure. Data quantifying transfer of arsenic to, and across, the human placenta are not available, though this process is known to occur. Also, there are not sufficient data available to allow recommendations to be made concerning modifications to this model for different ages, states of health, or types of medical treatment.

1.6 ILLUSTRATIVE CALCULATIONS

The model set out above has been used to calculate arsenic retention in the body following ingestion, or inhalation of a unit quantity of the element. Results of these calculations are shown in Figs. 17 and 18.

1.7 REFERENCES

Arnold, Von W., Kohlhaas, H.H. and Niewerth, E., 1970. Untersuchungen zum Arsen-Stoffwechsel mit As[74]. Beitr. Gerichtle. Med., 27, 339-351.

Axelson, O., 1980. Arsenic compounds and cancer. J. Toxicol. Environ. Health, 6, 1229-1235.

Bencko, V., Cmarko, V. and Palan, S., 1968. The cumulation dynamics of arsenic in the tissues of rabbits exposed in the area of the ENO plant. Cesk. Hyg., 13, 18-22.

Bencko, V., Beneo, B. and Cikrt, M., 1976. Biotransformation of As(III) to As(V) and arsenic tolerance. Arch. Toxicol., 36, 159-162.

Bertolero, F., Marafante, E., Edel Rade, J., Pietra, R. and Sabbioni, E., 1981. Biotransformation and intracellular binding of arsenic in tissues of rabbits after intraperitoneal administration of [74]As labelled arsenite. Toxicol., 20, 35-44.

Bettley, F.R. and O'Shea, J.A., 1975. The absorption of arsenic and its relation to carcinoma. Br. J. Dermatol., 92, 563-568.

Borgono, J.M., Vicent, P., Venturino, H. and Infante, A., 1977. Arsenic in the drinking water of the city of Antofagasta: epidemiological and clinical study before and after the installation of a treatment plant. Environ. Health Perspect., 19, 103-105.

Bowen, H.J.M., 1979. Environmental Chemistry of the Elements. Academic Press, London.

Braman, R.S. and Foreback, C.C., 1973. Methylated forms of arsenic in the environment. Science, 182, 1247-1249.

Buchet, J.P., Roels, H., Louwreys, R., Bruaux, P., Claeys-Thoreau, F., Lafontaine, A. and Verduyn, G., 1980. Repeated surveillance of exposure to cadmium, manganese, and arsenic in school-age children living in rural, urban, and non-ferrous smelter areas in Belgium. Environ. Res., 22, 95-108.

Charbonneau, S.M., Hollins, J.G., Tam, G.K.H., Bryce, F., Ridgeway, J.M. and Willes, R.F., 1980. Whole-body retention, excretion and metabolism of [74As] arsenic acid in the hamster. Toxicol. Lett., 5, 175-182.

Charbonneau, S.M., Spencer, K., Bryce, F. and Sandi, E., 1978. Arsenic excretion by monkeys dosed with arsenic-containing fish or with inorganic arsenic. Bull. Environ. Contam. Toxicol., 20, 470-477.

Cikrt, M. and Bencko, V., 1974. Fate of arsenic after parenteral administration to rats, with particular reference to excretion via bile. J. Hyg. Epidemiol. Microbiol. Immunol., 18, 129-136.

Coulson, E.J., Remington, R.E. and Lynch, K.M., 1935. Metabolism in the rat of the naturally occurring arsenic of shrimp as compared with arsenic trioxide. J. Nutr., 10, 255-270.

Crecelius, E.A., 1974. The geochemistry of arsenic and antimony in Puget Sound and Lake Washington, Washington. Thesis, Seattle, Washington, University of Washington.

Crecelius, E.A., 1977. Changes in the chemical speciation of arsenic following ingestion by man. Environ. Health Perspect., 19, 147-150.

Dinman, B.D., 1960. Arsenic: chronic human intoxication. J. Occup. Med., 2, 137-141, 1960.

Done, A.K. and Peart, A.J., 1971. Acute toxicities of arsenical herbicides. Clin. Toxicol; 4, 343-355.

Ducoff, H.S., Neal, W.B., Straube, R.L., Jacobson, L.O. and Brues, A.M., 1948. Biological studies with arsenic[76] II. Excretion and tissue localisation. Proc. Soc. Exp. Biol. (NY), 69, 548-554.

DuPont, O., Ariel, I and Warren, S.L., 1942. The distribution of radioactive arsenic in the normal and tumor-bearing (Brown-Pearce) rabbit. Am. J. Gonnorrhea Veter. Dis., 26, 96-118.

Dutkiewicz, T., 1977. Experimental studies on arsenic absorption routes in rats. Environ. Health Perspect., 19, 173-177.

Exon, J.H., Harr, J.R. and Claeys, R.R., 1974. The effects of long-term feeding of monosodium acid methanearsenate (MSMA) to rabbits. Nutr. Rep. Int., 9, 351-357.

Ferm, V.H., 1977. Arsenic as a teratogenic agent. Environ. Health Perspect., 19, 215-217.

Fowler, B.A., 1977. Toxicology of environmental arsenic. In: Goyer, R.A. and Mehlman, M.A. (Eds.). Advances in Modern Toxicology. Volume 2. Toxicology of Trace Elements, Hemisphere Publishing Co.

Fowler, B.A., Ishinishi, N., Tsuchiya, K. and Vahter, M., 1979. Arsenic. In: Friberg, L. et al. (Eds). Handbook on the Toxicology of Metals. Elsevier/North-Holland Biomedical Press.

Freeman, H.C., Uthe, J.F., Fleming, R.B., Odense, P.H., Ackman, R.G., Landry, G. and Musial, C., 1979. Clearance of arsenic ingested by man from arsenic contaminated fish. Bull. Environ. Contam. Toxicol., 22, 224-229.

Gabor, S. and Coldea, V., 1977. Some aspects of the environmental exposure to arsenic in Romania. Environ. Health Perspect., 19, 107-108.

Gerber, G.B., Maes, J. and Eykens, B., 1982. Transfer of antimony and arsenic to the developing organism. Arch. Toxicol., 49, 159-168.

Ginsburg, J.M., 1965. Renal mechanism for excretion and transformation of arsenic in the dog. Am. J. Physiol., 208, 832-840.

Gitter, M. and Lewis, G., 1969. Elimination of arsenic from pig tissues following arsinilic acid treatment. The Veterinary Record, 4 October.

Holland, R.H., McCall, M.S. and Lanz, H.C., 1959. A study of inhaled arsenic-74 in man. Cancer Res., 19, 1154-1156.

Hunter, F.T., Kip, A.F. and Irvine, J.W. Jr., 1942. Radioactive tracer studies on arsenic injected as potassium arsenite I. Excretion and localization in tissues. J. Pharmacol. Exp. Ther., 76, 207-220.

IARC, 1980. IARC Monographs on the Evaluation of the Carcinogenic Risk of Chemicals to Humans. Volume 23. Some Metals and Metallic Compounds. International Agency for Research on Cancer, Lyon.

ICRP, 1966. Deposition and retention models for internal dosimetry of the human respiratory tract. Health Phys., 12, 173-207.

ICRP, 1975. Report of the Task Group on Reference Man. International Commission on Radiological Protection, Publication 23, Pergamon Press, Oxford.

ICRP, 1981. Limits for Intakes of Radionuclides by Workers. ICRP Publication 30, Part 3. Annals of the ICRP, Vol. 6, No. 2/3.

Ishinishi, N., Kodama, Y., Nobotumo, K., Inamasu, T., Kunitake, E. and Suenaga, Y., 1977. Outbreak of chronic arsenic poisoning among retired workers from an arsenic mine in Japan. Environ. Health Perspect., 19, 121-125, 1977.

Iyengar, G.V., Kollmer, W.E. and Bowen, H.J.M., 1978. The Elemental Composition of Human Tissues and Body Fluids. Verlag Chemie, Weinheim.

Jelinek, C.F. and Corneliussen, P.E., 1977. Levels of arsenic in the United States food supply. Environ. Health Perspect., 19, 83-87.

Klaasen, C.D., 1974. Biliary excretion of arsenic in rats, rabbits and dogs. Toxicol. Appl. Pharmacol., 29, 447-457.

Kronenberg, J. and Hartung, R., 1981. The deposition of 10-10´ oxybisphenoxarsine (OBPA) in rats, rabbits and guinea pigs. Drug Chem. Toxicol, 4, 275-281.

Kyle, R.A. and Pearse, G.L., 1965. Hematologic aspects of arsenic intoxication. New England J. Med., 273, 18-23.

Lanz, N. Jr., Wallace, P.C. and Hamilton, J.G., 1950. The metabolism of arsenic in laboratory animals using As^{74} as a tracer. Univ. Calif. Pub. Pharmacol., 2, 263-282.

Lasko, J.U. and Peoples, S.A., 1975. Methylation of inorganic arsenic by mammals. J. Agric. Food Chem., 23, 674-676.

Lawton, A.H., Ness, A.T., Brady, F.J. and Cowie, D.B., 1945. Distribution of radioactive arsenic following intraperitoneal injection of sodium arsenite into cotton rats infected with Litomosoides Carinii. Science, 102, 120-122.

Léonard, A. and Lauwerys, R.R., 1980. Carcinogenicity, teratogenicity and mutagenicity of arsenic. Mutat. Res., 75, 49-62.

Levvy, G.A., 1947. A study of arsine poisoning. Q.J. Exp. Physiol., 34, 47-67.

Lisella, F.S., Long, K.R. and Scott, H.G., 1972. Health aspects of arsenicals in the environment. J. Environ. Health, 34, 511-518.

Mahieu, P., Buchet, J.P., Roels, H.A. and Lauwerys, R., 1981. The metabolism of arsenic in humans acutely intoxicated by As$_2$O$_3$. Its significance for the duration of BAL therapy. Clin. Toxicol., 18, 1067-1075.

Marafante, E., Rade, J., Pietra, R., Sabbioni, E. and Bertolero, F., 1980. Metabolic fate of inorganic arsenic in laboratory animals. International Symposium on Arsenic and Nickel, Jena, GDR.

McCabe, L.J., Symons, J.M., Lee, R.D. and Robeck, G.G., 1970. Survey of community water supply systems. J. Am. Water Works Assoc., 62, 670-687.

Mealey, J. Jr., Brownell, G.L. and Sweet, W.H., 1959. Radioarsenic in plasma, urine, normal tissues, and intracranial neoplasms. Arch. Neurol. Psychiatry, 81, 310-320.

NAS, 1977. Arsenic. National Academy of Sciences, Medical and Biological Effects of Environmental Pollutants, Division of Medical Sciences, Assembly of Life Sciences, National Research Council, Washington, D.C.

Nordberg, G.F., Pershagen, G. and Lauwreys, R., 1979. Inorganic arsenic. Toxicological and epidemiological aspects. Department of Health and Environmental Medicine, Odense University, Winslowsvej, 19, DK 5000 Odense, Denmark.

Overby, L.R. and Frost, D.V., 1960. Excretion studies in swine fed arsinilic acid. J. Anim. Sci., 19, 140-144.

Overby, L.R. and Frost, D.V., 1962. Nonavailability to the rat of the arsenic in tissues of swine fed arsinilic acid. Toxicol. Appl. Pharmacol., 4, 38-43.

Pershagen, G. and Vahter, M., 1979. Arsenic: a toxicological and epidemiological appraisal. Naturvardsverket Rapport SNV PM 1128.

Pershagen, G., 1981. The carcinogenicity of arsenic. Environ. Health Perspect., 40, 93-100.

Pomroy, C., Charbonneau, S.M., McCullough, R.S. and Tam, G.K.H., 1980. Human retention studies with ^{74}As. Toxicol. Appl. Pharmacol., 53, 550-556.

Schroeder, H.A. and Balassa, J.J., 1966. Abnormal trace metals in man: arsenic. J. chron. Dis., 19, 85-106.

Smith, H., 1964. The interpretation of the arsenic content of human hair. Forensic Sci. Soc. J., 4, 192-199.

Smith, H., 1967. The distribution of antimony, arsenic, copper and zinc in human tissue. Forensic Science Soc. J., 7, 92-102.

Smith, T.J., Crecelius, E.A. and Reading, J.C., 1977. Airborne arsenic exposure and excretion of methylated arsenic compounds. Environ. Health Perspect., 19, 89-93.

Stevens, J.T., Hall, L.L., Farmer, J.D., DiPasquale, L.C., Chernoff, N. and Durham, W.F., 1977. Disposition of ^{14}C and/or ^{74}As-cacodylic acid in rats after intravenous, intratracheal or peroral administration. Environ. Health Perspect., 19, 151-157.

Tam, K.H., Charbonneau, S.M., Bryce, F. and Lacroix, G., 1978. Separation of arsenic metabolites in dog plasma and urine following intravenous injection of [74]As. Anal. Biochem., 86, 505-511.

Tam, G.K.H., Charbonneau, S.M., Bryce, F., Pomroy, C. and Sandi, E., 1979. Metabolism of inorganic arsenic ([74]As) in humans following oral ingestion. Toxicol. Appl. Pharmacol., 50, 319-322.

Tseng, W-P., 1977. Effects and dose-response relationships of skin cancer and Blackfoot disease with arsenic. Environ. Health Perspect., 19, 109-119.

Tsuchiya, K., 1977. Various effects of arsenic in Japan depending on type of exposure. Environ. Health Perspect., 19, 35-42.

Tsutsumi, S., Nozaki, S. and Maehashi, H., 1975. Studies on arsenic metabolism. Report 15. Influence of arsenic antidotes on external absorption of arsenic trioxide (As_2O_3) in rabbits. Folia pharmacol. japon., 71, 545-551.

Underwood, E.J., 1977. Trace Elements in Human and Animal Nutrition, 4th edit., Academic Press, New York.

Vahter, M., 1981. Biotransformation of trivalent and pentavalent inorganic arsenic in mice and rats. Environ. Res., 25, 286-293.

Vahter, M. and Norin, H., 1980. Metabolism of [74]As-labelled trivalent and pentavalent inorganic arsenic in mice. Environ. Res., 21, 446-457.

Valentine, J.L., Kang, H.K. and Spivey, G., 1979. Arsenic levels in human blood, urine and hair in response to exposure via drinking water. Environ. Res., 20, 24-32, 1979.

Whanger, P.D., Weswig, P.H. and Stoner, J.C., 1977. Arsenic levels in Oregon waters. Environ. Health Perspect., 19, 139-143.

Appendix 2
Beryllium

CONTENTS

2.1   INTRODUCTION

Beryllium is an alkaline earth and one of the lightest of elements. It exhibits a 2+ oxidation state and compounds of interest with respect to metabolism include the oxide, hydroxide, sulphate, fluoride, chloride, citrate, phosphate and silicate. The oxide is amphoteric and, at pH values between 5 and 8, the element tends to form insoluble hydroxides or hydrated complexes. Reviews of beryllium in the environment include that by Hurlbut (1974) and, more recently, that of Reeves (1979). The information given here is drawn from the latter of these reviews.

Most beryllium is present as localised deposits of beryl, but about 30 other beryllium containing minerals are known. Some beryllium is mined as beryl, but other sources are bertrandite and helvite. Total world production is about 10^4 tonnes per annum and uses are mainly as the metal or its alloys, though beryllium oxides are used in some ceramics. An early major use of beryllia in fluorescent tube phosphors has now largely been abandoned. Production and uses of beryllium are discussed in detail by the IARC (1980).

The toxic effects of beryllium include skin reactions; pulmonary disease; beryllium rickets and osteoschlerosis with associated effects on haematopoiesis; liver necrosis; and cancer. A good general review of beryllium toxicology is that of Tepper (1972). Skin disease consists of an allergic- eczema following exposure to soluble salts and necrotizing granulomatous ulcerations deriving from insoluble beryllium embedded in the skin. Pulmonary disease occurs in acute and chronic form. The acute form follows inhalation of aerosols of soluble beryllium compounds in relatively high concentrations. All segments of the respiratory tract may become involved, while time-to-onset and severity appear to be related to the magnitude of exposure. In contrast, chronic lung disease ("beryllosis"), appears to be most often caused by insoluble beryllium compounds, particularly the oxide. In an advanced state, this disease is characterised by progessive pulmonary insufficiency, anorexia, weight loss, weakness, chest pain and constant hacking cough. In the earlier stages, only slight cough and fatigue are observed. A useful historical and clinical account of this disease is given by Hardy (1980).

Beryllium rickets appears to be caused by intestinal precipitation of beryllium phosphate and the resultant decrease in plasma phosphorus levels. However, data reviewed by Reeves (1979) suggest that inhibition of alkaline phosphatase activity could also be implicated in the etiology of this condition. Osteoschlerosis in rats and mice is discussed by Reeves (1979) and experiments on rabbits are described by Fodor (1977). It appears that beryllium oxide granules accumulate in bone marrow. Around these granules, haematopoietic elements decrease in number, fibrous foci develop and eventually medullary beryllium bone, which appears to arise independently of the endosteum, may fill the whole cavity (Fodor, 1977).

The carcinogenic effects of beryllium in animal experiments have recently been reviewed by the IARC (1980), Groth (1980) and Kuschner (1981). Beryllium compounds were the first non-radioactive chemicals found to cause osteogenic sarcomas in animals. Such tumours have been induced using a variety of compounds including zinc beryllium silicate, beryllium oxide, metallic beryllium, beryllium silicate and beryllium phosphate. Although the intravenous route of administration has been most common in these studies, osteogenic sarcomas have been induced as a

TABLE 1

CONCENTRATIONS OF BERYLLIUM IN   (1,2)
VARIOUS FOODSTUFFS

Food	Average concentration (μg g^{-1} w.w.)	
Beans	6.5×10^{-5}	(3)
Cabbage	2.3×10^{-4}	
Hens eggs (yolk)	1.8×10^{-4}	
(yolk and white)	6.1×10^{-5}	
(shell)	1.1×10^{-2}	
Milk	1.7×10^{-4}	(50)
Mushrooms	1.6×10^{-3}	
Peanut kernels	5.2×10^{-4}	(2)
Peanut shells	1.2×10^{-2}	(2)
Almond kernels	2.9×10^{-4}	
Almond shells	2.9×10^{-4}	
Tomatoes	2.1×10^{-4}	
Yeast (bakers)	3.2×10^{-4}	
Crabs	$1.5 - 2.6 \times 10^{-2}$	(7)
Eels	n.d.	
Mullet (whole)	1.1×10^{-2}	(8)
Blackfish (whole)	1.1×10^{-2}	(4)
Mullet (whole)	5.2×10^{-4}	
Mullet (gut)	5.0×10^{-2}	(6)
Blackfish (gut)	5.5×10^{-2}	(5)
Leather jacket (gut)	1.8×10^{-2}	(2)
Mullet (gut)	1.8×10^{-2}	(4)
Blackfish (gut)	5.9×10^{-2}	(2)
Mullet (fillet)	1.5×10^{-3}	(2)
Blackfish (fillet)	3.6×10^{-4}	
Perch and bream (fillet)	n.d.	
Blackfish (fillet)	4.4×10^{-4}	(2)
Bonita (fillet)	2.4×10^{-4}	
Perch (fillet)	1.6×10^{-4}	
Redfin (fillet)	5.7×10^{-4}	
Mullet (fillet)	6.6×10^{-4}	
Oyster (flesh)	6.0×10^{-4}	(59)
Scallops (Tasmanian)	3.4×10^{-4}	
Shellfish (flesh)	3.5×10^{-3}	
Shellfish (flesh)	6.5×10^{-3}	
Shellfish (flesh)	1.0×10^{-1}	

Notes: 1. From Meehan and Smythe (1967).
2. Where the number of samples is greater than one, it is given in parenthesis.

result of beryllium inhalation and direct intramedullary injection into bones. The tumour types observed appear to be osteosarcomas, chondrosarcomas and fibrosarcomas, but the distinctions between types are not completely clear, possibly because of the presence of multiple primary foci in individual animals, as observed by Fodor (1977). As with osteogenic sarcoma, a wide range of beryllium compounds has been found to produce lung cancer in a variety of animal models, both after inhalation and after intratracheal injection. Lung cancer induction in man has been studied by Mancuso (1980), Wagoner et al. (1980) and Infante et al. (1980). In the last of these studies, it was shown that the excess risk of lung cancer was associated with subjects who had been previously diagnosed with acute chemical pneumonitis or bronchitis secondary to short-term beryllium exposure. The authors point out that this may be due to a high non-neoplastic fatality rate in the group with chronic beryllium disease, so the association with the acute disease is not proven.

2.2   INTAKE RATES

2.2.1   Typical dietary intakes

Reeves (1979) summarised data for beryllium in foods in West Germany and concluded that total intakes of beryllium are $\sim$20 µg d^{-1} of which only a minor fraction is intake by inhalation. For comparison, the ICRP (1975) noted that in long-term balance studies of two individuals the daily intake was in the range 93-430 µg ($\bar{x}$ = 180 µg), but that an intake of 12 µg d^{-1} would be adequate for observed excretory losses.

Concentrations of beryllium in uncontaminated environmental materials have been discussed by Meehan and Smythe (1967), who reviewed earlier data and presented an extensive tabulation of their own measurements (see also Bowen, 1979). Concentrations relevant to foodstuffs have been converted to a fresh weight basis using the authors' listed conversion factors. The resulting concentrations are set out in Table 1. The data exhibit considerable variability, but typical concentrations are $\sim$5x10^{-3} µg g^{-1} for shellfish and $\sim$3x10^{-4} µg g^{-1} for other foodstuffs. Taken together with the food consumption data given by ICRP (1975), the concentrations derived from Meehan and Smythe (1967) represent an intake rate of 0.58 µg d^{-1}. However, the recorded concentrations are all for materials derived from uncontaminated areas in Southern Australia and may not be representative of other localities. Furthermore concentrations in general vegetation, including grasses, were $\sim$10^{-2} µg g^{-1}, suggesting that some plant foods could give daily intakes of a few µg. For comparison, Drury et al. (1978) quoted levels of 0.08 to 0.24 µg g^{-1} d.w. for potatoes, tomatoes, bread and rice.

Reeves (1979) has commented that ordinary agricultural soils contain beryllium in the µg kg^{-1} range, but Bowen (1979) gives the following concentrations in rocks and soils:

Material	Concentrations ($\mu g \ g^{-1}$)
Granite	5
Basalt	0.3
Soil	0.3
Shale	3
Limestone	<1
Sandstone	<1

These data might suggest that typical content in soil will not exceed 1 $\mu g \ g^{-1}$, considerably higher than the value given by Reeves (1979). At this level, an individual would have to ingest only a small amount of soil, either deliberately or as contamination on food, in order to take in several μg of beryllium per day and this could make a substantial difference to his total intake of the element.

In conclusion, the limited data currently available are not sufficient to define a typical dietary intake rate for beryllium, but this intake rate may be markedly affected by rates of ingestion of soil, either as contamination on food, or for other reasons.

2.2.2   Beryllium in drinking water

The ICRP (1975) estimated that the rate of intake of beryllium in drinking water is ~1 $\mu g \ d^{-1}$. Water concentrations of beryllium are listed by Meehan and Smythe (1967) as follows:

Source	Water concentration ($\mu g \ l^{-1}$)
Ocean water	5×10^{-4}
Oilfield waters	20-200
Rain	0.07
River - Lachlan (Forbes)	0.01
- Macquairie (Bathurst)	0.01
- Nepean (Emu plains)	n.d.
- Woronora (Discharge Pt.)	0.03
- Woronora (Tolofin)	0.02
Pacific Ocean	0.002
Indian Ocean	0.001
Storage tank	0.002

From these data, it appears that typical drinking water concentrations will be in the range of 0.001 to 0.1 $\mu g \ l^{-1}$, though much higher concentrations are possible in fossil waters. The IARC (1980) commented that less than 1 $\mu g \ l^{-1}$ of beryllium is found in freshwater and less than $6 \times 10^{-3} \ \mu g \ l^{-1}$ in seawater. These limits are consistent with the values given above. Typical water consumption rates are 1 to 2.4 $l \ d^{-1}$, therefore, water concentrations of 0.001 to 0.1 $\mu g \ l^{-1}$ correspond to beryllium ingestion rates of 0.001 to 0.24 $\mu g \ d^{-1}$, substantially less than the value given by the ICRP (1975).

2.2.3   Inhalation of beryllium

Concentrations of beryllium in ambient air have been discussed by Reeves (1979) and by the IARC (1980). Near beryllium plants, levels of 0.1 µg m^{-3} have been reported, but these values date from the late 1940s. Average beryllium levels in urban air (circa 1950) were as follows:

Location	Concentration (µg m^{-3})
Boston	$3x10^{-4}$
New York	$5x10^{-4}$
Brookhaven	$7x10^{-4}$
Cleveland	$1.3x10^{-3}$
Pittsburg	$3.0x10^{-3}$

Much of this beryllium probably originated from the burning of bitumous coal (Reeves, 1979). For comparison, Bowen (1979) estimated airborne levels of 10^{-4} to $4x10^{-3}$ µg m^{-3}. For a man inhaling air at a rate of 23 m^3 d^{-1} (ICRP, 1975), this corresponds to a rate of intake of $2.3x10^{-3}$ to 0.092 µg d^{-1}. This is consistent with the estimate of <0.01 µg d^{-1} given by ICRP (1975).

Reeves (1979) has reviewed data on the concentrations of beryllium in three brands of West German cigarettes, values were 0.47, 0.68 and 0.74 µg per cigarette, with 4.5, 1.6 and 10.0% of the beryllium content, respectively, being released into the smoke during smoking. For comparison, analysis of data presented by Meehan and Smythe (1967) gives the following data for concentrations of beryllium in tobacco:

Sample type	Concentration (µg g^{-1} w.w.) Range	Average	No. of samples
Cigarette tobacco	-	0.028	1
Pipe tobacco	-	0.027	1
Cigarettes (manufactured)	0.031-0.034	0.033	2

These concentrations are very similar to those obtaining for grasses and many other plants (∿0.01 µg g^{-1} w.w.). They indicate a content ∿0.03 µg per cigarette.

To obtain an upper estimate of beryllium intake by smoking it seems appropriate to assume that each cigarette contains 0.74 µg of beryllium, that 10% of this beryllium is inhaled and that 20 cigarettes are smoked per day. This gives a daily intake of 1.5 µg and demonstrate that cigarette smoking can be the dominant source of inhaled beryllium among the general population.

2.2.4   Summary

On the basis of data reviewed in this section the current state of information on typical intake rates for beryllium can be summarised as follows.

- Dietary intakes are not well known; reported values range from <1 µg d^{-1} to >100 µg d^{-1} and soil contamination of the diet may be a significant factor.

TABLE 2

DISTRIBUTION OF STABLE BERYLLIUM IN
HUMAN TISSUES (1)

Organ, tissue or fluid	Concentration in $\mu g \ g^{-1}$ (number of samples)
Blood (total)	3.8(5), <0.1(1)
Blood (plasma)	<0.004(1)
Bone	<0.0002(1),<0.001(2),0.011(1)
Breast	n.d.(?)
Hair	0.0063(3),0.021(6)
Nails	<0.01(1)
Skin	0.02(1)
Spleen	3.2(20)
Tooth (enamel)	<0.01(28)
Urine	n.d. (2)
Urine (24h) (2)	0.093 (?)

Notes: 1. Data are from Iyengar et al. (1978),
          but are converted to fresh weight using
          the dry and ash weight fractions given
          in that review.

       2. Based on excretion of 1400 ml d^{-1}
          (ICRP, 1975).

- Typical rates of intake in drinking water are estimated to be in the range 0.001 to 0.24 $\mu g\ d^{-1}$.

- Inhalation of ambient air results in intake rates which are typically $<0.01\ \mu g\ d^{-1}$, but the smoking of cigarettes could give rise to inhalation intake rates of as much as 1.5 $\mu g\ d^{-1}$.

2.3   DISTRIBUTION OF BERYLLIUM IN HUMAN TISSUES

Data on the distribution of beryllium in human tissues are very limited. Iyengar et al. (1978) reviewed relevant data that were available at that time; these data, which are summarised in Table 2, are derived from a wide variety of different publications and the values reported are not directly comparable. Reeves (1979) has commented that "in human pulmonary tissues, amounts less than 20 $\mu g\ kg^{-1}$ (dry weight basis) are not regarded as indicative of occupational exposure". With regard to blood and urine, Reeves (1979) commented that levels in unexposed persons were undetectable by the classic methods and that determination with the newer methods were yet to be made.

In occupationally exposed workers, pulmonary levels of beryllium may be as high as 1 to 100 $\mu g\ g^{-1}$ d.w. and various segments of the same lung may exhibit widely differing levels. Beryllium in blood and urine of exposed individuals is variable in the range 0.02 to 3 $\mu g\ l^{-1}$.

The ICRP (1975) gave some limited data for normal beryllium contents of organs and tissues of a reference man. The total content of blood was quoted as $<0.52\ \mu g$, corresponding to a concentration of $<10^{-4}\ \mu g\ g^{-1}$ (w.w.). All other data given by the ICRP were derived from the studies of Meehan and Smythe (1967).

Meehan and Smythe (1967) gave data for beryllium concentrations in several human organs and tissues. The following table has been derived from their results.

Organ or tissue	Concentration ($\mu g\ g^{-1}$ w.w.)	
	Range	Mean
Lung	3×10^{-4}-2×10^{-3}	1.3×10^{-3}
Brain	6.5×10^{-4}-1.3×10^{-3}	1.0×10^{-3}
Kidney	3.6×10^{-5}-4.2×10^{-5}	4.2×10^{-5}
Spleen	3.5×10^{-5}-6.3×10^{-5}	4.9×10^{-5}
Liver	3.3×10^{-4}-6.6×10^{-4}	4.4×10^{-4}
Muscle	4.0×10^{-5}-2.4×10^{-4}	1.6×10^{-4}
Vertebrae	9.1×10^{-4}-1.0×10^{-2}	3.6×10^{-3}
Heart	1.4×10^{-4}-8.4×10^{-4}	4.2×10^{-4}
Bone	-	4.2×10^{-3}
Hair	1.1×10^{-2}-2.4×10^{-2}	2.1×10^{-2}

Excluding hair, which was possibly externally contaminated, lung, brain and bone appeared to be the main accumulator tissues for beryllium. However, it is noted that the ash to fresh weight conversion factors for kidney and spleen are anomalously low and it may be that the concentrations listed above should be revised upward by at least an order of magnitude for these tissues.

TABLE 3

TISSUE DISTRIBUTION AND BALANCE OF BERYLLIUM IN RATS GIVEN BeSO₄ IN DRINKING WATER (1)

	Total quantity of beryllium (µg)							
	0.16 mg Be²⁺ ℓ⁻¹				1.66 mg Be²⁺ ℓ⁻¹			
	1	2	3	4	1	2	3	4
Consumption	157.90	446.00	639.50	862.90	2,069.60	3,891.10	5,830.80	10,344.60
Spillage	4.10	20.00	13.00	9.70	125.00	26.00	18.00	180.00
Total intake	153.80	426.00	626.50 (4)	853.20	1,944.60	3,865.10	5,812.80	10,164.60
Heart	0.01	0.01	0.00	0.01	0.01	0.01	0.00	0.00
Lungs	0.01	0.00	0.00	0.00	0.04	0.01	0.02	0.01
Kidneys	0.01	0.01	0.00	0.00	0.10	0.00	0.01	0.01
Spleen	0.01	0.00	0.00	0.00	0.01	0.01	0.00	0.00
GI tract	2.00	3.00	3.60	3.10	–	14.00	12.00	21.00
Skeleton (2)	1.08	1.24	2.86	0.77	0.73	1.94	0.95	1.12
Blood (2)	0.00	0.16	0.15	0.16	0.15	0.27	0.14	0.14
Liver (2)	0.20	–	0.00	0.07	0.01	0.02	0.16	0.04
Total body (3)	3.32	4.42	6.61	4.12	1.05	16.26	13.28	22.32
Faeces	116.00	318.00	528.10	738.00	1,160.00	3,180.00	5,280.00	7,380.00
Urine	1.00	1.60	2.20	2.80	2.80	3.60	4.20	4.80
Total output	117.00	319.60	530.20 (5)	740.80	1,162.80	3,183.60	5,284.20	7,384.80
Body plus output	120.32	324.02	536.81	744.92	1,163.85	3,199.86	5,297.48	7,407.12

Notes: 1. From Reeves (1965).   4. Incorrectly given as 626.00.
       2. Based on aliquot.   5. Differs by 0.1 from faeces plus urine.
       3. Sum of organs analysed.

More recently, Hurlbut (1978) has used flameless atomic absorption spectrometry to assay beryllium in a variety of tissue samples. He quotes a background beryllium level in urine of 0.05 µg l⁻¹, corresponding to a daily excretion ∿0.07 µg. Hair samples washed in acetone, rinsed with distilled water and boiled in detergent for 30 minutes exhibited beryllium concentrations of $<5 \times 10^{-4}$ µg g⁻¹. For comparison, samples washed only in acetone and water gave concentrations of 10^{-3} to 4×10^{-2} µg g⁻¹. From this, Hurlbut suggests that either the beryllium leached out of the hair during the wash or it was all surface beryllium. Hurlbut (1978) also estimated the background level of beryllium in faecal samples as 1 to 3 µg l⁻¹. Taking the rate of faecal excretion to be 0.135 kg d⁻¹ and the density of faeces to be ∿1 kg l⁻¹ (ICRP, 1975), these concentrations correspond to a beryllium loss in faeces of 0.14 to 0.41 µg d⁻¹. Thus, total excretory losses are estimated as 0.2 to 0.5 µg d⁻¹, suggesting that dietary intakes are typically toward the lower end of the recorded range (Section 2.2.1).

2.4   METABOLISM

2.4.1   Gastrointestinal absorption

The gastrointestinal absorption of beryllium has not been extensively studied. In experiments on rats, Bugryshev et al. (1974) estimated the fractional absorption of the element, administered as the chloride, to be between 0.0014 and 0.0021 and a similar value is indicated from experiments on dairy cows (Mullen et al., 1972). Reeves (1979), on the basis of his own experiments (Reeves, 1965), made the following comments. "At levels of 0.6 to 6.6 µg Be d⁻¹ in the drinking water, about 80% of the intake passed the gastrointestinal tract unabsorbed. The remainder was probably absorbed from the stomach, the pH of which (about 3.0-3.6 in the rat) allowed the beryllium sulfate to remain in ionised condition. Upon entering the alkaline milieu of the intestine, the beryllium became precipitated as the phosphate and was excreted in the faeces". This statement, which suggests a fractional absorption of 0.2 is not consistent with information given in the original paper (Reeves, 1965). Relevant data are shown in Table 3. These data demonstrate that total recovery of beryllium was typically ∿80%. Since beryllium which enters the systemic circulation is mainly excreted in the urine (Section 2.4.3), a reasonable estimate of fractional gastrointestinal absorption can be obtained by dividing total body content (excluding gastrointestinal tract) plus total urinary excretion by total intake. Results of this calculation are given below.

Beryllium Conc. in drinking water		Animal	Fractional absorption	Total intake (µg)
0.16 mg l⁻¹	)	1	0.015	153.80
	)	2	0.0071	426.00
	)	3	0.0083	626.50
	)	4	0.0045	853.20
1.66 mg l⁻¹	)	1	0.0020	1944.60
	)	2	0.0015	3865.10
	)	3	0.0009	5812.80
	)	4	0.0006	10164.60

It is noted that there appears to be a trend to lower fractional absorptions with higher intake, but in view of the low organ contents, poor recovery and different periods of exposure of the various animals, the significance of this trend cannot be easily assessed.

More recently, Furchner et al. (1973) have studied the retention of beryllium in mice, rats, monkeys and dogs following oral and intravenous administration. These experiments are discussed in detail in Section 4.3. Here it suffices to note that fractional gastrointestinal absorption can be estimated by comparison of the whole-body retention curves following oral and intravenous administration and also by using the values for total urinary excretion following oral dosing.   Relevant data are given below.

Animal	Fractional absorption	
	Based on retention	Based on urinary excretion
Mouse	<0.005	>0.0024
Rat	<0.011	>0.0011
Monkey	<0.010	>0.0371
Dog	<0.018	>0.0038

These results are self-consistent, except in respect of monkeys. Possible reasons for this inconsistency are contamination of urine samples or neglect of long-term components of retention after oral administration, but no additional data are available relevant to this comment.

In conclusion, the fractional absorption of beryllium from the gastrointestinal tract is typically less than 0.01, though somewhat higher values are not excluded for monkeys.   For comparison, typical values for the other alkaline earths are 0.3 for calcium (ICRP, 1980), 0.3 for strontium (ICRP, 1979) and 0.2 for radium (ICRP, 1979).   The reason for this distinction may be, as Reeves (1979) has suggested, the tendency for beryllium to precipitate as the phosphate in the alkaline mileiu of the small intestine (pH 7.6; Bell et al., 1972).   For the purpose of modelling, it is appropriate to adopt the recommendation of the ICRP (1981) and take the fractional absorption of all compounds of beryllium from the gastrointestinal tract to be 0.005.

2.4.2   Retention in the respiratory system

In view of the extensive data which are available concerning the deleterious effects of inhaled beryllium (Section 2.1), data on retention in, and translocation from, the lung are remarkably limited.   Van Cleave and Kaylor (1955) studied the retention of beryllium sulphate and beryllium citrate in the lungs of rats following intratracheal instillation and found evidence for a relatively long-term component of retention.   Results with the sulphate were very variable, but relatively long-term retention and significant uptake by the mediastinal lymph nodes was observed.   Citrate was lost rapidly from the lung and transferred to the skeleton with little accumulation in the mediastinal lymph nodes. However, a small component of intratracheally injected citrate was well retained in the lungs.

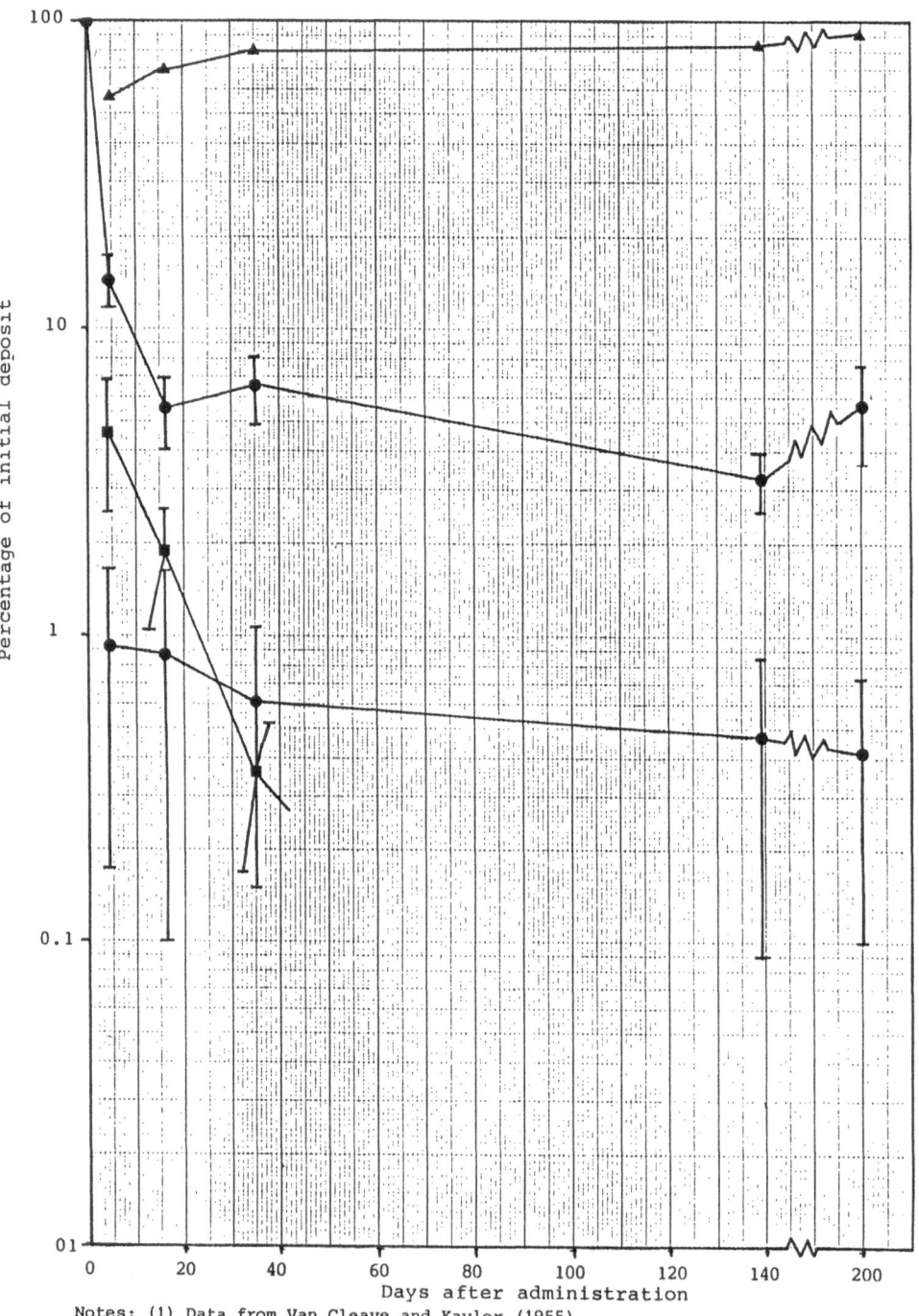

Notes: (1) Data from Van Cleave and Kaylor (1955)
       (2) Error bars are full ranges of recorded points

FIGURE 1. DISTRIBUTION OF CARRIER-FREE Be-7 IN FEMALE RATS AFTER
          INTRATRACHEAL INJECTION OF THE CITRATE.

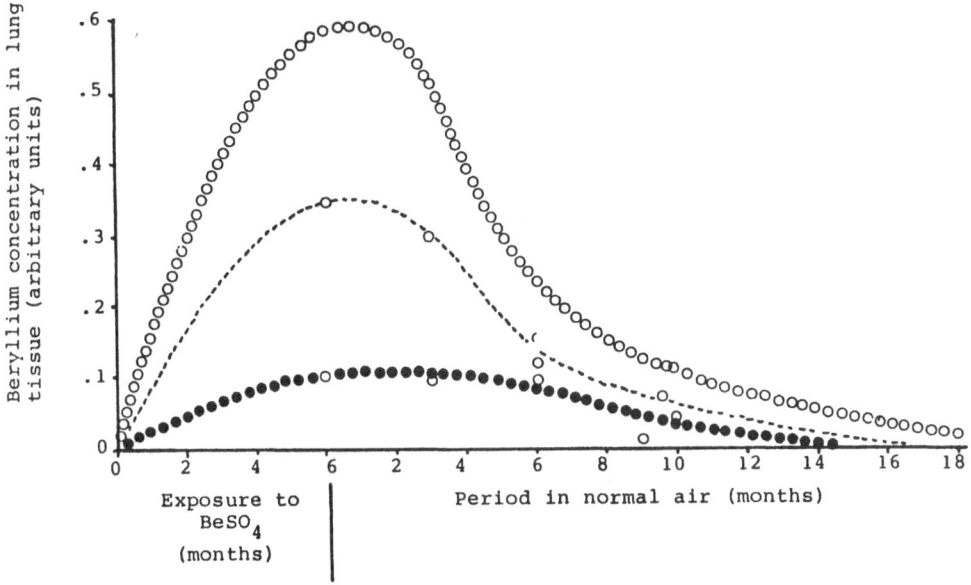

FIGURE 2.   ACCUMULATION AND EXCRETION OF BERYLLIUM
IN LUNG TISSUE OF RATS.

Kuznetsov and Matseev (1974) studied the retention of Be-7 in the lung after intratracheal injection and reported a pulmonary half-life of 20 days; 18% of the initial dose accumulated in the bones in 147 days.

With respect to inhalation studies, Shepers et al. (1957) reported in detail on pathological changes in the lungs of rats chronically exposed to beryllium sulphate over periods from one to 180 days. Although detailed metabolic information was not given, the authors do show some data for beryllium accumulation in and loss from lung tissue during and after the 180 d exposure period. These data are illustrated in Fig. 2 and are compatible with a long-term component of lung retention of about 120 d.

A more recent study of beryllium sulphate metabolism following inhalation is that of Reeves and Vorwald (1967). In this study, Sprague-Dawley rats were chronically exposed to a liquid aerosol of beryllium sulphate. Details of the pathological changes observed are given in the paper of Reeves et al. (1967). It should be noted that the lungs of exposed rats were much heavier than those of controls. This marked increase in lung weight was associated with visible changes in tissue texture and histopathologic examination suggested the existence of two distinct pathological processes, an inflammatory and a proliferative response. The inflammatory response occurred relatively late in the experiment, whereas a significant hyperplastic response appears to have been observed within four weeks of the commencement of exposure. These comments should be borne in mind when considering the data on beryllium accumulation and retention as shown in Fig. 3 and 4. The scatter on these data make the trend lines of limited significance, but lung contents do appear to have begun to saturate after 30 weeks of exposure, which would be compatible with a long-term retention half-life of about 100 d. Tracheobronchial lymph node contents appear to reach a maximum of about 1% of total lung contents after 40 to 60 weeks exposure. However, the decrease during the exposure period is not marked, the trend line in this region being defined mainly by the post-exposure data.

The retention of oxides of beryllium following inhalation has been studied by Sanders et al. (1978). About 30% of the initial alveolar deposition of beryllium was cleared from the lungs of rats during the first seven days after inhalation of high-fired oxide (calcination temperature 1000°C). After this early period of clearance, the residue of the lung deposit was cleared from the lungs with a half-life of about 325d. Approximately 25% of the beryllium cleared from the lung during the long-term clearance phase was translocated to the thoracic lymph nodes. The amount of beryllium in the thoracic lymph nodes at 23 months after exposure was about 10% of the initial alveolar deposition. It is noted that the lungs of rats exhibited striking differences in biological response to beryllium oxides calcined at different temperatures in the range 500 to 1600°C (Spencer et al., 1965).

Inhalation of beryllium nitrate by rats and beryllium chloride by humans has been studied by Stiefel et al. (1980). These studies demonstrate that some beryllium is transferred rapidly from lung to blood and urine, but the results are not useful in developing a quantitative metabolic model. The comparative toxicity of the beryllium ores bertrandite and beryl has been discussed by Wagner et al. (1969). These authors exposed male squirrel monkeys, rats and hamsters to the ores by inhalation for six hours per day, five days per week. The distribution of beryllium in various tissues at 6 to 23 months after the beginning of

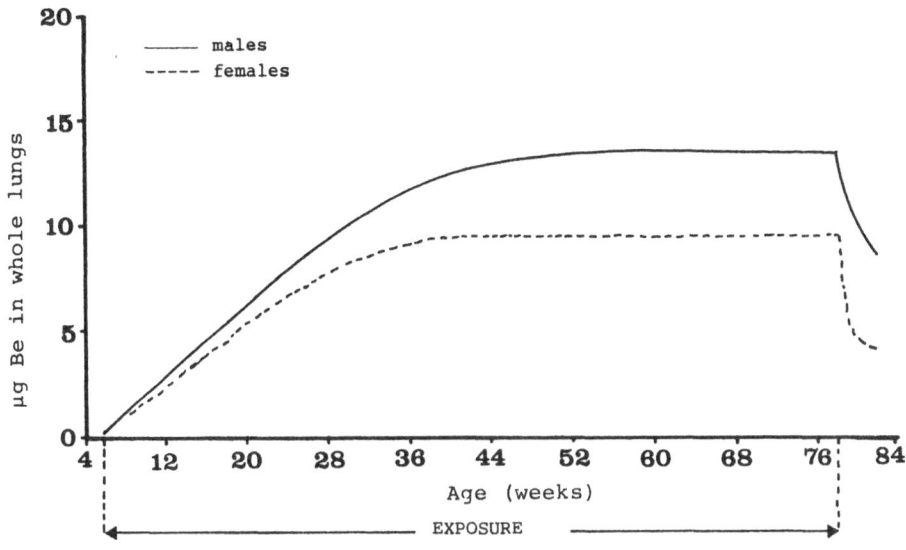

Note:
   (1) Data from Reeves and Vorwald (1967)

FIGURE 3. LUNG CONTENT OF BERYLLIUM IN RATS DURING
           AND AFTER EXPOSURE TO THE SULPHATE.

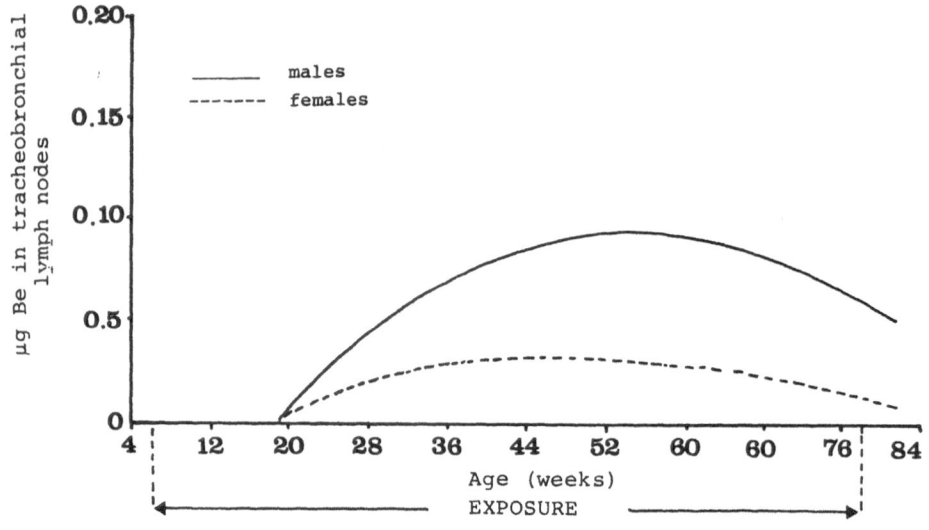

Note:

    (1) Data from Reeves and Vorwald (1967)

FIGURE 4.   TRACHEOBRONCHIAL LYMPH NODE CONTENT OF
               BERYLLIUM IN RATS DURING AND AFTER
               EXPOSURE TO THE SULPHATE.

TABLE 4

THE DISTRIBUTION OF BERYLLIUM IN THE TISSUES OF RATS, HAMSTERS AND MONKEYS AFTER VARIOUS PERIODS OF CHRONIC INHALATION EXPOSURE TO THE ORES BERTRANDITE AND BERYL

µg Be per gram of fresh tissue

Ore	Duration of exposure (months)	Lung			Femur			Liver			Kidney		
		Rat	Hamster	Monkey	Rat	Hamster	Monkey	Rat	Hamster	Monkey	Rat	Hamster	Monkey
Bertran-dite	6	–	–	8	–	–	0.003	–	–	0.01	–	–	0.003
	12	17.8	9.1	28	0.04	0.03	0.22	n.d.	0.004	0.06	n.d.	n.d.	0.03
	17	18.0	14.1	–	0.04	0.05	–	0.01	0.02	–	0.01	n.d.	–
	23	–	–	33	–	–	0.10	–	–	0.06	–	–	0.04
Beryl	6	–	–	100	–	–	–	–	–	0.18	–	–	0.10
	12	129	71.3	192	0.27	0.12	1.24	0.02	0.07	0.55	0.01	0.01	0.12
	17	83	77.4	–	0.37	0.14	–	0.04	0.16	–	0.02	0.04	–
	23	–	–	280	–	–	0.91	–	–	2.17	–	–	0.27
Control	6	–	–	0.02	–	–	–	–	–	0.01	–	–	0.03
	12	n.d.	n.d.	0.01	n.d.	n.d.	0.04	n.d.	n.d.	0.01	n.d.	n.d.	n.d.
	17	0.01	n.d.	–	n.d.	n.d.	–	n.d.	n.d.	–	n.d.	n.d.	–
	23	–	–	0.01	–	–	0.02	–	–	0.01	–	–	0.01

Notes: Data from Wagner et al. (1969)
n.d. = not detected.

exposure is shown in Table 4. These data indicate that both ores are retained in the lungs of hamsters and monkeys for several months. In particular, the data for beryl in monkeys are consistent with a half-life in lung of about 300 d. Much of the beryllium transferred from the lung to the systemic circulation appears to be deposited in bone, with a small additional fraction going to liver. Analysis of the data for monkeys suggests that <5% of beryllium was transferred from the lung to the systemic circulation.

The uptake of beryllium by macrophages and its cytotoxicity have been investigated in vitro. Hart and Pittman (1980) used suspensions of alveolar macrophages obtained by lavage from male rats and guinea pigs. The following conclusions were drawn:

- there was no measurable uptake of beryllium citrate, whereas there was rapid incorporation of insoluble complexes of the element;

- the rate of beryllium phosphate uptake was directly proportional to the number of particles present;

- beryllium phosphate uptake was reduced by inhibitors of glycolysis, inhibitors of cellular respiration, uncouplers of oxidative phosphorylation and by the inhibitor of microfilament formation cytochalasin B.

These observations indicate that phagocytosis may be the major mechanism by which the alveolar macrophage incorporates beryllium.

Data on the cytotoxicity of beryllium salts (Kang et al., 1979) are suggestive of the hypothesis that the release of lysosomal enzymes from macrophages may represent an important non-specific inflammatory mechanism.

The ICRP, when it reviewed the retention of compounds of beryllium in the lung (ICRP, 1981), assigned oxides, halides and nitrates of the element to inhalation class Y (half-life in the pulmonary region 500 d) and other commonly occurring compounds of the element to inhalation class W (half-life in the pulmonary region 50 d). The data reviewed above suggest that beryllium sulphate retention in, and translocation from, the lung is well-modelled by the ICRP class W model, but with the long-term component of retention given a half-life of 100 d instead of the standard 50 d value. Compounds of beryllium which are present in colloidal or particulate form, such as the phosphate and oxide, as well as ores such as beryl and bertrandite, are likely to be mobilised mainly by phagocytosis and cellular transport. For such compounds, the ICRP class Y model is thought to be appropriate. For citrate, the class D model may be most appropriate, but exposure to the citrate is unlikely to be a significant practical problem.

2.4.3   Systemic metabolism

The distribution and retention of beryllium in the body following its entry into the systemic circulation has been studied relatively extensively.

Reeves (1979) discussed the transport of beryllium in body fluids on the basis of earlier studies by Feldman et al. (1953), Reeves and Vorwald (1961), and Vacher and Stoner (1968). He concluded that the consensus of

TABLE 5

WHOLE-BODY RETENTION OF BERYLLIUM IN VARIOUS SPECIES   (1)

Mode of adminis-tration	Species	Retention parameters (2)					
		A_1 (%)	$\lambda_1 (d^{-1})$	A_2 (%)	$\lambda_2 (d^{-1})$	A_3 (%)	$\lambda_3 (d^{-1})$
Intra-gastric	Mouse	97.28	6.71	2.72	1.29	–	–
	Rat	100.00	2.34	–	–	–	–
	Monkey	99.08	2.05	0.92	0.18	–	–
	Dog	99.35	1.78	0.65	0.25	–	–
Intra-peritoneal	Mouse	53.15	2.72	9.08	0.092	37.77	4.0E-4
	Rat	45.23	2.55	13.25	0.068	41.52	6.0E-4
Intra-venous	Mouse	46.67	4.04	7.73	0.071	45.60	6.0E-4
	Rat	39.71	3.05	10.04	0.086	50.24	6.0E-4
	Monkey	22.18	2.35	18.83	0.019	58.99	2.0E-4
	Dog	43.00	1.38	16.63	0.058	40.37	4.0E-4

Notes: 1. Data taken from Furchner et al. (1973) and corrected for radioactive decay of Be-7.

2. Whole-body retention represented by $\sum_{i=1}^{3} A_i \, e^{-\lambda_i t}$ where

A_i is the percent of administered activity associated with component i.   Note that values of λ_3 are very small compared with the radioactive decay constant (0.013 d^{-1}) and are subject to considerable uncertainty.

these studies was that the bulk of circulating beryllium is in the form
of a colloidal phosphate, probably absorbed on plasma α-globulin, while
minor portions are carried as citrate or hydroxide. As Vacher et al.
(1973) have noted, the distribution of beryllium depends not only on the
dose, but also on its form. The lower the dose the greater the fraction
excreted in urine or retained in bone. Both injected sulphate and phosphate can give rise to blockade of the reticuloendothelial system, but
the sulphate is much less effective per unit dose (Vacher et al. 1973).
It is probable that the sulphate blockade is attributable to in vivo
sulphate to phosphate conversion.

More recently, Stiefel et al. (1980) have given the following data
for the distribution of beryllium in the blood of three species.

Sample		Weight percent contribution		
	Cellular constituents	Constituents of low molecular weight M<10^4	Pre-albumin	γ-globulin
Human:				
ubiquitous	33.2	7.3	8.0	51.5
additions	17.9	9.2	69.9	3.5
Guinea pig:				
ubiquitous	25.8	------------------74.2----------------		
additions	23.2	1.7	73.2	1.9
inhalation	18.3	9.8	70.9	1.0
Rat:				
ubiquitous	34	------------------66----------------		
inhalation	35	------------------65----------------		

These data again indicate the substantial binding of beryllium to blood
proteins.

Stiefel et al. (1980) also gave data for the clearance of beryllium
from blood. Two components were found, but their relative magnitude and
half-lives cannot be estimated from the data presented.

The whole body retention of carrier-free beryllium, administered as
the chloride, has been studied most extensively by Furchner et al.
(1973). Whole-body retention was studied in mice, rats, monkeys and dogs
following intragastric, intraperitoneal and intravenous injection.
Following intraperitoneal or intravenous injection, whole-body retention,
R(t), was well described by a function of the form:

$$R(t) = a_1 \exp(-\lambda_1 t) + a_2 \exp(-\lambda_2 t) + a_3 \exp(-\lambda_3 t)$$

The λ values given by Furchner et al. (1973) were not corrected for the
radioactive decay of the Be-7 used. Corrected values are given in
Table 5 and the various whole-body retention functions are plotted in
Fig. 5. These data demonstrate that there is little difference in
beryllium retention, except in respect of monkeys, which, in intravenous
injection studies, appear to exhibit a component of long-term retention
with a half-life substantially in excess of that recorded for other
animals. However, it should be emphasised that radioactive decay of Be-7
made it difficult to define the biological half-life of this component.

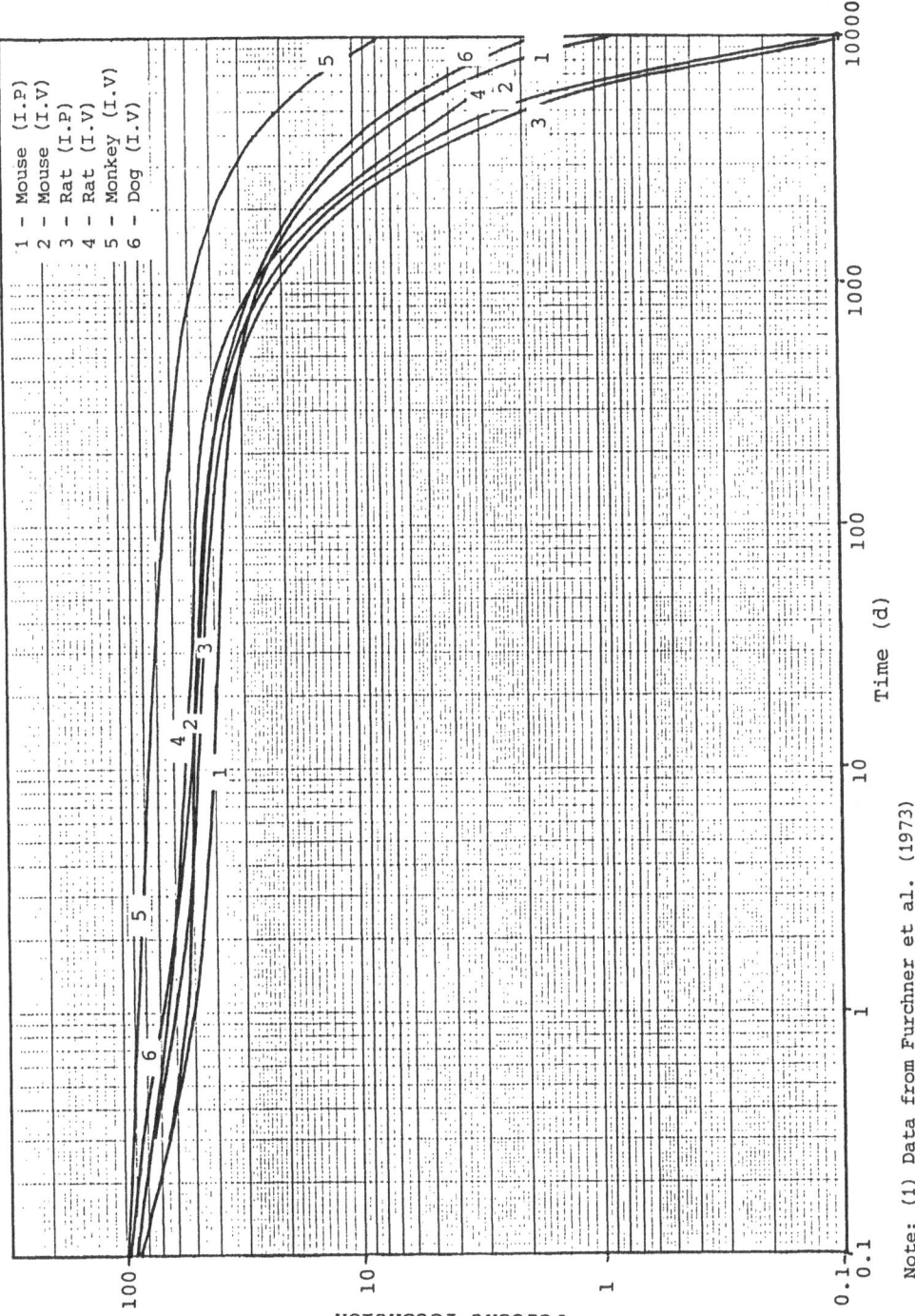

Note: (1) Data from Furchner et al. (1973)

FIGURE 5.   THE WHOLE BODY RETENTION OF BERYLLIUM IN VARIOUS MAMMALS.

TABLE 6

DISTRIBUTION OF BERYLLIUM IN THE RAT AT VARIOUS TIMES
AFTER INTRAPERITONEAL INJECTION

Tissue	Percent injected activity						
	0.25d	1d	3d	6d	10d	30d	71d
Whole body	57.04	55.86	52.47	46.83	44.30	30.17	16.86
Carcass	40.26	42.11	41.45	39.32	38.89	28.65	16.49
Pelt	2.09	1.70	1.40	0.98	0.73	0.31	0.16
Liver	4.38	4.40	4.16	2.49	1.30	0.31	0.12
Gut	3.84	3.10	2.44	1.57	1.13	0.39	0.13
Remains	1.17	1.13	0.96	0.75	0.64	0.24	0.17
Blood	0.47	0.53	0.48	0.33	0.28	0.082	0.044
Kidney	3.54	3.18	1.62	0.85	0.51	0.12	0.10
Spleen	0.16	0.17	0.18	0.17	0.13	0.18	0.12
Lung	0.26	0.17	0.28	0.14	0.10	0.082	0.092
Testis	0.07	0.08	0.08	0.05	0.05	0.041	0.12
Bone	34.72	36.01	36.62	34.63	36.00	25.93	15.65
Muscle	5.03	3.31	3.38	3.77	2.32	2.01	6.64

Tissue	Percent residual body burden						
	0.25d	1d	3d	6d	10d	30d	71d
Carcass	70.58	75.38	79.00	80.85	87.79	94.96	97.80
Pelt	3.66	3.04	2.67	2.02	1.65	1.03	0.95
Liver	7.68	7.88	7.93	5.12	2.93	1.03	0.71
Gut	6.73	5.55	4.65	3.32	2.55	1.29	0.77
Remains	2.05	2.02	1.83	1.54	1.44	0.80	1.01
Blood	0.82	0.95	0.91	0.68	0.63	0.27	0.26
Kidney	6.21	5.69	3.09	1.75	1.15	0.40	0.59
Spleen	0.28	0.30	0.34	0.35	0.29	0.60	0.71
Lung	0.46	0.30	0.53	0.29	0.23	0.27	0.54
Testis	0.12	0.14	0.15	0.10	0.11	0.14	0.71
Bone	60.87	64.46	69.79	71.21	81.26	85.95	92.82
Muscle	8.82	5.92	6.44	7.75	5.24	6.66	9.73

Note: from Furchner et al. (1973)

TABLE 7

CONCENTRATION OF Be-7 IN VARIOUS ORGANS AND TISSUES
OF THE RAT AT VARIOUS TIMES AFTER INTRAPERITONEAL
INJECTION

Tissue	Concentration (% I.A. g^{-1})						
	0.25d	1d	3d	6d	10d	30d	71d
Whole body	0.148	0.154	0.160	0.128	0.114	0.079	0.043
Carcass	0.179	0.200	0.197	0.185	0.170	0.127	0.070
Pelt	0.028	0.023	0.021	0.014	0.010	0.0045	0.0022
Liver	0.315	0.333	0.338	0.186	0.087	0.022	0.0086
Gut	0.120	0.127	0.093	0.055	0.036	0.013	0.0043
Remains	0.060	0.053	0.054	0.037	0.026	0.011	0.0083
Blood	0.042	0.056	0.048	0.031	0.029	0.0085	0.0041
Kidneys	1.204	1.209	0.628	0.295	0.176	0.040	0.031
Spleen	0.188	0.191	0.220	0.189	0.165	0.212	0.129
Lung	0.103	0.075	0.081	0.051	0.045	0.030	0.030
Testis	0.019	0.022	0.022	0.014	0.013	0.010	0.030
Bone	1.322	1.403	1.376	1.426	1.361	0.941	0.566
Muscle	0.027	0.018	0.018	0.020	0.011	0.010	0.032

Note: from Furchner et al. (1973)

Integrating the whole-body retention function with time allows comparison of the predicted build-up of beryllium in the body. Results are given below for the intravenous route only.

	Integrated retention function (d)			
Time(d)	Mouse	Rat	Monkey	Dog
0.1	0.092	0.094	0.098	0.097
1	0.644	0.722	0.862	0.798
10	5.215	5.813	7.702	5.602
100	45.46	50.06	66.93	42.74
1000	344.1	379.1	544.7	335.9
3000	635.6	700.2	1341	708.4

This table illustrates the limited extent of inter-species differences in the whole-body retention of beryllium. On the basis of these data, a reasonable whole-body retention function for man is given by:

$$R(t) = 0.4 \exp(-2.0t) + 0.16 \exp(-0.046t) + 0.44 \exp(-0.00046t)$$

where t is in days.

This function is very similar to that recommended by the ICRP (1981).

The distribution of beryllium between different organs and tissues has been studied by various authors. The data of Furchner et al. (1973) are listed in Tables 6 and 7. These data demonstrate that beryllium injected as carrier-free chloride is strongly concentrated in bone and slightly concentrated in the liver and kidneys.

The distribution of Be-7 in female rats intravenously injected with beryllium sulphate has been studied by Van Cleave and Kaylor (1953). Data from this study are summarised in Table 8 and 9. These data indicate that, even in the absence of carrier, beryllium sulphate is rapidly and efficiently taken up by the reticuloendothelial system. Data on beryllium chloride given in the same paper indicate that this compound is also accumulated by the liver (Table 10) whereas the citrate is deposited mainly in bone (Table 11). However, following intratracheal instillation the skeleton was invariably the main tissue of deposition (Van Cleave and Kaylor, 1955).

The distribution of beryllium in rats, following oral intakes of the sulphate in drinking water, has been studied by Reeves (1965). Data from this study, which are summarised in Table 3, indicate that the skeleton is the main tissue of deposition and probably contains more than 75% of the total systemic body content.

Skilleter and Price (1978) studied the distribution of beryllium in various organs and tissues after intravenous injection of beryllium phosphate or beryllium sulphate into rats. Beryllium phosphate was cleared from the blood with a half-life of a few minutes, whereas beryllium sulphate clearance had a half-life of ∿1h. Of beryllium entering the systemic circulation, ∿50% was deposited in the liver in the case of beryllium sulphate and ∿90% in the case of beryllium phosphate. Further papers by Skilleter and Price (1979; 1980) consider details of deposition and cellular interaction, but are of limited relevance with respect to exposure via inhalation or ingestion.

TABLE 8

THE DISTRIBUTION OF BERYLLIUM IN FEMALE RATS FOLLOWING
INTRAVENOUS INJECTION OF THE SULPHATE IN CARRIER-FREE FORM (1)

Organ or tissue	Content (% I.A.) (2)						
	30min.	2h	1d	3d	8d	28d	62d
Liver	8.89	42.84	56.75	67.20	14.19	2.25	1.23
Spleen	1.15	10.19	12.41	5.06	0.51	0.31	0.23
Kidneys and adrenals	1.72	0.80	0.53	0.23	0.38	0.17	0.02
Striated muscle	6.28	8.70	0.39	<0.009	1.38	<0.004	1.14
Skeleton	5.20	8.19	11.98	6.81	22.60	24.8	19.21
Blood	29.60	9.35	0.17	0.09	0.02	–	0.02
Lung	–	0.50	0.12	0.02	<0.005	<0.004	<0.004
Remaining carcass (3)	82.60	36.29	15.11	12.65	36.71	35.92	36.10
Remaining carcass less skeleton and muscle.	72.00	20.49	3.34	6.20	14.01	12.48	17.29

Notes: 1. from Van Cleave and Kaylor (1953)
       2. only one animal at each time.
       3. remaining carcass is not defined in the original paper.

TABLE 9

THE DISTRIBUTION OF BERYLLIUM IN FEMALE RATS FOLLOWING (1)
INTRAVENOUS INJECTION OF TOXIC AMOUNTS OF THE SULPHATE

Organ or tissue	Content (% I.A.)			
	1d	2d	3d	10d
Liver	28.49	45.18	34.53	30.38
Spleen	5.26	6.79	7.18	6.32
Kidneys and adrenals	1.16	1.28	1.02	0.47
Blood	<0.009	–	0.22	–
Remaining carcass	56.79	37.22	40.63	43.58

Note: 1. from Van Cleave and Kaylor (1953)

TABLE 10

THE DISTRIBUTION OF BERYLLIUM IN FEMALE RATS FOLLOWING INTRAVENOUS INJECTION OF THE CHLORIDE   (1)

Organ or tissue	Content (% I.A.)							
	2h	11h	1d	3d	10d	25d	52d	102d
Liver	18.50	28.85	19.54	18.30	11.38	3.97	4.49	1.82
Spleen	0.77	0.76	0.80	0.42	0.57	0.30	0.83	0.98
Kidneys and adrenals	3.41	1.68	2.61	2.45	1.09	<0.005	0.41	<0.004
Striated muscle	<0.01	<0.007	<0.008	<0.007	<0.006	<0.005	3.88	–
Lung	<0.01	<0.007	<0.008	<0.007	0.24	–	–	–
Skeleton	31.90	34.59	25.63	32.16	35.06	32.75	32.31	–
Blood	0.77	0.19	0.38	0.42	0.30	0.17	0.06	0.08
Remaining carcass	75.40	39.96	48.92	42.17	47.11	48.04	36.67	32.72
Remaining carcass less skeleton and muscle	43.50	5.52	23.30	10.01	13.04	15.18	3.35	–

Note: 1. data from Van Cleave and Kaylor (1953)

TABLE 11

THE DISTRIBUTION OF BERYLLIUM IN FEMALE RATS
FOLLOWING INTRAVENOUS INJECTION OF THE CITRATE (1)

Organ or tissue	Content (% I.A.)	
	2d	9d
Liver	1.31	0.38
Spleen	0.25	0.24
Kidneys and adrenals	0.51	0.10
Striated muscle (sample)	0.76	0.10
Femur	2.08	0.79
Remaining carcass	27.64	29.48

Note: 1. data from Van Cleave and Kaylor (1953).

Mullen et al. (1972) have studied the distribution of beryllium in a dairy cow and three calves after oral or intravenous administration of the chloride. In the cow, which was killed 119 hours after intravenous injection, blood contained 9.44% of the injected activity, compact bone 21.6%, kidney 1.41%, liver 14% and muscle 1.43%. Total retention was 50.9% of the injected activity. Data from the orally dosed calves are summarised below.

Organ or tissue	Total content (% dose)		
	71 h	190 h	454 h
Blood	<0.001	0.012	0.001
Bone (compact)	<0.001	0.142	0.264
Kidney	0.002	0.002	<0.001
Liver	0.006	0.005	0.006
Muscle	0.026	<0.001	<0.001

In general, beryllium injected in the presence of carrier deposits primarily in the reticuloendothelial system including liver, spleen and bone marrow. However, carrier-free beryllium or beryllium entering the body by ingestion or inhalation deposits primarily in the skeleton. The one exception to this is the work of Van Cleave and Kaylor (1953), where carrier-free beryllium was taken up by the organs and tissues of the reticuloendothelial system. It is not clear from the original paper whether the experiments protocols used would have excluded the possibility of colloid formation prior to injection.

Overall, it is preferrable to estimate the distribution of beryllium in the body on the basis of the comprehensive and consistent set of data presented by Furchner et al. (1973), as set out in Table 6. These suggest that of beryllium entering the systemic circulation $\sim$0.04 is deposited in the liver, $\sim$0.04 in the kidneys, $\sim$0.05 in muscle and $\sim$0.35 in mineral bone. Of the remainder, $\sim$0.4 goes rapidly to excretion, leaving $\sim$0.12 for distribution among other organs and tissues. Beryllium appears to be well retained in bone and muscle whereas it is lost relatively rapidly from other tissues (see the distribution of residual body burden given in Table 6). On the basis of these considerations, the whole-body retention function derived above can be partitioned as follows:

$$R_{BONE}(t) = 0.03 \exp(-2.0t) + 0.35 \exp(-0.00046t)$$

$$R_{LIVER}(t) = 0.01 \exp(-2.0t) + 0.03 \exp(-0.046t) + 0.01 \exp(-0.00046t)$$

$$R_{KIDNEY}(t) = 0.002 \exp(-2.0t) + 0.03 \exp(-0.046t) + 0.01 \exp(-0.00046t)$$

$$R_{MUSCLE}(t) = 0.16 \exp(-2.0t) + 0.02 \exp(-0.046t) + 0.03 \exp(-0.00046t)$$

$$R_{OTHER}(t) = 0.198 \exp(-2.0t) + 0.08 \exp(-0.046t) + 0.04 \exp(-0.00046t)$$

The time-dependent rate of excretion of beryllium, $E(t)$, following the instantaneous entry of a unit quanitity of the element into the systemic circulation, can be estimated by differentiating the whole-body retention function. This yields:

$$E(t) = 80 \exp(-2.0t) + 0.74 \exp(-0.046t) + 0.020 \exp(-0.00046t) \% \, d^{-1}$$

where t is in days.

Furchner et al. (1973) have measured urinary to faecal excretion ratios at different times after intravenous and intraperitoneal injection. Their results are summarised below.

Mode of injection	Species	\multicolumn{4}{c}{Urinary/Faeces ratio}
		1d	2d	7d	14d
I.V.	Mouse	3.50	0.51	0.96	1.17
	Rat	21.34	1.00	1.51	1.44
	Monkey	4.03	0.52	-	-
	Dog	48.61	4.62	-	-
I.P.	Mouse	3.21	0.80	0.91	0.62
	Rat	10.20	0.75	1.13	1.17

Thus urinary/faecal ratios are typically >∿ 3 on the first day after injection, but drop to ∿1 at later times. This is presumably because the short-term component of retention can be attributed to circulatory beryllium being mainly cleared by the kidneys. On the basis of the above figures, urinary and faecal excretion rates, E_u and E_f, are probably best modelled by;

$$E_u(t) = 64 \exp(-2.0t) + 0.41 \exp(-0.046t) + 0.011 \exp(-0.00046t) \% \, d^{-1}$$
$$E_f(t) = 16 \exp(-2.0t) + 0.33 \exp(-0.046t) + 0.009 \exp(-0.00046t) \% \, d^{-1}$$

Urine to faecal ratios calculated from these curves are 3.94, 3.63, 2.59, 1.25 and 1.29 at days 0, 1, 2, 7 and 14 respectively.
    It is of interest to note that a daily intake of 10 µg of beryllium coupled with fractional gastrointestinal absorption of 5×10^{-3} and the organ retention and excretion functions given above would give a urinary excretion rate of 0.03 µg Be d^{-1}, a faecal excretion rate of 9.97 µg Be d^{-1} and the following tissue concentrations of Be at $10^4 d$ (27y) after the commencement of intake.

Organ or tissue	Concentration ($\mu g \, g^{-1}$ w.w.)
Bone	7.6×10^{-3}
Liver	6.2×10^{-4}
Kidney	3.6×10^{-3}
Muscle	1.2×10^{-4}
Other	1.3×10^{-4}

These results demonstrate that this model, based primarily on animal experiments, is reasonably consistent with the fragmentary human data reviewed in Section 2.2.

2.4.4   Other metabolic information

2.4.4.1   Skin absorption

Most beryllium salts do not remain soluble at physiological pH and there is ordinarily no ready systemic diffusion following skin contact (Reeves, 1979). Ionic beryllium applied to the skin becomes largely bound to epidermal constituents, mainly alkaline phosphatase and nucleic acids (Reeves, 1979). From these considerations, it is concluded that absorption of beryllium through the intact skin does not need to be included in a metabolic model, though skin reactions from contact exposure can occur (Section 1).

2.4.4.2   Placental transfer

No data have been found concerning transfer of beryllium to the placenta or developing foetus. In view of the affinity of beryllium for bone, and similarities between its chemistry and that of the other alkaline earths, this is a topic deserving of study.

2.4.4.3   Loss in milk

No data on the transfer of beryllium to human milk are available, but Mullen et al. (1972) have studied transfer of beryllium to the milk of cows following oral and intravenous administration. These data indicate that milk concentrations over the first 120h following intravenous injection of the chloride are well described by:

$$U(t) = 2.2 \times 10^{-4} \exp(-0.42t) \ l^{-1}$$

where t is in days; and

U(t) is the fraction of the beryllium excreted per litre of milk.

For a cow excreting 10 l of milk per day, this indicates that ∿0.5% of an injected dose of beryllium will be excreted in the milk.

2.5.   MODEL SUMMARY

The following model is recommended for beryllium on the basis of data discussed in previous sections of this review.

2.5.1   Fractional gastrointestinal absorption

For the purpose of modelling, the fractional gastrointestinal absorption of all compounds of beryllium can be taken as 0.005.

2.5.2   Retention in, and translocation from, the lung

For retention in, and translocation from, the lung it is appropriate to use the ICRP lung model, but changing the long-term component of class W retention from a 50 to 100 day half-life. With this modification, beryllium sulphate can be assigned to inhalation class W, whereas compounds of beryllium which are present in colloidal or particulate form, such as the phosphate and oxide, as well as ores such as beryl and bertrandite, should be assigned to inhalation class Y. Beryllium citrate should probably be assigned to class D, but exposure to this compound is unlikely to be a significant practical problem.

2.5.3   Systemic metabolism

Following instanteneous entry of a unit quanitity of beryllium into the systemic circulation, the following retention functions can be taken to apply:

$$R_{WHOLE\ BODY}(t) = 0.4\ exp(-2.0t) + 0.16\ exp(-0.046t) + 0.44\ exp(-0.00046t)$$

$$R_{BONE}(t) = 0.03\ exp(-2.0t) + 0.35\ exp(-0.00046t)$$

$$R_{LIVER}(t) = 0.01\ exp(-2.0t) + 0.03\ exp(-0.046t) + 0.01\ exp(-0.00046t)$$

$$R_{KIDNEY}(t) = 0.002\ exp(-2.0t) + 0.03\ exp(-0.046t) + 0.01\ exp(-0.00046t)$$

$$R_{MUSCLE}(t) = 0.16\ exp(-2.0t) + 0.02\ exp(-0.046t) + 0.03\ exp(-0.00046t)$$

$$R_{OTHER}(t) = 0.198\ exp(-2.0t) + 0.08\ exp(-0.046t) + 0.04\ exp(-0.00046t)$$

where t is time in days.

2.5.4   Excretion

Following the instantaneous entry of a quality of beryllium into the systemic circulation, the time dependence of urinary and faecal excretion can be taken to be described by:

$$E_u(t) = 64\ exp(-2.0t) + 0.41\ exp(-0.046t) + 0.011\ exp(-0.00046t)$$

$$E_f(t) = 16\ exp(-2.0t) + 0.33\ exp(-0.046t) + 0.009\ exp(-0.00046t)$$

where $E_u(t)$ is the urinary excretion rate (% introduced beryllium d^{-1});

$E_f(t)$ is the faecal excretion rate (% introduced beryllium d^{-1});

t is time in days.

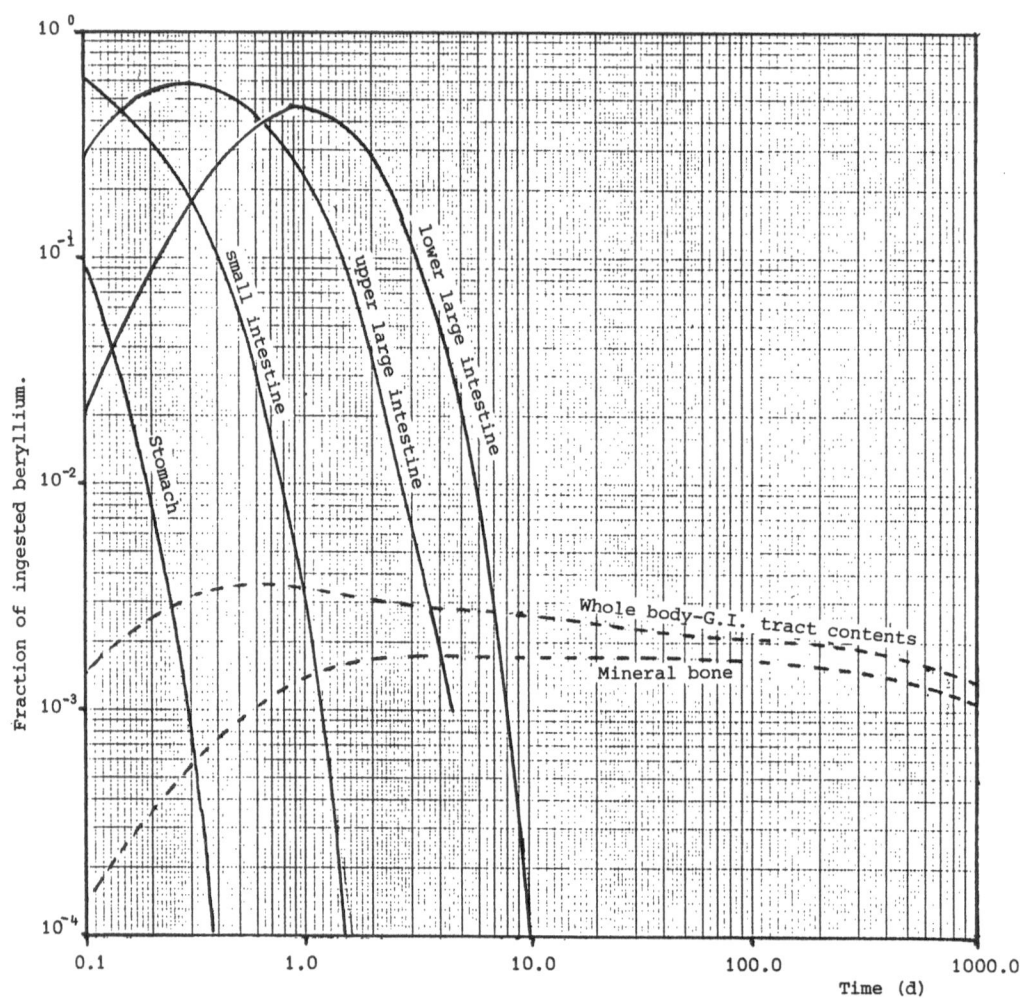

FIGURE 6.   RETENTION OF BERYLLIUM IN VARIOUS ORGANS AND TISSUES AFTER
A SINGLE ORAL INTAKE.

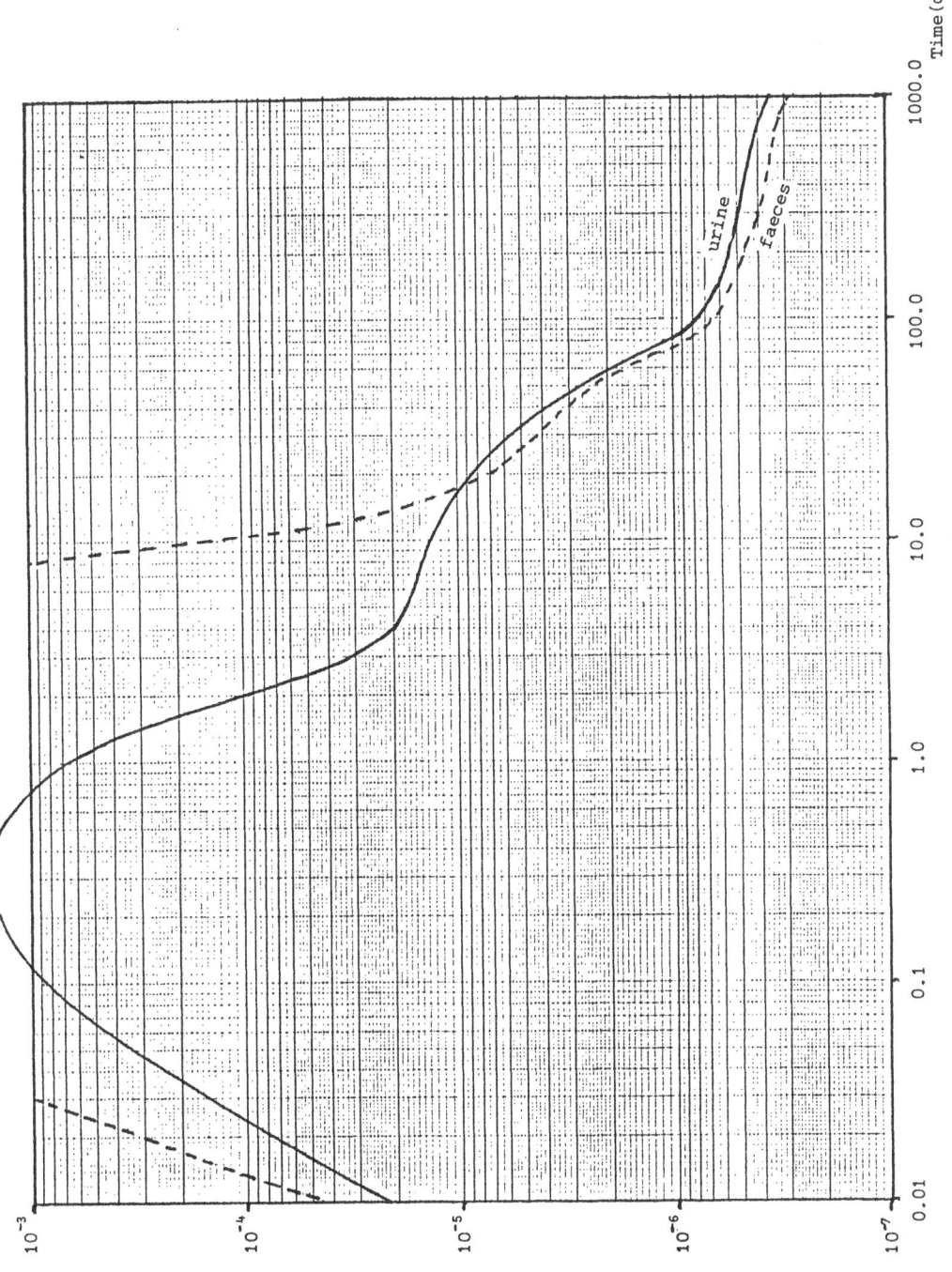

FIGURE 7.   EXCRETION OF BERYLLIUM FOLLOWING A SINGLE ORAL INTAKE

2.5.5   Skin absorption

Absorption of beryllium through the intact skin does not need to be included in a metabolic model, though skin reactions from contact exposure can occur.

2.5.6   Placental transfer and transfer via milk

No data have been found concerning transfer of beryllium to the placenta or developing foetus, or for transfer to human milk.

2.6   ILLUSTRATIVE CALCULATIONS

To illustrate the proposed model, the distribution of beryllium in the body and its excretion in urine and faeces following a single instantaneous oral intake is shown in Figs. 6 and 7.

2.7   REFERENCES

Bell, G.H., Davidson, J.N. and Emslie-Smith, D.; 1972. Textbook of Physiology and Biochemistry, 8th edit., Churchill Livingstone, Edinburgh, 1972.

Bowen, H.J.M., 1979. Environmental Chemistry of the Elements. Academic Press, London.

Bugryshev, P.F., Moskalev, Yu.I. and Nozarova, V.A., 1974. Effect of an isotope carrier (^{9}Be) on the distortion of the ^{7}Be in the organs and tissues of rats. Gig. Sanit., 6, 43-47.

Drury, J.S., Shriner, C.R., Lewis, E.G., Towill, L.E. and Hammons, A.S., 1978. Reviews of the Environmental Effects of Pollutants: VI. Beryllium. Report No. EPA-600/1-78-028, US Environmental Protection Agency, Cincinnati, OH.

Feldman, I., Havill, J.R. and Neuman, W.F., 1953. The state of beryllium in blood plasma. Arch. Biochem. Biophys., 46, 443-453.

Fodor, I., 1977. Histogenesis of beryllium-induced bone tumours. Acta Morphologica Acad. Sci. Hung., 25, 99-105.

Furchner, J.E., Richmond, C.R. and London, J.E., 1973. Comparative metabolism of radionuclides in mammals. VIII. Retention of beryllium in the mouse, rat, monkey and dog. Health Phys., 24, 293-300.

Groth, D.H., 1980. Carcinogenicity of beryllium: review of the literature. Environ. Res., 21, 56-62.

Hardy, H.L., 1980. Beryllium disease: a clinical perspective. Environ. Res., 21, 1-9.

Hart, B.A. and Pittman, D.G., 1980. The uptake of beryllium by the alveolar macrophage. J. Reticuloendothel. Soc., 27, 49-58.

Hurlbut, J.A., 1974. History, Uses, Occurrences, Analytical Chemistry, and Biochemistry of Beryllium. A Review. US Atom. Ener. Comm. Rep. RF 2152.

Hurlbut, J.A., 1978. Determination of beryllium in biological tissues and fluids by flameless atomic absorption spectroscopy. At. Absorpt. Newsl., 17, 121-124.

ICRP, 1975. Report of the Task Group on Reference Man. ICRP Publication 23. Pergamon Press, Oxford.

IARC, 1980. Beryllium and beryllium compounds. IARC Monographs on the Evaluation of the Carcinogenic Risk of Chemicals to Humans, Vol. 23, Some Metals and Metallic Compounds, International Agency for Research on Cancer, Lyon.

ICRP, 1979. Limits for Intakes of Radionuclides by Workers. Part 1. Annals of the ICRP, 2, No. 3/4.

ICRP, 1980. Limits for Intakes of Radionuclides by Workers, Part 2. Annals of the ICRP, 4, No.3/4.

ICRP, 1981. Limits for Intakes of Radionuclides by Workers. Part 3. Annals of the ICRP, 6, No. 2/3.

Infante, P.F., Wagoner, J.K. and Sprince, N.L., 1980. Mortality patterns from lung cancer and nonneoplastic respiratory disease among white males in the beryllium case registry. Environ. Res., 21, 35-43.

Iyengar, G.V., Kollmer, W.E. and Bowen, H.J.M., 1978. The Elemental Composition of Human Tissues and Body Fluids. Verlag Chemie, Weinheim.

Kang, K-Y., Bice, D., D'Amato, R., Ziskind, M. and Salvaggio, J., 1979. Arch. Environ. Health, 25, 133-140.

Kuschner, M., 1981. The carcinogenicity of beryllium. Environ. Health Perspect., 10, 101-105.

Kuznetsov, A.V. and Matseev, O.G., 1974. Differences in the distribution of labelled beryllium chloride with or without carrier in rats following intratracheal administration. Gig. Sanit., 10, 113-114.

Manucuso, T.F., 1980. Mortality study of beryllium industry workers' occupational lung cancer. Environ. Res., 21, 48-55.

Meehan, W.R. and Smythe, L.E., 1967. Occurrence of beryllium as a trace element in environmental materials. Envir. Sci. Tech., 1, 839-844.

Mullen, A.L., Stanley, R.E., Lloyd, S.R. and Moghissi, A.A., 1972. Radioberyllium metabolism by the dairy cow. Health Phys., 22, 17-22.

Reeves, A.L., 1965. The absorption of beryllium from the gastrointestinal tract. Arch. Environ. Health, 11, 209-214.

Reeves, A.L., 1979. Beryllium. In Friberg, L. et al. (Eds.). Handbook on the Toxicology of Metals. Elsevier/North-Holland Biomedical Press.

Reeves, A.L., Deitch, D. and Vorwald, A.J., 1967. Beryllium carcinogenesis I. Inhalation exposure of rats to beryllium sulfate aerosol. Cancer Res., 27, 439-445, 1967.

Reeves, A.L. and Vorwald, A.J., 1961. The humoral transport of beryllium. J. Occup. Med., 3, 567-574.

Reeves, A.L. and Vorwald, A.J., 1967. Beryllium carcinogenesis II. Pulmonary deposition and clearance of inhaled beryllium sulphate in the rat. Cancer Res., 27, 446-451.

Sanders, C.L., Cannon, W.C. and Powers, G.J., 1978. Lung carcinogenesis induced by inhaled high-fired oxides of beryllium and plutonium. Health Phys., 35, 193-199.

Spencer, H.C., Jones, J.C., Sadek, S.E., Dodson, K.B. and Morgan, A.H., 1965. Toxicological studies on beryllium oxides. Toxicol. Appl. Pharmacol., 7, p. 498.

Shepers, G.W.H., Durkan, T.M., Delahant, A.B. and Creedon, F.T., 1957. The biological action of inhaled beryllium sulfate. A preliminary chronic toxicity study on rats. Arch. Ind. Health, 15, 32-58.

Skilleter, D.N., and Price, R.J., 1978. The uptake and subsequent loss of beryllium by rat liver parenchymal and non-parenchymal cells after the intravenous administration of particulate and soluble forms. Chem.-Biol. Interactions, 20, 383-396.

Skilleter, D.N. and Price, R.J., 1979. The role of lysosomes in the hepatic accumulation and release of beryllium. Biochem. Pharmacol., 28, 3595-3599.

Skilleter, D.N. and Price, R.J., 1980. Apparent two phase beryllium labelling of hepatic cell nuclei isolated after intravenous administration of beryllium compounds to rats. A possible explanation. Arch. Toxicol., 45, 75-80.

Stiefel, Th., Schulze, K., Zorn, H. and Tolg, G., 1980. Toxicokinetic and toxicodynamic studies of beryllium. Arch. Toxicol., 45, 81-92.

Tepper, L.B., 1972. Beryllium. CRC Clinical Reviews of Toxicology. 235-259.

Vacher, J., Deraedt, R. and Benzoni, J., 1973. Compared effects of two beryllium salts (soluble and insoluble): toxicity and blockade of the reticuloendothelial system. Toxicol. Appl. Pharmacol., 24, 497-506.

Vacher, J. and Stoner, H.B., 1968. The transport of beryllium in rat blood. Biochem. Pharmacol., 17, 93-107.

Van Cleave, C.D. and Kaylor, C.T., 1953. Distribution and retention of carrier-free radioberyllium in the rat. AMA Arch. Ind. Hyg. Occup. Med., 7, 367-375.

Van Cleave, C.D. and Kaylor, C.T., 1955. Distribution, retention and elimination of ^{7}Be in the rat after intratracheal injection. AMA Arch. Ind. Health, 11, 375-392.

Wagner, W.D., Groth, D.H., Holtz, J.L., Madden, G.E. and Stokinger, H.E., 1969. Comparative chronic inhalation toxicity of beryllium ores, bertrandite and beryl, with production of pulmonary tumors by beryl. Toxicol. Appl. Pharmacol., 15, 10-29.

Wagoner, J.K., Infante, P.F. and Bayliss, D.L., 1980. Beryllium: an etiologic agent in the induction of lung cancer, nonneoplastic respiratory disease, and heart disease among industrially exposed workers. Environ. Res., 21, 15-34.

Appendix 3
Cadmium

CONTENTS

3.1   INTRODUCTION

Cadmium is a bluish-white metallic element in group IIb of the period table, chemically similar to zinc and, to a lesser extent, mercury. The metal is of considerable ductility, with a melting point of 320.9°C and a boiling point of 767°C. Its atomic number is 48 and its atomic weight 112. Only the divalent form of cadmium is stable, although highly unstable, strongly reducing Cd^+ ions can be obtained by irradiation of aqueous Cd^{2+} solutions (Cotton and Wilkinson 1972). From biological and toxicological considerations, two main groups of compounds of the element may be defined:

-    inorganic compounds, principally the oxide (CdO), sulphate ($CdSO_4$), nitrate ($Cd(NO_3)_2$) and the chloride ($CdCl_2$);

-    biologically incorporated or organic compounds of cadmium.

Cadmium is a well known industrial and environmental toxicant (Suzuki 1980), produced largely by mining or as a by-product of smelting zinc, and to a lesser extent copper and lead (Piotrowski and Coleman 1980). In a review of literature pertaining to cadmium, Underwood (1977) stated that "cadmium is toxic to virtually every system in the animal body, whether ingested, injected or inhaled". Present world production of refined cadmium is estimated to be ~15,000 to 18,000 te per year (Piotrowski and Coleman 1980). Although cadmium has a relatively short history of industrial use (Carmichael et al. 1982) it has found a wide variety of industrial applications including electroplating, manufacture of batteries, stabilization of plastics and use as a pigment additive (Piotrowski and Coleman 1980). As a result of human utilisation of cadmium and of zinc, with associated cadmium pollution, it is probable that, as with lead, the cadmium burdens of all flora and fauna have risen significantly (Nriagu 1980).

The possibility of acute cadmium poisoning has long been recognized and accounts of cadmium related illnesses can be traced back to the 19th century (see Friberg 1959; Yasamura et al. 1980). Probably the first account of acute cadmium toxicity in man was that of Sovet (1858), although cadmium poisoning was not definitely identified until 1920 (see Yasamura et al. 1980). The question of chronic cadmium poisoning was not studied in detail until the 1940's, when Friberg and co-workers produced the first series of studies relating specific symptoms and death to cadmium oxide exposure in Swedish workers (Friberg 1949, 1950; and see reviews of Friberg 1959 and Yasamura et al. 1980). A brief summary of the literature relating to chronic toxicity in man up to the late 1950's is provided in the review by Friberg (1959). Early data relating to cadmium concentrations in the environment may be subject to uncertainty in the light of analytical difficulties, and emphasis has been placed on more recent data in this review.

Over the last 20 to 25 years, a vast literature has emerged concerning many aspects of cadmium in the environment, including distribution, metabolism, and toxicity in man and animals. A large number of reviews have also been published covering these topics, and, although the original literature has been referred to whenever possible, much of the information in this chapter has been drawn from some of the more recent reviews (Anon 1981; Bremner and Campbell 1980; Calabrese 1981; Fox et al. 1980; Friberg 1978; Friberg et al. 1979;

Kwast 1981; Nriagu 1980, 1981; Piscator 1981; Travis and Haddock 1980; Yasamura et al. 1980; Fielder and Dale 1983; Korte 1983). The production of, and estimated levels of human exposure to, cadmium in the member countries of the European Economic Community (EEC) have been reviewed in two recent reports by the Monitoring and Assessment Research Centre (Hutton 1982; Piotrowski et al. 1980). Several reviews are also available outlining exposure to cadmium and dietary intakes in other parts of the world (e.g. Kobayashi 1978; Meranger et al. 1981; Travis and Haddock 1980). A review of particular interest is that of Nriagu (1980), which states as its objective: "to provide a comprehensive picture of the current biological, chemical, geochemical and clinical research pertaining to cadmium in the environment", describing primarily the "sources, distribution, mechanisms of transport, transformations, and flow of cadmium in the environment", and also covering biological and toxicological aspects of cadmium.

The quantities of cadmium derived from 'natural' sources are generally considered to be relatively small, and the largest sources of atmospheric cadmium in the EEC are from the iron and steel industries, together with refuse incineration. Waste disposal results in the largest single input to land and the manufacture of cadmium-containing articles probably results in the largest aquatic input (Hutton 1982). Underwood (1977) also identified cadmium contamination in phosphate fertilizers and sewage sludges as potentially important routes into the biosphere.

The metabolic and toxicologic interactions of cadmium with other elements and compounds, such as calcium, zinc, iron, vitamin D, amino acids, and metallothionein have been studied in some considerable detail (e.g. Bernard and Lauwerys 1981; Bonner et al. 1979; Cantilena and Klaasen 1980; Johnson and Foulkes 1980; Jones and Fowler 1980; Oh et al. 1981) and much of this work has been reviewed recently (Calabrese 1981). Several reviews and reports have considered specifically the potential carcinogenicity of cadmium and its compounds (e.g. Kjellström and Nordberg 1978, Kolonel 1976; Löser 1980) and the International Agency for Research on Cancer concluded that whilst the specific compounds responsible have not been identified there is 'sufficient' evidence for the carcinogenic effect of cancer in animals and 'limited' evidence for man (IARC 1980). The relative risk of cancer following occupational exposure may be doubled in cigarette smokers (Kolonel 1976), and this effect is apparently synergistic rather than additive. Details of the clinical and pathological manifestations of cadmium poisoning in man and animals are readily available from a number of sources (e.g. Boisset and Boudene 1981; Daston and Grabowski 1979; Kobayashi 1978; Kolonel 1976; Nakamura et al. 1981; Piscator 1981; Sabbioni et al. 1978) from which it is seen that the kidney is generally regarded as the critical organ for risk assessment (FAO/WHO 1972; Fox et al. 1980; Friberg 1978; Lauwerys et al. 1979). In a review of the literature, Underwood (1977) noted that it has been claimed by Fox (1976) that "5 mg Cd/kg are usually required" to produce adverse physiological effects on an otherwise adequate diet. In view of its interactions with a variety of dietary components (e.g. Zn, Cu, Fe, Se), this is clearly subject to wide variation. However, given that Reference Man (ICRP 1975) has a body weight of 70 kg, the above value is in reasonable accord with the estimate noted by Anderson and Danylchuk (1978), that 50 mg Cd d^{-1} will result in clinical symptoms of toxicity.

TABLE 1

CADMIUM CONCENTRATIONS IN ROCKS, SOILS ($\mu g\ g^{-1}$) AND
WATER SAMPLES ($\mu g\ l^{-1}$), UNCONTAMINATED AREAS

Material	Concentration	Reference
Rocks:		
Continental crust	0.15	Coughtrey and
Igneous rocks, average	0.20	Thorne (1983):
Metamorphic rocks, average	0.42	review
(excluding sphalerite)		
Sedimentary rock, average	1.02	
(excluding peat, oil, coal,		
phosphate		
Sandstones	0.05	
Limestones	0.035	
Soils:		
Common concentration	0.06 (0.01-7.0)	
Average content	0.5	
World average	<1.0	
Freshwater:		
Open lakes	0.1	
Lowland rivers, urban lakes	0.5	
Seawater:		
Offshore waters	0.02	
Coastal waters	0.2	

TABLE 2

CADMIUM CONCENTRATIONS IN FOODSTUFFS ($\mu g\ g^{-1}$ d.w. unless
otherwise specified), FROM UNCONTAMINATED AREAS

Material	Concentration ($\mu g\ g^{-1}$)	Reference
Grain and cereal products	0.032	Travis and Etnier (1982)
Fruits	0.042	
Potatoes	0.045	
Dairy products	0.005	
Vegetables	0.026	
Meat, fish and poultry	0.009	
Most foodstuffs	<0.05	Coughtrey and Thorne (1983): review
Edible portions of fruits nuts and vegetables	0.04–0.08	
13 fruits and vegetables	rarely >0.05	
Vegetables	0.01–0.45	
Grains and cereals: Various	0.028	
	0.021	
	0.01–0.57	
	<0.03	
	0.002–0.008	
	>0.05	
	0.057(0.008–0.12)	
	0.1–0.19	
	0.068(0.018–0.136)	
	0.035(0.005–0.077)	
	1.2	
	0.05	
	0.10±0.02	
	0.07±0.02	
	0.022	
	0.05	
	0.01–0.07	
	0.06	
	0.05	
	0.035–0.148	
	<0.1	
	<0.05	
	0.3–0.5	
	n.d.–0.63	
	0.046(0.035–0.062)	
	0.1	
	0.055±0.032	
	0.03–0.11	
	0.25	
	0.25	
	0.1	

TABLE 2   (Cont.)

Materials	Concentration ($\mu g\ g^{-1}$)	Reference
Root vegetables cont.		Coughtrey and Thorne (1983): review
Potatoes, median (w.w.)	0.047	
Potatoes, (w.w.)	<0.01-0.67	
Potatoes, (w.w.)	0.01-0.17	
Potatoes, whole	0.5	
	n.d.-0.63	
Potatoes, washed	0.33-0.55	
Potatoes, peeled	0.08-0.75	
Potato peel	1.13, 1.25	
Carrots, as prepared (w.w.)	0.09	
Carrots, root	0.05	
Carrots (w.w.)	<0.01-0.22	
Carrots (w.w.)	0.03-0.22	
Carrots	0.2	
	n.d. - 2.0	
Radishes	0.1	
Radishes (ash)	6.5	
Red beet (w.w.)	0.01-0.25	
Red beet	0.50	
Parsnips (w.w.)	0.01-0.09	
Parsnips	0.30-0.50	
Swedes (w.w.)	0.01-0.08	
Swedes (w.w.)	0.01-0.08	
Turnips (w.w.)	0.01-0.23	
Turnips	n.d. - 2.1	
Onions (w.w.)	0.01-0.09	
Leeks (w.w.)	0.02-0.23	
Leeks (w.w.)	0.02-0.09	
Leeks	0.2-1.5	
Fruit vegetables:		
Legume vegetables, prepared (w.w)	0.006	
Legume vegetables, median (w.w.)	0.005	
Phaseolus fruits	0.03-0.1	
Peas	0.04	
Runner beans	0.1-0.25	
Phaseolus leaves	0.1-<0.5	
Pea leaves	0.06	
Fruits:		
Garden fruits, as prepared (w.w.)	0.019	
Garden fruits, median (w.w.)	0.013	
Fruits, as prepared (w.w.)	0.042	
Fruits, median (w.w.)	0.003	
Fruits, (w.w.)	0.01-0.03	
Fruits and preserves (w.w.)	<0.01	
Nuts	0.03-0.07	

TABLE 2   (Cont.)

Materials	Concentration ($\mu g\ g^{-1}$)	Reference
Corn shoots	<0.4	Coughtrey and Thorne (1983): review
Corn leaf	0.03	
Corn leaf	0.8	
Rye shoots	0.8	
Wheat straw	0.39(0.21-0.64)	
Barley straw	0.43(0.22-0.70)	
Barley leaf	<0.1	
Rice leaf	0.1	
Rice straw	0.1-0.3	
Swedish flour	0.033	
Swedish bran	0.148	
Patent flour	0.05±0.01	
White bread	0.16, 0.19	
Leafy vegetables:		
General (w.w.)	0.07	
(ash)	1.2	
(w.w.)	0.051	
(w.w.)	0.039	
(w.w.)	0.05(0.01-0.15)	
Cabbage, kale, sprouts, lettuce, as prepared, >8 mi. from smelter	0.09(0.02-0.25)	
Cabbage	0.05	
Cabbage (w.w.)	0.01-0.25	
Cabbage (w.w.)	0.01-0.15	
Cabbage	0.10	
Spinach	0.83	
Broccoli (w.w.)	0.13-0.19	
Spring greens (w.w.)	0.02-0.28	
Green vegetables (w.w.)	<0.01	
Kale (w.w.)	0.05-0.25	
Kale	0.1, 2.8	
Sprouts (w.w.)	0.01-0.15	
Sprouts (w.w.)	0.01-0.11	
Sprouts	0.70, 0.95	
Glycine max., shoots	0.301	
Lettuce (w.w.)	0.01-1.81	
Lettuce	0.8, 2.9	
Root vegetables:		
General, as prepared (w.w.)	0.021	
General, median (w.w.)	0.03	
General, (w.w.)	<0.02	
Beetroot, carrots, onions, parsnips, potatoes, >8 mi. from smelter (w.w.)	0.07(0.02-0.10)	
Retail, GB (w.w.)	0.08(0.01-0.22)	
Potatoes, as prepared (w.w.)	0.046	
Potatoes, as prepared (w.w.)	0.080	

TABLE 2 (Cont.)

Materials	Concentration	Reference
Tomatoes (w.w.)	0.01-0.08	Coughtrey and
Tomatoes (w.w.)	0.01-0.08	Thorne (1983):
Tomatoes	0.03	review
Plums (w.w.)	0.01-0.04	
Pears, whole (w.w.)	0.01-0.09	
skin (w.w.)	0.01-0.04	
flesh (w.w.)	0.01-0.09	
Mushrooms (w.w.)	0.01-0.04	
Mushrooms	2.2-2.4	
Porphyra sp.	0.05-0.97	
Crabmeat, UK, brown (w.w.)	6.0	
raw (w.w.)	5.4(0.17-9.7)	
raw, brown (w.w.)	6.4(2.5-8.6)	
raw, dressed (w.w.)	5.9(3.9-10)	
Shrimps, UK average (w.w.)	0.73(0.28-0.55)	
Lobster, UK average (w.w.)	0.09(<0.03-0.23)	
Cancer pagurus, brown meat (w.w.)	0.03-3.42	
Mussels, UK (w.w.)	0.57(<0.05-2.3)	
Scallops, UK (w.w.)	0.82(0.36-1.4)	
Oysters,UK (w.w.)	1(0.48-1.9)	
Winkles, UK (w.w.)	0.64(<0.03-1.7)	
Whelks, UK (w.w.)	0.66(0.38-1)	
Pleuronectes platessa (w.w.):		
UK, middle waters	<0.05-0.40	
UK, distant waters	<0.05-0.35	
>40km distance, North Sea	0.12	
>40km distance, Irish Sea	0.07	
North Sea	0.12	
Cod, Trondheinsfjord (w.w.)	0.2, 0.2	
Haddock,Trondheinsfjord (w.w.)	0.1, 0.1	
Cod, Hardangerfjord (w.w.)	0.10-0.35	
Cod, Strathcona Sound	0.62(0.26-1.5)	
Cod, Artic	<0.5	
Brooktrout, whole fish	0.044±0.006	

TABLE 3

CADMIUM CONCENTRATIONS IN FOODSTUFFS GROWING ON OR NEAR
CONTAMINATED SITES (μg g^{-1} d.w. unless otherwise specified)

Material	Concentration	Comments	Reference
Vegetables	0.1-0.45	Urban areas	Coughtrey and
Rice (w.w.)	0.5-1.0		Thorne (1983):
Radishes (ash)	1.5-15	Mining area	review
Wheat grain	1.03		
Barley grain	0.2, 0.3		
Corn	0.7, 1.6		
Rye	1.6		
Corn grain	0.1-0.59		
Corn leaf	3.5-22.1	Sewage sludge	
Cabbage	1.2	and fertiliser	
Carrots	5.3	applications	
Parsnips	5.2		
Red beet	3.5		
Leeks	5.7		
Potatoes, whole	0.3-0.8		
Potatoes, peeled	0.08		
Potato peel	0.4-1.1		
Soya beans	2.0		
Runner beans	0.2		
Mushrooms	4.5-33.7		
Wheat grain (w.w.)	0.081-0.108		
Rice grain	0.72-4.17		
Rice grain	0.02-1.82		
Rice straw	0.7-3.6		
Barley	0.25(0.14-0.35)		
Vegetables	7.2-62.3		
Leafy vegetables (w.w.)	0.14(<0.02-0.5)		
	-0.44(0.05-0.95)		
Cabbage	0.5(0.26-1.05)	Smelting and	
Lettuce	2.09(0.60-4.60)	industrial	
Parsley	1.28(0.30-3.20)	sources	
Root vegetables	0.08(<0.02-0.17)		
	-0.19(0.04-0.43)		
Potatoes	0.26(0.19-0.42)		
Carrots	0.91(0.27-3.95)		
Winkles (w.w.)	3.8(3.2-8.6)	Bristol	
Mussels (w.w.)	4.1(3.7-9.1)	Channel	
Mussels (w.w.)	17(4.8-27)		
Whelks (w.w.)	20(14-31)		
Shrimps (w.w.)	4.8(4.3-5.7)		
Shrimps (w.w.)	3.7(2.5-4.9)		
Brooktrout, whole fish	0.059±0.004	Gottingen	

3.2   INTAKE RATES

3.2.1   Typical dietary intakes

As a result of local industrial, or natural, emissions the
concentration of cadmium may vary widely.   Thus, the 'background'
concentration of cadmium in British soils has been estimated at 0.75 µg
g^{-1} d.w. (DoE 1980), whereas a value of 998 µg g^{-1} d.w. has been recorded
at a single site in Shipham, Somerset (DoE 1980) and up to 9040 µg g^{-1}
d.w. in dust from the yard of a smelting works in Missouri, USA (Gale and
Wixson 1978).   Bowen (1979) listed the following mean or median
concentrations:

Geosphere

Granite and basalt	0.09-0.13	µg g^{-1}
limestone and sandstone	0.028-0.05	µg g^{-1}
Shale	0.23	µg g^{-1}
Soil	0.35	µg g^{-1}
Air	<0.8	ng m^{-3}
Freshwater	0.1	µg l^{-1}
Seawater	0.11	µg l^{-1}

Biosphere

Land plants	0.02-2.4	µg g^{-1} d.w.
Edible vegetables	0.85	µg g^{-1} d.w.
Mammalian muscle	0.14-3.2	µg g^{-1} d.w.
Marine fish	0.1-3	µg g^{-1} d.w.

Literature pertaining to the distribution and transfer of cadmium,
and its radioisotopes, through the terrestrial and aquatic environments
was reviewed by Coughtrey and Thorne (1983), which can be consulted for
further information on cadmium concentrations in the environment.
Tables 1 to 3 present some of the data available concerning cadmium
concentrations in rocks, soils and foodstuffs growing in contaminated or
uncontaminated areas. With regard to human diet, it appears that marine
molluscs, crustaceans and grain are the principal sources of cadmium
(ICRP 1975; see also Tables 1-3). A wide range in dietary intakes may be
expected, due both to dietary preference and local environmental cadmium
levels.   Thus, the ICRP (1975) estimated that a vegetarian diet might
provide about 100 µg Cd d^{-1}, whereas a diet high in seafood, meat and
cereals could provide 1 mg Cd d^{-1}.   Several estimates of average daily
intake are available for different areas of the world, see Table 4, and
indicate a wide range in values, from <18 µg Cd d^{-1} in the UK, up to 215
or 600 µg Cd d^{-1} in Japan depending on the area considered.   The ICRP
(1975, 1981) estimated a 'typical' total dietary intake to be in the
order of 150 µg d^{-1}, but on the basis of data presented in Table 4 a
better estimate for areas not known to be contaminated may be ~20 to 100
µg d^{-1}; a value which is similar to the FAO/WHO provisional total
tolerable intake level of 57-72 µg d^{-1} (FAO/WHO 1972).   Travis and
Haddock (1980) suggested that a normal dietary intake of around 50 µg Cd
d^{-1} could be assumed, and noted that dietary intake varies with age in a
manner correlated with calorific intake.   In general, it was suggested

TABLE 4

ESTIMATED DAILY AVERAGE DIETARY INTAKE OF CADMIUM

Country/ Area	Daily Cd intake ($\mu g.d^{-1}$)	Method of estimation	Authority
U.K.	<18	Standard diet	Hubbard and Lindsay (1979)
U.K.	15-30		MAFF (1973)
U.K.	64±30	Standard diet	Hamilton and Minski (1972/1973)
W. Germany	31	Faecal analysis	Essing et al. (1969)
W. Germany	48	Standard diet	Essing et al. (1969)
France	20-30	Standard diet/ duplicate meal	CEC (1978)
Denmark	<30	Standard diet	Milj0ministriat (1980)
Holland	29	Standard diet	Ministry of Health (1980)
Sweden	10-20		Cited in: Drury and Hammons (1979)
Canada	67(52-80)	Standard diet	Meranger and Smith (1972)
Canada	67		Kirkpatrick and Coffin (1974)
New Zealand (woman only)	69-92		Robinson et al.(1973)
Japan	up to 215		Cited in: Drury and Hammons (1979)
Japan	up to 600		Kobayashi (1978)(1)
U.S.A	26	Market basket survey	Duggan and Lipscomb (1969)
U.S.A.	13-16	Faecal analysis	Kowal et al.(1979)
U.S.A.	26-61	Standard diet	FDA (1977)
U.S.A.	26-51		Mahaffey et al. (1975)
U.S.A.	~22-30	Standard diet	Travis and Etnier (1982)
Children in institutions	27-64		Murthy et al. (1971)
General	150	Review/Balance study	ICRP (1975): from Tipton and Stewart (1969)
Provisional total toler- able intake, all sources.	57-72	Recommendation	FAO/WHO (1972)

Note:

(1) Value associated with areas of known high cadmium concentration in Japan, where incidences of 'Itai-itai' disease have been reported.

that an intake of 1 kilo-calorie can be equated with an intake of 0.02 μg Cd. This is consistent with the ICRP (1975) recommended energy expenditure estimate of 3000 kcal d^{-1} for Reference Man, assumed in energy balance.

It is of note that Travis and Etnier (1982) estimated US dietary cadmium intakes for the period 1945-1975, assuming (i) constant cadmium levels in foodstuffs, or; (ii) slowly increasing cadmium levels in foodstuffs due to industrial contamination. Because of dietary changes over the 30 year period of estimation, assumption (i) resulted in a 20% decline in cadmium intake, whereas assumption (ii) resulted in dietary intakes remaining constant over the period, at around 22-30 μg d^{-1}. Diets containing in excess of 100 to 200 μg Cd d^{-1} appear to be uncommon, unless local land contamination is present, as at sites in Somerset and Derbyshire (UK) or areas of Japan where 'itai-itai' disease has been prevalent (e.g. Cole 1979; Tsuchiya 1978). This statement is not in agreement with the ICRP (1975) conclusion that 150 μg Cd d^{-1} represents a typical dietary intake, which estimate was based on a long-term balance study by Tipton and Stewart (1969), but is in accord with the majority of data presented in Table 4.

3.2.2   Cadmium in drinking water

Concentrations of cadmium in drinking water are generally relatively low compared with dietary concentrations and the predominant chemical form is expected to be Cd^{2+}. American drinking water has been estimated to exhibit a cadmium concentration of about 6.0 μg l^{-1} (cited in; ICRP 1975), which represents an average daily intake of about 12 μg Cd. In most freshwaters which are not known to be contaminated, cadmium levels are generally <1 μg l^{-1} (Piotrowski and Coleman 1980). In a study of the intake of metals from drinking water amongst residents of Seattle, USA, Sharrett et al. (1982) found a high correlation between daily intake and the material used for plumbing. Their results can be summarised as follows (μg Cd d^{-1}):

Percentile	Copper plumbing		Galvanized plumbing	
	standing water	running water	standing water	running water
25	0.0	0.0	0.5	0.2
50	0.1	0.0	1.3	0.5
75	0.4	0.2	2.6	1.2
mean	0.5	0.1	2.2	1.0

Much higher concentrations, up to 100 μg l^{-1}, have also been recorded, (Travis and Haddock 1980) and as early as 1945 concern was expressed at the use of cadmium as a plating material, since it was known that acidic drinks such as fruit juices or lemonade could dissolve toxic quantities of this metal (Klein and Wickmann 1945). More recently, several cases of cadmium poisoning in American children were diagnosed and traced to a cooled soft-drinks vending machine on school premises (Nordberg et al. 1973). In this case, cadmium reached a concentration of 16 mg l^{-1} in solution and 40 mg l^{-1} in precipitate. If it is assumed

TABLE 5

CONCENTRATION OF CADMIUM IN AIR SAMPLES

Period of study	Concentration of cadmium (μg m^{-3})	Location and comments	Reference
Annual average	0.006	San Francisco } Range for 20	Friberg et al
Annual average	0.036	St. Louis } largest US cities 1969	(1974): R
Annual average	0.12	El Paso, Texas: 1964, highest average recorded	
Annual average	0.23	Manhatten, New York	
Annual average	0.14	Bronx, New York	
Annual average	0.003	Non-urban site, USA	
Annual average	0.014	New York	
Annual average	<0.003	26 non-urban sites, USA[1]	
24-hr	<0.005–0.08	Chicago	
24-hr	0.33	Houston, Texas	
3-mo (geom. mean)	0.0032–0.0034	Cincinatti-urban	
3-mo (geom. mean)	0.0017–0.0021	Cincinatti-suburban	
Annual average	0.002–0.05	Poland–10 cities	
Several months	0.010–0.053	Tokyo–1969 to 1971	
24-hr max. value	0.53	Tokyo–1969 to 1971	
7 days	0.005	Stockholm	
7 days (2)	0.0009	Rural area–Sweden	
—	0.0015	Erlangen–W. Germany	
—	0.08	Cincinatti-downtown	
—	0.02	Cincinatti-suburbs	
—	0.01	St. Louis	
—	0.026	Missouri-industrial area	Dorn (1979): R
—	0.002	Missouri-non-industrial area	
—	∿0.025	Estimated normal air level	Yasamura (1980): R

TABLE 5 (Cont.)

Period of study	Concentration of Cadmium ($\mu g\ m^{-3}$)	Location and comments	Reference
-	>0.5	Zn, Cu, Pb smelters . near vicinity	Piotrowski and Coleman (1980) : R
Annual average	0.002-0.09	Highly urbanized areas,[3] Europe	Piotrowski et al (1980) : R

Notes:

(1) 0.003 $\mu g\ m^{-3}$ was the lowest detectable level by method used.
(2) Period of study unknown or not reported in review article.
(3) Typically, values in range 0.01-0.02 $\mu g\ m$ 3.
(4) R = Review

that the daily fluid intake is ~2 litres (ICRP 1975) and an intake of 35-50 mg d^{-1} over an extended period results in the manifestation of clinical symptoms (cited in: Underwood 1977; Anderson and Danylchuk 1978), then a cadmium concentration in water of 15-20 mg l^{-1} could be expected to give rise to toxic effects. This is in accord with the review of Friberg (1978), which notes that in water, a concentration of 15 mg Cd l^{-1} will cause vomiting and stomach cramps. It is unlikely that levels would normally rise as high as 15 mg l^{-1}, since, even in contaminated areas of Japan, associated with "itai-itai" disease, relatively low levels of cadmium have been recorded in the water, although much higher levels were associated with the underlying sediments (e.g. Kobayashi 1978). Thus, in general the cadmium content of drinking water will form an insignificant source of human intake, in comparison to Cd ingestion in food (Travis and Haddock 1980). In this context·milk, which may have higher levels of cadmium than water (see Section 3), is included in the term 'food'.

3.2.3   Inhalation of cadmium

It is generally accepted that, in the majority of areas unaffected by local contamination the main source of cadmium intake is via ingestion rather than inhalation (e.g. Oberdoerster et al. 1979). However, inhalation may represent a significant further burden, particularly for occupationally exposed workers, and hence airborne concentrations require evaluation (Adamsson et al. 1979; Oberdoester et al. 1979). Recorded levels of airborne cadmium are presented in Table 5 and it can be seen that airborne concentrations vary between ~0.002 and ~0.10 µg Cd m^{-3}, with substantial variation occurring at a single site. Generally, values are higher in urban and heavily industrialised areas, and lower in rural areas, but typically the average concentration is <0.05 µg m^{-3} in all locations. For purposes of comparison with dietary intakes, a typical air concentration of 0.03 µg m^{-3} can be assumed and an average individual taken to inhale around 20 to 23 m³ air per day (ICRP 1975; Yasamura et al. 1980). This implies a daily atmospheric cadmium intake of ~0.6 to ~0.7 µg, compared with an estimated total daily ingestion of ~20 to 100 µg Cd in areas not known to be contaminated (Section 2.1 and ICRP 1975, 1981).

Tobacco typically contains 0.5 to 3.5 µg Cd g^{-1}, and smoking, particularly of cigarettes, may form a further significant source of cadmium intake (Carmichael et al. 1982). It may be assumed, as for arsenic (Appendix 1, Sections 1.2.3 and 1.4.2), that approximately 10% of the available cadmium in tobacco smoke is inhaled, which represents about 0.1 to 0.2 µg Cd per cigarette or 2-4 µg Cd d^{-1} for a smoker of twenty cigarettes per day (Carmichael et al. 1982; Yasamura et al. 1980; Travis and Haddock 1980). Pipe and cigar smoking are reported to result in only a small rise in body Cd levels (Yasamura et al. 1980). In one study of 15 male workers in a Swedish nickel-cadmium battery producing factory, Adamsson et al. (1979) reported the following faecal excretions of cadmium (µg d^{-1}):

	Smokers	Non-smokers
$\bar{x}$	619	268
(range)	(97-2577)	(31-1102)

In these workers, cadmium intakes in food and drink contributed only 100 μg Cd d^{-1}. Thus, contamination must have occurred (even in non-smokers) and direct oral contact with contaminated cigarettes or pipes probably contributed to the intakes by smokers.

Marek et al. (1981) reported that cadmium air levels in a Polish Cd-accumulator plant were 2 to 7 times the acceptable working value although the actual level was not quantified. Lauwerys et al. (1979) reported a Cd concentration of 110 to 2125 μg m^{-3} in a small cadmium-salt producing factory. Assuming an 8 hour working day, engaged in 'light activity' for which the ICRP (1975) estimate a respiration rate of 0.02 m^3 min^{-1}, this implies a maximum daily inhalation of 1100 to 20000 μg Cd. Engaged in heavy activity, with an 8 hour working day, a respiration rate of 0.043 m^3 min^{-1} (ICRP 1975) and an atmospheric concentration of 110 to 2125 μg m^{-3} within the factory (Lauwerys et al. 1979), up to 2300 to 44000 μg Cd may be inhaled. In practice, no single worker would be expected to be exposed to these conditions for long continous periods, and face masks are available, although apparently not frequently used (Lauwerys et al. 1979). Nonetheless, it is clear that for exposed workers the inhalation of contaminated air may be a major source of cadmium intake.

3.2.4   Summary

From the information presented in this section, the following ranges for normal daily intakes of cadmium can be estimated.

Route of intake	Typical intake (μg Cd d^{-1})	Comments
Diet	20-100	The ICRP (1975, 1981) estimated an intake of 150 μg d^{-1}; however, except in areas of high known contamination, values in excess of 100 μg d^{-1} are not commonly reported. Typical intakes in Europe are likely to be less than or around 50 μg d^{-1}.
Drinking water	<20	Generally around 12 μg d^{-1} in USA, although substantially higher water concentrations have been reported.
Air	0.6-0.7	Concentrations in local areas of contamination, especially if enclosed, may result in an intake equivalent to, or much greater than, the dietary intake noted above.
Smoking	∿2-4	Based on a daily consumption of 20 cigarettes (∿20 g tobacco) and inhalation of 10% of Cd in tobacco.

Cadmium has not been demonstrated to be an essential element and has no reported medicinal value. Groups or individuals at high risk are principally those living near, or working in, cadmium producing factories. As is apparently the case with lead (Piotrowski and Coleman 1980; O'Brien et al. 1980; and see Appendix 4) children in areas with high environmental cadmium contamination may also form a high risk group.

3.3   DISTRIBUTION OF CADMIUM IN HUMAN TISSUES

In a recent review of the distribution of cadmium in human tissues, amounting to more than 400 pages of text and tables and including around 400 references, Cherry (1981) noted that, "it is inevitable that references have been missed, and that relevant material from the references cited has been overlooked or reported inaccurately." The scope of the present review is more limited and hence many primary references could not be included. Where more detailed information is required, including a consideration of analytical techniques, reference should be made to the above review. There is general agreement that cadmium is primarily concentrated in the liver and kidneys of man and other animal species (e.g. Meranger et al. 1981; Kowal et al. 1979; Friberg 1978; Carmichael et al. 1982; Buhler et al. 1981; Fielder and Dale 1983). Available data for cadmium concentrations in tissues and organs of man, not known to be unduly exposed to cadmium, are presented in Table 6, and it is clear from

TABLE 6

CADMIUM CONCENTRATIONS IN VARIOUS ORGANS AND TISSUES OF MAN, NOT KNOWN TO BE OCCUPATIONALLY EXPOSED TO HIGH LEVELS OF CADMIUM

Tissue, organ or fluid		Cadmium concentration ($\mu g\ g^{-1}$ w.w.) (1)		
		(2)	(3)	(4)
Adrenal		0.35(15)	1.41(44)	
Aorta		0.75(105)	0.29 to 0.68 (247)	
Bile			2.09(63)	
Blood:	total	0.006	0.0052(352)	0.006–0.12
	plasma	<0.1	0.0026(2)	
	serum		0.0069(60)	
Bone:	whole	<2.4(91)	0.41 to 1.00(284)	
Brain		<0.79	<0.75(234)	
G.I. tract:	whole	<0.39	<0.4 to 1.21(621)	
Heart		<0.48(140)	0.048 to 0.56(292)	
Kidney		31.9(145)	20.87 to 21.22(1125)	35 to 40(26) (5)
Liver		2.2(150)	2.43(902)	1.00
Lung		0.35	0.20 to 0.56(439)	
Lymph node		0.064	0.06(6)	
Milk			0.002 to 0.019(51)	
Muscle		0.61(137)	0.59(156)	0.052
Oesophagus		0.45(68)	0.45(68)	
Ovary			0.20 to 0.46(34)	
Pancreas		0.96(139)	1.31 to 1.34(253)	0.49
Prostate		0.6(50)		
Skin		0.35(22)	0.16 to 0.28(64)	

TABLE 6 (Cont.)

Tissue, organ or fluid	Cadmium concentration (μg g^{-1} w.w.)[1]		
	(2)	(3)	(4)
Spleen	0.72(143)	0.48 to 0.89(385)	
Testis	0.54(72)	0.25 to 0.59(145)	
Thyroid	0.70(21)	0.70(45)	
Tongue	0.16(8)	0.16(8)	
Urine	0.0016	0.0021(795)	
Urine: 24 hr. collection[6]		0.0039 to 0.0073(109)	

Notes:

(1) Where available, numbers in parenthesis indicate the number of subjects analysed.

(2) Data collected by Iyengar et al.(1978) and evaluated by Coughtrey and Thorne (1981).

(3) Data compiled in ICRP Publication 23 (1975), on Reference Man.

(4) Data obtained from original articles published from 1978, and compiled in this review (Kowal et al.1979; Méranger et al.1981).

(5) Values for adults age 30 to 50 years, male and female.

(6) Based on an assumed excretion rate of 1.4 l d^{-1} (ICRP 1975).

these data that kidney has the highest concentration of cadmium, with the liver approximately an order of magnitude lower. On the basis of data presented in Table 6, the following distribution of cadmium in human tissues and organs can be obtained.

Organ	Geom. mean conc. ($\mu g \ g^{-1}$ w.w.)	Total organ content (mg)	% of whole body content
bone	<1.1	5.50	14.7
brain	<0.76	1.06	2.85
G.I. tract	0.8	1.20	3.21
kidney	23.0	7.13	19.1
liver	2.3	4.14	11.1
lung	0.36	0.36	0.96
muscle	0.60	16.8	44.9
skin	0.25	0.65	1.74
all other tissues	0.04	1.19	1.44
Total:		37.38	100.0

From the above, it appears that of cadmium deposited in the body, ~20% is located in the kidney, 15% in the bone and 11% in the liver. However, available animal data deriving from the experimental administration of cadmium (Table 7), suggest that the fraction of total body content local-ised in bone may be lower than the upper limit value of 0.147 calculated for man. It is noted that some distinctions exist between distributions of cadmium following acute and chronic exposure. Following acute oral or injected administration of Cd, ~75% of the body content is equally divided between the kidney and liver, whereas following long-term low level exposure less than 50% is located in these two organs, with approximately twice as much in the kidneys as the liver (Friberg 1978). Within the kidney, the cadmium concentration is generally appreciably higher within the cortex than the medulla (e.g. Fox et al. 1980; Kowal et al. 1979; Yasamura et al. 1980).

It is notable that, in man, cadmium accumulates in the body at least to the age of ~55 years, when dietary changes may result in a net loss of cadmium (e.g. Friberg 1978; Kowal et al. 1979). Renal dysfunction in elderly subjects may also contribute to the decrease in body burden, but the absence of a noticeable increase in urinary cadmium levels (see Section 5) suggests that tubular dysfunction is unlikely to be of import-ance in this respect for most 'normal' people. Considerable variation in renal concentration occurs, coupled with a long-term transfer of hepatic cadmium to the liver (e.g. Carmichael et al. 1982). Meranger et al. (1981) recorded kidney cortex cadmium concentrations in Canadians, cate-gorised by age, and compared the result with values reported for Swedish individuals. Their results are presented below:

TABLE 7

DISTRIBUTION OF CADMIUM IN ORGANS AND
TISSUES OF ANIMALS OTHER THAN MAN

Organ	Species (% whole-body content)					
	Monkey			Dog		Mouse
	(1)	(2)	(3)	(4)	(5)	(6)
bone	1.08	0.43	0.28	0.06	7.07	2.05
brain	∿0.03	0.25	0.27	0.06	0.88	0.28
G.I. tract	33.9	2.49	6.60	2.40	1.03	1.61
kidney	17.2	26.9	38.4	9.79	38.4	24.5
liver	25.7	47.1	37.5	74.7	38.8	55.7
lung	0.16	0.81	0.42	1.25	0.56	3.91
muscle	3.84	0.84	0.46	0.45	9.2	
skin	2.42					
all other tissues	15.67	21.18	16.07	11.29	4.06	11.95

Notes:

(1)   Suzuki & Taguchi (1980); 19 to 25 days following
       a single oral dose of 1mg Cd-109.

(2)   Thomas et al. (1980); 409 to 410 days following
       intravenous injection.

(3)   Thomas et al. (1980); 409 to 410 days following
       oral administration.

(4)   Thomas et al. (1980); 534 to 535 days following
       intravenous injection.

(5)   Thomas et al. (1980); 534 to 535 days following
       oral administration.

(6)   Bhattacharjee et al.(1979); 3 hours to 10 days
       following intravenous injection of 0.25 μCi Cd.

TABLE 8

SUBCELLULAR DISTRIBUTION OF CADMIUM IN
THE LIVER AND KIDNEY OF RATS AND MICE

Fraction	% Incorporation		
	kidney	liver	
	rat[1]	rat[1]	mouse[2]
Nuclear (+ cell debris)	9.71	6.59	4.15
Mitochondrial	8.75	10.43	2.39
Microsomal	Nt[3]	Nt	4.52
Post-microsomal supernatant	81.54	82.98	87.92

Notes:

(1)   Kanwar et al. (1979). Rats killed 8 hours
      to 7 days following a single oral dose of
      50 μCi Cd-115m. No time dependence in distri-
      tion was found.

(2)   Bhattacharjee et al. (1979). Mice killed 3 hours
      to 10 days after injection with 0.25 μCi Cd.
      No time dependence in distribution was found.

(3)   Nt - Not tested.

Age (yr)	n	Canada Conc. (µg g^{-1} d.w.) mean±s.e.	n	Sweden Conc. (µg g^{-1} d.w.) mean±s.e.
5-19	5	40±7	6	33±5
20-29	4	115±35	8	55±7
30-39	11	192±36	12	127±11
40-49	10	190±33	10	140±22
50-59	9	232+28	5	118±15
60-69	12	163+27	11	70±12
70-79	11	135±34	9	63±12
80+	10	111±20	6	72±14

Both data sets indicate a pattern of increasing renal concentration to middle age, followed by a decrease thereafter. In the Canadian sample, this decrease appears to be progressive. Values obtained from Canadian samples are consistently higher than the corresponding values for Swedes and indicate the inter-population variability of mean cadmium levels. They may also reflect differing environmental concentrations of cadmium and data presented in Table 4 do indicate higher dietary intakes of cadmium by Canadians relative to Swedes. Data presented by Meranger et al. (1981) indicate no significant (p>0.05) differences in concentration between males and females, and consequently all results were pooled in each age class. For the purposes of metabolic modelling following chronic intake, it is probably appropriate to assume that of cadmium entering the systemic circulation, fractions of 0.20 and 0.30 are initially deposited in the liver and kidney respectively. The remainder of cadmium entering the systemic circulation can probably be assumed to be uniformly distributed throughout all other organs and tissues. These assumptions differ slightly from those of the ICRP (1981), which assigned fractions of 0.3 to both the liver and kidney, but are in accord with data presented for both man and animals (Tables 6 and 7) and with the review of Friberg (1978), for long-term low level exposure, noted above. It is also noted that the concentration of cadmium in human milk and blood is typically more than 10 times lower than the corresponding values in organs and tissues other than liver and kidney. Urinary levels of cadmium are also generally low, but will depend to some extent upon age and state of health as well as body burden of cadmium.

Limited data are available for the sub-cellular distribution of renal and hepatic cadmium in rats and mice, and are presented in Table 8. Data for both species are similar, and indicate that the major fraction of the cadmium is associated with the post-mitochondrial supernatant.

On the basis of data presented in Tables 6 to 8, and from the above discussions, the following conclusions can be drawn.

- Cadmium is primarily concentrated in the liver and kidneys, where it is typically found at levels of 2.3 and 23.0 µg g^{-1} (w.w.) respectively. Fractions of 0.2 and 0.3 of cadmium entering the systemic circulation can be assumed to be deposited initially in the liver and kidneys respectively. Within the kidneys, concentrations are higher in the cortex than in the medulla.

- Cadmium is relatively uniformly distributed throughout all other organs and tissues, with a mean concentration around 0.4 µg g^{-1} (w.w.). Typical concentrations in milk, blood and urine are of the order of 0.002 to 0.01 mg l^{-1}.

TABLE 9

FRACTIONAL GASTROINTESTINAL ABSORPTION OF COMPOUNDS OF CADMIUM

Species	Compound	Fractional absorption	Reference	Comments
Rat	$CdCl_2$	0.006–0.01	Coughtrey and Thorne (1983): R	Estimated from long term retention in liver and kidneys.
Rat	$CdCl_2$	0.023		Estimated by a comparison of oral and intravenous retention studies.
Rat		<0.01		Estimated from the rate of accumulation in the kidneys.
Rat	$CdCl_2$	∿0.02		Administered to suckling rats.
Rat	Cadmium nitrate	0.026		Absorption based on liver and kidney uptake.
Rat	$CdCl_2$	∿0.01		Based on whole-body retention.
Rat	$109-CdCl_2$	0.0192 (0.0099–0.0333)	Taguchi and Suzuki (1979c)	Based on retention in carcass 24 hrs. post-administration.
Rat		0.015 to 0.052	Rabai and Kostial (1981)	Based on retention in carcass 6 days post-administration; given a variety of diets.
Mouse	$109-CdCl_2$	0.02 to 0.05	Coughtrey and Thorne (1983): R	The higher uptake was noted on a milk diet.
Mouse	Cadmium sulphate	0.005 to 0.08		4 to 8 week old animals.
Mouse		0.007		Animals on a high iron diet.
Mouse		0.005		Animals on a low iron diet.

TABLE 9 (Cont.)

Species	Compound	Fractional absorption	Reference	Comments
Mouse		~0.01		Estimated by extrapolation of the whole-body retention curve.
Mouse and Monkey		0.005 to 0.03		Retention of a single oral dose.
Mouse		0.0025 to 0.005	Bhattacharyya et al. (1981)	Pregnant and lactating mice; varying Fe and Ca intakes.
Mouse		0.0056 to 0.0094	Taguchi and Suzuki (1979a)	Cd administered in drinking water for 3 to 32 days. G.I. absorption declined with prolonged exposure.
Rabbit	$CdCl_2$	0.003	Coughtrey and Thorne (1983)	Estimated from daily intake and kidney content after 6 months.
Goat	$CdCl_2$	0.004 to 0.01		Based on a comparison of liver after oral and intravenous dosing. Estimated from liver and kidney uptake.
Sheep	$CdCl_2$	0.05 to 0.11		Based on faecal excretion in lambs.
Cow		0.008		Absorption in a 3 year old lactating jersey cow.
All animal species	any compound	<0.1	Thomas et al. (1980): R	Typically, absorption is estimated to be less than 0.05.
All animal species	any compound	0.02	Dorn (1979): R	Estimated value.

TABLE 9 (Cont.)

Species	Compound	Fractional absorption	Reference	Comments
Man		0.06	Coughtrey and Thorne (1983): R	Estimated from the long term component of retention for protein bound cadmium in a calf kidney suspension.
Man		0.023±0.003 0.089±0.02	Fox et al. (1980): R	Normal diet. Low Fe diet or low Fe body store.
Man	CdCl₂	0.011 to 0.041 0.015 to 0.07	Shaikh and Smith (1980)	Males. Females.
Man	all compounds	∿0.06	Dorn (1979): R	Estimated value.
Man	all compounds	∿0.05	Friberg et al.(1979): R	Estimated value.
Mouse	CdCl₂	∿0.03	Cherian et al. (1978)	Estimated by extrapolation of the whole-body retention curve.
Mouse	Cd-metall-othionein	∿0.03		
Mouse	CdCl₂	0.005 to 0.032	Engström and Nordberg (1979)	Administered dose of 1μg to 37.5mg kg⁻¹ body weight. The highest uptake was found with the largest dose.
Man and domestic animals	all compounds	0.02	Coughtrey and Thorne (1983): R	Estimated mean value, although noted that this may vary by a factor of 5 depending on a variety of dietary and other circumstances.
Man	all inorganic compounds	0.05	ICRP (1980): R	Recommended mean value for purposes of metabolic modelling.

TABLE 9 (Cont.)

Species	Compound	Fractional absorption	Reference	Comments
Man	all compounds	0.03 to 0.08	Underwood (1977): R	Range of typical values for dietary intakes.
Rat	$Cd(No_3)_2$	<0.10	Thomas et al. (1980): R	
Rat	$CdCl_2$	0.023	Thomas et al. (1980): R	
Mouse	$CdCl_2$	0.081 to 0.092	Thomas et al. (1980): R	
Man	Environmental-Cd	0.03 to 0.08	Thomas et al. (1980): R	
Man	Environmental-Cd	0.02 to 0.05	Thomas et al. (1980): R	
Man	Environmental-Cd	0.005 to 0.12	Thomas et al. (1980): R	
Lamb	dietary-Cd	0.11	Thomas et al. (1980): R	Intake of 180 μg Cd d^{-1}.
Lamb	dietary-Cd	0.05	Thomas et al. (1980): R	Intake of 119mg Cd d^{-1}.

- The total body burden increases with age to a peak at about 50-60 years. Thereafter, concentrations decline as urinary excretion rises, possibly as a result of reductions in renal efficiency or the development of renal dysfunction.

- Subcellular analysis of animal liver and kidney indicates that the majority of the cadmium is associated with the post-mitochondrial supernatant.

3.4   METABOLISM

3.4.1   Gastrointestinal absorption

The gastrointestinal absorption of cadmium has been studied in a variety of species, including man, rats, mice and dogs, and under differing dietary regimes (see Table 9). Gastrointestinal absorption, principally in man has been discussed in several reviews (e.g. Underwood 1977, Travis and Haddock 1980, Friberg et al. 1979, ICRP 1980, Coughtrey and Thorne 1983), and generally the fractional gastrointestinal absorption (f_1) is considered to be less than 0.1 under most dietary conditions. Fielder and Dale (1983) noted that the metabolism of cadmium is similar in rodents and other mammalian species, with poor absorption of oral intakes of cadmium, but much higher absorption following inhalation. Typically, the ICRP (1980) recommended an f_1 value of 0.05 for purposes of metabolic modelling in man. Coughtrey and Thorne (1983) suggested an f_1 value of 0.02 for man and domestic animals, but noted that it may be appropriate to assume a range of 0.004 to 0.10 to take account of individual variations deriving from intrinsic or extrinsic, including dietary, factors. A range of 0.005 to 0.05 for f_1 in adult rats, mice and monkeys was noted by Fielder and Dale (1983) in a review of cadmium toxicity.

On the basis of data presented in Table 9, and in agreement with the comment of Dorn (1979), it is suggested that for most dietary regimes, an f_1 value of 0.05 can be assumed for man, compared with 0.02 for all other animals.

It is generally assumed that gastrointestinal absorption is not under homeostatic control (e.g. Coughtrey and Thorne 1983), although limited data available for mice (Taguchi and Suzuki, 1979a) suggest that the absorption of cadmium may decline during long-term exposures. However, it is notable that apparently contradictory data have been obtained by Engström and Nordberg (1979) who found, in mice, that the gastrointestinal absorption of a single oral dose is higher with increased dosage administered. A similar effect was also noted in respect of cadmium absorption by chickens (Koo et al. 1978), but data reviewed by Thomas et al. (1980) indicated, that absorption in lambs decreased with increased oral doses. For the purpose of metabolic modelling, it is probably appropriate to assume that the fractional gastrointestinal absorption of cadmium by man remains constant over a typical range of dietary intakes (see Section 3.2.1) and with time.

Few data are available for direct comparison of gastrointestinal absorption of different cadmium compounds. However, data for sulphates, nitrates and protein complexes in mice and rats (presented in Table 9) indicate a similar uptake for all compounds. Accordingly, in the absence of more detailed data, the f_1 value of 0.05 suggested for man, is taken to be appropriate for all compounds of cadmium.

It has been reported that cadmium absorption and toxicity may be enhanced by diets low or deficient in iron, zinc, calcium, phosphorus or selenium (e.g. Calabrese 1981, Koo et al. 1978). Also, the presence of vitamin D may increase absorption (Koo et al. 1978). However, data obtained by Kostial and co-workers (1979, 1980a, 1980b, 1981) suggest that if such a relationship does exist, it is neither simple nor readily predictable. In a series of experiments on suckling and adult rats, they demonstrated that enhanced uptake does occur in the sucklings, but this is not due to iron, zinc, manganese or copper deficiencies in the milk diet, as addition of these elements failed to alter cadmium absorption. Additions of 100 µg Fe ml^{-1} in a milk diet administered to adult rats did reduce Cd uptake (Kostial et al. 1980a) and this was apparently due to decreased gut absorption.

In view of the uncertainties relating to the influence of other dietary factors on Cd absorption, and the range of values observed or estimated for typical diets (Table 9), no recommendation is made regarding alteration of the gastrointestinal absorption of cadmium by various dietary regimes. However, it is noted that absorption will be higher in juveniles of all species, including man.

In vivo and in vitro experiments on rat and chicken guts suggest that cadmium uptake occurs in two stages; uptake and binding to the outer or inner membrane surfaces or intracellular substance of the intestinal tissue; and the transport of Cd out of the tissue into the fluid bathing the serosal surface (e.g. Chertok et al. 1979). Koo et al. (1980) noted, in studies on chickens, that an initial rapid uptake (presumably to the intestinal surfaces) occurs in the first 20 minutes following ingestion and that this is followed by a subsequent slower phase. Chertok et al. (1979) noted that in vitro total uptake (intestinal tissue and serosal fluid) after 30 minutes increased linearly with the cadmium concentration in the medium bathing the gut such that:

$$y = 0.0835 + 0.961 \ x \qquad (r^2 = 0.99)$$

where;   y is the total uptake, µmol g^{-1} w.w.
          x is the concentration of cadmium, x 10^{-4} M.

Tissue levels approached a steady state within 30 minutes of incubation with mucosal concentrations greater than 1.2×10^{-4} M and it thus appears that uptake of Cd is a relatively rapid process.

It is of note that Taguchi and Suzuki (1979b) reported that although transport from mucosal to serosal fluid increases with higher Cd concentrations, wall uptake in rat guts is limited and can be saturated at relatively low concentrations. A similar finding was noted by Foulkes (1980) where Cd uptake by rat tissues was reported to obey saturation kinetics, with km ∼0.1 mM and V_{max} ∼0.01 µmol min^{-1}. Thus, from the Michaelis-Menten equation, the initial rate (V_o) of gut uptake can be related to the cadmium concentration ([Cd]) by:

$$V_o = \frac{V_{max} \ [Cd]}{[Cd] + k_m} \qquad \mu mol \ min^{-1}$$

A detailed explanation of the Michaelis equation and the terms v_{max} and k_m can be found in most standard physical chemistry reference books (e.g. Morris 1974).

3.4.2   Retention in the respiratory system

Although it has been recognized that inhalation of cadmium may result in a significant body burden in excess of that due to dietary intakes, especially in exposed workers (e.g. Adamsson et al. 1979, Oberdoester et al. 1979), there has been comparatively little direct work on the metabolism of cadmium following inhalation or intratracheal instillation.

It is generally assumed, on the basis of limited experimental data for animals that, of cadmium deposited in the human lung, a fraction of 0.1 to 0.5 is absorbed (e.g. Underwood 1977; Dorn 1979: Travis and Haddock 1980; Yasamura et al. 1980; Coughtrey and Thorne 1983). On the basis of the amount of cadmium in tissues of cigarette smokers, it has been calculated that up to a fraction of 0.6 of cadmium deposited in the lungs is absorbed (EEC 1978). Fielder and Dale (1983) concluded that "from the limited data available, it appears that cadmium compounds deposited in the lungs are rapidly absorbed". For workers exposed to radioactive cadmium, the ICRP (1966) has assigned oxides and hydroxides to inhalation class Y, sulphides, halides and nitrates to class W and all other compounds to class D, representing a biological half-life of retention in the deep lung in the order of years, weeks and days respectively. However, exceptions to the above generalisation do occur, and the ICRP (1980) noted that in one experiment, where dogs inhaled a near lethal dose of $CdCl_2$, an element of long-term retention was exhibited. This was subsequently confirmed in rats (see discussion in Coughtrey and Thorne 1983) and indicates that the long-term component of retention of this compound in the human lung may exhibit a biological half-life in excess of 100 days. Hardley et al. (1980) demonstrated that Cd-109, intratracheally instilled into rats as CdO, had an initial half-life in the lung of 4 h and that by 24 h after intracheal instillation 80% of the CdO had left the lung. However, in the next 2 weeks, little further loss occurred from the lungs. Similarly, in a comparison of the clearance rates of CdO and $CdCl_2$ from the rat lung following inhalation, Oberdoester et al. (1979) demonstrated a long term component of retention of 67 days for both compounds. However, whilst $CdCl_2$ exhibited no clear component of short-term retention, CdO was initially cleared at a much faster rate. A subsequent study by Oberdoester et al. (1980) compared lung clearance rates of $CdCl_2$ in rats following inhalation or intratracheal instillation. Airborne $CdCl_2$ was administered at a concentration of 660 ng l^{-1} (0.34 μm AMAD), and by instillation as 0.3 ml of 0.9% NaCl solution containing 27 μg Cd ml^{-1}. Data obtained for 100 days post-administration indicate that lung retention [R_{lung}] can be modelled by:

$$R_{lung}(t) - \text{inhalation} = 0.45e^{-0.693t/1.1} + 0.58e^{-0.693t/61} \quad (r = 0.98)$$

$$R_{lung}(t) - \text{instillation} = 0.47e^{-0.693t/0.7} + 0.50e^{-0.693t/66} \quad (r = 0.99)$$

where   t is the time in days, and
          r is the correlation coefficient.

The short-term component of retention, apparently absent in the previous study (Oberdoester et al. 1979) is clearly apparent from the above functions, while the agreement between the retention functions following instillation and inhalation is remarkable.

From the above discussion, it thus appears that considerable uncertainty is associated with the classification of cadmium lung clearance rates, and it may be appropriate to consider oxides, and possibly hydroxides, with halides in inhalation class W of the ICRP lung model. This model, which is used to describe clearance from the respiratory system has been presented in ICRP Publication 30 (1980). For an aerosol with an AMAD of 1 μm and a gastrointestinal absorption of 0.05, the model implies that following inhalation approximately 85% of the deposited material will be lost from the body in the order of weeks. This prediction is similar to the experimental results obtained by Oberdoester et al. (1979) for rats inhaling CdO, reported above. However, it is noted that the particle size distribution of respirable dust is of considerable importance in the rate of lung clearance, and following environmental or occupational exposure the particle size may not follow a log-normal distribution, as assumed in the ICRP model.

If short-term dynamics of cadmium lung clearance are not of concern, it is reasonable to assume that 0.1 to 0.5 of cadmium deposited in the lungs is eventually transferred to the systemic circulation. A best estimate for this fraction is 0.25 (see also Travis and Haddock, 1980).

It is notable that Friberg et al. (1974) stated that no data exist for the chemical state in which cadmium is present in air. However, it may be reasonable to assume that CdO is the major form of airborne cadmium, and thus the implied and measured greater solubility of CdO, noted above, is of some consquence in assessing the potential transfer of airborne cadmium to organs other than the lung. Sulphurous cadmium may also be of importance in releases to atmosphere (e.g. Hutton 1982).

3.4.3   Systemic metabolism

Several studies have considered the concentration and accumulation of cadmium in blood following ingestion or inhalation in man and animals (e.g. Kjellstrom 1979; Ikebuchi et al. 1979; Lauwerys et al. 1979; Kowal et al. 1979). The chemical form and binding of cadmium in blood have also received attention (e.g. Hildebrand and Cram 1979; Suzuki and Yamamura 1979; Shaikh and Smith 1980; Tanaka 1982).

In general, blood concentration levels are below 0.1 μg Cd ml^{-1}, and a typical value in man appears to be of the order 0.01 μg ml^{-1} (Section 3.3 and Table 6). Data obtained for rats suggest that cadmium transferred in the blood is complexed with metallothionein (MT) to form cadmium-metallothionein (Suzuki and Yamamura 1979; Tanaka 1982), and results suggest that hepatic metallothionein is released to the blood in the same manner as hepatic enzymes (Tanaka 1982). Cadmium has been shown to induce the synthesis of metallothionein in many tissues including liver, kidneys, stomach, small intestine, spleen, pancreas and testes (Fielder and Dale 1983). Since its discovery in 1957, metallothionein has been the subject of considerable investigation. It is a low molecular weight protein (about MW 10,000) containing a very high proportion of cysteine residues (Ridlington et al. 1979), and cadmium readily binds to the thio-groups in the cysteine moieties, as do other

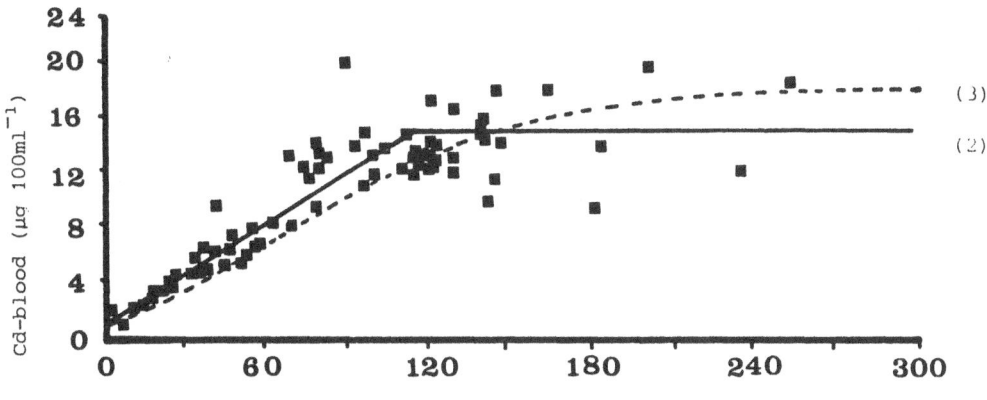

Notes:

1. Data points for different individuals have not been distinguished.
2. Line fitted to data by Lauwerys et al. (1979); method of fit not stated.
3. Line fitted by eye in this review.

FIGURE 1. CHANGES IN CADMIUM LEVELS IN HUMAN BLOOD DURING THE FIRST 250 DAYS OF OCCUPATIONAL EXPOSURE TO CADMIUM (LAUWERYS ET AL. 1979) (1)

heavy metals (Fielder and Dale 1983), but much of its biological function remains uncertain and it is not clear whether thionein, without a metal complex exists (e.g. Shaikh 1979). It is known that MT is produced de novo and has biological half-lives of 5 days and 2.8 days in the kidney and liver respectively (Shaikh 1979). In the liver it can be resolved into two fractions of molecular weights 10,000 and 12,000 (Shaikh 1979). Cadmium may complex with thionein to form a metallothionein, but in rats Ridlington et al. (1979) have suggested that within each tissue Cd^{2+} is complexed predominantly by thionein as Cd,Zn-thionein. In vivo and in vitro experiments on rabbits indicated that by day 19 following intra peritoneal injection 98.1% of the cadmium in the blood was in the erythrocytes; of this cadmium more than 90% existed in the stroma-free haemolysate and ~70% of that was bound to thionein (Ikebuchi et al. 1979). However, MT was never incorporated into the blood cells by incubating red blood cells with [Cd-115m] MT, and it was presumed that the MT in the red blood cells originated from some source other than the liver (Ikebuchi et al. 1979). At high levels of cadmium concentration in the liver and kidneys of experimental animals, some binding to high molecular weight proteins may occur, and tissue damage is thought to result when the concentration of this fraction of cadmium reaches a critical level (Fielder and Dale 1983). Thus, in situ binding of cadmium to MT may be an important mechanism in protecting against cellular damage.

In vitro experiments with human blood (Hildebrand and Cram 1979) indicated that, following 3 days exposure to $CdCl_2$ at a concentration of 2×10^{-7} M, erythrocytes accumulated a cadmium concentration 5x that of the medium, whereas lymphocytes accumulated 3000x the medium concentration. Furthermore, whereas Cd in the lymphocytes was associated with MT, that in the erythrocytes was not. However, in vivo, cadmium is probably bound to MT in the erythrocytes as well as to MT in lymphocytes (e.g. Coughtrey and Thorne 1983). It is also notable that high levels of dietary cadmium have been shown to cause anaemia, with lower levels of haemoglobin, erythrocyte count and haematocrit values, in man and a variety of other animals including rats, cattle and Japanese quail (Fox et al. 1980; Marek et al. 1981). Data recorded by Marek et al. (1981), for exposed workers in a Polish cadmium accumulator production factory, suggest that the low haemoglobin count is a direct consequence of the loss of erythrocytes and does not represent a lowering of the haemoglobin content per erythrocyte.

Several studies and reviews on man have considered that the cadmium concentration in blood is potentially a good indicator of the average cadmium intake over the previous month or so (e.g. Kjellstrom 1979; Kowal et al. 1979). This is in accord with the findings of Lauwerys et al. (1979), which reported that in workers exposed to high levels of airborne cadmium, the concentration in blood rose linearly for 120 days and thereafter became constant. However, the data of Lauwerys et al. (1979) appear to be more consistent with the suggestion that cadmium levels in blood rise approximately linearly for 120 days, but thereafter the evidence for saturation, or equilibrium concentration, of cadmium is limited, and a curvelinear response over 250 days may equally be indicated (see Fig. 1). Data presented by Welinder et al. (1977), for 11 occupationally exposed solderers, indicated a biological half-life of cadmium in blood of 25 to 146 days, with a median value of 41 days. Following intraperitoneal injection of $CdCl_2$ in rabbits, Ikebuchi et al. (1979) estimated the half-life of cadmium in blood to be ~158 days. It is possible that the half-life in blood is mainly determined by the lifespan of mature erythrocytes (~110 d).

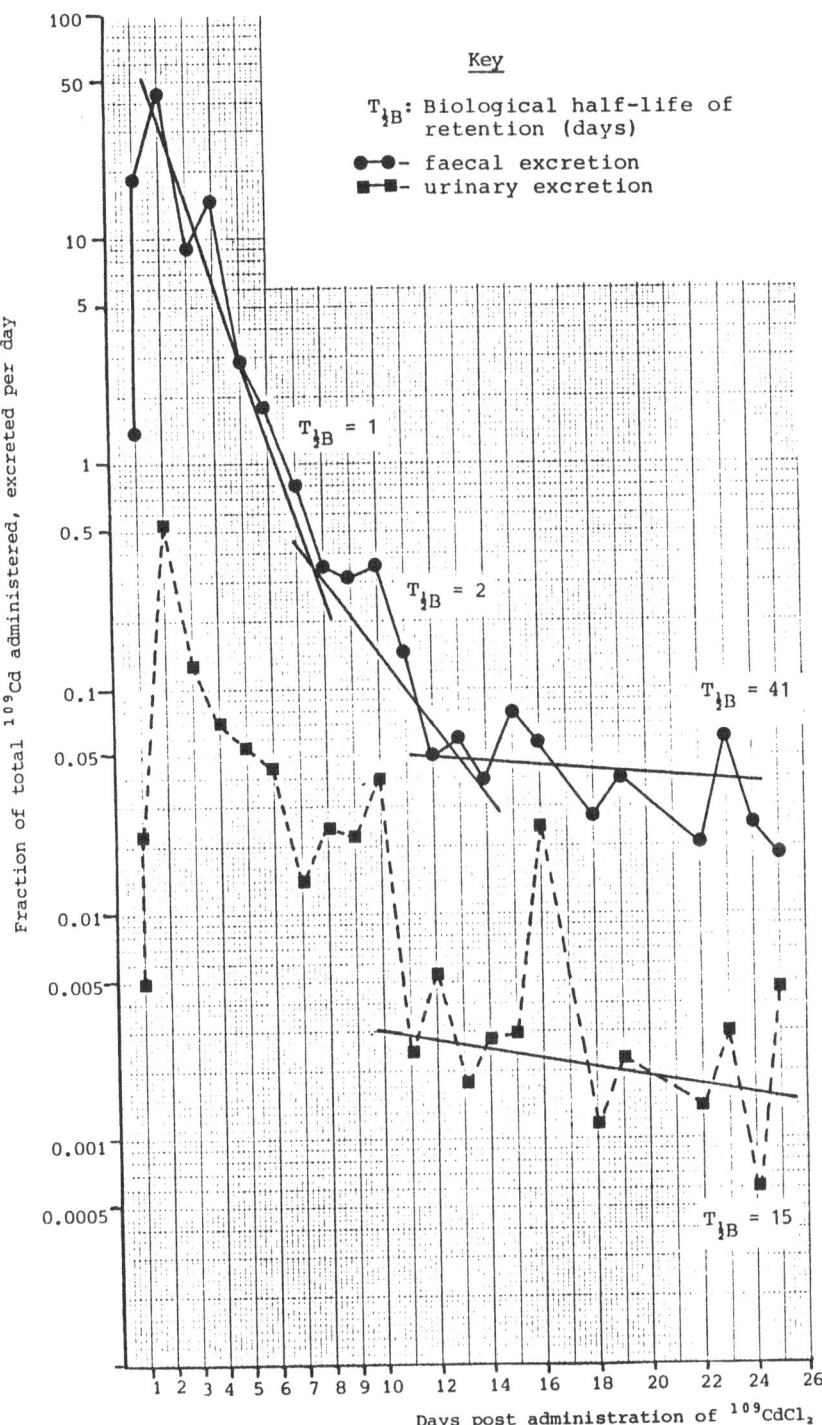

FIGURE 2. DAILY EXCRETION OF CADMIUM AFTER A SINGLE ORAL DOSE OF $^{109}CdCl_2$ IN WATER SOLUTION (FROM SUZUKI & TAGUCHI 1980)

From the above, it is concluded that cadmium in the blood of man is mainly localised in the erythrocytes where it is bound to metallothionein, which may not be of hepatic origin. The biological half-life of cadmium in blood is probably in excess of 100 days, and in the absence of more detailed data is assumed to be 150 days, which is consistent with findings in rabbits (Ikebuchi et al. 1979). Although the cadmium level of blood may be a good indicator of recent average dietary intakes in man, it is noted that Pietrzak-Flis et al. (1978) did not find this to be the case in rats. However, it is noted that the binding of cadmium to rat erythrocytes may differ from that of man and rabbits. Following chronic intake of $CdCl_2$ in contaminated water, cadmium was only detectable in the blood of rats when its concentration in the water was in excess of 5.0 μg ml^{-1}. Data for rats thus suggest that for long-term low level exposure to cadmium, blood levels may be a very poor indicator of intake, and this is a reflection of the low concentration normally found in blood, noted above and in Section 3. Blood levels of cadmium in man may provide an estimate of average cadmium intake, but it is evident from the above discussion that data must be interpreted with caution.

3.4.3.1   Whole-body retention

The ICRP (1980) do not recommend assigning any fraction of absorbed cadmium to early excretion. However, considerable uncertainty exists as to whether cadmium, ingested chronically at sub-toxic levels, exhibits an early phase of rapid excretion following entry to the systemic circulation, or whether it is rapidly bound in tissues and thereafter released only slowly. Coughtrey and Thorne (1983) in their review of the literature pertaining to cadmium in man and animals, noted that while some cadmium may be rapidly excreted before it becomes firmly bound to any body tissue, this effect is not always observed.

Following a single oral dose of $^{109}CdCl_2$ to monkeys, Suzuki and Taguchi (1980) found a rapid early excretion in faeces, which would be expected because of the limited gastrointestinal absorption of cadmium, but also found an initial elevation in urinary levels of cadmium (Fig. 2). Following subcutaneous injection of 5 μmol $CdCl_2$ kg^{-1} into rats, Shaikh and Hirayama (1979) did not note any early increase in urinary levels. Nevertheless, during the 14 week study period a total of 22% of the injected dose was excreted, mainly in the faeces. This represents an elevated rate of excretion compared to estimates for long-term excretion of 0.005 to 0.01% of total cadmium body burden per daily in man (Friberg, 1978; Friberg et al. 1979).

It is possible that the form of cadmium ingested will influence the magnitude of the component of early clearance. Following injection or ingestion of Cd-MT in rats the whole-body retention has been reported to be similar to that of $CdCl_2$ (Cherian et al. 1978; Johnson and Foulkes, 1980), although rather more Cd-MT is deposited in the kidney. However, since Cd-MT appears to be the principal form of cadmium involved in metabolic transport and tissue retention (Suzuki et al. 1980) it may be more rapidly incorporated and hence less available for early excretion than some other compounds or complexes of the element. It has been claimed that MT is not destroyed by cooking (Cherian et al. 1978), and if true, this compound may represent a substantial contribution to dietary intake, especially in diets with a high content of liver or kidney.

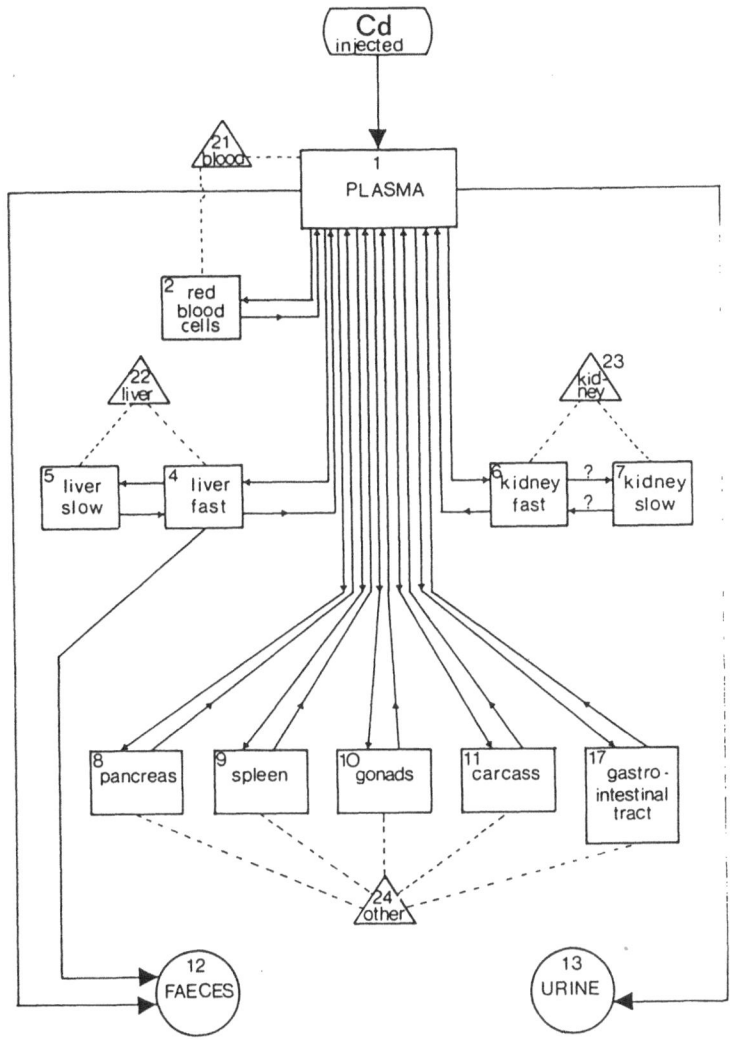

FIGURE 3. MULTI-COMPARTMENT MODEL, AND COEFFICIENTS, OF CADMIUM METABOLISM IN MICE (FROM MARCUS 1982; BASED ON DATA OF SHANK ET AL. 1977).

| Para-meter (1) | Estimate (from/to) | Cadmium (only) (2) | | Cadmium (zinc) |
		Shank (SS = 3688) (3)	Marcus (SS = 2.67) (3)	Marcus (SS = 3.38) (3)
L(2,1)	Blood plasma/cells	–	2.74 ± 0.78	*6.34 ± 2.40
L(1,2)	Blood cells/plasma	–	24.90 ± 0.63	25.98 ± 0.64
L(4,1)	Blood/liver	950.4	397.0 ± 8.31	*260.6 ±18.6
L(1,4)	Liver/blood	2.30	3.82 ± 0.14	*3.17 ± 0.14
L(5,4)	Liver fast/slow	–	5.34 ± 1.03	*11.03 ± 1.00
L(4,5)	Liver slow/fast	–	3.83 ± 0.94	? 6.62 ± 0.75
L(6,1)	Blood/kidney	96.48	29.52 ± 1.08	*22.67 ± 1.34
L(1,6)	Kidney/blood	2.02	0.976± 0.019	*0.744± 0.024
L(8,1)	Blood/pancreas	43.2	13.47 ± 0.37	*8.92 ± 0.68
L(1,8)	Pancreas/blood	2.88	1.47 ± 0.05	*1.11 ± 0.04
L(9,1)	Blood/spleen	4.32	2.37 ± 0.09	1.85 ± 0.14
L(1,9)	Spleen/blood	5.47	5.18 ± 0.25	4.57 ± 0.21
L(10,1)	Blood/gonads	3.60	1.62 ± 0.05	1.41 ± 0.11
L(1,10)	Gonads/blood	3.02	2.42 ± 0.10	2.95 ± 0.13
L(11,1)	Blood/carcass	561.6	388.9 ± 8.55	396.4 ±29.2
L(1,11)	Carcass/blood	6.05	7.03 ± 0.30	7.78 ± 0.31
L(17,1)	Blood/GI tract	345.6	98.96 ± 1.64	*80.86 ± 5.17
L(1,17)	GI tract/blood	8.64	5.94 ± 0.17	5.26 ± 0.18
L(12,4)	Liver/faeces	–	0.044± 0.006	0.063± 0.006
L(12,1)	Blood/faeces	1.04	6.74 ± 0.45	7.00 ± 0.53
L(13,1)	Blood/urine	0.14	1.18 ± 0.14	1.18 ± 0.14

Notes: 1. Rate parameters L(i,j) in units of days^{-1} were estimated by SAAM 27 program. Statistically very significant differences, as reported by Marcus (1982), due to zinc treatment are marked with an astetisk (*): significance level not recorded.
2. All data reported by Marcus (1982) but Shank, column 3, based on Shank et al. (1977). Cadmium (zinc), column 5, represents rate parameters for zinc treated mice.
3. SS is the residual sum of squares.

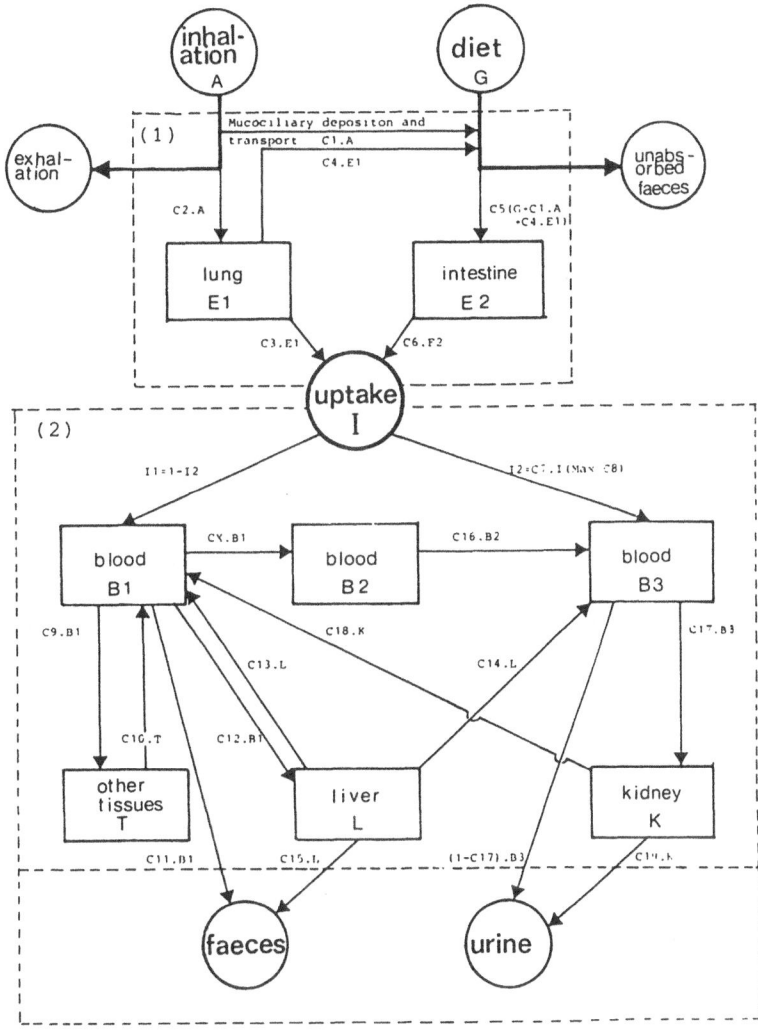

Notes: 1.   Based on previous models proposed
              by the ICRP (1980).
         2.   Based on empirical data collated
              by Nordberg & Kjellstrom (1979).

FIGURE 4.   FLOW DIAGRAM, COEFFICIENTS OF TRANSFER AND
            MATHEMATICAL FORMALISM OF WHOLE-BODY METABOLIC
            MODEL OF CADMIUM PROPOSED BY NORDBERG &
            KJELLSTROM (1979).

Coefficient	Initially assumed ranges (1)	Values fitting empirical data (corresponding biological half-time).
C_1	0.1-0.2 (cigarette smoke) 0.4-0.9 (factory dust)	0.1 0.7
C_2	0.4-0.6 (cigarette smoke) 0.1-0.3 (factory dust)	0.4 0.13
C_3	0.01-1, day^{-1}	0.05
C_4	0.1 x C_3 = 0.001-0.1, day^{-1}	0.005
C_5	0.03-0.1	0.048
C_6	0.05, day^{-1}	0.05
C_7	0.2-0.4	0.25
C_8	0.5-5, μg	1
C_9	0.4-0.8	0.44
C_{10}	0.00004-0.0002, day^{-1}	0.00014 (13 yr)
C_{11}	0.05-0.5	0.27
C_{12}	0.1-0.4	0.25
C_{13}	0-0.0001, day^{-1}	0.00003
C_{14}	0.0001-0.0003, day^{-1}	0.00016 (7.5 yr)
C_{15}	0-0.0001, day^{-1}	0.00005
C_{16}	0.004-0.015, day^{-1}	0.012 (54 day)
C_{17} (2)	0.8-0.98	0.95
C_{18}	0-0.0001, day^{-1}	0.00001
C_{19} (3)	0.00002-0.0002, day^{-1}	0.00014 (12 yr)
C_x	0.01-0.05	0.04
C_{20}	0.05-0.5	0.1
C_{21}	0-0.000002, day^{-1}	0.0000011

Notes: 1. If no unit is given, it means that the coefficient is a unitless proportion.
2. C_{17} decreases from age 30 to age 80 by 33%.
3. C_{19} increases from age 30 with C_{21} each year.

When considering the above discussion and results presented for early excretion, two points must be considered. First, since early clearance (of unabsorbed cadmium) is predominantly in the faeces, very little contamination of urinary samples is required to give the impression of an early clearance of absorbed cadmium following an oral dose. Second, cadmium is known to be highly nephrotoxic (e.g. Johnson and Foulkes 1980) and following an acute dose, renal damage may result in an elevated level in urine. However, even taking the above into account, it is suggested that following chronic sub-toxic ingestion, of cadmium entering the systemic circulation a fraction of up to 0.1 may be available for early excretion, with a biological half-life of about 1.5 days.

Several multicompartment models of cadmium metabolism have been proposed (e.g. Marcus 1982; Nordberg et al. 1979; Shank et al. 1977; Whanger et al. 1980). Figs. 3 and 4 outline the models of Nordberg et al. (1979) and Marcus (1982). In essence the model proposed by Marcus (1982) is based on that of Shank et al. (1977), while that of Whanger et al. (1980) is concerned primarily with interactions between cadmium and other elements. It can be seen from Figs. 3 and 4 that the basic conceptual model is very simple, with cadmium entering the blood and transferred to liver, kidney and other tissues from the plasma fraction (Marcus 1982; and blood compartment 1 of Nordberg et al. 1979) or directly from metallothionein bound cadmium in the whole blood (blood compartment 3 of Nordberg et al. 1979). In both models, material can be relocated after transfer to each compartment. The main difference between the models proposed is the introduction of fast and slow transfer compartments within the liver and kidney in the model of Marcus (1979). However, it is noted that the model of Marcus (1982) has been developed specifically for mice (on the basis of data from Shank et al. (1977)) and whilst this distinction may be appropriate for rodents, available data do not indicate the need for it in human models. In this context, it is noted that the model of Nordberg et al. (1979), in common with the majority of models which have been developed for man, is also based largely on animal data and several of the transfer coefficients may be subject to considerable uncertainty.

On the basis of data reviewed herein, a generalised conceptual model of cadmium metabolism is presented in Fig. 5. It can be seen from this, that of cadmium entering the systemic circulation, that present as Cd-MT is assumed to be preferentially taken up by the kidneys (e.g. Suzuki and Yamamura 1979). For the remainder, the liver forms the main target organ (e.g. Suzuki and Yamamura 1979). Once located in the liver, the cadmium is bound to metallothionein and may be available for reflux to the systemic circulation and thence for transfer to other organs and tissues. This is consistent with the indication of long term hepatic-renal transfer, noted by Carmichael et al. (1982), and the suggestion of hepatic Cd-MT release to blood in rats (Tanaka, 1982).

The whole body retention of cadmium in man has been reviewed in several articles (e.g. Friberg et al. 1979; Friberg 1978; Shaikh and Smith 1980; ICRP 1980). There is general agreement that the biological half-life of whole-body retention falls in the range 10 to 50 years (e.g. Friberg et al. 1979; Coughtrey and Thorne 1983) and for the purposes of radiological protection the ICRP (1980) have modelled whole-body retention [R(t)] by:

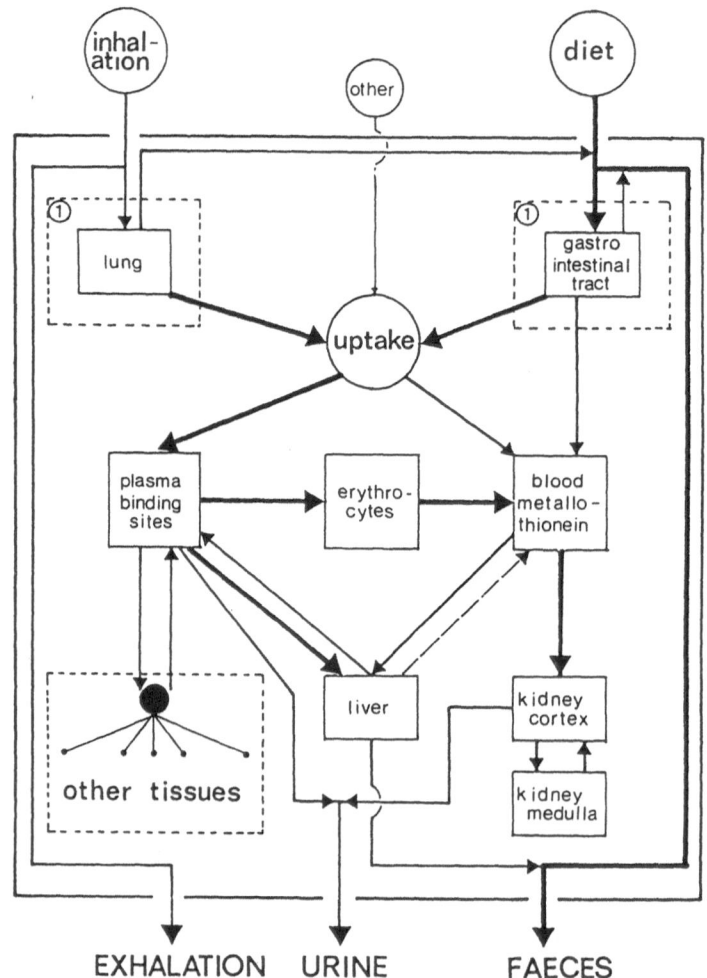

Notes: (1)   organs of input based on ICRP (1980) model

FIGURE 5.   CONCEPTUAL FLOW DIAGRAM OF CADMIUM
            METABOLISM IN MAN.

$$R(t) = e^{-0.693t/9125}$$

where t is in days.

Data presented by Shaikh and Smith (1980), following ingestion of $^{109}CdCl_2$ in beef kidney cortex homogenate by humans, indicated three components of retention with half-lives of 1.58, 33.7 and 9605 days. From data reviewed herein a three compartment model with half-lives of 1.5, 150 and 9125 days could be proposed, where the compartments represent respectively, early excretion, the half-life of cadmium in the blood system (or the 'body exchangeable pool') and the half-life of long term retention in other tissues and organs. However, the middle term is of dubious statistical and physiological validity, as the blood carries very little cadmium at any time (Section 3) and of this most is transferred to other tissues, rather than excreted directly. Furthermore, the last term is subject to some uncertainty, and whilst a long-term biological half-life of 9125 days (25 years) appears to be the best estimate (e.g. ICRP 1980; Underwood 1977) values of 3650 days (10 years) to 10950 days (30 years) may occur in different individuals (e.g. Friberg et al. 1979; Shaikh and Smith 1980; Coughtrey and Thorne 1983; Fielder and Dale 1983).

Taking the above into account, it appears that the whole-body retention of cadmium in man can best be approximated by:

$$R(t) = 0.1e^{-0.693t/1.5} + 0.9e^{-0.693t/9125}$$

where t is in days.

It is noted that the above retention function has been developed primarily on the basis of data available for the transport and retention of cadmium complexed as metallothionein. The retention and early excretion of some cadmium compounds may differ somewhat as noted previously in this section. However, insufficient data are available to justify the proposal of a separate retention function for inorganic compounds or complexes. Of cadmium deposited in tissues and organs, fractions of 0.2, 0.3, 0.1 and 0.01 can be assumed to be deposited in the liver, kidneys, bone and blood respectively. The remainder can be assumed to be uniformly distributed amongst all other tissues and organs (see also Section 3.3). By integrating the above retention function for periods 10 to 85 years in conjunction with an f_1 of 0.05 (Section 3.4.1) and a daily dietary intake of 60 µg (Section 3.2.1) the following whole-body cadmium contents and kidney concentrations are obtained.

Time integral (years)	Whole-body content (mg)	Kidney concentration (µg g^{-1} w.w.)
10	8.6	8.3
25	17.8	17.3
35	22.0	21.4
45	25.3	24.5
55	27.8	26.9
65	29.6	28.6
75	31.0	29.9
85	32.1	31.0

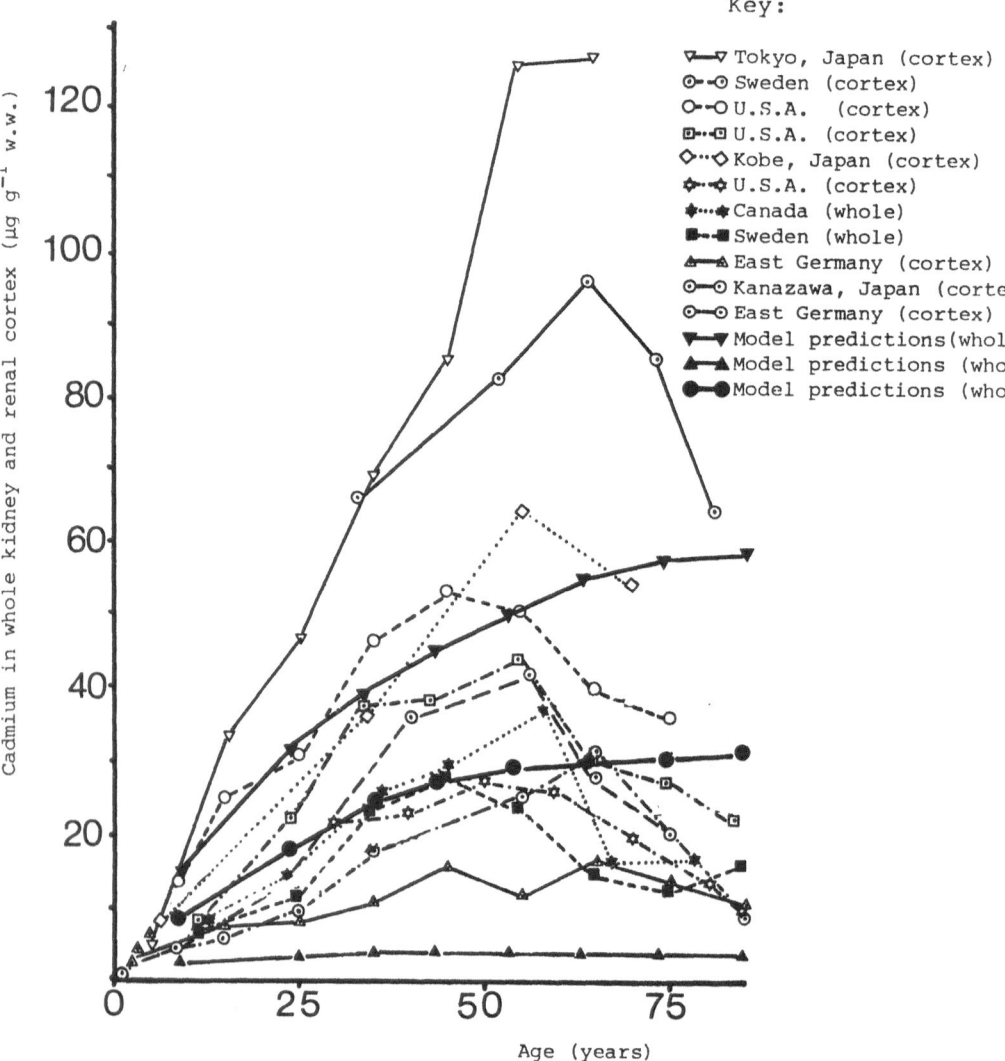

Key:

▽—▽ Tokyo, Japan (cortex)
⊙-⊙ Sweden (cortex)
O-O U.S.A. (cortex)
◨··◨ U.S.A. (cortex)
◇···◇ Kobe, Japan (cortex)
✧-✧ U.S.A. (cortex)
✦···✦ Canada (whole)
◪-◪ Sweden (whole)
▲-▲ East Germany (cortex)
⊙—⊙ Kanazawa, Japan (cortex)
⊙-⊙ East Germany (cortex)
▼—▼ Model predictions(whole)
▲—▲ Model predictions (whole
●—● Model predictions (whole

Notes: 1. Assuming the half-life of long term retention is 10950 days;
           and mean daily intake is 100μg cd.
        2. Assuming the half-life of long term retention is 3650 days,
           and mean daily intake is 20 μg.
        3. Assuming the half-life of long term retention is 9125 days,
           and mean daily intake is 60μg.

FIGURE 6.   COMPARISON OF MEASURED AND DERIVED VALUES
            FOR CADMIUM CONCENTRATIONS IN THE HUMAN
            KIDNEY WITH AGE.

Integrating over 55 years also indicates concentrations of 3.1, 0.005, 0.6 and 0.14 μg g^{-1} w.w. in liver, blood, bone and all other tissues respectively. It can be seen from Section 3.3 that these provide a reasonable approximation to available, average, concentration values from autopsy data (assumed typical age at death 50-60 y for individuals likely to be subject to autopsy).

Concentrations of cadmium in the kidney obtained from the above equation are plotted in Fig. 6 with experimental data obtained from 11 studies. It can be seen that the model tends to overestimate cadmium concentration in juveniles (below ~15 yrs) and ·above the age of ~60 years. In the latter case, experimental data indicate that renal levels decline at ages above ~55 years in the majority of cases. With respect to elderly subjects it may be necessary to revise the proposed model, both with regard to dietary intake and long-term retention of cadmium, but the latter modification will clearly be subject to considerable variation between individuals depending largely upon state of health.

Following long-term low level exposure to cadmium, with no evidence of acute cadmium toxicity, several changes in the physiology of organs can be expected. Renal dysfunction may be accompanied by hepatic dysfunction and changes in gut absorption may occur. Dietary intake usually declines after ~55-60 years, and this will tend to be associated with a decline in cadmium intake (e.g. Travis et al. 1980). In cases of kidney damage associated with chronic cadmium toxicity, as evidenced by victims of 'itai-itai' disease, renal levels of cadmium may also be low (e.g. Friberg 1978) although hepatic levels typically remain high. For juveniles, the intake of cadmium may be lower than for adults, and an assumed daily intake of 40 μg d^{-1} up to the age of 10 years would result in a kidney concentration of 5.5 μg g^{-1} w.w. which is in good agreement with data presented in Fig. 6. It is also notable that, from the above function, if daily intake is taken to vary between 20 to 100 μg d^{-1} and the component of long term retention is taken to vary with a biological half-life between 3650 to 10950 days, then at 65 years a range of 4.5 to 53.3 μg g^{-1} w.w. is predicted for renal cadmium concentration. This range indicates the considerable degree of uncertainty in modelling retention and metabolism of cadmium. On the basis of the best-estimate model proposed for retention of cadmium in man, a renal concentration of 28.6 μg g^{-1} w.w. is predicted at 65 years, and this value falls well within the limits for autopsy data presented in Fig. 6.

In view of the above discussion, and taking into account the uncertainties associated with metabolic data for man, the retention function proposed is taken to adequately represent the retention and distribution of cadmium in man. However, it is noted that when inhalation of cadmium forms the major route of exposure, as is likely to be the case in industrial exposure, the f_1 value must be modified accordingly (Section 3.4.2).

3.4.4   Other metabolic information

3.4.4.1   Skin absorption

No data have been found concerning skin absorption of cadmium, or skin reactions from contact, and it is widely reported that ingestion and

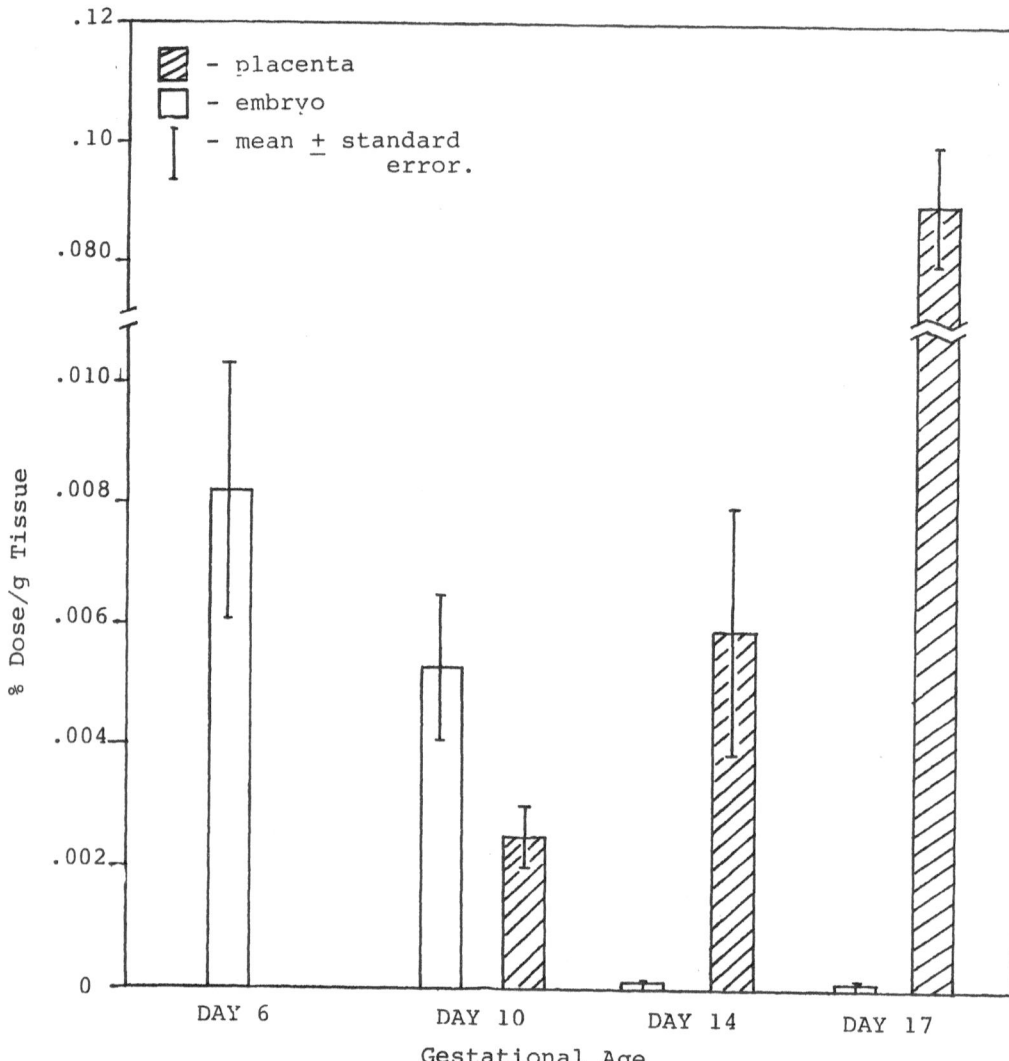

FIGURE 7.   EMBRYO AND PLACENTAL LEVELS OF CADMIUM 24 HOURS
AFTER MATERNAL INTRAGASTRIC ADMINISTRATION OF A
SINGLE 100μg DOSE ON DAYS 6, 10, 14 AND 17 OF
GESTATION (AHOKAS & DILTS 1979).

inhalation of the element account for all or nearly all of the cadmium entering the systemic circulation (e.g. Friberg et al. 1979; Underwood 1977). No ready systemic diffusion of cadmium following skin contact would be expected, and absorption of cadmium through the intact skin need not be included in a metabolic model.

3.4.4.2   Cross-placental transfer

Several studies and reviews have given consideration to cross-placental transfer of cadmium from the mother to foetus (e.g. Ahokas and Dilts 1979, Dorn 1979; Lucis et al. 1972; Samarawickrama and Webb 1979), from foetus to mother (e.g. Kelman and Walter 1980), the placental blood circulation (e.g. Copius Peereboom-Stegeman and Jongstra-Saapen, 1979), the binding of cadmium to the placenta (e.g. Hanlon et al. 1979), and the mutagenicity of cadmium on mammalian oöcytes (e.g. Watanabe et al. 1979).

It is generally reported that the placenta forms an effective barrier to cadmium, and correspondingly cadmium levels in newborn and foetal humans are very low (e.g. Friberg et al. 1979, Lucis et al. 1972). In one experiment on rats Ahokas and Dilts (1979) demonstrated that 24 hours after injecting rats with 10 to 1000 µg Cd per rat, very little cadmium entered the foetus after formation of a functional placenta (∼day 12 of gestation). However, prior to day 10 of gestation a significant transfer to the foetus did occur (Fig. 7).

It has also been noted by Dorn (1979), in a review of the literature, that whilst the placental barrier is effective at relatively low doses, the foeto-placental unit may be destroyed at high doses. Breakdown of placental discrimination may occur at a well-defined level. This is indicated by the observation that in rats 9-15 days into gestation a single injection of 1.1 mg Cd kg^{-1} was not teratogenic or embryocidal, but a single injection of 1.35 mg Cd kg^{-1} killed all embryos (Samarawickrama and Webb 1979). It is of note, however, that following an injection of 5 mg CdCl$_2$ kg^{-1} in prepubertal rats, Copius Peereboom-Stegeman and Jongstra-Spaapen (1979) reported that uterine damage was maximal at 24 hours post injection, with extruded red cells observed in the interstitial tissue, but by 48 hours a marked recovery had started.

Hanlon et al. (1982) studied the chemical status of cadmium in the mouse placenta following a teratogenic dose of 12 µmol CdSO$_4$ kg^{-1} at gestation day 9. The yolk sac and chorioallantoic placenta were removed on day 10 of gestation. Data obtained from gel-filtration and disc electrophoresis suggest that the Cd-binding macromolecule of the chorioa-lantois (which binds 61% of the cadmium content of the tissue) is a metallothionein dimer. It is unlikely that the primary function of this cadmium chelator is to sequester Cd^{2+} (thus sparing embryos teratogenic insult). It probably participates in the storage and transfer of Zn^{2+} in the foetal system and, in a sense, its affinity for cadmium is an una-voidable concommitant of its role as a heavy metal ion chelator.

Finally, it may be noted that whereas no dose-dependent uptake was observed in foetal rats by Ahokas and Dilts (1979), a positive corre-lation between the cadmium level in human material and newborn hair was reported by Huel et al. (1981). Furthermore, Huel et al. (1981) noted that cadmium transfer across the placenta could be likened to simple diffusion and is more marked during the early part of the pregnancy.

From the above discussion it is concluded that at levels of cadmium likely to be found in the environment, it is the dose to the mother which will be a limiting factor of concern and not the potential dose to foetus. It is unlikely that pregnancy will substantially modify the metabolic model presented. With regard to women exposed to high levels of cadmium, Copius Peereboom-Stegeman et al. (1983) have noted that the placental cadmium content is elevated by comparison with other women, and a reduction in birth weight of newborns from women occupationally exposed to cadmium has been observed (Tsvetkova 1970). Data relating to the accumulation of cadmium in human placentas have been summarized by Van Hattam et al. (1981) and Copius Peereboom and Copius Peereboom-Stegeman.

3.4.4.3   Loss in milk

In a review of the literature, Underwood (1977) reported a mean concentration of 26 µg Cd l^{-1} in US cows milk, with a range of 20-37 µg Cd l^{-} in 37 individual cows and 17-30 µg Cd l^{-1} in US market milk from a number of locations. In a survey of human milk, Murthey and Rhea (1968, 1971) reported a mean concentration of 19±2.7 µg Cd l^{-1} on the basis of 22 samples. These data are consistent with the observation of Lucis et al. (1972) that the mammary gland effectively limits cadmium transport to milk. If, on the basis of data presented in Table 6, concentrations of 0.02 and 0.01 µg Cd ml^{-1} are assigned as typical values for blood plasma and milk respectively, then a concentration ratio for cadmium in milk:blood plasma of 0.5 may be assigned. However, it is clear that on the basis of the limited data available (Table 6) this ratio may vary from around 0.02 to considerably greater than 1. Additionally, it is notable that Bhattaryya et al. (1981) recorded an increased fractional gastrointestinal absorption in lactating mice.

For cows, Ng (1982) assigned a forage to milk transfer coefficient, f_m, of 1.5×10^{-3} d l^{-1}. However, two experiments cited by Ng et al. (1977) measuring stable and radioactive isotopes of cadmium in the milk and forage of cows, estimated f_m values of $<3.3 \times 10^{-5}$ d l^{-1} and $<2.7 \times 10^{-6}$ d l^{-1}. On the basis of this wide range of reported values, and in the absence of time dependent data, Coughtrey and Thorne (1983) were unable to propose a model for transfer of cadmium to the milk of domestic animals. Currently, this is also the position with respect to man.

3.5   URINARY AND FAECAL EXCRETION OF CADMIUM

The rate of cadmium excretion has been studied extensively and reviewed for both man and animals (e.g. Friberg et al. 1979; Nomiyama et al. 1979; Shaikh and Smith 1980, Carmichael et al. 1982), although few studies have reported the form of cadmium excreted (but note work of Bernard and Lauwerys (1981) on the urinary excretion of Cd^{2+}). Some dispute exists as to whether urine or faeces form the major excretory pathway. In a review of cadmium and its compounds, Fielder and Dale (1983) noted that in man, excretion is mostly in the urine. However, following a single oral dose to monkeys, Suzuki and Taguchi (1980) reported that by day 25 post-administration 75% of the dose had been excreted in the faeces and <1.0% in urine. Clearly, a large part of the

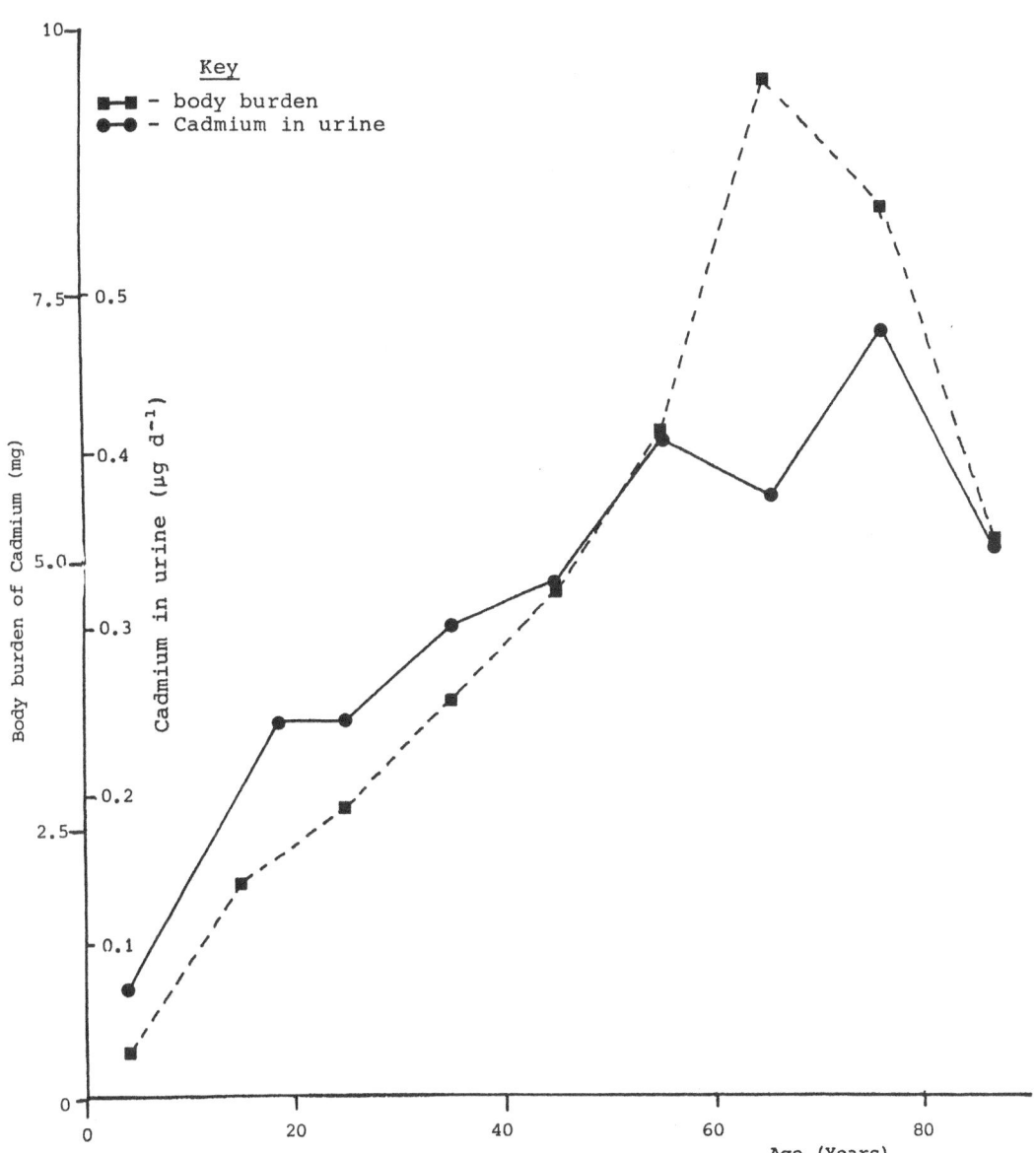

FIGURE 8.   DAILY EXCRETION OF CADMIUM IN RELATION TO TOTAL
BODY BURDEN FOR NON-SMOKING SWEDES
(FROM FRIBERG 1978)

faecal excretion represents material and such excretion may persist for a relatively long period. For example, following an oral dose of $CdCl_2$ to man, it was reported that while the majority of unabsorbed cadmium was excreted in the faeces during the first 7 days, the element was still detectable some 2 to 4 weeks after ingestion (Shaikh and Smith 1980). The persistence of cadmium in the faeces, for up to 28 days following ingestion, is consistent with cadmium uptake by the mucosal cells of the gastrointestinal tract followed by their shedding and subsequent excretion.   It is also notable that rats injected subcutaneously with $CdCl_2$, excreted a total of 22% of the injected dose within 14 weeks, mostly in the faeces (Shaikh and Hirayama 1979).   Furthermore, in the above mentioned study on man, Shaikh and Smith (1980) specifically noted that recovery of cadmium in urine was negligible.

Conversely, Carmichael et al. (1982) reported that for non-occupationally exposed non-smokers, excretion is mainly via the urine, although it was noted that faecal excretion may be important, especially in cases of long-term exposure prior to the onset of renal damage. Following a single intravenous injection of cadmium, biliary excretion may account for 0.8 to 5.7% of the dose (Carmichael et al. 1982), although pre-treatment with cadmium or metallothionein tends to decrease biliary excretion (Kiyozumi and Kojima 1978). Kiyozumi and Kojima (1978) also reported that excretion through the gastrointestinal mucosa remained unaffected by pre-treatment, and following an intraperitoneal injection, in rats, excretion was predominantly in the faeces.

Suzuki and Taguchi (1980) have proposed a three component function to model the fraction of a single oral dose of cadmium excreted in faeces, i.e.:

$$Y = 0.622e^{-0.70t} + 0.031e^{-0.31t} + 0.0003e^{-0.017t}$$

where Y is the fractional daily excretion at t days (normalised to a fractional excretion of 1 over all time).

By integration of this function, it can be determined that the long-term component of excretion accounts for 0.018 of the ingested cadmium, which represents a minimum estimate for absorption, and falls within the range noted in Section 3.4.1.

Urinary excretion of cadmium was also reported by Suzuki and Taguchi (1980), and is presented in Fig. 2. At times of more than 10 days after administration, it can be seen that daily urinary excretion falls in the range 0.001 to 0.01% of the ingested dose. However, the remarkable parallel between urinary and faecal excretion, and the potential difficulty of avoiding cross contamination when using female monkeys, suggests that some faecal contamination of the urine samples may have occurred.

In man it is generally accepted that daily excretion of cadmium represents 0.005 to 0.01% of the body burden (Friberg et al. 1979; Kjellstrom 1979). Kowal et al. (1979) reported that urinary excretion tends to increase with age, from $\sim$0.5 µg l^{-1} at age 0 t0 19 years, to $\sim$1.0 µg l^{-1} at age 60-90 years, which reflects the increasing body burden. In a review of the literature, Friberg (1978) also reported an increase in urinary excretion throughout life, paralleling the increasing body burden (see Figs. 8 and 9). It is, however, notable from Figs. 8 and 9 that urinary excretion of cadmium may decline slightly from the age

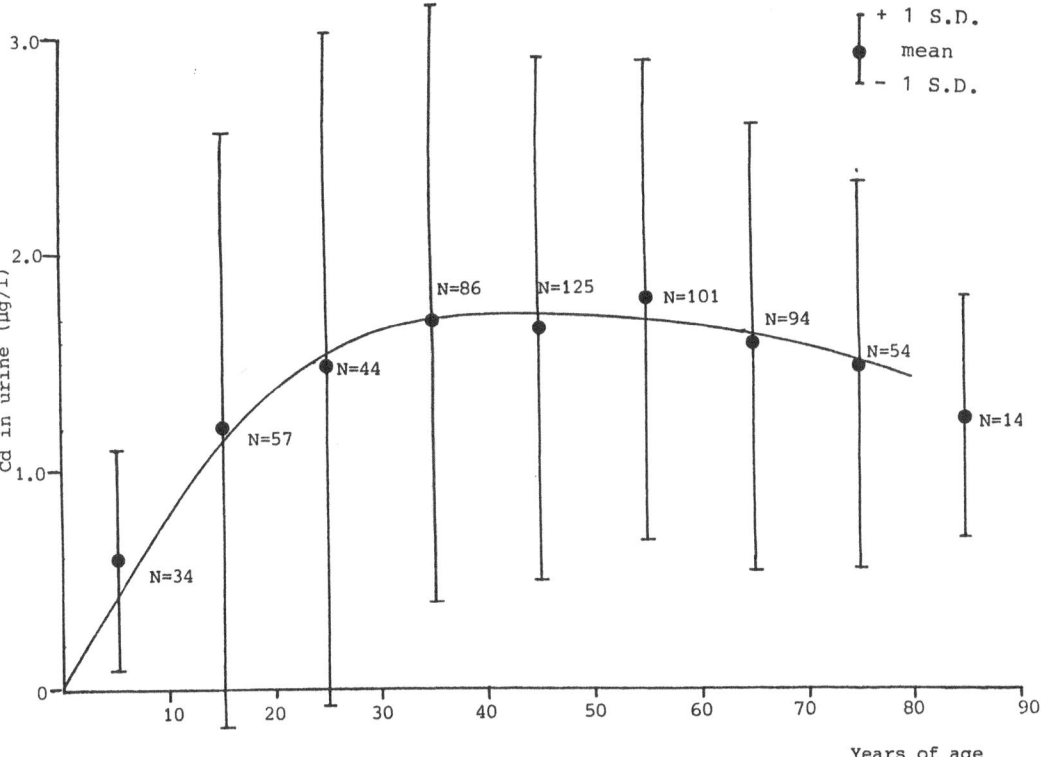

FIGURE 9.   AVERAGE CADMIUM CONCENTRATION IN URINE
             WITHIN DIFFERENT AGE CLASSES, IN TOKYO
             (FROM FRIBERG 1978)

of about 55 years. It is probable that this reflects a decrease in dietary intake and suggests that the decline in body burden observed from about 55 years may be mainly attributable to factors other than renal dysfunction (see also Sections 3.3 and 3.4.3.1). This is particularly taken to be the case, since urinary cadmium levels increase markedly if tubular dysfunction occurs (Fielder and Dale 1983) and this is not generally present (e.g. Figure 9).

Cadmium excreted after absorption has been reported to be detected either as the free ion Cd^{2+} or bound to metallothionein (e.g. Bernard and Lauwerys 1981; Suzuki and Yamamura 1978). Bernard and Lauwerys (1981) administered cadmium to rats in drinking water for 4 months at 200 µg ml^{-1} avoiding kidney damage, and reported a progressive increase in the Cd^{2+} content of the urine. They also reported that administration of Na_2ClO_4 (a known nephrotoxin) resulted in a sharp, albeit transitory, increase in Cd^{2+} secretion. Bernard and Lauwerys (1981) concluded that:

- liver cytolysis alone results in Cd^{2+} transfer to the kidneys with relatively little increase in urinary Cd^{2+};

- kidney damage alone results in increased urinary Cd^{2+}, either due to a release of Cd^{2+} accumulated in the kidney, or due to a reduction in the reabsorption of circulating Cd^{2+};

- liver damage and kidney damage result in a marked increase in urinary Cd^{2+}, due to reduced renal uptake.

It is noted that following kidney damage, either alone or in combination with liver damage, increased urinary levels of cadmium may be due to a decrease in resorption of released cadmium, as well as to reduced renal uptake. Suzuki and Yamamura (1979) reported that in rats ingesting Cd-MT, especially at high doses, the cadmium is detected in urine still bound to metallothionein. This is in accord with the observations of Tanaka (1982) that, whilst some MT released from rat liver is reabsorbed by the kidney, most is excreted in the urine. On the basis of several experiments in rabbits, Foulkes (1978) concluded that renal reabsorption of Cd-MT is a completely saturable process, and is depressed by exposure to cadmium, due to its specific nephrotoxicity. Shaikh and Hirayama (1979) have stated that the presence of MT in urine may be taken as evidence of specific cadmium poisoning.

From the above, it may be concluded that early excretion of ingested cadmium is predominantly in the faeces. At later times very little cadmium is lost relative to the body burden (<0.01% d^{-1}; Friberg et al. 1979) and the dominant pathway of excretion may depend on the level of renal or hepatic damage (e.g. Carmichael et al. 1982). Cadmium can be present in the urine either as the free ion or bound to MT, though presence of the latter may be indicative of cadmium poisoning (Shaikh and Hirayama 1979). Data presented by Friberg (1978) and Kowal et al. (1979) indicate that urinary levels of cadmium can be used to estimate total body burden except presumably in the case of cadmium poisoning. Excretion of cadmium via hair, skin, sweat or saliva can be detected but is considered to be of minor importance (see Carmichael et al. 1982). The concentration of cadmium in hair is not reported to be a good indicator of the body burden (e.g. Kobayashi 1978; Kowal et al. 1979).

3.6   EFFECTS OF STATE OF HEALTH, ADMINISTRATION OF TOXIC LEVELS AND
       THERAPEUTI: PROCEDURES

Tsuchiya (1981) has noted that although both acute and chronic cadmium poisoning has been reported in industrially developed countries such as the United States, Great Britain, France and Japan, improvements in the working environment has resulted in an emphasis on the aspects of chronic poisoning. Acute cadmium poisoning of occupationally exposed workers is generally via inhalation, and workers in areas of high atmospheric cadmium concentration or cadmium dust are the main group at risk. Amongst the general population ingestion in food is more likely, although reports of such food poisoning have become rare in recent years (Tsuchiya 1981).

Paterson (1947) distinguished three stages of acute cadmium poisoning following inhalation: lung oedema, proliferation, and fibrosis. Lung oedema reaches a peak within 4 to 48 hours after exposure and begins to disappear within 72 hours. Subsequently, interstitial cells swell, body fluids permeate the alveoli and fibrin is deposited. This stage lasts from 7 to 10 days and may be fatal. Survivors may suffer permanent lung fibrosis. Friberg et al. (1974) reported on two cases of fatal cadmium inhalation by man and calculated the exposure to be 2500 mg m^{-3} for 1 minute.

Fielder and Dale (1983) have summarized much of the data relating to acute and chronic toxicity of cadmium in man and animals. The following discussion is based largely upon their review of findings of chronic effects and is limited to consideration of those effects likely to significantly modify the metabolism of cadmium.

Following repeated oral administration in the rat, nephrotoxicity is the first clinical effect; limited to the proximal tubules. The 'critical concentration' of cadmium in the renal cortex at which tubular dysfunction first occurs is thought to be 150 mg g^{-1} in the rat. Primates appear to have a similar sensitivity to nephrotoxic effects, although data are limited. Rhesus monkeys fed a diet containing 10-30 μg g^{-1} for 130 weeks exhibited tubular damage, and a 'no-effect' level was determined to be 3 μg g^{-1} over the same period (Nomiyama et al. 1979; Nomiyama et al. 1982). The estimated 'critical concentration' in that case was 600 μg g^{-1} in the renal cortex. In addition to nephrotoxicity, osteoporosis may also be noted in rats administered 10 to 30 μg g^{-1} or more for three weeks (Nomiyama et al. 1982). This bone disorder may be due to the tubular dysfunction resulting in disturbance to calcium metabolism.

At levels of administration stated to be low (e.g. 5 μg Cd ml^{-1} as cadmium acetate in drinking water for 1 year) hypertension may be noted in rats (Schroeder et al. 1965; Schroeder 1964, 1967; Schroeder and Vinton 1962; Schroeder and Balassa 1965; Kanisawa and Schroeder 1969), although available data are to some extent contradictory (e.g. Kopp et al. 1982; Fingerle et al. 1982; Stowe et al. 1972). Parenteral administration of cadmium produces similar effects.

Limited data are available for the toxic effects of cadmium following inhalation by animals. Lung appears to be the most sensitive organ, with marked lesions in rats exposed to 25 μg m^{-3} for 90 days (Prigge 1978). A 'no-effect' level was not established. Nephrotoxicity was not noted in that study, but a further study in which rabbits were exposed to 4 mg m^{-3} (3 hours a day, 21 days a month) for 9 months, identified both lung and kidney damage (Friberg 1950).

In man, various authors have identified the symptoms of exposure to cadmium dust or fumes of 0.5 mg m^{-3} or more to be: coughing, shortness of breath, irritation of the upper respiratory tract, runny nose and loss of sense of smell (e.g. Friberg 1950; Baader 1951, 1952; Lane and Campbell 1954; Buxton 1956; Kazantis 1963; Adams et al. 1969). At levels of exposure of 3-15 mg Cd m^{-3}, exposed workers may develop emphysema over a period of 20 years or more (Townshend 1982). Signs of renal dysfunction generally precede lung damage, and, as with animals, the kidney appears to be the most sensitive organ in man (Fielder and Dale 1983). Proteinuria (the excretion of low molecular weight proteins in urine), and at later stages glucosuria, are generally believed to be caused by impairment of the reabsorption capacity of the renal tubuli (Tsuchiya 1981). Proteinuria was first reported among alkaline battery workers by Friberg (1950) and many subsequent studies have confirmed these findings (e.g. Baader 1951; Smith et al. 1955; Bonnell et al. 1959; Potts 1965; Suzuki et al. 1965; Tsuchiya 1967; Adams et al. 1969; Harada 1973; Lauwerys et al. 1979), suggesting that tubular dysfunction may be widespread among workers exposed to moderately high levels of cadmium in respirable dust (e.g. 1 mg m^{-3} for 10 years or more). The critical concentration in the renal cortex is taken to be ~300 µg g^{-1} (Fielder and Dale 1983). Proteinuria may be reversible in the early stages, but not after a long period (Tsuchiya 1981). Tsuchiya noted that "chronic cadmium poisoning with renal tubular dysfunctions is almost symptom-free. Those with chronic cadmium poisoning will probably reach old age, although there is a possibility that symptoms of osteomalacia may develop during the long subclinical course if and when certain other factors, especially nutritional deficiency and multiple pregnancies, are involved."

In general, Tsuchiya (1981) noted that no specific therapy exists for either chronic or acute cadmium poisoning and treatment is based on alleviation of symptoms. Vitamin D has been found to be of benefit in cases of osteomalacia, otherwise known as 'itai-itai' or 'ouch-ouch' disease, resulting from ingestion of cadmium (Nogawa 1981). For acute exposures following inhalation, treatment of pulmonary oedema is most important. The lack of symptoms resulting from renal tubular dysfunction due to chronic cadmium poisoning, does not suggest that therapy is required. In his monograph on the diagnosis and treatment of poisoning, Driesbach (1966) recommended the use of calcium edetate for both acute and chronic cadmium poisoning. However, more recently, Friberg et al. (1974) and Tsuchiya (1981) have disputed the use of this drug. The use of Ca-EDTA is not recommended mainly on the grounds that in one worker identified by Tsuchiya (1976) to be suffering from chronic cadmium poisoning, whilst Ca-EDTA increased the level of cadmium in urine it also increased proteinuria. No favourable effects on renal functions could be discerned.

3.7   MODEL SUMMARY

The following summary of recommendations and models for the metabolism of cadmium in man is based on data presented and discussed in previous sections of this review.

3.7.1 Intake of cadmium

Considerable geographical and individual variation in the dietary intake of cadmium is apparent. Daily intakes generally lie within the range 50-100 µg Cd d^{-1}, though up to 600 µg Cd d^{-1} has been recorded in areas of Japan where 'itai-itai' disease is endemic. Where local contamination is not known to have occurred, an intake of 12 µg Cd d^{-1} may be expected from water and up to 4 µg Cd d^{-1} may be inhaled in air or from tobacco smoke. A typical total daily intake, for non-occupationally exposed individuals, is taken to be 75 µg Cd d^{-1}.

3.7.2 Fractional gastrointestinal absorption

Reported values for the fractional gastrointestinal absorption (f_1) of cadmium in man are normally <0.1 and fall in the range 0.004 to 0.1. An appropriate value for all compounds and complexes of cadmium, over recorded ranges of dietary intake, is taken to be 0.05.

3.7.3 Retention in, and translocation from, the lungs

Of cadmium deposited in the human lung, between 0.1 and 0.5 is absorbed, with values for absorption typically around 0.25. Oxides, halides, sulphides and nitrates of cadmium are assigned to ICRP inhalation class W and all other compounds, apart from hydroxides, are assigned to class D. The position of cadmium hydroxide is unclear, due to insufficient data and it may be properly assigned to class W or class Y.

3.7.4 Retention in the body

Of cadmium entering the systemic circulation a fraction of about 0.1 is apparently available for early excretion with a biological half-life of 1.5 days. The remainder of the cadmium is apparently retained in all organs and tissues with a biological half-life of about 25 years, though a range of 20 to 30 years can be expected. On this basis, a reasonable representation of the whole-body retention of cadmium, following entry of a unit quantity of the element into the systemic circulation, is:

$$R(t) = 0.1e^{-0.693t/1.5} + 0.9e^{-0.693t/9125}$$

where t is in days.

Data for the distribution of cadmium in man suggest that fractions of 0.2, 0.3, 0.1 and 0.01 of cadmium deposited in the body be assigned to the liver, kidneys, bone and blood respectively.

3.7.5 Excretion

Cadmium is generally excreted primarily in the faeces, although urinary excretion has been reported to be the main route of loss in some cases.   In the absence of clinical manifestations of cadmium poisoning, associated with renal and/or hepatic dysfunction, the daily excretion of cadmium typically represents some 0.005 to 0.01% of the total body burden.   Loss of cadmium in hair, sweat or saliva is detectable, but not significant compared with urinary or faecal excretion.   In general, for man, several reviews suggest that urinary levels of cadmium can be taken to reflect the total body burden, and blood levels of cadmium to reflect the average daily intake for the preceeding few months.   However, more data are required before such values can be interpreted unambiguously.

3.7.6   Skin absorption

No data have been found concerning the skin absorption of cadmium, and this does not appear to require inclusion in the metabolic model.

3.7.7   Cross-placental transfer and transfer in milk

At cadmium levels likely to be encountered in the environment, the placenta apparently forms an effective barrier to the transport of cadmium to the foetus and it is unlikely that pregnancy will substantially modify the metabolic model proposed.   At higher levels of exposure, the placenta itself may be affected and some data available suggest that following high level exposure to the mother the newborn have a lower birth weight compared with those from non-exposed mothers.   Data concerning the loss of cadmium in milk are very variable.   In view of the degree of uncertainty with respect to loss in milk, no recommendations are made concerning the effect of lactation on the metabolism of cadmium, or on transfer of the element via this route.

3.8   REFERENCES

Adams, R.G., Harrison, J.F. and Scott, P., 1969.   The development of cadmium-induced proteinurea, impaired renal function and osteomalacia in alkaline battery workers.   Quart. J. Med., 38: 425-443.

Adamsson, E., Piscator, M. and Nogawa, K., 1979.   Pulmonary and gastrointestinal exposure to cadmium oxide dust in a battery factory. Environ. Health Perspect., 28: 219-222.

Ahokas, R.A. and Kilts, P.V. Jr., 1979.   Cadmium uptake by the rat embryo as a function of gestational age.   Am.J. Obstet. Gynacol., 135: 219-222.

Anderson, C. and Danylchuk, K.D., 1978.   Effect of chronic low-level cadmium intoxication on the haversian remodelling system in dogs. Calcif. Tiss. Res., 26: 143-148.

Anon, 1981.   Attualita del cadmio negli organismi vivienti: conside+razioi fisiopatalogiche, cliniche e terapertiche.   Cl. Therap., 98: 545-560.

Baader, E., 1951. Die chronische Kadmium vergiftung. Dtsch. Med. Wochenschr., 76: 864.

Baader, E., 1952. Chronic cadmium poisoning. Ind. Med. Surg., 21: 427-430.

Bernard, A.M. and Lauwerys, R.R., 1981. The effects of sodium chromate and carbon tetrachloride on the urinary excretion and tissue distribution of cadmium in cadmium pretreated rats. Toxicol. Appl. Pharmacol., 57: 30-38.

Bhattacharjee, D., Shatty, T.K. and Sundaram, K., 1979. Studies on the distribution of 115m-cadmium in mice tissues. Ind. J. Exp. Biol., 17: 74-76.

Bhattarcharyya, M.H., Whelton, B.H. and Peterson, D.P., 1981. Gastrointestinal absorption of cadmium in mice during gestation and lactation 1. Short-term exposure studies. Toxicol. Appl. Pharmacol., 61: 335-342.

Boisset, M. and Boudene, C., 1981. Effect of a single exposure to cadmium oxide fumes on rat lung microsomal enzymes. Toxicol. Appl. Pharmacol., 57: 335-345.

Bonnell, J.A., Kazantzis, G. and King, E., 1959. A follow-up study of men exposed to cadmium oxide fume. Br. J. Ind. Med., 16: 135-147.

Bonner, F.W., King, L.J. and Parke, D.V.L., 1979. The tissue deposition and urinary excretion of cadmium, zinc, copper and iron, following repeated parenteral administration of cadmium to rats. Chem.-Biol. Interactions, 27: 343-351.

Bowen, H.J.M., 1979. Environmental Chemistry of the Elements. Academic Press, London.

Bremner, I. and Campbell, J.K., 1980. The influence of dietary copper intake on the toxicity of cadmium. Ann. N.Y. Acad. Sci., 355: 319-332.

Buhler, D.R., Wright, D.C., Smith, K.L. and Tinsley, I.J., 1981. Cadmium absorption and tissue distribution in rats provided low concentrations of cadmium in food and drinking water. J. Toxicol. Environ. Health, 8, 185-197.

Buxton, R. St. J., 1956. Respiratory function in men casting cadmium alloys. II: the estimation of the total lung volume, its subdivisions and the mixing coefficient. Br. J. Ind. Med., 13: 36-40.

Calabrese, E.J., 1981. Nutrition and Environmental Health, The Influence of Nutritional Status on Pollutant Toxicity and Carcino-genicity: Vol. 2, Minerals and Macronutrients. John Wiley and Sons, New York.

Cantilena, L.R. Jr. and Klaassen, C.D., 1980. The effect of ethylenediaminetetraacetic acid (EDTA) and EDTA plus salicylate on acute
cadmium toxicity and distribution. Toxicol. Appl. Pharmacol., 53:
510-514.

Carmichael, N.G., Backhouse, B.L., Winder, C. and Lewis, P.D., 1982.
Teratogenicity, toxicity and perinatal effects of cadmium. Human
Toxicol., 1: 159-162.

CEC, 1978. Criteria (Dose/Effect Relationships) for Cadmium.
Report of a Working Group of Experts prepared for the Commission of
the European Communities. Pergamon Press, Oxford.

Cherian, M.G., Goyer, R.A. and Valverg, L.S., 1978.
Gastrointestinal absorption and organ distribution of oral cadmium
chloride and cadmium metallothionein in mice. J. Toxicol. Environ.
Health, 4, 861-868.

Cherry, W.H. 1981. Distribution of cadmium in human tissues. In:
Nriadu, J.O. (Ed.) Cadmium in the Environment Part II: Health
Effects. John Wiley & Sons, New York: 69-536.

Chertok, R.J., Sasser, L.B., Callaham, M.F. and Jacobs, G.E., 1979.
Intestinal absorption of Cd in vitro. Environ. Res., 20: 125-132.

Cole, J.F., 1979. Cadmium toxicity (letter), 1979. Lancet, 1
(8130): 1345.

Copius Peereboom, J.W. and Copius Peereboom-Stegeman, J.H.J. (1981).
Exposure and health effects of cadmium. Part 2. Toxic effects of
cadmium to animals and man. Toxicol. Environ. Chem. Reviews, 4:
67-178.

Copius Peereboom-Stegeman, J.H.J. and Jongstra-Saapen, E.J., 1979.
The effect of a single sublethal administration of cadmium chloride
on the micro circulation in the uterus of the rat. Toxicol., 13:
199-213.

Copius Peereboom-Stegeman, J.H.J., van der Velde, W.J. and Dessing,
J.W.M., 1983. Influence of cadmium on placental structure.
Ecotoxicol. Environ. Safety, 7: 79-86.

Cotton, F.A. and Wilkinson, G., 1972. Advanced Inorganic Chemistry:
A Comprehensive Text. Interscience Pub., New York.

Coughtrey, P.J. and Thorne, M.C., 1983. Radionuclide Distribution
and Transport in Terrestrial and Aquatic Ecosystems. Volume 2.
A.A. Balkema, Rotterdam.

Daston, G.P. and Grabowski, C.T., 1979. Toxic effects of cadmium on
the developing rat lung. 1. Altered pulmonary surfactant and the
induction of respiratory distress syndrome. J. Toxicol. Environ.
Health, 5: 973-983.

DoE, 1980. Cadmium in the Environment and its significance to Man. An Inter-department Report. Pollution Paper, 17, HMSO, London.

Dorn, C.R., 1979. Cadmium and the food chain. Cornell Vet., 69: 323-343.

Engstrom, B. and Nordberg, C.F. 1979. Dose dependence of gastrointestinal absorption and biological half-time of cadmium in mice. Toxicol., 13: 215-222.

FAO/WHO, 1972. Evaluation of certain food additives and the contaminants mercury, lead and cadmium. Sixteenth report of the Joint FAO/WHO Expert Committee on Food Additives. Technical Report Series, no. 505.

Fielder, R.J. and Dale, E.A., 1983. Toxicity Review 7. Cadmium and its Compounds. Health and Safety Executive. HMSO, London.

Fingerle, H., Fischer, G. and Classen, H.G., 1982. Failure to produce hypertension in rats by chronic exposure to cadmium. Food Chem. Toxicol., 20: 301-306.

Foulkes, E.C., 1980. Some determinants of intestinal cadmium transport in the rat. J. Environ. Pathol. Toxicol., 3: 417-481.

Fox, M.R.S., Jacobs, R.M., Lee Jones, A.O., Fry, B.E. Jr. and Stone, C.L., 1980. Effects of vitamin C and iron on cadmium retention. Ann. N.Y. Acad. Sci., 355: 249-261.

Fox, M.R.S., 1976. In: Prasad, A.S. (Ed.) Trace Elements and Human Disease, Vol.2. Academic Press, New York: 401-406.

Friberg, L., 1949. Proteinuria and emphysema among workers exposed to cadmium and nickel dust with special reference to chronic cadmium poisoning. In: Proceedings of the 9th International Congress on Industrial Medicine, pp. 641-644.

Friberg, L., 1950. Health hazards in the manufacture of alkaline accumulators with special reference to chronic cadmium poisoning. Acta Med. Scand., 138 (Suppl. 240): 1-241.

Friberg, L., 1959. Chronic cadmium poisoning. A.M.A. Arch. Ind. Health, 20: 401-407.

Friberg, L., 1978. The toxicology of cadmium. In: Proceedings, First International Cadmium Conference, San Francisco, 31 Jan - 2 Feb. 1977: 167-175.

Friberg, L., Piscator, M., Nordberg, G.F. and Kjellström, T., 1974. Cadmium in the Environment, 2nd Edit. CRC Press, Cleveland, Ohio.

Friberg, L., Kjellström, T., Nordberg, G. and Piscator, M., 1979. Cadmium, Chapter 21 of: Friberg, L., Nordberg, G.F. and Vouk, V.B. (Eds.). Handbook on the Toxicology of Metals. Elsevier/North-Holland Biomedical Press, Amsterdam.

Gale, N.L. and Wixson, B.C., 1978. Cadmium in forest ecosystems around lead smelters in Missouri. Environ. Health Perspect., 28: 23-27.

Hanlon, D.D., Specht, C. and Ferm, V.H., 1982. The chemical status of cadmium ion in the placenta. Environ. Res., 27:89-94.

Harada, A., 1973. Medical examination of workers in a cadmium pigment factory. Kankyo Hoken Rep., 24: 16-22.

Hardley, V.G., Conklin, A.W. and Sanders, C.L., 1980. Rapid solubilization and translocation of 109-CdO_2 following pulmonary deposition. Toxicol. Appl. Pharmacol., 54: 156-160.

Hattum, B. van, Voogt, P. de, and Copius Peereboom, J.W., 1981. Cadmium content of human placenta. Int. J. Environ. Anal. Chem., 10: 121-133.

Hilderbrand, C.E. and Cram, L.S., 1979. Distribution of cadmium in human blood cultured in low levels of $CdCl_2$ accumulation of Cd in lymphocytes and preferential binding to metallothionein. Proc. Soc. Exp. Biol. Med., 161: 438-443.

Huel, G., Ibrahim, M.A. and Boudene, C., 1981. Cadmium and lead content of maternal and newborn hair, relationship to parity, birth weight and hypertension. Arch. Environ. Health, 36: 221-227.

Hutton, M., 1982. Cadmium in the European Community. A Prospective Assessment of Sources, Human Exposure and Environmental Impact. MARC Report no. 26, London.

IARC Working Group Report, 1980. An evaluation of chemicals and industrial processes associated with cancer in humans based on human and animal data: IARC monographs volumes 1-20. Cancer Res., 40: 1-12.

ICRP Task Group on Lung Dynamics, 1966. Deposition and retention models for internal dosimetry of the human respiratory tract. Health Phys., 12: 173-207.

ICRP Publication 23, 1975. Report of the Task Group on Reference Man. Pergamon Press, Oxford.

ICRP Publication 30, 1980. Limits for Intakes of Radionuclides by Workers. Annals of the ICRP, 4 (3 and 4).

Ikebuchi, H., Kido, Y and Urakubo, G., 1979. Behaviour of cadmium in rabbit blood. Chem. Pharm. Bull., 27: 1034-1038.

Iyengar, G.V., Kollmer, W.S. and Bowen, H.J.M., 1978. The Elemental Composition of Human Tissues and Body Fluids: A compilation of Values for Adults. Verlag Chemie, New York.

Johnson, D.R. and Foulkes, E.C., 1980. On the proposed role of metallothionein in the transport of cadmium. Environ. Res., 21: 360-365.

Jones, H.S. and Fowler, B.A., 1980. Biological interactions of cadmium with calcium. Ann. N.Y. Acad. Sci., 355: 309-318.

Kanisawa, M. and Schroeder, H.A., 1969. Renal areteriolar changes in hypertensive rats given cadmium in drinking water. Exp. Mol. Pathol., 10: 81-98.

Kanwar, K.C., Kaushal, S.C. and Mehra, R.K., 1980. Temporal distribution of orally administered 115m-Cd in subcellular fractions of liver and kidney of rat. Ind. J. Exp. Biol., 18: 664.

Kazantis, G., 1978. Some long term effects of cadmium on the human kidney. In: Cadmium 77: Edited Proceedings of the First International Cadmium Conference, San Francisco. Cadmium Association, London: 194-198.

Kelman, B.J. and Walter, B.K., 1980. Foetal to maternal cadmium movements across the perfused hemochorial placenta of the guinea pig. Toxicol. Appl. Pharmacol., 52: 400-406.

Kirkpatrick, D.C. and Coffin, D.E., 1974.

Kiyozumi, M. and Kojima, S., 1978. Studies on poisonous metals in excretion of cadmium through bile and gastrointestinal mucosa and the effect of chelating agents on its excretion in cadmium-pretreated rats. Chem. Pharm. Bull., 26: 3410-3415.

Kjellström, T., 1979. Exposure and accumulation of cadmium in populations from Japan, the United States, and Sweden. Environ. Health Perspect., 28: 169-197.

Kjellström, T. and Nordberg, G.F., 1978. A kinetic model of cadmium metabolism in the human being. Environ. Res., 16: 248-269.

Klein, A.K. and Wichmann, H.J., 1945. Report on cadmium. Ass. Offic. Agric. Chem., 28: 257-269.

Kobayashi, J., 1978. Pollution by cadmium and the itai-itai disease in Japan. In: Oehme, F.W. (Ed.) Toxicity of Heavy Metals in the Environment, Part 1. Marcel Dekker Inc., New York: 199-260.

Kolonel, L.N., 1976. Association of cadmium with renal cancer. Cancer (Phila.), 87: 1782-1789.

Koo, S.I., Fullmer, C.F. and Wasserman, R.H., 1978. Intestinal absorption and retention of 109-Cd: Effects of cholecalciferol, calcium status and other variables, J.Nutr., 108: 1812-1822.

Kopp. S.J., Glonek, T., Perry, H.M., Erlanger, M and Perry, E.F., 1982. Cardiovascular actions of cadmium at environmental exposure levels. Science, 217: 837-839.

Korte, F., 1983. Ecotoxicology of cadmium: general overview. Eco-toxicol. Env. Safety, 7: 3-8.

Kostial, K., Rabar, I., Blanusa, M. and Ciganovic, M., 1980b. Influence of trace elements on cadmium and mercury absorption in sucklings. Bull. Environ. Contam. Toxicol., 25: 436-440.

Kostial, K., Rabar, I., Blanusa, M. and Landeka, M. 1979. Effect of age on heavy metal absorption. Proc. Nutr. Soc., 38: 251-256.

Kostial, K., Simonovic, I., Rabor, I and Landeka, M., 1981. Effect of rats diet on 85-Sr, 115m-Cd and 203-Hg absorption in suckling rats. Environ. Res., 25: 281-285.

Kostial, K., Rabar, I., Blanusa, M. and Simonovic, I., 1980a. The effect of iron additive to milk on cadmium, mercury and manganese absorption in rats. Environ. Res., 22: 140-145.

Kowal, N.E., Johnson, D.E., Kraemer, D.F. and Pahren, H.R., 1979. Normal levels of cadmium in diet, urine, blood and tissues of inhabitants of the United States. J. Toxicol. Environ. Health, 5: 995-1014.

Kwast, M., 1981. The role of cadmium in the development of osteopathy. Przeg. Epid., 35: 511-516.

Lane, R.E. and Campbell, A.C.P., 1954. Fatal emphysema in two men making a copper-cadmium alloy. Br. J. Ind. Med., 11: 118-122.

Lauwerys, R., Roels, H., Regniers, M., Buchet, V.P., Bernard, A. and Goret, A., 1979. Significance of cadmium concentration in blood and in urine in workers exposed to cadmium. Environ. Res., 20: 375-391.

Löser, E., 1980. A 2 year oral carcinogenicity study with cadmium on rats. Cancer Lett., 9: 191-198.

Lucis, O.J., Lucis, R. and Shaikh, Z.A., 1972. Cadmium and zinc in pregnancy and lactation. Arch. Environ. Health, 25: 14-22.

Marcus, A.M., 1982. Multicompartment kinetic models for cadmium 1: effects of zinc on cadmium retention in male mice. Environ. Res., 27: 46-51.

Marek, K., Klopotowski, J., Wocka-Marek, T., Zuchoka, B. and Krol, B. 1981. Cadmium exposure effect on the haemopoietic system. Polski Tygoduik Lekarski, 36: 1329-1331.

Meranger, J.C., Conacher, H.B.S., Cunningham, H.M. and Krewski, D.L., 1981. Levels of cadmium in human kidney cortex in Canada. Can. J. Pub. Health, 72: 269-272.

Morris, J.G., 1974. A Biologist's Physical Chemistry. 2nd edit. Edward Arnold. London.

Murphy, G.K. and Rhea, U. (1968). Cadmium and silver content of market milk. J. Dairy Sci., 51: 610-613.

Murphy, G.K. and Rhea, U. (1971). Cadmium, copper, iron, manganese, and zinc in evaporated milk, infant products and human milk. J. Dairy Sci., 54: 1001-1005.

Nakamura, K., Takata, T., Suzuki, E., Sugiura, Y. and Kobayashi, T., 1981. Effects of calcium deficiency on the in vivo interaction of cadmium and zinc. Jpn. J. Hyg., 35: 851-857.

Ng, Y.C., 1982. A review of transfer factors for assessing the dose from radionuclides in agricultural products. Nuclear Saf., 23: 57-71.

Ng, T.C., Colsher, C.S., Quinn, D.J. and Thompson, S.E., 1977. Transfer coefficients for the prediction of the dose to man via the forage-cow-milk pathway from radionuclides released to the biosphere. University of California, UCRL-51939.

Nogawa, K., 1981. Itai-itai disease and follow up studies. In: Nriagu, J. (Ed.). Cadmium in the Environment. Part II: Health Effects. John Wiley & Sons, New York: 1-37.

Nomiyama, K., Nomiyama, H., Akahori, F. and Masaoka, T., 1982. Cadmium health effects in monkeys with special reference to the critical concentration of cadmium in the renal cortex. In: Cadmium 81. Proceedings of the Third International Cadmium Conference, Miami. Cadmium Association, London.

Nomiyama, K., Nomiyama, H., Nomura, Y. et al., 1979. Effects of dietary cadmium in rhesus monkeys. Environ. Health Perspect., 28: 223-243.

Nordberg, F. and Kjellstrom, T., 1979. Metabolic model for cadmium in man. Environ. Health Perspect., 28: 211-217.

Nordberg, G.F., Slorach, S. and Stenstrom, T., 1973. Cadmium poisoning caused by a cooled soft-drink. Lakartidningen, 70: 601-604.

Nriagu, J.O., 1980a. Cadmium in the Environment, Part I. Ecological Cycling. John Wiley and Sons, New York.

Nriagu, J.O., 1980b. Global cadmium cycle. In: Nriagu, J.O. (Ed.). Cadmium in the Environment, Part I. Ecological Cycling. John Wiley and Sons, New York; pp. 1-12.

Nriagu, J.O., 1981. Cadmium in the Environment. Part II: Health Effects. John Wiley and Sons, New York.

Oberdoerster, G., Baumert, H.P., Hochrainer, D. and Stoeber, W., 1979. The clearance of cadmium aerosols after inhalation exposure. Am. Ind. Hyg. J., 40: 443-450.

Oberdorster, G., Oldiges, H. and Zimmerman, B., 1980. Lung deposition and clearance of cadmium in rats exposed by inhalation or by intratracheal instillation. Zbl. Bakt. I. Abt. Orig. B. 170: 35-43.

O'Brien, B.J., Smith, S and Colemen, D.O., 1980. Lead Pollution of the Global Environment. MARC Report No.16, London.

Oh, S.H., Whanger, P.D. and Deagen, J.T., 1981. Tissue metallothionein, dietary interaction of cadmium and zinc with copper, mercury and silver. J. Toxicol. Environ. Health, 7: 547-560.

Paterson, J.C., 1947. Studies on the toxicity of inhaled cadmium III: the pathology of cadmium smoke poisoning in man and in experimental animals. J. Ind. Hyg. Toxicol., 29: 294-?.

Pietrzak-Flis, Z., Rehnberg, G.L., Favor, M.J., Cahill, D.F. and Laskey, J.W., 1978. Chronic ingestion of cadmium and/or tritium in rats I. Accumulation and distribution of cadmium in two generations. Environ. Res. 16: 9-17.

Piotrowski, J.K. and Coleman, D.O., 1980. Environmental Hazards of Heavy Metals: Summary Evaluation of Lead, Cadmium and Mercury. MARC Report no. 20, London.

Piscator, M., 1981. Role of cadmium in carcinogenesis with special reference to cancer of the prostate. Environ. Health Perspect., 40: 107-120.

Prigg, E., 1978. Early signs of oral and inhalative cadmium uptake in rats. Arch. Toxicol., 40: 231-237.

Rabar, R. and Kostial, K., 1981. Bioavailability of cadmium in rats fed various diets. Arch. Toxicol., 47: 63-66.

Ridlington, J.W., Winge, D.R. and Fowler, B.A., 1981. Long-term turnover of cadmium metallothionein in liver and kidney following a single low dose of cadmium in rats. Biochim. Biophys. Acta, 673: 177-183.

Sabbioni, E., Marafante, E., Amantini, L., Ubertalli, L. and Pietra, R., 1978. Cadmium toxicity studies under long-term low-level exposure (LLE) conditions. 1. Metabolic patterns in rats exposed to present environmental dietary levels of Cd for two years. Sci. Tot. Environ., 10: 135-161.

Samarawickrama, G.P. and Webb, M., 1979. Acute effects of cadmium on the pregnant rat and embryo-fetal development. Environ. Health Perspect., 28: 245-249.

Sato, M. and Nagai, Y., 1980. Form of cadmium in rat liver subcellular particles. Toxicol. Lett., 7: 119-123.

Schroeder, H.A. 1964. Cadmium hypertension in rats. Am. J. Physiol., 204: 62-66.

Schroeder, H.A., 1967. Cadmium, chromium and cardiovascular disease. Circulation, 35: 570-582.

Schroeder, H.A., Balassa, J.J., 1965. Influence of chromium, cadmium and lead on rat aortic lipids and circulating cholesterol. Am. J. Physiol., 209: 433.

Schroeder, H.A., Balassa, J.J. and Vinton, W.H., 1965. Chromium, cadmium and lead in rats. Effects on life span, tumours and tissue levels. J, Nutr., 86: 51-66.

Schroeder, H.A. and Vinton, W.H., 1962. Hypertension induced in rats by small doses of cadmium. Am. J. Physiol., 202: 515-518.

Shaikh, Z.A., 1979. The low molecular weight cadmium-, mercury-, and zinc- binding proteins (metallothioneins), biosynthesis, metabolism, and possible role in metal toxicity. Experienta, 34 (Suppl.): 281-291.

Shaikh, Z.A. and Hirayama, K., 1979. Metallothionein in the extracellular fluids as an index of cadmium toxicity. Environ. Health Perspect., 28: 267-271.

Shaikh, Z.A. and Smith, J.C., 1980. Metabolism of orally ingested cadmium in humans. Dev. Toxicol. Environ. Sci., 8: 569-574.

Shank, K.E., Vetter, R.J. and Ziemer, P.L., 1977. A mathematical model of cadmium transport in a biological system. Environ. Res., 13: 209-214.

Sharrett, A.R., Carter, A.P., Orheim, R.M. and Feinleib, M., 1982. Daily intake of lead, cadmium, copper and zinc from drinking water: the Seattle study of trace metal exposure. Environ. Res., 28: 456-475.

Smith, J.C., Kench, J.E. and Lane, R.E., 1955. Determination of cadmium in urine and observations on urinary cadmium and protein excretion in men exposed to cadmium oxide dust. Biochem. J., 61: 698-701.

Sovet, Dr, 1858. Poisoning by a powdered silver-polishing agent. Presse Med. (Bel.), 10: 69-70.

Stowe, H.D., Wilson, M. and Goyer, R.A., 1972, Clinical and morphological effects of oral cadmium toxicity in rabbits. Arch. Pathol., 94: 389-405.

Suzuki, Y., 1980. Cadmium metabolism and toxicity in rats after long-term subcutaneous administration. J. Toxicol. Environ. Health. 6: 469-482.

Suzuki. S., Suzuki, T and Ashizawa, M., 1965. Proteinuria due to inhalation of cadmium stearate dust. Ind. Health, 3: 73-85.

Suzuki, S., and Taguchi, T., 1980. Retention, organ distribution and excretory pattern of cadmium orally administered in a single dose to monkeys. J. Toxicol. Environ. Health, 6: 783-796.

Suzuki, K.T., and Yamamura, M., 1979. Distribution of cadmium in liver and kidneys by loadings of various Cd-complexes and relative metal ratios in the induced metallothioneins. Biochem. Pharmacol., 28: 3643-3649.

Suzuki, K.T., Yamamura, M., Yamada, Y.K. and Shimizv, F., 1980. Distribution of cadmium in heavily cadmium-accumulated rat liver cytosols: metallothionein and related cadmium binding proteins. Toxicol. Lett., 8: 105-114.

Taguchi, T. and Suzuki, S., 1979a. The metabolism of 109-Cd administered to mice previously given an oral dose of cadmium. Jap. J. Hygiene, 34: 382-386.

Taguchi, T. and Suzuki, S., 1979b. The transport mechanism of cadmium by the small intestine of rats. Jap. J. Hyg., 34: 371-375.

Taguchi, T. and Suzuki, S., 1979c. Absorption rates of cadmium orally administered in a single dose to rats, and the sites in the digestive canal primarily concerned in absorbing Cd. Jap. J. Hyg., 34: 376-381.

Tanaka, K., 1982. Effects of hepatic disorder on the fate of cadmium in rats. Dev. Toxicol. Environ. Sci., 9: 237-249.

Thomas, R.G., Wilson, J.S. and London, V.E., 1980. Multispecies retention parameters for cadmium. Environ. Res., 23: 191-207.

Tipton, I.H. and Stewart, P.L., 1969. Patterns of elemental excretion in long-term balance studies: II. Health Physics Division Annual Progress Report for Period Ending July 31, 1969. ORNL-4446: 303-305.

Townshend, R.H., 1982. Acute cadmium pneumontis: a 17 year follow up. Brit. J. Ind. Med., 39: 411-412.

Travis, C.C. and Etnier, C.L., 1982. Dietary intake of cadmium in the United States, 1920-1975. Environ. Res., 27: 1-9.

Travis, C.C. and Haddock, A.G., 1980. Interpretation of the observed age-dependency of cadmium body burden in man. Environ. Res., 22: 46-60.

Tsuchiya, K., 1967. Proteinuria of workers exposed to cadmium fume: the relationship to concentration in the working environment. Arch. Environ. Health, 4: 875-880.

Tsuchiya, K., 1976. Proteinuria of cadmium workers. J. Occup. Med., 18: 463-466.

Tsuchiya, K., 1978.   Cadmium Studies in Japan - A Review, Elsevier, Amsterdam.

Tsuchiya, K., 1981.   Clinical signs, symptoms, and prognosis of cadmium poisoning.   In: Nriagu, J. (Ed.).   Cadmium in the Environment.   Part II: Health Effects.   John Wiley and Sons, New York: 39-54.

Tsvetkova, R.P., 1970. Gig, Truda, Prof. Zabolevanij, 12: 31-34.

Underwood, E.J., 1977.   Trace Elements in Human and Animal Nutrition. 4th edit. Academic Press, New York.

Watanabe, T., Shimada, T. and Endo, A., 1979. Mutagenic effects of cadmium on mammalian oocyte chromosomes.   Mutation Res., 67: 349-356.

Whanger, P.D., Riddlington, J.W. and Holcomb, C.L., 1980. Interactions of zinc and selenium on the binding of cadmium to rat tissues proteins. Ann. N.Y. Acad. Sci., 355: 333-346.

Yasamura, S., Vartsky, D., Ellis, K.J. and Cohn, S.H. 1980.   An overview of cadmium in human beings.   In: Nriagu, J.O. (Ed.). Cadmium in the Environment, Part I. Ecological Cycling, Wiley, New York: pp. 12-34.

Appendix 4
Lead

4.1   INTRODUCTION

Lead is a member of the group of elements commonly referred to as 'heavy metals' (Piotroswki and Coleman 1980; Martin and Coughtrey 1983). It is a soft, easily fusible, dull bluish-grey metallic element with a melting point of 327.5°C and a boiling point of 1744°C. Lead is in group IVa of the periodic table, but in many properties resembles the alkaline earths more than other members of this group, except that its halides, hydroxides and phosphates are insoluble (Gerber et al. 1980). The atomic number of lead is 82 and its atomic weight is 207.2 (Cotton and Wilkinson 1972). Lead is a well known industrial and environmental pollutant, and has been identified by Piotrowski and Coleman (1980) as an element of 'potential environmental concern'. Lead occurs naturally as 'relatively abundant' in the environment (Piotrowski and Coleman, 1980) and is the most abundant of the heavy metals (O'Brien et al. 1980). As a result of man's activity, global levels of lead have risen in several parts of the physical environment (WHO 1977; UNEP 1978). Long-range transport of atmospheric lead contributes to lead deposition, even in remote areas (Piotrowski and Coleman 1980). In particular, UNEP (1978) noted that analysis of lead in Greenland ice indicates an increase in concentration by a factor of 25 between 800 BC and 1750 AD. Current levels of lead in Greenland snow are approximately 0.2 μg kg^{-1}, which probably represents a factor of 500 above 'natural' levels.

The use of lead by man has been recorded from around 2500 BC (Patterson 1971), and O'Brien et al. (1980) speculated that the early use of lead, and its subsequent pollution of the environment, may have had some effect on 'baseline' levels. It was reported in Metallgesellschaft (1978), that, between 1968 and 1977, world production of refined lead rose from 3.55 to 4.27 million tonnes, of which approximately half came from recycling of lead products, particularly pipes, roofing and batteries. Roskill Information Service (1979) reported the following end uses for refined lead in 1976.

- 45% manufacture of batteries.
- 7% alkyl lead fuel additives.
- 9.5% cable sheathing.
- 15% chemicals.
- 6.5% alloys.
- 15% semi-manufactures etc.

The remaining 2% was not accounted for. It was noted by Piotrowki and Coleman (1980) that the use of lead as a fuel additive is relatively greater in the USA than Europe, but, as a result of national regulations, an overall decrease in its use has become apparent in recent years.

Nriagu (1979) estimated that the natural rate of emission of lead to atmosphere is 24,500 t y^{-1}, compared with an emission of 449,000 t y^{-1} due to man's activities. The greatest single source of lead to atmosphere is from combustion of lead alkyls in motor fuels; global emission from this source in 1974-1975 was estimated to be 267,000 t y^{-1}, which is equivalent to about 60% of total man-made release to atmosphere (Nriagu 1978, 1979; O'Brien et al. 1980). Other major sources of man-made lead emission to atmosphere in 1975 were listed by Nriagu (1979) as:

- iron and steel production (50,000 t);

TABLE 1

SUMMARY OF LEAD CONCENTRATIONS IN FOODSTUFFS

Material, location	Concentration ($\mu g \cdot g^{-1}$)	Reference and comments
Lean meat	0.2 (f.w.)	MAFF (1975)
Fresh fish	0.9 (f.w.)	
Shellfish	0.5-4 (f.w.)	Goldberg et al. (1978)
Mussels, USA	3.1 (f.w.)	
Atlantic and Pacific coasts		
Vegetables	0.2-56 (d.w.)	Warren and Delavault (1971)
England and Canada		
Wheat (hard), USA	0.5±0.22 (d.w.)	
Wheat (soft), USA	1.00±0.61 (d.w.)	
Flour (bakers patent), USA	0.92±0.43 (d.w.)	Zook et al. (1970)
Flour (soft patent), USA	1.02±0.59 (d.w.)	
Bread (white), USA	0.41±0.29 (d.w.)	
Tinned fruit	0.94	Thomas et al. (1975)
	(0.02-8.16)	
Condiments	0-1.5 (f.w.)	
Fish and seafood	0.2-2.5 (f.w.)	
Meat and eggs	0-0.37 (f.w.)	UNEP/WHO (1977)
Grains	0-1.39 (f.w.)	
Vegetables	0-1.3 (f.w.)	
Bottled milk, USA	<0.04	Angle et al. (1974)
Market milk, USA	0.049	Murthy et al. (1967)
	(0.023-0.079)	
Milk direct from cows, USA	0.009	IARC (1980), R
Market milk, USA	0.02-0.04	

TABLE 1 (Cont.)

Wine, various	0.060-0.255	}	UNEP/WHO (1977), cited
	0.130-0.190	}	in IARC (1980): R
	0.299	}	

Note:

(1) Specific items were listed by Warren and Delavault (1971) but have been considered together in this review.

- copper production (27,000 t);
- lead smelting (31,000 t);
- zinc production (17,000 t);
- combustion of coal (14,000 t).

The commonest ore of lead is galena, which is polymetallic and also represents a source of several other metals (O'Brien et al. 1980). Piotrowski and Coleman (1980) and O'Brien et al. (1980) noted that a mean concentration for lead in rock is around 20 μg g^{-1}, but that considerable variability exists, and even in uncontaminated areas the concentration may be an order of magnitude higher than this. Soils tend to reflect the composition of the parent material, and there is little agreement on the mean lead concentration or range. Bowen (1979) listed the following mean, median, or ranges, of values for the concentration of lead in the environment.

Geosphere

Granite	24 μg g^{-1}
Basalt	3 μg g^{-1}
Soil (contaminated)	35 μg g^{-1}
	(range 2-300)
Shale	23 μg g^{-1}
Limestone	5.7 μg g^{-1}
Sandstone	10 μg g^{-1}
Seawater	0.00003 μg l^{-1}
Freshwater (contaminated)	0.003 μg l^{-1}
Air (range)	0.0006-13.2 μg m^{-3}

Biosphere

Land plants	1-13 μg g^{-1} d.w.
Edible vegetables	0.2-20 μg g^{-1} d.w.
Mammal muscle	0.23-3.3 μg g^{-1} d.w.
Mammal bone	3.6-30 μg g^{-1} d.w.
Marine algae	2-40 μg g^{-1} d.w.
Marine fish	0.001-15 μg g^{-1} d.w.

Detailed discussions of lead in soil were given by Khan (1980) and Davis (1983). Considerable variability exists for estimated ranges of lead concentrations in soil. WHO (1973b) reported a range of 0.04 to 1.0 μg Pb g^{-1} soil, whereas, on the basis of 752 samples collected from several hundred UK farms (Archer 1977, unpublished report), it was suggested by O'Brien et al. (1980) that a mean concentration for lead in agricultural soils of temperate countries is around 50 μg g^{-1}. Summary mean estimates, ranges or recorded levels of lead in atmosphere, drinking water and food products are presented in Table 1.

4.1.1   Evidence of the carcinogenicity of lead

During the late 1930's and early 1940's, Fairhall and Miller (1941) maintained rats for two years on laboratory diets containing 0.1% lead arsenate or 0.1% lead carbonate. The mortality for the group fed lead carbonate was similar to that of the controls, but at the end of the two year period, the kidneys of rats in this experimental group were found to have many swollen cells with large vesicular nuclei and brown granules. The granules were most prominent in cells of the proximal convoluted tubules. No neoplasms were reported. Zollinger (1953) reported on the long-term effects of large doses of lead, and described tumours of the kidneys induced by repeated injections of lead phosphate. This finding was confirmed later by Walpole (personal communication, in Matthews and Walpole 1958). Van Esch et al. (personal communication, in Boyland et al. 1962) fed rats a diet containing 1% basic lead acetate for 2 years, and reported that many of the surviving rats had malignant tumours of the kidney. These findings were subsequently confirmed by Boyland et al. (1962) and van Esch et al. (1962) for dietary regimes containing 0.1% to 1.0% lead acetate. In view of the known toxicity of lead compounds, Boyland et al. (1962) expressed some surprise that rats should be able to survive for 2 years on a diet containing 1% lead acetate. Coogan et al. (1972) reported the occurrence of renal cortical adenomas and renal cortical carcinomas in rats given lead subacetate in the diet (1%), or by intraperitoneal or subcutaneous injection in aqueous solution. An equal incidence was noted, irrespective of route of administration of lead, as follows.

Period of administration	% Incidence	
	Adenomas	Carcinomas
20 to 40 weeks	10 to 20	2 to 4
40 to 60 weeks	70 to 75	8 to 10
60 to 90 weeks	50 to 60	30 to 35

Furst et al. (1976) demonstrated the carcinogenic potential of aqueous solutions of lead chromate injected intramuscularly in mice and rats. Three rats, from 50 tested, developed renal tumours, despite the very low solubility of lead chromate in water. Sixty-four per cent of rats developed malignant tumours at the site of injection. Powdered elemental lead administered to rats perorally or by intramuscular injection "did not seem to produce any appreciable number of tumours" (Furst et al. 1976). On the basis of these findings, Furst (1977) concluded that, in animals, certain compounds of lead are carcinogenic, but that elemental lead is not.

The IARC concluded that there is 'sufficient evidence' for the carcinogenicity of lead compounds, notably acetate, subacetate and phosphate, in experimental animals (IARC 1979; 1980). They also concluded that there are inadequate data with respect to the carcinogenicity of compounds of lead in man (IARC 1979), but: "in the absence of adequate human data, it is reasonable, for practical purposes, to regard these compounds as if they presented a carcinogenic risk to humans" (IARC 1980). The carcinogenicity of lead has also been reviewed by Moore and Meredith (1979) and Gerber et al. (1980).

Moore and Meredith (1979) noted that several studies (Azar et al. 1973; Fouts and Page 1942; van Esch and Kroes 1969) had failed to demonstrate a pathological effect of lead on renal function in hamsters and dogs, and in one instance (Babenko et al. 1977) organic lead was shown to inhibit the growth of Brown-Pierce carcinoma of the eye. Manuel (personal communiciation in Moore and Meredith 1979) never observed any carcinogenic effects of lead, in all of his studies of pathological effects of lead in primates. Moore and Meredith (1979) concluded as follows:

> "In the search for the various compounds that might
> cause cancer in man it is easy to be deluded by the
> chimera of potential carcinogenicity and upon this
> basis to make unwarranted extrapolations from animal
> studies to man. It is clear even from the animal
> studies that considerable species and sex differences
> exist in the carcinogenicity of lead. The evidence to
> date has not proven that lead can cause cancer in man."

Gerber et al. (1980) commented that evidence for the carcinogenicity of lead in man is inadequate, and, where available, often contradictory. In so far as lead does have a carcinogenic effect in at least some animal species, the mechanism of carcinogenicity is unknown (Furst et al. 1976; Gerber et al. 1980). Furst et al. (1976) suggested, with respect to renal cancer, that the disturbance of porphyrin synthesis by lead may be a contributory factor. Gerber et al. (1980) noted that lead can be concentrated in nuclei, and Sirover and Loeb (1976) have shown that lead chloride concentrations of 20 to 150 mM affect the fidelity of DNA synthesis in vitro.

4.1.2   Symptoms of lead poisoning

As far as is known, lead has no beneficial or desirable nutritional effects in man or animals (WHO 1973a), and is one of the few metals which seems to have toxic effects, but no essential function, in the organism (Gerber et al. 1980). Evidence for the toxicity of lead in man and experimental animals is extensive and the toxic properties of lead have been recognised for many centuries and probably since the second century BC (e.g. Lauer 1955; Green et al. 1978; Damstra 1977 and Gerber et al. 1980). The first scientific description of lead poisoning was given by Tanquerel des Planches (1839).

Lead is unusual among toxic agents in that the concentration which can cause symptoms is less than an order of magnitude above normal body levels (Gerber et al. 1980; Piotrowski and O'Brien 1980). Gerber et al. (1980) cited as an example that a normal blood lead concentration is around "200 ppb; subclinical changes are noted in particularly sensitive persons at 400 to 600 ppb; and clinical symptoms can arise at more than 600 ppb". This small margin presents problems in setting attainable guidelines for acceptable levels of lead in the human environment (Piotrowski and O'Brien 1980). The symptoms and pathology of lead poisoning (also referred to as 'plumbism' or 'saturnism') lie somewhat outside the scope of this review, except in so far as they affect metabolism of the element. Extensive reviews of the literature pertaining to clinical aspects of lead poisoning are available (e.g. Gerber et al. 1980; Piotrowski and O'Brien 1980; Green et al. 1978; Damstra 1977; Smith 1976; Goyer and Mushak 1977), and data relating to the causes of mortality of workers occupationally exposed to lead have been analysed in several studies (e.g. Malcolm and Barnett 1982; Tokudome and Kuratsune 1976;

Robinson 1976; Cooper and Gaffey 1975). The following simplified descriptions of the symptoms of chronic and acute lead intoxication are based largely upon the above mentioned sources.

4.1.2.1   Chronic intake

The following have been reported as being among the most commonly encountered sources for lead poisoning:
- lead based paints;
- lead water-storage vessels, or lead water-pipes;
- illictly stilled spirits, such as whisky;
- industrial exposure.

Excepting industrial exposure, young children appear to be at particular risk, and this is associated with their tendancy to pica, which may result in ingestion of large amounts of lead from lead based paints. Green et al. (1978) estimated that 'one small paint chip' may contain up to 100 μg of lead. In further statement, Green et al. (1978) noted that " a paint chip the size of a thumb nail may contain 100 μg of a lead salt." Newsprint, ink, lead soldering on cans, or lead from toothpaste tubes may also contribute to the intake of children with a tendency to chew objects (Smith 1976). Direct inhalation of automobile exhaust fumes is also likely to be of some importance, particularly in urban areas (Goyer and Mushak 1977).

Early symptoms of lead poisoning identified by Green et al. (1978) include the following:
- anorexia;
- recurrent sporadic vomiting;
- colic;
- anaemia;
- irritability;
- constipation.

Severe encephalopathic symptoms have been identified by Green et al. (1978) to include:
- hyperirritability;
- agitation;
- ataxia;
- weakness;
- paralysis of the upper motor neurons;
- stupor;
- convulsion;
- coma, associated with a high mortality rate.

It should be noted that lead has been called a great imitator, with respect to its clinical manifestations. Onset of lead poisoning may be insidious and the symptoms can be confused with those of other causes of intoxication (Lauer 1955).

Clinical evidence currently suggests that 'lead' poisoning is more prevalent in summer months, but the causative agent has not been conclusively identified, nor should lead poisoning be considered a 'summertime disease' (Green et al. 1978; Goyer and Mushak 1977). The biological and physiological changes which accompany symptoms of lead poisoning have been reviewed by Gerber et al. (1980).

4.1.2.2   Acute intakes

In contrast with lead poisoning in children, cases of intoxication in adults usually derive from acute ingestion and are related to industrial exposure (Green et al. 1978). Industrial workers, or occupations, noted by Ziegfeld (1964) and summarised by Green et al. (1978) to be at particular risk with regard to lead poisoning are those involved with; lead mining, smelting and refining, storage battery manufacture, ship breaking, automobile body and other painting, pottery glazing and ceramics, petroleum products, cable construction, munitions, preventive shielding and noise and vibration control.

Green et al. (1978) noted that the distinction between symptoms of chronic and acute ingestion is vague. Ingestion of metallic lead does not result in acute intoxication, but the lead is retained as a source of chronic poisoning. An acute symptomatic episode may occur days to weeks after ingestion and is indistinguishable from chronic poisoning. Treatment is the same as for chronic poisoning (Green et al. 1978). Following acute ingestion, symptoms are primarily related to the gastrointestinal tract and include a 'metallic taste', dry mouth, nausea, vomiting and abdominal pain. Systemic symptoms may include anaemia, proteinuria, weakness, headache, paraesthesias, pain and cramp in legs, depression, coma and death. In the case of acute exposure to tetraethyl lead (TEL) or tetramethyl lead (TML), which are used as additives to automobile petrol, Chisolm (1971) and Sanders (1964), estimated that a 20% mortality rate accompanies severe symptoms of the disease. If a patient does not succumb sequelae are reported to be rare.

Industry is required to control and monitor lead exposure, and a safe level for lead, as TEL, was cited by Green et al. (1978) to be 75 μg Pb m^{-3}, for a 40 hour working week at 8 hours per day. The recommended limit of exposure to soluble particulate inorganic compounds of lead was cited as 200 μg m^{-3}. This level is reported to result at most in mild intoxication (Kehoe 1967). Green et al. (1978) cited the following as 'well tolerated' limits for different durations of exposure in the workplace.

Duration of exposure (h)	Upper limit for lead in air (μg m^{-3})
1	1000
2	600
3	400
4	280

Monitoring of workers with known potential exposure is also undertaken, and levels of urinary coproporphyrin (UCP) and δ-aminolevulinic acid are stated by Green et al. (1978) to be "[probably]

the most reliable indicators of body lead load and soft tissue
concentrations of lead." At UCP levels of 110 µg l^{-1} a worker should be
placed on a watch list, at 150 µg l^{-1} transferred to a low-exposure area,
and at 200 µg l^{-1} a medical doctor should be consulted and treatment
initiated if necessary (Fleming 1964; Karpatkin 1961; cited in Green
et al. 1978).

4.2   INTAKE RATES

4.2.1   Dietary intake

It is commonly reported that the major intake of lead by members of
the general public is from food (e.g. Goyer and Mushack 1977; Angle and
McIntire 1979). In this context, the ICRP (1975) noted that between 44%
and 100% of lead intake is by way of food. Data presented in Table 1
indicate that lead is detectable in all foodsources which have been
analysed, and this is in accord with the ICRP (1975) statement that,
"lead is a common contaminant of the human environment." There is limited
evidence that shellfish and selected vegetables concentrate lead, but it
was noted by Underwood (1977) that "published values for lead content of
individual food items are so variable that it is difficult to provide a
meaningful classification into high, medium and low groups". Although
some of this variability may be due to differing analytical techniques it
is likely that considerable intrinsic variability also exists. On the
basis of data presented in Table 1 a 'typical' value for lead in fresh
food items is <1 µg g^{-1} f.w. Milk generally has a lower concentration of
lead (<0.05 µg ml^{-1}) than other food items. However, it is notable that
tinned evaporated milk has been reported to contain 0.202 µg Pb ml^{-1}
(Mitchell and Aldous 1974; Underwood 1977), which is somewhat higher than
bulk milk samples. The elevated level of lead in tinned milk, and other
tinned food items, may derive from the lead solder in the seams and caps
of tins (UNEP/WHO 1977; IARC 1980). Mitchell and Aldous (1974) have drawn
attention to the potential health hazard arising from lead in tinned baby
foods. They reported that of 256 baby foods tested, mostly fruit juices,
62% of those in metal (non-aluminium) containers had lead levels of
0.1 µg ml^{-1} or more, 37% contained 0.2 µg ml^{-1} or more, and 12% contained
0.4 µg ml^{-1} or more. Of products in glass or aluminium containers, only
1% had levels in excess of 0.2 µg ml^{-1}. Results obtained by Thomas et al.
(1975) demonstrated a range of lead levels in samples of tinned fruits,
obtained from the UK, of 0.02 to 8.16 µg g^{-1}. Of the 168 samples tested,
16 were above the statutory limit of 2 µg g^{-1}
      Food wrappings, other than metal containers, have also been reported
to contain high levels of lead. Watkins et al. (1976) reported
concentrations ranging from 1400 µg g^{-1} in an ice-cream bar wrapping to
28700 µg g^{-1} in a bread wrapping. Vegetables grown in contaminated soils
can accumulate high levels of lead. Davies (1978) reported finding lead
in radishes (1.1 to 56.7 µg g^{-1} d.w.) and potatoes (1.91 to
3.91 µg g^{-1} d.w.) grown in soils containing high lead levels, but no
consistent correlation was observed between plant and soil concentrations
of lead.
      With respect to the above statements on the variability of lead
content in individual food items, it is notable that estimated total

TABLE 2

ESTIMATED DIETARY INTAKES OF LEAD

Diet	Daily intake of lead (µg)	Comments	Reference
Food Fluids	0.15-0.44[1]	Typical intake estimated be 0.44 mg d^{-1}	ICRP (1975, 1980): R
Total diet	0.14[2]	UK	MAFF (1975)
Total food and beverages	0.32[3]	UK	Monier-Williams (1949)
Total food and beverages	0.32±0.15	UK	Hamilton and Minski (1972/1973)
Total food and beverages	0.28	USA	Schroeder and Tipton (1968)
Total food and beverages	0.239-0.318	Japan	Horiuchi (1965)
Total food and beverages	0.105	Holland	Reith et al. (1974)
Average total	0.10-0.50	Adults	IARC (1980): R
	0.13	Children under 3	
General population	0.10-0.30	USA, adults	Goyer and Mushak (1977): R
	0.1	USA, children	
Diet, individuals site close to a smelter	0.67-2.64		UNEP/WHO (1977), cited in IARC (1980): R
General diet	0.085[2]	USA	O'Brien et al. (1980): R from Bogen et al. (1975)

Notes:

(1) ICRP (1975) noted that no data are available which are directly applicable intake by children, but that a value of 0.035-0.15 mg d^{-1} can be calculated.

TABLE 2 (Cont.)

(2) A summarised breakdown of values was listed by O'Brien et al. (1975) as follows:

Dietary intake of lead ($\mu g \ y^{-1}$)

Foodsource	UK	USA
Cereals	11.7	5.8
Meat and fish	10.6	6.5
Fruit	10.2	8.3
Root vegetables	6.9	3.8
Green vegetables	7.6	3.5
Milk	2.9	3.2
Total	49.9	31.1

(3) Estimated value for "normal, healthy individuals".

daily average dietary lead intakes are generally in good agreement, particularly with regard to estimates for individuals not known to be occupationally or environmentally exposed to high lead levels. Data presented in Table 2 indicate a range of values between 0.1 and 0.5 mg d^{-1}. The ICRP (1975; 1980) defined a total mean daily lead intake of 0.44 mg for Reference Man. It is clear from data presented in Table 2 that this estimate is at the upper end of the range of reported values, and a more representative estimate is taken to be 0.3 mg d^{-1}. However, daily intakes may be up to an order of magnitude larger than this for individuals in areas exposed to smelter emissions; thus it was reported by UNEP/WHO (1977) that people in one locality near a smelter had lead intakes ranging between 0.67 and 2.64 mg d^{-1}. For the purposes of, modelling an estimated range of intakes of 0.2 to 0.4 mg Pb d^{-1} is taken to represent most localities.

4.2.2   Ingestion of lead from non-edible sources

Lead may be present at very high concentrations in substances normally considered to be non-edible, such as soil, dust and lead-based paint (Table 3). The tendency for young children to place non-edible objects or materials into their mouths may give rise to intakes of lead from these sources which can be in excess of intakes derived from diet. Largely on the basis of potential for ingestion of lead from non-edible sources, the US government has defined as hazardous products any objects for consumer use, particularly if accessible to children, which contain more than 0.06% lead by weight in the surface paint or other similar surface coatings (IARC 1980).

For 15 high school children, in urban and suburban areas, Angle et al. (1974) reported correlations between blood lead and lead in soil ($r = 0.31$) or house dust ($r = 0.29$). Samples obtained for 16 urban school children aged 10-12 years indicated a significant correlation between blood lead and lead in soil ($r = 0.49$, $p<0.05$) but no correlation between blood lead and house dust ($r = 0.01$). In a study conducted in Hartford, USA, Lepow et al. (1975) commented that ingestion of 0.25 g street dirt (mean lead concentration 1200 µg g^{-1}) or house dust (mean lead concentration 11000 µg g^{-1}) could result in an extra daily intake of 300 or 2750 µg lead respectively. In addition, they noted a lead in dirt-on-hands concentration of 2400 µg g^{-1}. Given that approximately 10 mg of dirt-on-hands can be ingested by sucking or licking the fingers or hand, they estimated that a small child playing in such a contaminated environment and putting his hands or fingers in his mouth ten times a day could theoretically ingest 240 µg lead. Leaded paints were recognised as a further potential source of ingestion by small children and Lepow et al. (1975) summarised an estimated potential daily lead intake for a two-year-old child as follows.

Source	Potential daily intake of lead (µg)
Inhalation	6-60
Ingestion:	
paint	50000
dust	2750
dirt	300
dirt-on-hands	240
food and water	130-170

Smith (1976) and Green et al. (1978) also identified paint chips and other non-edible lead containing materials as potential sources of ingestion of lead by young children.

Angle and McIntire (1979) demonstrated a simple Peirson correlation between the concentration of lead in blood and lead in house dust for children 1-5 years (r = 0.29) and 6-18 years (r = 0.29). A significant bivariate correlation (p<0.001) was fitted to the data for all children, 1-18 years, as follows.

$$PbB = 8.2 \ PbHD^{0.16}; \ n = 1074, \ r = 0.29$$

where   PbB is the concentration of lead in blood and,

PbHD is the concentration of lead in house dust.

A further Peirson correlation was calculated between the concentrations of lead in blood and lead in soil for children 1-5 years (r = 0.27) and 6-18 years (r = 0.4). For all children in the study, aged 1-18 years, a significant bivariate correlation (p<0.001) was calculated as follows.

$$PbB = 9.5 \ PbS^{0.15}; \ n = 1074, \ r = 0.38$$

where   PbS is the concentration of lead in soil.

Angle and McIntire (1979) suggested that there may have been a steeper slope for the line of regression for the 1-5 year olds, but this was not commented upon further. Considerable within- and between-individual variability was found in analysis of samples, but this was considered, by Angle and McIntire (1979), to compare favourably with the variance reported for other studies by Lucas (1977).

Roels et al. (1980) reported high correlations between the amount of lead on hands of Belgian school children and the concentration of lead in dust collected from their respective school yards, which were within 1 km of a lead smelter, as follows.

TABLE 3

CONCENTRATION OF LEAD IN DUST SAMPLES

Location	Concentration	Reference
USA 1963-1971; three geographically separate sites	1-34 mg m^{-2}	Angle and McIntire (1979)
Belgian school yards		Roels et al. (1980)
rural areas	0.122 mg g^{-1}	
urban areas >2.5 km from smelter	0.114 mg g^{-1}	
urban areas 2.5 km from smelter	0.466 mg g^{-1}	
urban areas <1 km from smelter	2.56 mg g^{-1}	
Hartford, USA		Lepow et al. (1975)
outdoor dirt	1.2 mg g^{-1} (95% conf. limits, 0.7-1.7 mg g^{-1})	
household dust	11.0 mg g^{-1} (95% conf. limits, 4.9-17.0 mg g^{-1})	
Omaha, USA[1]		Angle et al. (1974)
dustfall suburban areas	~3.0 mg m^{-2} mo^{-1}	
dustfall urban areas	11.4-32.96 mg m^{-2} mo^{-1}	
housedust suburban areas	0.335±0.0068-0.340±0.078 mg g^{-1}	
housedust urban areas	0.361±0.036-0.572±0.147 mg g^{-1}	
USA housedust	GM[2] Range	Angle and McIntire (1979)
site C	479 76-5571 mg g^{-1}	
site M	300 76-860 mg g^{-1}	
site S	211 81-845 mg g^{-1}	

Notes:

(1) Self-collected environmental samples by elementary-school children (age 10-12 years) and high-school children (age 14-18 years).

(2) GM; geometrical mean.

Boys:

$$PbH = -5.9 + 0.172 \; PbD;$$

$$n = 4, \; r = 0.999, \; p < 0.001.$$

Girls:

$$PbH = -6.8 + 0.097 \; PbD;$$

$$n = 4, \; r = 0.994, \; p < 0.01.$$

where   PbH is the amount of (µg) on each hand;
               PbD is the concentration of lead in dust ($\mu g \; g^{-1}$).

They also reported a very high correlation between the amount of lead on hands and the concentration of lead in blood. For boys and girls tested, this was shown to be:

$$PbB = -4.33 + 11.54 \; \log(PbH);$$

$$n = 8, \; r = 0.976, \; p < 0.001.$$

where   PbB is the concentration of lead in blood ($\mu g \; ml^{-1}$)

All children in the above study were stated to be past the age of pica, hence it was inferred by Roels et al. (1980) that "lead particles deposited by the smelter in the environment are ingested mainly via excessively lead-contaminated hands". No general estimate can be provided for the amount of lead likely to be ingested from non-edible sources, since this will clearly be highly site-specific and dependent upon the habits of the individual. However, it is clear that this may be a significant source of lead which can be absorbed systematically. Haley (1977) reported that pica is the most important source of lead in pediatric plumbism, followed by lead-based window putty and earth contaminated with lead-based paint chips. Several other non-edible sources were also recognised. A summary of data reported for the concentration of lead in household and external dust is presented in Table 3. It is noted that data presented are not exhaustive, but indicate the range of values which may be found.

4.2.3   Lead in drinking water

The WHO International Standard (WHO 1971) and WHO European Standard (WHO 1970) for lead in drinking water are both set at 100 µg l^{-1}. More stringent controls have been adopted in the USA and for the European Community, with the maximum contaminant level of lead in drinking water established at 50 µg l^{-1} (US Environmental Protection Agency 1976; European Economic Community, EEC 1975a). In the European Community, a limit of 50 µg l^{-1} is also set for surface waters intended for the abstraction of drinking water (EEC 1975b). In Japan, the content of lead in drinking water must not exceed 100 µg l^{-1} (Ministry of Health and Welfare 1978).

The concentration of lead in drinking water may vary markedly (Table 4) on occasion exceeding the statutory limits noted above. The

TABLE 4

CONCENTRATION OF LEAD IN DRINKING WATER

Location	Concentration (µg l^{-1})	Reference
USA, Omaha	<10	Angle et al. (1974)
USA, Seattle		
25th percentile (1)	0.7 , 2.9	
50th percentile (1)	2.8, 5.5	
75th percentile (1)	5.9, 15.3	Sharrett et al. (1982)[3]
25th percentile (2)	0.8, 1.7	
50th percentile (2)	1.9, 3.7	
75th percentile (2)	3.5, 8.6	
USA	13.1 (max. 64)	
USA; two cities with	30	Safe Drinking Water Committee (1977)
lead service system piping	(13–1510)	

Notes:

(1) Running water and standing water respectively: houses with copper piping at the house shut-off valve
(2) Running water and standing water respectively: houses with galvanized piping at the house shut-off valve
(3) On the basis of data obtained, Sharrett et al. (1982) estimated the following daily intakes of lead from drinking water by Seattle employees:

	Intake (mg d^{-1})	
	Houses < 5 years old	Houses > 5 years old
Running water	0.031	0.006
Standing water	0.111	0.014

observed variation reflects the original water concentration, water treatment, pH and distribution system (Safe Drinking Water Committee 1977; IARC 1980). A study of raw (untreated) and finished (ready for distribution) water by the US National Academy of Sciences (Safe Drinking Water Committee 1977) demonstrated concentrations of lead in finished water ranging between 1 and 139 μg l^{-1}, with a mean of 33.9 μg l^{-1}. The range for raw water was reported to be 2 to 140 μg l^{-1}, with a mean of 23 μg l^{-1}. Tap water from 969 water systems in the USA contained an average lead concentration of 13.1 μg l^{-1}, with a maximum recorded concentration of 64 μg l^{-1}. Comparison between finished water (chlorination treatment only) and slightly acidic tap water in two USA cities using lead piping showed that in every one of the 383 household samples the lead concentration was higher at tap than at the treatment plant. The lead concentration in tap water ranged between 13 and 1510 μg l^{-1}, with a mean of 30 μg l^{-1} (Safe Drinking Water Committee 1977). On the basis of a review of these data, the International Agency for Research on Cancer (IARC 1980) concluded that lead appears to enter drinking water chiefly in the distribution system, including household plumbing. In addition to the above noted variability, concentrations of lead in drinking water have been observed to be increased following storms, as a result of metals present in surface runoff and storm-water collection systems entering urban watersheds (Pfaender et al. 1977).

Estimates of the daily intake of lead from drinking water have been reported by the ICRP (1975) to range between 0.01 mg and 0.024 mg, but data presented by Sharrett et al. (1982) indicate a range of 0.006 mg to 0.111 mg. The range of values reported by Sharrett et al. (1982) reflects the different materials used for water pipes and consumption of either 'running' or 'standing' water. It is clear from the variability of data presented in Table 4 that no single estimate can be assigned as a 'typical value' to the concentration of lead in drinking water. However, the range of mean values is generally between 5 and 30 μg l^{-1}. On this basis, and assuming a daily intake of 1.6 l of drinking water (ICRP 1975), it is estimated that between 0.008 mg d^{-1} and 0.048 mg d^{-1} of lead is ingested in drinking water. By comparison with dietary intakes or ingestion of lead from non-edible sources, the intake due to drinking water is generally small, being less than or approximately equal to 5% of dietary intake (Section 4.2.1). At the highest recorded concentration of lead in drinking water, 1510 μg l^{-1} (Table 4), the corresponding daily intake would be 2.4 mg of lead, which is considerably more than the mean daily dietary intake estimated in Section 4.2.1.

Greathouse et al. (1977) reported that in a survey of 969 community water systems in the US, only 1.4% of the 2995 drinking water samples exceeded the US Public Health Service limit of 50 μg Pb l^{-1}. However, they also noted that when corrosive water is distributed, as for instance in some geographic areas of the northeast and northwest USA, the problem may be locally widespread, particularly where lead service lines are used to convey the water. McCabe et al. (1970) studied tap water quality in the Beacon Hill area of Boston and showed that 65% of the 54 households sampled had in excess of 50 μg Pb l^{-1}, with some samples 5-6 times this value. In that area, the source water has a low initial concentration of lead, but is soft and slightly acidic.

TABLE 5

CONCENTRATIONS OF LEAD IN ATMOSPHERE

Locality	Concentration (ng m^{-3})	Comments	Reference
Uncontaminated samples 1971-1977	0.63-21		Bowen (1979)
Contaminated samples	28-2700	Maximum reported value of 13000 ng m^{-3} for USA	
USA, 1970-1977	40-1660	Three geographically separate sites	Angle and McIntire (1979)
USA, mean values	1000-7700 (95% conf. limits 700-9900)		Lepow et al. (1975)
Belgian school yards			
rural areas	300		Roels et al. (1980)
urban areas >2.5 km from smelter	450		
urban areas 2.5 km from smelter	800		
urban areas <1 km from smelter	3670		
Remote areas	0.1-1		IARC (1980): R
UK: 7 rural sites, 1974	33-245 (27-200 ng kg^{-1})		Cawse (1975)
European: mean values	400-7500		Fishbein (1976)
Tokyo: 10 sites, annual average	650		
Urban, average	1100		NAS (1972)
Non-urban (near cities), average	210		
Rural	20		
USA, Omaha:			
urban	430-630		Angle et al. (1974)
suburban	290		
USA, Lead smelters	6670-2.9x10^6		Constant et al. (1977)
USA	6-300	Organic lead concentration	Harrison and Perry (1977)
Stockholm, Sweden	400-3370		
London, UK	40-110		

4.2.4   Inhalation of lead

The concentrations of lead in air can be highly variable, particularly due to the influence of local contamination. Data for the concentration of lead in air are summarised in Table 5, which is intended only as a guide to atmospheric lead levels and is not an exhaustive listing of all data available. In order to facilitate consideration of data, intake by inhalation can be divided into two broad categories, environmental and occupational.

4.2.4.1   Inhalation of environmental lead

It has been estimated, on the basis of geochemical data, that naturally occurring levels of lead in the atmosphere are approximately 0.5 to 0.6 ng m^{-3} (Patterson 1965; UNEP/WHO 1977). The natural concentration arises from airborne dust and from gases diffusing through the earth's crust (IARC 1980). As noted in Section 4.1, emissions of lead to the atmosphere deriving from man-made sources are considerably greater than natural emissions. It has been reported by the International Agency for Cancer Research (IARC 1980) that approximately 98% of the total releases of lead to atmosphere in the USA are from the combustion of leaded petrol. The US National Academy of Sciences (NAS 1972) recorded that concentrations of lead in ambient air are closely related to the density of vehicular traffic. Lead concentrations measured along a highway in Los Angeles were as high 54300 ng m^{-3}. Harrison and Parry (1977) reported that urban air concentrations of organic lead in the US varied between 6 and 300 ng m^{-3}. Corresponding values for Stockholm and London were 400 to 3370 ng m^{-3} and 40 to 110 ng m^{-3} respectively. Levels reported for petrol stations varied from 210 to 1540 ng m^{-3} and, in an underground car park, levels of 1900 to 2200 ng m^{-3} were recorded.

Other major sources of lead emissions to atmosphere are lead smelting and solid waste disposal (NAS 1972; Faoro and McMullen 1977; IARC 1980). Constant et al. (1977) recorded lead-in-air concentrations of 6.67 to 2990 µg m^{-3} at two primary lead smelters in the USA. Solid wastes remelted in secondary smelters, or burned in municipal incinerators, also result in large localised inputs of lead to atmosphere (UNEP/WHO 1977). Coal and oil burning have also been identified as minor local sources of atmospheric lead (UNEP/WHO 1977). However, their global contribution to atmospheric lead may be significant.

In the USA, an ambient air quality standard has been established, limiting the concentration of lead in air to 1.5 µg m^{-3} as an arithmetic mean averaged over a calendar quarter (Environmental Protection Agency 1978; IARC 1980). From information presented in Table 5, and discussed above, it is likely that this limit is exceeded in several instances.

Depending upon locality, the daily inhalation of environmental lead may vary markedly. The ICRP (1975) estimated a mean inhalation of 10 µg d^{-1}, whereas Goyer and Mushak (1977) concluded that up to 20 µg d^{-1} may be inhaled. However, in a study at Hartford, USA, Lepow et al. (1975) estimated that a two-year-old child could inhale between 6 and 60 µg d^{-1}, assuming a daily respiration of 6 m^3 and a lead-in-air concentration of 1 to 10 µg m^{-3}. Data presented in Table 5 indicate that average atmospheric concentrations of lead in urban areas generally do not exceed 5 µg m^{-3}. On this basis, and assuming an inhalation rate of 23 m^3 d^{-1} (ICRP 1975) up to 115 µg Pb d^{-1} could be inhaled. In the vicinity of lead smelters the value could be considerably higher. For the purposes of metabolic modelling, it may be assumed that atmospheric lead concentrations vary between 0.05 and 5 µg m^{-3}, implying a range of approximately 1 to 100 µg Pb d^{-1} inhaled, with the majority of individuals, particularly in non-urban areas, exposed at the lower end of this range.

Angle and McIntire (1979) calculated a bivariate correlation between lead in blood and lead in air for 1-18 year olds. A significant and positive correlation was obtained only for 6-18 year olds, as follows.

$$PbB = 23.2 \ PbA^{0.08};$$

$$n = 832, \ r = 0.31, \ p<0.001.$$

where   PbB is the concentration of lead in blood (µg 100 ml^{-1}) and

PbA is the concentration of lead in air (µg m^{-3}).

In a more recent study on Belgian school children, Roels et al. (1980) demonstrated that blood lead and atmospheric lead levels were not corre-lated directly, although atmospheric lead levels were highly correlated with lead-on-hands, which in turn was highly correlated with the concen-tration of lead in blood.

In addition to atmospheric concentrations of lead a further source of inhaled lead derives from the smoking of cigarettes. The International Agency for Research on Cancer (IARC 1980) reviewed data relating to the level of lead in tobacco and the concentration in mainstream smoke. Several brands of cigarettes from the USA were sampled in 1957 and found to contain between 21 and 84 µg of lead per cigarette, with 1.0 to 3.3 µg per cigarette transferred to mainstream smoke. It is believed that these concentrations resulted from residues of the insecticide lead arsenate, which was at one time commonly used in tobacco fields. More recent find-ings have suggested that cigarettes contain 10.4 to 12.15 µg of lead per cigarette, of which 0.48 µg per cigarette is transferred to total smoke. UNEP/WHO (1977) estimated that 2% of lead in cigarettes is transferred to mainstream smoke and that direct inhalation of lead from smoking twenty cigarettes per day could be as high as 5 µg d^{-1}.

4.2.4.2   Inhalation of lead due to occupational exposure

An air quality standard, limiting the maximum permissible exposure at work to 50 µg m^{-3} averaged over an 8 hour period has been adopted in the USA (Occupational Safety and Health Administration 1979). A comparable recommendation, of 100 µg m^{-3}, has been made by the MAK committee of West Germany (Senatskommission 1977). The time-weighted average allowable concentrations for lead as inorganic fumes and dusts are 150 µg m^{-3} in East Germany, 100 µg m^{-3} Sweden and 50 µg m^{-3} in Czechoslovakia. In Russia, a maximum permissible concentration is established at 10 µg m^{-3} (Winell 1975; IARC 1980). A concentration of 100 µg m^{-3} corresponds to an intake of ∿960 µg over an 8 h shift.

TABLE 6

THE DISTRIBUTION OF STABLE LEAD IN HUMAN TISSUES[1]

Organ, tissue or tissue fluid	Concentration in μg g^{-1} (number of samples)	Weighted mean[2] (μg g^{-1})	Unweighted mean[2] (μg g^{-1})	Number of samples
Adrenal	1.04(6), 0.16(29), 0.18(16), 2.27(15)	0.72	0.91	66
Aorta	3.6(2), 1.05(5), 1.25(19), 1.89(10), 1.27(39), 2.24(104), 1.25(16), 2.52(15), 1.26(66), 0.85(5)	1.72	1.72	281
Bile	21(50)(3)	21	21	50
Blood (total)	0.26(502), 0.255(6151), 0.19(430), 0.119(2000), 0.177(47), 0.339(140), 0.196(28), 0.3(200), 0.29(115), 0.28(103), 0.40(100), 0.284(15), 0.11(244), 0.22(2849), 0.30(226), 0.17(897), 0.17(801), 0.182(2456), 0.37(30), 0.088(1)	0.214	0.235	17335
Blood (erythrocytes)	0.374(79), 0.51(30), 0.61(16), 0.69(25), 0.15(?), 0.45(200)	0.46	0.46	>350
Blood (plasma)	0.024(30), 0.039(17), 0.125(17), 0.108(16), 0.158(25), 0.18(200), 0.012(1), 0.155(11), 0.034(63)	0.13	0.093	380
Blood (serum)	0.035(170), 0.13(105), 0.016(1), 0.3(39), <0.04(1)	0.099	0.104	316
Bone	34(1), 23.2(258), 37.3(341), 35(5), 18.8(?), 17.2(44), 71(106), 10.8(30), 19(60), 42.5(19), 10(19), 23.2(31), 30(1)	25.7	28.6	>1175

TABLE 6 (Cont.)

Organ, tissue or tissue fluid	Concentration in µg g^{-1} (number of samples)	Weighted mean [2] (µg g^{-1})	Unweighted mean [2] (µg g^{-1})	Number of samples
Brain	0.50(191), 0.075(5), 0.075(5), 0.21(17), 0.15(51), 0.09(8), 0.084(61), 0.18(97), 0.31(7), 0.13(?), 0.30(10), 0.40(?)	0.31	0.208	>452
Cerebrospinal fluid	0.025–0.60(?)			?
Diaphragm	0.121(91)[4]	0.121	0.121	91
Gastrointestinal tract:				
unspecified	0.23(?), 0.78(22), 0.12(34)	0.77	0.38	>56
caecum	0.216(31), 0.13(34)	0.171	0.173	65
colon	0.104(13), ND(?)	0.104	<0.104	>13
duodenum	0.2(68)	0.2	0.2	68
ileum	0.16(84)	0.16	0.16	84
jejunum	0.103(104)	0.103	0.103	104
rectum	0.16(42)	0.16	0.16	42
stomach	0.096(131), 0.22(?), 0.23(11), 0.115(33)	0.108	0.165	>175
Hair[5]	16.5(293), 51(166), 30.2(426), 18.2(164), 9.4(200), 16(178), 14.4(147), 25.4(40), 9.9(?), 70(18), 12.2(121), 20.4(29), 8.9(20), 3(1), 30(2)	22.5	22.4	>1805
Heart	0.2(140), 0.055(43), 0.26(19), 0.46(63), 0.218(8), 0.53(186), 0.082(66), 0.38(?), 0.98(23), 0.075(64), 0.40(?)	0.32	0.33	612

TABLE 6 (Cont.)

Organ, tissue or tissue fluid	Concentration in µg g^{-1} (number of samples)	Weighted mean[2] (µg g^{-1})	Unweighted mean[2] (µg g^{-1})	Number of samples
Kidney	0.54(25), 0.59(39), 1.15(2), 1.32(145), 0.4(48), 0.81(31), 1.54(66), 0.55(9), 0.82(315), 1.31(119), 4.06(6), 1.02(64), 0.27(?), 1.27(24), 1.4(8), 0.51(114), 0.79(23), 1.0(8), 0.50(?), 1.24(?)	0.97	1.05	>1046
Larynx	2.82(50)	2.82	2.82	50
Liver	1.46(39), 1.15(11), 1.92(150), 1.20(45), 1.22(33), 1.28(67), 1.28(9), 2.77(6), 1.45(313), 3.39(5), 2.72(87), 1.3(?), 2.0(24), 2.3(11), 0.81(64), 1.20(2), 2.00(?)	1.72	1.73	>866
Lung	0.43(30), 1.0(2), 0.74(141), 0.31(44), 0.90(34), 0.50(69), 0.40(7), 0.33(68), 0.59(10), 1.21(23), 0.28(?), 0.4(11), 0.21(64), 0.20(?)	0.546	0.536	>503
Lymph node	0.4(6)	0.4	0.4	6
Milk (mature)	0.012-0.03(137)			137
Muscle (skeletal)	0.10(?), 0.71(22), 0.05(6), 0.055(34), 0.30(?), 0.22(8)	0.23	0.24	>84
Nails	168[7](18), 13.8(17), 39(1), 19.8(18)	17.5	24.2	36
Oesophagus[8]	0.16(68)	0.16	0.16	68
Omentum[4]	0.36(74)	0.36	0.36	74

TABLE 6 (Cont.)

Organ, tissue or tissue fluid	Concentration in µg g^{-1} (number of samples)	Weighted mean [2] (µg g^{-1})	Unweighted mean [2] (µg g^{-1})	Number of samples
Ovary	0.13(16), 0.40(2), 0.71(11), 0.10(5)	0.33	0.34	34
Pancreas	2.81(2), 0.83(138), 0.34(6), 0.59(26), 0.80(59), 0.61(4), 0.82(64), 1.32(22), 0.34(60)	0.75	0.94	383
Placenta [4]	0.5(234), 0.35(55), 1.4(6)	0.49	0.75	295
Prostate	1.60(4), 0.13(50), 0.29(8), 0.32(29)	0.27	0.59	91
Skin	0.12(39), 0.32(22), 306(18), 0.10(13)	60.0	76.6	92
Spleen	0.38(143), 0.29(40), 0.79(34), 0.44(62), 0.82(8), 0.72(67), 0.61(97), 1.38(3), 1.74(83), 1.33(24), 0.3(?), 0.22(63), 0.3(?)	0.69	0.72	>624
Sweat	0.07(14), 0.079(30), 2.74(30), 0.051(33), 0.118(15)	0.73	0.61	122
Testis	0.13(72), 0.32(2), 0.72(17), 0.65(38), 0.29(4), 0.67(13), 0.09(6), 0.09(16)	0.35	0.37	168
Thyroid	0.11(21), 0.13(9), 0.21(49)	0.17	0.15	79
Tooth (dentine)	21.9(200), 7.3(?), 23.2(40), 10.7(?), 52(7)	23.0	23.0	>247
Tooth (enamel)	3.6(28), 36(7)	10.1	29.8	35
Trachea	0.93(60)	0.93	0.93	60
Urinary bladder	0.104(112), 0.39(4)	0.11	0.25	116

TABLE 6 (Cont.)

Organ, tissue or tissue fluid	Concentration in µg g^{-1} (number of samples)	Weighted mean[2] (µg g^{-1})	Unweighted mean[2] (µg g^{-1})	Number of samples
Urine	0.047(10), 0.046(8), 0.11(6), 0.03(36), 0.0063(368), 0.0157(81), 0.031(122), 0.047(10), 0.031(64), 0.069(8), 0.082(3), 0.023(20), 0.035(829), 0.107(6), 0.04(16), 0.044(3), 0.029(10)	0.027	0.047	1600
Urine 24 h[9] collection	0.039(44), 0.0069(40), 0.028(18), 0.075(24), 0.018(20), 0.011(6), 0.014(3), 0.024(15), 0.027(1), 0.019(?), 0.019(?)	0.030	0.026	>171

Notes:

(1) Data are from Iyengar et al. (1978), but are all converted to fresh weight using the dry and ash weight fractions given in that publication.

(2) Weighted means are based on all studies where the number of subjects is specified and a mean value is given. Unweighted means are based on all studies.

(3) Possible influence of gallbladder.

(4) Ash to fresh weight conversion based on muscle.

(5) Concentrations are not specified as ash, dry or fresh weight. This could imply concentrations a factor of two lower, since fresh weight has been assumed.

(6) Concentrations are not specified as ash, dry or fresh weight. Fresh weight has been assumed.

(7) Possible outlier not used in calculating mean.

(8) Ash to fresh weight conversion based on trachea.

(9) Assuming a daily mean excretion of 1.6 l (ICRP 1975).

4.2.5   Summary

Based on the information presented in this section, the following ranges for normal daily intakes of lead can be estimated.

Route of intake	Typical intake (μg Pb d^{-1})	Comment
Diet	200-400	The ICRP (1975; 1980) estimated a value of 440 μg d^{-1}, but this appears to be at the upper end of the range of reported intakes.
Drinking water	8-48	In localised areas, particularly with acidic water and lead service pipes, in excess of 2000 μg d^{-1} could potentially be ingested in drinking water.
Ingestion of non-edible substances	-	No 'typical' value can be presented, but in excess of 2000 μg d^{-1} could be ingested from this source, and for urban children it is likely to result in intakes similar to those from diet.
Air	1-100	Estimated for non-occupationally exposed individuals. The majority of individuals will be exposed at lower end of the range.
Smoking	5	Estimated intake on the basis of a smoker of twenty cigarettes per day (UNEP/WHO 1977).

4.3   DISTRIBUTION OF LEAD IN HUMAN TISSUES AND FLUIDS

Several studies are available presenting information on the distribution and concentration of lead in human tissues and fluids obtained from healthy individuals, autopsy samples and patients with clinical symptoms of illness (e.g. Barker et al. 1977; Mackie et al. 1977; Rica and Kirkbright 1982; Conradi et al. 1977; Shapiro et al. 1972; Manton and Malloy 1983; Henderson and Inglis 1957). Iyengar et al. (1978) reviewed and summarised the lead content of a wide range of human tissues and body fluids, and data presented in Table 6 have been derived from that review. For convenience of comparison, all concentrations have been converted to μg lead per gram fresh tissue. Dry weight and ash weight fractions for each organ, listed by Iyengar et al. (1978), have been used to derive fresh weight equivalents. Data for humans, which have been presented since 1978, or were not included in the review of Iyengar

TABLE 7

RECORDED CONCENTRATIONS OF LEAD IN HUMAN TISSUES[1]

Tissue, organ of fluid	Concentration in $\mu g\ g^{-1}$ f.w. (number of samples)	Comments	Reference
Rib Vertebrae	2.95-6.70 2.20-5.14	Range of mean values for 9 males, aged 17-81 years at death	Forbes et al. (1977)
Rib Vertebrae	2.70-7.51 1.89-6.39	Range of mean values for 6 females, aged 45-82 years at death	
Skull Rib	35.2 17.0	Autopsy samples from patient with Bight's disease of known aetiology	Henderson and Inglis (1957)
Skull Rib	34.5 22.2	Subjects without chronic Bight's disease	
Skull Rib	84.5, males: 86.6, females 40.9, males: 45.3, females	Subjects with chronic Bright's disease but with- out known aetiology	
Hair	71.90±30.8 (50)[2] 33.13±17.8 (50) 7.16±4.41 (40) 3.76±2.30 (30)	Lead smelter workers Inhabitants around lead plant City inhabitants Farmers	Stankovit et al. (1977)
Hair	GM[3] 3.9 AM 5.05±4.34 GM 6.92 AM 9.37±7.88	Males, 16-25 years old, village inhabitants: India Males, 16-25 years old, college students: India	Barker et al. (1977)
Nail (toe)	0.4±0.01	From five adult males	Hislop et al. (1977)

TABLE 7 (Cont.)

Tissue, organ of fluid	Concentration in µg g^{-1} f.w. (number of samples)	Comments	Reference
Tooth (dentine)	15–982	Permanent teeth: range for all samples	Shapiro et al. (1972)
	14–379	Deciduous teeth: range for all samples	
Tooth (enamel)	13–70	Permanent teeth: range for all samples	
	11–500	Deciduous teeth: range for all samples	
Tooth (whole, deciduous)	10.7	Mean value, children living in Birmingham, UK	Mackie et al. (1977)
Skeletal muscle	0.146	Patients with amytrophic lateral sclerosis	Conradic et al. (1978)
	0.119	Control subjects	
Blood	0.234±0.017	Males, control samples	Clausen and Rastogi (1977)
	0.121±0.011	Females, control samples	
	0.448±0.228	Autoworkers (all)	
	0.446±0.298	Mechanics	
	0.400±0.256	Apprentice mechanics	
	0.383±0.191	Smiths	
	0.428±0.223	Painters	
	0.420±0.172	Miscellaneous workers	

TABLE 7 (Cont.)

Tissue, organ of fluid	Concentration in µg g^{-1} f.w. (number of samples)	Comments	Reference
Blood	0.180±0.120(88)	1. Males, mean age 33.1 years, non-occupationally exposed	P'An (1981)
	0.268±0.240(114)	2. Males, mean age 33.0 years, occupationally exposed 1-15 years	
	0.668±0.134(31)	3. Males, mean age 33.1 years, occupationally exposed 1-6 years	
	0.818±0.130(83)	4. Males, mean age 37.7 years, occupationally exposed 1-35 years	
Saliva	0.055±0.027(88)	1. as above	
	0.043±0.067(114)	2. as above	
	0.947±1.012(31)	3. as above	
	2.221±1.413(33)	4. as above	
Milk	0.13(16), 0.14(22), 0.14(32)	Mean values, three countries: poor urban conditions	Rica and Kirkbright (1982)
	0.11(31), 0.12(31)	Mean values, two countries: urban areas, high living standard	
	0.15(23), 0.12(24)	Mean values, two countries: rural areas	

Notes:

(1) All data are presented as fresh weight. Where it has been necessary to convert data the dry weight and ash weight fractions presented by authors have been used. If these data were not available the dry weight and ash weight fractions listed by Iyengar et al. (1978) were used.

(2) Mean ± 1 standard deviation.

(3) GM; geometric mean
     AM; arithmetic mean

et al. (1978), are summarised in Tables 7 and 8. In addition to the studies noted above and listed in Tables 7 and 8, many studies are available for laboratory animals (e.g. Bjorklund et al. 1981; Jugo 1980; Lloyd et al. 1975; Cohen 1970). On the basis of data presented in Tables 6 and 7, the following conclusions can be drawn.

- Lead is concentrated to a considerable extent in bone, but the health status of the individual can markedly influence the lead concentration in that tissue.
- Lead may be highly concentrated in skin.
- Lead is concentrated in hair, nails and teeth, but is present at very low levels in milk, sweat and urine.
- There is an indication that lead may be present at elevated levels in organs of the reticulo-endothelial system, principally the liver and kidneys.

It cannot be determined on the basis of data presented, whether high levels of lead recorded for skin and hair reflect external contamination, although it is notable that the high value attributed to skin arises from the influence of one study only. The ICRP (1975) reported data indicating a concentration of 0.3 $\mu g\ g^{-1}$ f.w. for skin, which is consistent with three of the studies reviewed by Iyengar et al. (1978) and presented in Table 6. Accordingly, a value of 0.3 $\mu g\ g^{-1}$ f.w. is considered to be 'typical' for the purpose of assessing total body content. The concentration of lead in lung tissue is not elevated by comparison with other tissues. Weighted mean concentrations of lead in human tissues, organs and fluids (Table 6), in conjunction with anatomical data for Reference Man (ICRP 1975), have been used to estimate the following tissue lead contents for adults.

Organ	Weighted mean concentration ($\mu g\ g^{-1}$ f.w.)	Total organ content (mg)	% of whole-body content
Bone	25.7	128.5	86.6
Blood	0.214	1.18	0.8
Kidney	0.97	0.30	0.2
Liver	1.72	3.10	2.1
Muscle	0.23	6.44	4.3
Pancreas	0.75	0.08	0.05
Spleen	0.69	0.12	0.08
All other tissues	0.3	8.73	5.88
Total		148.4	

The total body content of lead estimated above is in good agreement with the ICRP (1975) estimate of 120 mg. More than 85% of the total body lead is calculated to be present in bone, and this is also in accord with data reviewed by the ICRP (1975). Posner (1961) demonstrated that lead can be substituted in the calcium positions of apatite, and it is, therefore, probable that the element distributes fairly rapidly throughout the volume of mineral bone (see also ICRP 1980). Lloyd et al. (1975) and Cohen (1970) demonstrated for dogs and baboons respectively, that Pb-210 is primarily deposited in bone, liver and kidneys, but is retained tenac-

TABLE 8

BLOOD LEAD CONCENTRATIONS OF ADULTS ACCORDING TO SMOKING CATEGORY
AND LEVEL OF OCCUPATIONAL EXPOSURE TO LEAD[1]

Smoking category (cigarettes d⁻¹)	Occupational exposure	Blood lead concentration (μg ml^{-1})	Number of samples
≥21	None	0.108±0.04	30
1-20	None	0.114±0.048	141
Stopped smoking	None	0.108±0.051	49
Never smoked	None	0.102±0.042	135
≥21	Slight	0.227±0.125	95
1-20	Slight	0.225±0.131	270
Stopped smoking	Slight	0.207±0.111	99
Never smoked	Slight	0.193±0.115	150
≥21	Moderate	0.291±0.148	124
1-20	Moderate	0.263±0.137	479
Stopped smoking	Moderate	0.251±0.120	202
Never smoked	Moderate	0.246±0.133	313
≥21	Heavy	0.558±0.327	50
1-20	Heavy	0.477±0.309	198
Stopped smoking	Heavy	0.438±0.343	54
Never smoked	Heavy	0.384±0.271	74

Note: data from Tola and Nordman (1977)

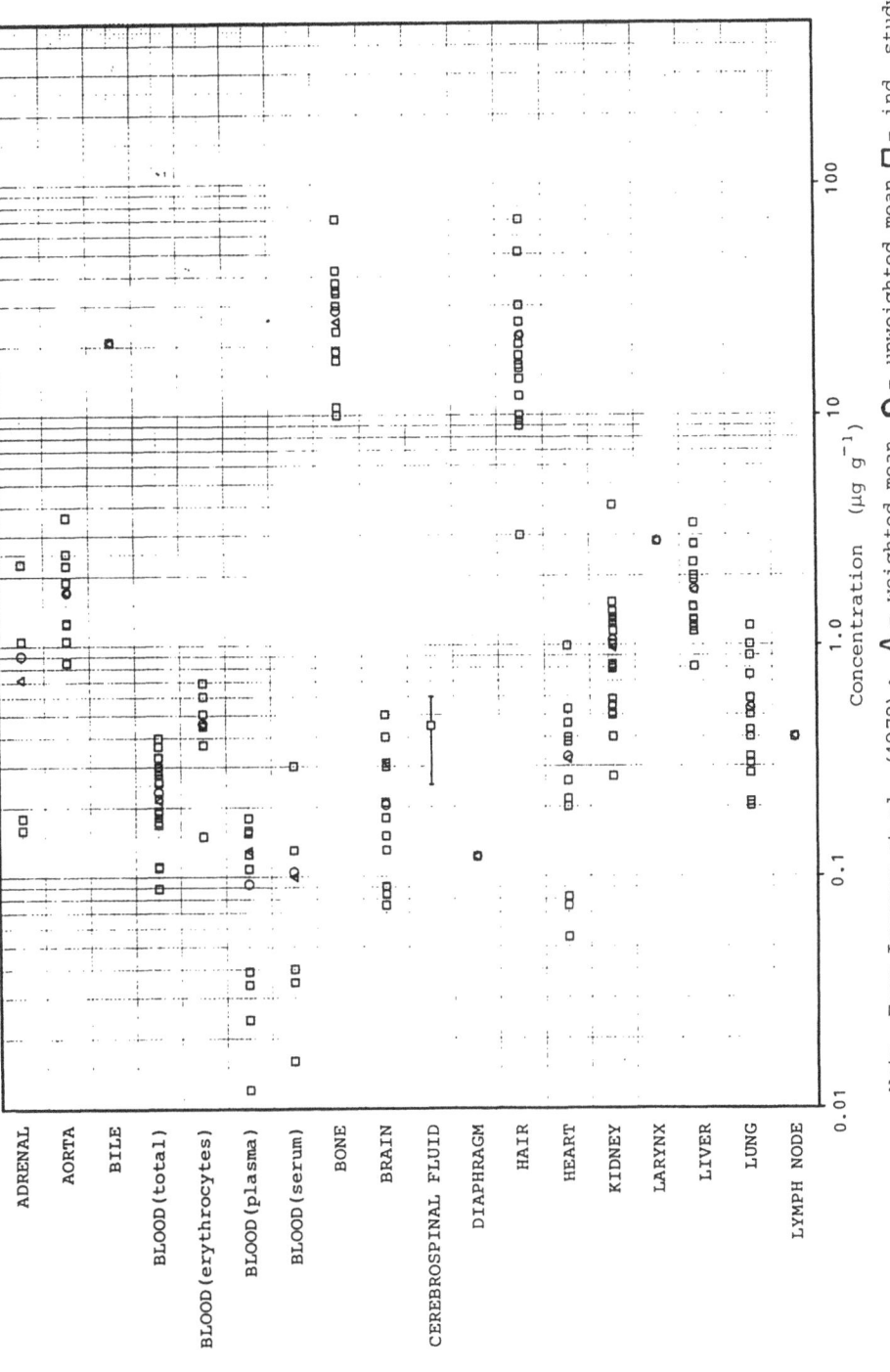

Note: From Igengar et al. (1978) : △ - weighted mean ○ - unweighted mean ☐ - ind. study

FIGURE 1. DISTRIBUTION OF STABLE LEAD IN HUMAN TISSUES

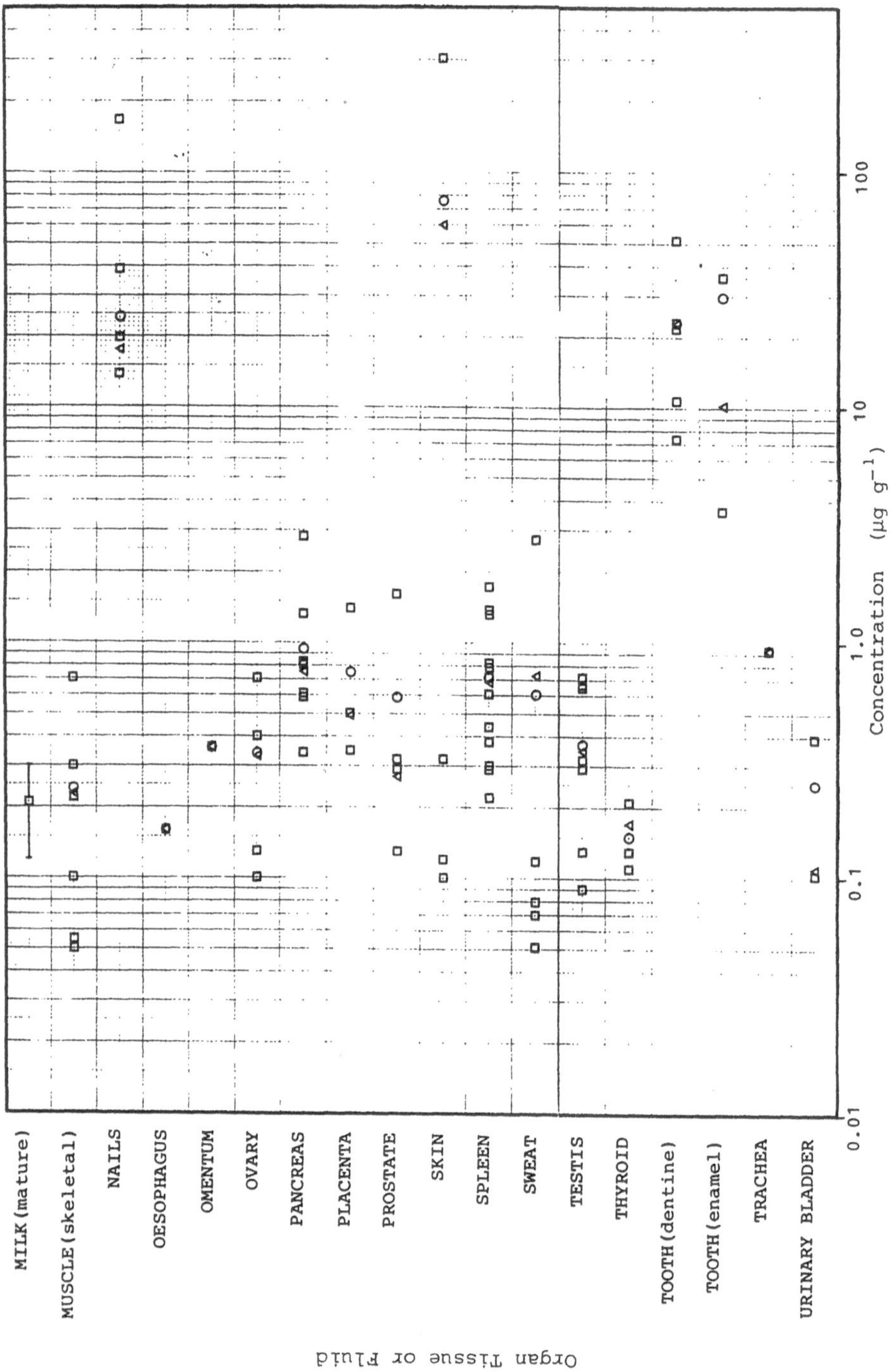

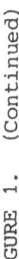

FIGURE 1.   (Continued)

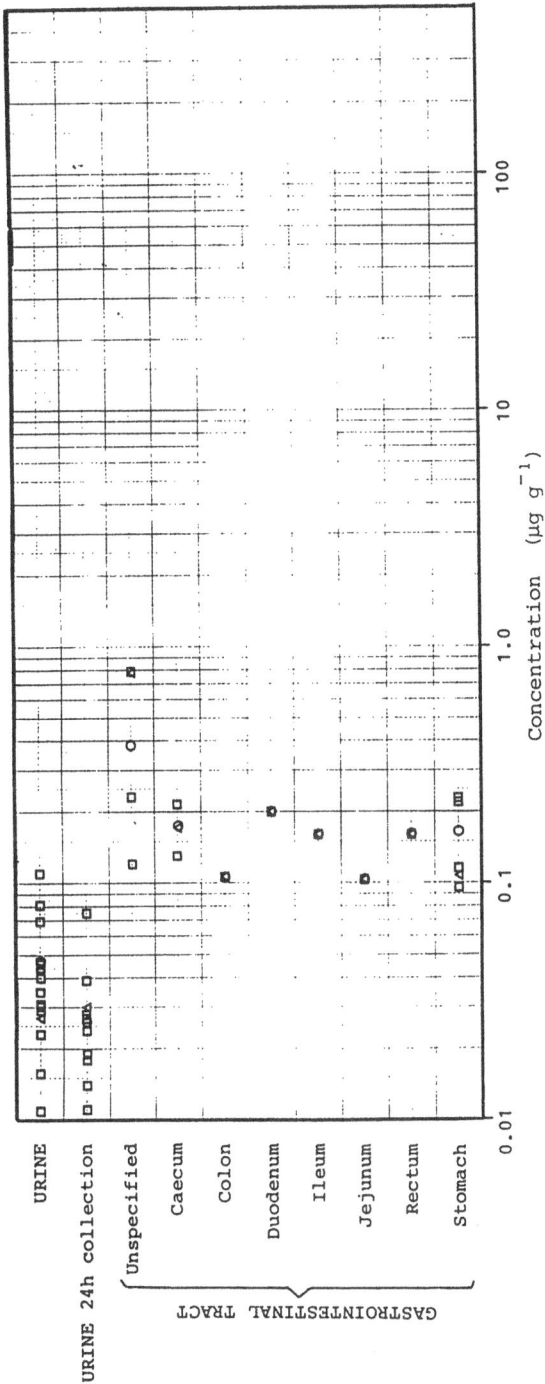

FIGURE 1. (Continued)

iously only by mineral bone. These findings are consistent with the data reviewed by Iyengar et al. (1978) and presented in Table 6.

Within the rat kidney, Oskarsson et al. (1982) demonstrated the presence of two lead-binding components in the postmitochondrial fraction, in addition to lead-binding components binding in the void volume and total volume regions. Binding of lead to the two postmitochondrial components, with molecular weights of 11500 and 63000 Daltons, was markedly decreased in lead pre-treated rats. It was suggested by Oskarsson et al. (1982), on the basis of ^{14}C-leucine binding data, that the 11500 Dalton lead-binding component of the postmitochondrial fraction is a preformed constituent of the kidney. In vitro incubation of postmitochondrial supernatants of brain, liver and lung of rat with lead-203, disclosed that these two binding components are also present in brain, but not in liver or lung. In this context, it is relevant to note that Osheroff et al. (1982) reported the presence of intranuclear lead inclusion bodies in the anterior horn cells of the cervical spinal cord, neurons of the substantia nigra and renal proximal convoluted tubule cells of adult rhesus monkeys. However, other tissues and organs do not appear to have been analysed.

4.4   METABOLISM

4.4.1   Gastrointestinal absorption

A great many factors have been demonstrated to affect the fractional gastrointestinal absorption, f_1, of lead in man and experimental animals, including the following.

-     Physical and chemical form of lead ingested (e.g. Barltrop and Meek 1979).
-     Associated dietary intakes (e.g. Anders et al. 1982; Bushnell and Deluca 1981; Bell and Spickett 1981; Aungst and Fung 1981; Quarterman et al. 1980).
-     Period of fasting or undernourishment preceeding intake of lead (e.g. Aungst and Fung 1981; Rabinowitz et al. 1980).
-     Total body content of calcium and iron (e.g. Watson et al. 1980; Hart and Smith 1981; Gerber et al. 1980).
-     Circadian rhythm and drugs altering gastric emptying (e.g. Aungst and Fung 1981).

A summary of values obtained for f_1 is presented in Table 9. The ICRP (1980) noted values for f_1 ranging between 0.05 and 0.65, depending upon state of fasting. The ICRP (1980) commented that values of f_1 considerably greater than 0.1 have been reported in several studies, and concluded that 0.2 is "a value thought to be appropriate for compounds of lead ingested between meals". For occupational exposure, it is probably appropriate to assume a limited period of fasting prior to ingestion of lead. For other individuals, diet is likely to be the main source for intake, and hence this assumption will not be valid. Human data indicate that an f_1 value of at least 0.1 and up to 0.37, depending upon preceeding period of fast, may be appropriate for dietary intakes of lead (Table 9). In addition, data presented in Table 9 for the gastro-

TABLE 9

FRACTIONAL GASTROINTESTINAL ABSORPTION OF LEAD

Chemical/physical form of lead	Species	Fractional absorption	Comments	Reference
All forms	Man	0.05 to 0.65 'typical' value 0.2	Range of reported values, and estimate for absorption of lead ingested between meals	ICRP (1980): R
Lead present in food	Man	0.103±0.022		
Lead nitrate	Man	0.088±0.018		
Lead nitrate	Man	0.081±0.040	Lead ingested in food	Rabinowitz et al. (1980)
Lead cysteine	Man	0.064		
Lead nitrate	Man	0.37±0.061		
Lead sulphide	Man	0.308±0.194	Lead ingested during fasting	
Lead cysteine	Man	0.30		
Lead in water	Rat	0.387±0.051	4.0 μCi of Pb-210 administered to all rats in 10 ml intubation solution of varying sugar content. Rats 26 days old, fasted for 24 hrs prior to intubation and killed after 18-22 hours	
Lead in glucose soln.1 mg g^{-1}	Rat	0.408±0.072		
3 mg g^{-1}	Rat	0.445±0.027		
6 mg g^{-1}	Rat	0.427±0.036		
Lead in lactose soln.1 mg g^{-1}	Rat	0.400±0.052		Bushnell and Dehuca (1981)
3 mg g^{-1}	Rat	0.747±0.036		
6 mg g^{-1}	Rat	0.691±0.030		
Lead in glucose soln.	Rat	0.458±0.049	As above. All rats intubated with solutions containing 3 mg g^{-1} of sugar	
Lead in galactose soln.	Rat	0.489±0.063		
Lead in mallose soln.	Rat	0.409±0.099		
Lead in lactose soln.	Rat	0.706±0.049		
Lead in human 'baby foods'	Rat	0.030±0.003 to 0.198±0.037		Kostial and Kello (1979)
Lead in commercially obtained rat foods	Rat	0.44±0:09	Food contained high calcium (1%) and iron (0.4%)	

intestinal absorption of lead administered in sugar solutions to pre-fasted rats suggest an f_1 value of 0.4 to 0.5. In view of the many uncertainties influencing gastrointestinal absorption of lead, it is not clear whether a real distinction can be made between values of f_1 for fasting and non-fasting individuals, and it is suggested that a single f_1 value is adopted. An appropriate value for f_1 is taken to be 0.3 for adults, although it is noted that considerable variability exists between individuals.

Gerber et al. (1980) noted, in a review of factors affecting the metabolism of lead, that the fractional gastrointestinal absorption of lead has been reported to be substantially higher in children compared with adults. Values of up to 0.5 were reported for f_1 in children by Gerber et al. (1980). Although these values are within the range previously noted for adults, it is considered appropriate to use a conservative value of 0.5 when assessing uptake by children.

4.4.2   Retention in the respiratory system

In a study of the deposition in the human lung and uptake to blood of motor exhaust labelled with Pb-203 Wells et al. (1977) demonstrated that deposition in the lung was dependent upon particle size of inhaled material, but that uptake from the lung was in all cases rapid and vir-tually complete. Little or no ciliary clearance was observed. Under two differing inhalation regimes, Wells et al. (1977) demonstrated that for all subjects approximately 90% of the lead was cleared from the lung with a half-life of 6.6 (± 1.3) hours. The remaining 10% was cleared more slowly, with a half-life of at least 70 hours. In a more recent study, Russell et al. (1978) concluded that, in rats continuously exposed to airborne lead, there is a rapid removal of the metal from lung. These remarks are in agreement with the recommendations of the ICRP (1980) that all commonly occurring compounds of lead should be assigned to inhalation class D. This recommendation represents a change from that previously proposed by the ICRP Task Group on Lung Dynamics (1966), which had assigned all commonly occurring compounds of lead to inhalation class W.

It was also recommended by the ICRP (1980) that lead inhaled and cleared to the gastrointestinal tract should be assigned an f_1 value equal to that assigned to ingested lead. However, data reviewed by Oehme (1978) indicate that inhaled lead is better absorbed than ingested lead. In view of the observations of Wells et al. (1977) that little or no muco-ciliary clearance of lead from the lungs occurs, and that virtually all lead deposited in the lung is directly absorbed to the systemic circulation, the gastrointestinal absorption of inhaled lead is of limited concern.

It is also of note that Morrow et al. (1980) concluded that "the collective evidence supports the view that atmospheric lead is rapidly and completely absorbed from the human lungs." Morrow et al. (1980) exposed 17 human volunteers to aerosols of [Pb-203]chloride or [Pb-203]hydroxide. The lead chloride was used in picogram amounts, the lead hydroxide at microgram levels. These two chemical species of lead were used to simulate the range of physicochemical properties found in atmospheric lead. Both aerosols were of comparable aerodynamic size (MMAD = 0.25 ± 0.1 μm), and about 25% of aerosolised lead was deposited in both exposure groups, following brief mouth breathing exposures. The biological half-lives for lead retention in the lungs of both groups were reported to be approximately 1 hour for 10% of the deposited lead, and 14 hours for the remaining 90%. Data was obtained to 3.9 d after exposure and the possibility of a small, longer-term, component of retention cannot be discounted.

4.4.3   Uptake and binding to blood

It has been noted by Rosen et al. (1982) that lead can substitute for iron in the synthesis of haem, and it is known that lead can inhibit the enzymatic processes leading to haem synthesis (Smith 1976). Lead may bind preferentially to the HbA_2 component of haemoglobin in normal human erythrocyte haemolysates. As saturation of lead binding to HbA_2 occurs, the lead binds more to HbA (Bruenger et al. 1973). Raghavan et al. (1980) demonstrated that lead also binds preferentially to a low-molecular-weight protein (molecular weight 10000) in occupationally exposed individuals. It was suggested that production of this protein is inducible by exposure to lead and represents a mechanism for reducing the toxicity of lead. Once the lead-binding capacity of HbA and the low molecular weight protein are exceeded, excess lead can bind to the erythrocyte membrane and to the high molecular-weight proteins within the cytoplasm. Critical, lead-sensitive, systems are found in both of those fractions (e.g. Na-K-ATPase in the membrane fraction and ALA dehydrase in the high-molecular-weight fraction of the cytoplasm). Consequently, the increased content of lead in these fractions could be associated with symptoms of toxicity (Raghavan et al. 1980). Since it has been suggested by Raghavan et al. (1980) that the inducibility of the low-molecular-weight protein and the lead-binding capacity of HbA_2 varies markedly between individuals, this may account for considerable variations in susceptibility to lead poisoning.

4.4.4   Systemic metabolism

As discussed in Section 4.3, lead is deposited primarily in bone, liver and kidneys, but is tenaciously retained only by mineral bone. The systemic metabolism of lead in humans and animals has been studied extensively (e.g. Rabinowitz et al. 1973; Lloyd et al. 1975; Domanski and Trojanowska 1980; Mahaffey and Rader 1980; Hill 1980; Williams et al. 1978; Hamilton 1978; Momcilovic and Kostial 1974; Rosen et al. 1982) and modelled or reviewed (e.g. Abdelnour et al. 1974; Smith 1976; Jugo 1977; Bernard 1977; Hammond 1978; Batschelet et al. 1979; ICRP 1980). The physiological and dietary status of the individual can have a marked effect on the whole-body retention of lead. Hamilton (1978) demonstrated that lead is retained more tenaciously in iron-deficient mice than in iron-replete mice. Calcium, vitamin C, vitamin D and chelating agents have all been investigated and reported to influence the uptake and retention of lead in the body (e.g. Hart and Smith 1981; Rosen et al. 1977; Hill 1980; Rosen et al. 1982; Sorrell et al. 1977). Quarterman et al. (1980) studied the influence of dietary amino acids on lead absorption. Dietary supplements of a number of amino acids (~ 5 g kg^{-1}) increased tissue lead concentrations in newly weaned rats but decreased them in older animals. The uptake of Pb-203 by tissues was reduced when

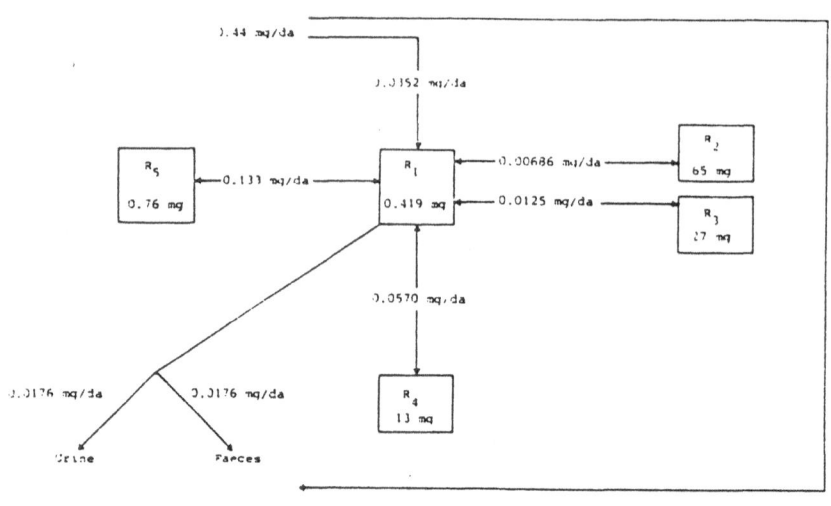

$R_1(t) = 0.00027e^{-\mu_1 t} + 0.000826e^{-\mu_2 t} + 0.00774e^{-\mu_3 t}$
  $+ 0.165e^{-\mu_4 t} + 0.826e^{-\mu_5 t}$

$R_2(t) = 0.176e^{-\mu_1 t} - 0.0561e^{-\mu_2 t} - 0.06515e^{-\mu_3 t}$
  $- 0.0390e^{-\mu_4 t} - 0.0195e^{-\mu_5 t}$

$R_3(t) = 0.0167e^{-\mu_1 t} + 0.226e^{-\mu_2 t} - 0.135e^{-\mu_3 t}$
  $- 0.0717e^{-\mu_4 t} - 0.0356e^{-\mu_5 t}$

$R_4(t) = 0.00654e^{-\mu_1 t} + 0.0278e^{-\mu_2 t} + 0.475e^{-\mu_3 t}$
  $- 0.346e^{-\mu_4 t} - 0.063e^{-\mu_5 t}$

$R_5(t) = 0.000373e^{-\mu_1 t} + 0.00149e^{-\mu_2 t} + 0.0142e^{-\mu_3 t}$
  $+ 0.492e^{-\mu_4 t} - 0.508e^{-\mu_5 t}$

In the above, with t in days,

$\mu_1 = 0.0000866$
$\mu_2 = 0.000347$
$\mu_3 = 0.00217$
$\mu_4 = 0.0693$
$\mu_5 = 0.693.$

Also, the retention equations for tissues obtained from the mammillary model are:

Bone $= 0.636R_5(t) + 0.800R_4(t) + 0.899(R_3(t) + R_2(t))$

Liver $= 0.2R_5(t) + 0.02R_4(t) + 0.02(R_3(t) + R_2(t))$

Kidneys $= 0.1R_5(t) + 0.002(R_3(t) + R_2(t))$

Tissues $= 0.0636R_5(t) + 0.0800R_4(t) + 0.0889(R_3(t) + R_2(t))$

Blood $= R_1(t) + R_4(t).$

Notes:

1.   Model redrawn from Bernard (1977).

methionine was given in the diet over a period of 5 weeks. Tissue uptake was also reduced when either methionine or ethionine was orally administered 24 h before Pb-203 activity was measured. In the liver, the fraction of the total activity found in the nuclei and mitochondria was increased by methionine, but in the kidney only the fraction found in the nuclei was increased. The mechanisms' by which various substances affect lead metabolism vary, but have been given some consideration by Rosen et al. (1982). Depletion of essential trace elements from bone may affect bone cell metabolism. A reduction of zinc in extracellular fluids leads to increased bone resorption, thereby enhancing the efflux of lead. At sites distant from the bone, Rosen et al. (1982) commented that interactions of trace elements are likely to be complex. Metal-metal interactions may occur in any of the metabolic pathways of trace metals. For instance, lead may substitute for iron in the synthesis of the haem moiety (Section 4.4.3) and Smith (1976) noted that the "best known effect of lead is the inhibition of nearly all the enzymatic steps that lead to haemsynthesis". Mahaffey and Racler (1980) noted that a number of similarities exist between the metabolism of lead, calcium, strontium and barium.

Abdelnour et al. (1974) developed a compartmental model of lead uptake by blood, liver, kidney and bone in mature and young adult rats. The model proposed for mature rats was found not to be applicable to young adult rats. A better fit to the data was obtained by assuming that growing tissue has a higher uptake rate from the blood than does mature tissue. Bernard (1977) presented a mathematically detailed model for the metabolism of lead in man, which is illustrated in Fig. 2. The model was based on data given by ICRP (1975) for Reference Man, and experimental studies on baboons. Following a single injection of lead into blood, the whole-body retention, R(t) was described by a five component retention function.

$$R(t) = 0.1e^{-0.693t/1} + 0.2e^{-0.693t/10} + 0.3e^{-0.693t/320}$$

$$+ 0.2e^{-0.693t/2000} + 0.2e^{-0.693t/8000}$$

where t is in days.

Assuming a total daily ingestion of 350 μg lead, together with an f_1 value of 0.3, and integrating over all time, leads to a calculated whole-body lead content of ∿320 mg. This is somewhat higher than the estimate of 148.4 mg of lead, presented in Section 4.3. However, it should be noted that Bernard (1977) assigned f_1 a value of 0.08, which would give a value of ∿85 mg for the total body content of lead. Bernard (1977) noted that long-term retention of lead occurs in all organs and tissues, with the exception of blood, but that the bulk of long-term retention is in bone. On the basis of the retention functions presented in Fig. 2, and making the same assumptions as noted above, the following contents of lead in man are estimated.

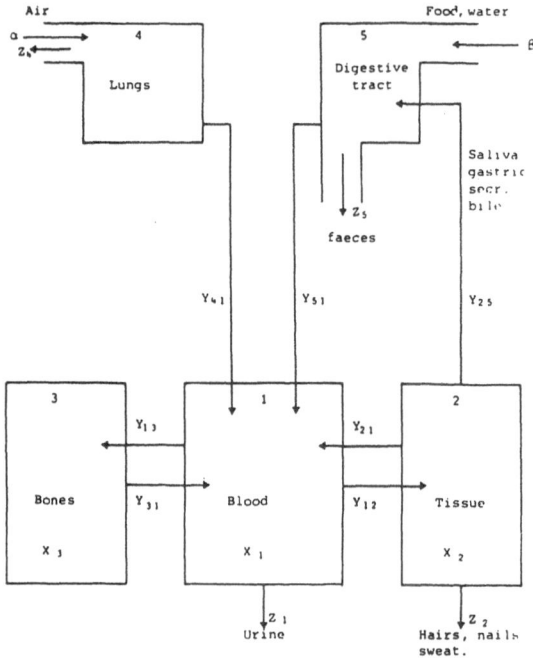

Notes:

1.   From Batschelet, E. et al. (1979)
2.   Coefficients for the above figure are:

$X_1 = 1.8 \times 10^3$ µg, $Y_{12} = 20$ µg/d, $Z_1 = 38$ µg/d,

$X_2 = 0.7 \times 10^3$ µg, $Y_{21} = 8$ µg/d, $Z_2 = 4$ µg/d,

$X_3 = 200 \times 10^3$ µg, $Y_{13} = Y_{31} = 7$ µg/d, $Z_4 = 32$ µg/d,

$\alpha = 49$ µg/d, $Y_{41} = 17$ µg/d,

$\beta = 367$ µg/d, $Y_{51} = 33$ µg/d,

$Y_{25} = 8$ µg/d.

3.   The daily lead inputs are α (air), β (food, water). The daily
      lead outputs are Z_1 (urine), Z_2 (hairs, nails, sweat), Z_4 (air,
      mucus), Z_5 (faeces). The amount of lead stored are X_1 (blood),
      X_2 (tissues), X_3 (bones). The daily exchange portions of lead
      are denoted by Y_{ik}, numbers i,k meaning the compartments of
      origin and destination respectively. All quantities are measured
      in µg or µg/d.

FIGURE 3   A THREE COMPARTMENT MODEL FOR THE KINETICS OF LEAD

Organ	Estimated content (mg)	Content based on data of Iyengar et al. (2978)
Skeleton	279.8	128.5
Liver	6.8	3.1
Kidneys	0.8	0.3
Blood	5.6	1.18
All other tissues	28.0	15.32

A three compartment model for the kinetics of lead in humans was proposed by Batschelet et al. (1979) and is illustrated in Fig. 3. On the basis of data presented by Lloyd et al. (1975) for dogs, and Rabinowitz et al. (1973) for humans, the ICRP (1980) proposed a whole body retention function for lead in man as follows.

$$R(t) = 0.69e^{-0.693t/12} + 0.191e^{-0.693t/180} + 0.119e^{-0.693t/10000}$$

where   t is in days

Fractions of 0.55, 0.25, 0.02 and 0.18 were assumed to be translocated to the skeleton, liver, kidneys and all other tissues respectively. Of lead translocated to the skeleton, fractions of 0.6, 0.2 and 0.2 were assumed to be retained with biological half-lives of 12, 180 and 10000 days respectively. Of lead translocated to any organ or tissue other than skeleton, fractions of 0.8, 0.18 and 0.02 were assumed to be retained with biological half-lives of 12, 180 and 10000 days respectively. On this basis and making the same assumptions for intake and fractional gastrointestinal absorption of lead noted above, the following organ and tissues contents are estimated.

Organ	Estimated content (mg)	Content based on data of Iyengar et al. 1978) (mg)
Skeleton	169.9	128.5
Liver	9.1	3.1
Kidneys	0.7	0.3
All other tissues	6.6	16.5

This comparison of models for the retention of lead in man suggests that both the Bernard (1977) and ICRP (1980) models provide a reasonable approximation to the organ and whole-body retention of lead in man, although the ICRP (1980) model provides a somewhat better fit to the data available. Bearing in mind that the long-term component would not equilibrate in a lifetime of 70 y, the ICRP (1980) model gives results in reasonable agreement with the stable element data and it is adopted here.

4.4.5   Other metabolic information

4.4.5.1   Skin absorption

It has been noted by Oehme (1978) that metallic lead is "slowly, but constantly, absorbed by most routes except the skin". However, skin lesions or abrasions will allow some absorption of lead, and Oehme (1978) commented that lead particles buried subcutaneously or intramuscularly are absorbed, and that a sufficient systemic concentration has been reported from this source to cause poisoning within one month.

4.4.5.2   Effects of pregnancy and lactation, and transfer to the foetus and newborn

It is known that lead can be transferred from mother to offspring through milk, at levels sufficient to cause symptoms of lead toxicity (Kostial and Momcilovic 1974). Brain damage can be induced in suckling rats at doses tolerated by their mothers, indicating that infants are a high risk group in respect of lead exposure (Schroeder et al. 1971). Momcilovic (1979) demonstrated a two-fold increase in lead absorption in lactating rats receiving 2 mg Pb l^{-1} in drinking water. About half of the absorbed lead was transferred to the litter. Using Pb-203 as a tracer, the retention of lead by suckling and adult mice was demonstrated by Keller and Doherty (1980b) to be independent of dose over a range of 4 to 445 mg kg^{-1}. Hackett et al. (1982a) reported that neither pregnancy nor the stage of gestation was found to affect Pb-210 clearance from the blood of rats. Also, with the exception of the reproductive system, the partition of Pb-210 was independent of the stage of gestation.
Engelhardt et al. (1979) noted for humans that the placental unit forms a limited barrier to the transfer of maternal blood lead to the foetus at environmental levels of exposure. For 148 normal births, 19 premature births and 12 abortions they reported that, on average, maternal blood lead levels were 1.4 times those of the newborn. Similarly, McClain and Becker (1975) demonstrated in pregnant rats given single intravenous doses of 25 to 70 mg Pb kg^{-1} as lead nitrate, that 'significant' quantities of lead were transferred to the foetus. However, the placenta acted to limit the passage of lead, since large maternal-foetal lead gradients existed. Kelman and Walker (1980) noted that organic lead generally gains easy access to the developing foetus of species containing haemochorial placentas. Perfusion of the guinea-pig foetal circulation (at 60 days gestation) indicated that the clearance of lead from mother to foetus is linearly related to umbilical flow rate. Measurements indicated a lead clearance rate of 0.047±0.004 ml min^{-1} at an umbilical flow rate of 2.5 ml min^{-1}. It has been demonstrated in several studies (e.g. Hackett et al. 1982b; Roels et al. 1977) that lead uptake to the foeto-placental unit is dependent upon dose level, and at higher doses progressively more lead is detectable in the foetus; although lead retention is not similarly affected (Keller and Doherty 1980b; Hackett et al. 1982a). Dose-dependent alterations of maternal lead distribution (e.g. deposition in organs of the reticulo-endothelial system at high dose levels) may influence foetal response to dose, since these maternal organs could serve as pools for metal translocation (Hackett et al. 1982a).

TABLE 10

TISSUES LEAD LEVELS IN NEONATAL RATS[1]

Tissue	Concentration ($\mu g\ g^{-1} \pm$ s.e.) at various times post-partum		
	7 d (n = 15)	14 d (n = 14)	21 d (n = 32)
Intestinal contents[2]	$8.31\pm1.16^{d[3]}$	441.26 ± 23.77^{e}	1.03 ± 0.02^{f}
Intestine	129.07 ± 20.09^{d}	45.87 ± 4.93^{e}	4.22 ± 1.68^{f}
Femur	undetectable	20.86 ± 1.05^{d}	43.85 ± 1.18^{e}
Kidney	1.21 ± 0.20^{d}	2.51 ± 0.08^{e}	2.38 ± 0.07^{e}
Liver	1.48 ± 0.14^{d}	2.59 ± 0.22^{e}	1.03 ± 0.02^{f}
Brain	undetectable	0.14 ± 0.03^{d}	0.31 ± 0.02^{e}
Blood	undetectable	0.87 ± 0.07^{d}	0.29 ± 0.02^{e}

Notes:

(1) Data from Miller et al. (1983). Lead acetate (containing
     lead-210) was intragastrically administered to rats on
     day 6 post-partum, and at 3 day intervals to day 18:
     50 mg kg^{-1} of lead was administered on each occasion.
(2) Expressed as total lead.
(3) Comparisons are made for each tissue across days;
     values with the same letter are not significantly
     different, p<0.05.

Miller et al. (1983) reported a study of the tissue distribution of lead in neonatal rats exposed to multiple intragastrically administered, 50 mg kg^{-1} doses of Pb-210 labelled lead acetate. Doses were administered at day 6 post-partum and thereafter at 3 day intervals until day 18. A time dependent pattern of uptake was observed in bone, kidney, liver and brain. Stomach, lung, heart and spleen did not exhibit accumulation of lead (Table 10). By day 21 the bone contained the highest concentration of lead. These results are consistent with the data reviewed in Section 4.3. Body weight was not significantly affected by the level of lead exposure employed.

Lead is highly embryo- and foeto-toxic, and these subjects have been given considerable attention (e.g. McClain and Becker 1974; Roels et al., 1977; Kuhnert et al. 1977; Grant et al., 1980; Kimmel et al. 1980). McClain and Beckman (1974) reported a urorectocaudal syndrome of malformations in embryos of rats administered 25-70 mg kg^{-1} of lead nitrate on day 9 of gestation. Lead nitrate was increasingly embryo- and foeto-toxic when administered on later days of gestation (days 10 to 15), but was not teratogenic. Roels et al. (1977) administered 0, 1, 10 and 100 mg Pb l^{-1} to lactating rats up to day 21 after delivery, when both mothers and young were killed. Values of blood lead concentration (Pb-B), haematocrit (Htc), haemoglobin (Hb), free erythrocyte porphyrin concentration (FEP) and δ-aminolevulinate dehydratase activity (ALAD) were determined. Tissue ALAD activity, free tissue porphyrin concentration (FTP) and lead concentration (Pb-T) were also determined. In mothers, a significant increase of Pb-B and a reduction in ALAD activity of blood were found in the 100 mg l^{-1} group. In tissues, Pb was significantly increased in both liver and kidney of the 100 mg l^{-1} group, but only the kidney of the 10 mg l^{-1} group. None of the biochemical parameters measured in tissues was significantly modified. In the suckling rats, an increase in Pb-B and a reduction of ALAD activity in blood were observed in the 10 mg l^{-1} and 100 mg l^{-1} groups. Lead concentrations were significantly increased in liver, kidney and brain of the 100 mg l^{-1} group, but were elevated only in the kidney of the 10 mg l^{-1} group. Lead storage in the kidney of the 100 mg l^{-1} was associated with a marked increase in FTP and a slight reduction in ALAD activity. Kuhnert et al. (1977) reported that clinical studies on urban pregnant women and their foetuses indicated erythrocyte levels of lead, in both mother and foetus, high enough to inhibit ALAD activity. Approximately 27% inhibition was observed in the mothers and 11% in the foetuses. Mean levels of ALAD activity were 1040 nmol porphobilinogen (PBG) formed per ml of erythrocytes per hour in mothers, and 1230 nmol PBG ml^{-1} of erythrocytes h^{-1} in foetuses. Mothers who smoked cigarettes were found to have higher blood-lead levels, with lower maternal and foetal ALAD activities than reported for non-smoking individuals.

Kimmel et al. (1980) and Grant et al. (1980) reported growth retardation in foetuses derived from rats exposed chronically to lead. Exposure to lead has also been demonstrated to impair calcium metabolism, and Edeus et al. (1976) noted that Japanese quail hens exposed to levels of lead which did not cause any other overt signs of chronic plumbism had a decreased reproductive capacity. The concentration of lead in milk is in proportion to the concentration of lead in blood cells and probably never exceeds 1.0 μg ml^{-1} (Oehme 1978, see also Table 6).

4.5   EXCRETION OF LEAD

4.5.1   Urinary and faecal excretion

Inorganic lead is excreted from the body primarily in faeces and urine; concentrations being dependent upon duration and level of exposure and degree of absorption of the metal. In addition to non-absorbed lead, the faeces also contain lead excreted in the bile and from the intestinal mucosa. In cases of high lead exposure levels, bile excretion may represent a major pathway of elimination (Oehme 1978). Most of the systemic uptake of lead is excreted by the kidneys at rates directly proportional to the rate of absorption. Industrial workers in lead smelter plants have been reported to exhibit excretion rates of between 0.05 and 7.36 µg of lead per ml of urine (Oehme 1978). After discontinuance of lead exposure, the concentration of lead in urine declines rapidly at first and then more slowly, to reach a normal range of urinary-lead concentrations after a period which ranges from a few weeks to 18 months or longer (Oehme 1978). Data presented in Table 6 indicate a normal concentration of lead in urine of about 0.03 µg ml^{-1}.

Hammond et al. (1980) noted that the concentration of lead in faeces is a good indicator of current exposure to lead and should be used in place of lead-in-blood measurements to determine intake rates. Concentrations of lead in urine reflect the blood-lead level and, following a single oral administration of lead to mice, Keller and Doherty (1978) reported a long term component of excretion which was related to the skeletal retention of lead. Keller and Doherty (1980a) also reported that over the period 15 to 50 d after administration of lead to mice, excretion rates in urine and faeces were of similar magnitude.

5.5.2   Other pathways of excretion

The concentration of lead in sweat is the same or higher than that reported for urine (Oehme 1978, and see Table 6). The ICRP (1975) estimated, on the basis of sweat production of 0.65 l d^{-1} and a urinary production of 1.6 l d^{-1}, that loss of lead is roughly the same by each route. Data presented in Table 6 for the concentration of lead in sweat are influenced by a single set of high values. If a 'typical' concentration of 0.1 µg ml^{-1} is assumed, then it is estimated that about 65 µg lead per day will be lost via sweat. This compares with an estimated urinary loss of 43.2 µg lead per day. It is of interest to note that this implies a total daily loss of systemically absorbed lead of a little over 100 µg. Given a typical dietary intake of 300 µg or total daily intake of 350 µg, this implies an f_1 value of approximately 0.3.

Hair may form a further measurable route for loss of lead. If it is assumed, on the basis of data presented for Reference Man (ICRP 1975), that a total of 50 µg of hair is produced per day (facial, scalp and body hair), this represents a daily loss of approximately 1 µg Pb. This value is somewhat lower than the range of 3 to 30 µg Pb d^{-1} estimated by ICRP (1975).

TABLE 11

VARIATION OF LEAD CONCENTRATIONS ($\mu g\ g^{-1}$ f.w.)
IN TISSUES OF MAN WITH AGE

Decade (y)	20-29	30-39	40-49	50-59	60-69	70-79
Number in group	6	4	8	9	11	6
Tibia	6.61 ±0.92	9.37 ±4.64	10.77 ±5.09	9.68 ±4.43	18.57 ±8.34	28.36 ±21.37
Skull	7.27 ±1.76	9.07 ±4.31	12.85 ±5.12	10.13 ±4.21	19.60 ±8.17	21.76 ±18.06
Rib	4.06 ±1.92	5.48 ±3.82	8.04 ±4.13	4.83 ±1.55	9.77 ±4.69	9.42 ±4.65
Vertebrae	3.48 ±1.50	2.98 ±1.84	4.98 ±1.52	2.88 ±1.20	6.66 ±3.24	4.17 ±2.26
Aorta	0.40 ±0.18	0.86 ±0.71	0.75 ±0.16	1.14 ±0.46	2.83 ±2.55	3.32 ±2.18
Liver	1.59 ±0.62	0.87 ±0.58	0.98 ±0.60	0.87 ±0.38	0.84 ±0.32	0.98 ±0.61
Kidney cortex	1.16 ±0.54	1.28 ±0.62	0.83 ±0.22	0.68 ±0.33	0.61 ±0.24	0.63 ±0.31

Notes:
    Data from Gross and Pfitzer (1974), presented as $\mu g\ g^{-1}$ f.w.
    ± standard deviation.

4.6   EFFECTS OF STATE OF HEALTH, TOXIC LEVELS AND THERAPEUTIC
       PROCEDURES

Lead present in soft tissues is readily mobilised by chelating agents such as EDTA and penicillamine, whereas lead stored in bones is less easily released by such means (Underwood 1977). Information reviewed by Underwood (1977) also indicates that increased levels of circulating corticosteroids and of parathyroid hormone enhance the mobilisation of lead from bone. Release of lead from bone into the blood stream has also been reported to occur in some types of physiological stress, including trauma of pregnancy and infection (e.g. Aug et al. 1926; Cantarow and Trumper 1944). Gross and Pfitzer (1974) reviewed some of the pathological conditions which can alter tissue concentrations of lead. They summarised their findings by stating that, "some of the more obvious changes were reduced [lead] concentrations associated with osteoporosis in the rib and vertebrae, fatty change in the liver, and nephrosclerosis in the kidney. Elevated concentrations in the aorta were associated with atherosclerotic disease. Alterations in skeletal calcification, fatty changes and fibrosis are often observed during the ageing process. Such changes need to be considered when assessing the significance of environmental or occupational exposure to lead. Data reviewed by Gross and Pfitzer (1974) for the content of lead in organs and tissues of man at various ages are reported in Table 11.

As noted in Section 4.4.4, the physiological status of the individual may modify the metabolism of lead. Levander et al. (1980) demonstrated that the lead-induced inhibition of δ-aminolevulinic acid dehydrase (ALAD) is exacerbated by a deficiency of vitamin-E, causing an anaemia in rats more severe than that produced by either insult alone. It is noted that a pronounced reticulocytosis was observed by Levander et al. (1980), suggesting that the anaemia was haemolytic in nature, rather than due to impaired red cell production. Enlargement of the spleen was noted in the vitamin E deficient lead poisoned rats, which is consistent with increased splenic trapping of defective red blood cells. Also, in vitro mechanical fragility of erythrocytes was demonstrated in blood from these rats. Levander et al. (1980) noted that the rat may not be a good model for the study of haemolytic congestive hypersplenism, since in this species, the spleen becomes an active centre of haematopoiesis in severe anaemias and the 'filtering' function of the organ may be obscured by the haematopoietic response.

Tetraethyl lead (TEL), which is the form of lead added to petrol to reduce 'knocking' is a known potential risk to human health and renal damage is a prominent finding in human TEL intoxication. Urinary analysis typically reveals erythrocyte casts, proteinuria, polyuria and oliguria (Robinson 1978). Chang et al. (1980) intraperitoneally injected rabbits with 100 to 200 mg of TEL, and killed the animals at the onset of toxic symptoms (hyperirritation, tremor and convulsion). Pathological changes in the renal cortex were not remarkable under the light microscope, but electron microscopic examination revealed marked cytological changes in the epithelial cells of the proximal tubules. It was observed that honeycomb-like bodies were formed, and Chang et al. (1980) suggested that this may represent a hyperplastic, hypoactive form of the rough endoplasmic reticulum and denote a disruption of protein synthesis.

Therapeutic treatment of patients with lead poisoning has been debated for many years. In the early 1950's Hardy et al. (1951) concluded that oral doses of sodium citrate can control the symptoms of lead poisoning, but data obtained from four case studies did not indicate an increased excretion of lead due to such treatment. More recently, Lilis et al. (1977) reported that, in cases of chronic or acute occupational exposure at lead smelters, it was usual practice to intravenously administer chelating agents such as versenate (CaNa$_2$ EDTA). Less often, oral versenate or penicillamine had been given. Chelating agents principally mobilise lead present in soft tissues (Underwood 1977).

4.7   SUMMARY

4.7.1   Intake of lead

    For non-occupationally exposed individuals, the major route for intake of lead is likely to be via diet. A typical rate of ingestion is about 300 µg Pb d^{-1}, with a range of approximately 200 to 400 µg Pb d^{-1} in most localities. An additional intake of 8-48 µg Pb d^{-1} is estimated to arise from consumption of drinking water, but it is noted that considerable variability occurs. In areas with lead service pipes, estimates of daily lead intake from drinking water have been reported in excess of 2000 µg. Lead can also be ingested from sources normally considered to be non-edible, and this is likely to be particularly prevalent amongst children. No 'typical' value for ingestion of lead from these sources can be estimated, but values may be in excess of 2000 µg Pb d^{-1} in extreme cases. For urban children, such sources are likely to result in intakes similar to those from diet. Atmospheric levels of lead vary widely between localities and between 1 µg and 100 µg of lead inhaled daily by the non-occupationally exposed. For the majority of individuals, particularly in non-urban localities, it is likely that exposure will be at a lower end of this range. An additional inhalation of ∿5 µg Pb d^{-1} can arise from smoking of cigarettes.

4.7.2   Distribution of lead

    Lead is primarily deposited in bone, liver and kidney Approximately 87% of the total body content of lead is present in bone. Lead is also concentrated in nails and teeth. High concentrations of lead recorded in hair and skin may reflect external contamination, but insufficient data are available to determine this.

4.7.3   Gastrointestinal absorption

    The fractional gestrointestinal absorption, f_1, of lead is influenced by a great many factors and a range of values have been reported, between 0.05 and 0.65. A representative value of 0.3 is assumed for all compounds of lead in adults. A value of 0.5 is taken to be appropriate for children.

4.7.4   Retention in the respiratory system

Lead deposited in the lungs is rapidly, and almost completely, absorbed from that organ. Clearance from the lungs exhibits at least two components. It is probable that 90% of deposited lead is absorbed with a biological half-life of 7 to 14 hours. The remainder is thought to be absorbed with a half-life of about 70 hours. Some data obtained for man have also indicated a shorter-term component of retention, applying to about 10% of deposited lead and exhibiting a biological half-life in the lung of 1 hour.

4.7.5   Uptake and binding to blood

Lead binds preferentially to the HbA_2 component of haemoglobin, and to a low-molecular-weight protein, which is apparently inducible by exposure to lead. Binding to this protein may act to reduce lead toxicity, and variability between the capacity of individuals to produce the low-molecular-weight protein may account for some of the variability in lead-susceptibility detected among workers.

4.7.6   Systemic metabolism

The whole-body retention of lead in man is well represented by the retention function.

$$R(t) = 0.69e^{-0.693t/12} + 0.191e^{-0.693t/180} + 0.119e^{-0.693t/10000}$$

where   t is in days.

The following functions are taken to represent the retention of lead in individual organs.

$$R_{BONE}(t) = 0.55 [0.6e^{-0.693t/12} + 0.2e^{-0.693t/180} + 0.2e^{-0.693t/10000}]$$

$$R_{LIVER}(t) = 0.25[0.8e^{-0.693t/12} + 0.18e^{-0.693t/180} + 0.02e^{-0.693t/10000}]$$

$$R_{KIDNEY}(t) = 0.02[0.8e^{-0.693t/12} + 0.18e^{-0.693t/180} + 0.02e^{-0.693t/10000}]$$

$$R_{OTHER}(t) = 0.18[0.8e^{-0.693t/12} + 0.18e^{-0.693t/180} + 0.02e^{-0.693t/10000}]$$

where t is in days.

4.7.7   Other metabolic information

Essentially no absorption of metallic lead occurs through intact skin, though some absorption can occur through skin lesions or abrasions. Placental transfer of lead is related to unbilical flow rate and it has been demonstrated that foeto-toxic levels of lead can be transferred. On the basis of data for rats, it is suggested that that infants are a high risk group in respect of effects resulting from exposure to lead.

4.7.8   Excretion

Urine, faeces and sweat can all form significant pathways for the excretion of lead, and a detectable loss occurs in hair. Of dietary lead taken up into the systemic circulation, it is likely that about 65 μg per day will be lost in sweat and 43 μg per day in urine. Losses in faeces are primarily dependent upon intake, and may be used as an indicator of recent exposure to lead in preference to blood-lead levels.

4.7.9   Effects of state of health, toxic levels and therapeutic procedures

Several pathologic conditions alter lead deposition and retention. Physiological status of the individual can modify the effects of exposure to lead. Thus, vitamin-E deficiency exacerbates the tendancy of lead to cause anaemia. Toxic levels of tetraethyl lead may result in disruption of protein synthesis by renal cortex cells, and alter excretion of lead. Treatment in cases of lead poisoning generally involves administration of chelating agents and removal from the source of exposure. Chelation principally reduces the soft tissue content of lead.

4.8   REFERENCES

Abdelnour, J., Wheeler, G.L. and Forbes, R.M., 1974. A compartment model of lead uptake in mature and young adult male rats. In: Hamphill, D.D. (Ed.) Trace Substances in Environmental Health, VIII. University of Missouri Press, Columbia, Mo., 411-416.

Anders, E., Bagnell, C. R. Jr., Krigman, M.R. and Mushak, P., 1982. Influence of dietary protein composition on lead absorption in rats. Bull. Environ. Contam. Toxicol., 28, 61-67.

Angle, C.R. and McIntire, M.S., 1964. Lead poisoning during pregnancy. Am. J. Dis. Child., 108, 436-439.

Angle, C.R. and McIntire, M.S., 1979. Environmental lead and children: the Omaha study. J. Toxicol. Environ. Health, 5, 855-870.

Angle, C.R., McIntire, M.S. and Colucci, A.V., 1974. Lead in air, dust-fall, soil house dust, milk and water: correlation with blood lead of urban and suburban school children. In: Hemphill, D.D. (Ed.) Trace Substances in Environmental Health, VIII. University of Missouri Press, Columbia, Mo., 23-29.

Archer, F.C., 1977. Trace elements in soils in England and Wales. ADAS Conference on Inorganic Pollution and Agriculture, April 4-6, 1977, London (unpublished).

Aug, J., Fairhall, L., Minot, A. and Reznikoff, P., 1926. In: Medicine Monographs, Vol.7. Williams and Wilkins, Baltimore, Maryland.

Aungst, B.J. and Fung, H.-L., 1981. Intestinal lead absorption in rats: effects of circadian rhythm, food, undernourishment and drugs which alter gastric emptying. Res. Comm. Chem. Pathol. Pharmacol., 34, 515-530.

Azar, A., Trochimowicz, H.J. and Maxfield M.E., 1973. Review of lead studies in animals carried out at Haskell Laboratory. Two year feeding study and response to haemorrage study. In: Proc. Int. Symp. Environmental Health Aspects of Lead, Amsterdam. Commission of the European Communities, Luxembourg, 199-210.

Babenko, G.A., Tsok, R.M. and Shkromida, M.I., 1977. Experimental studies of the action of organic lead preparations 5PA on the growth of Brown-Pirse carcinoma implanted on to the iris and under the conjunctiva of the eyeglobe. Oftalmol., 32, 45-49.

Barker, D.H., Rencker, A.C., Mittal, B.M. and Shanbhag, S.V., 1977. Metal concentrations in human hair from India (Pilani, Rajasthan). In: Hemphill, D.D. (Ed.) Trace Substances in Environmental Health, X. University of Missouri Press, Columbia, Mo., 71-81.

Barltrop, D. and Meek, F. 1979. Effect of particle size on lead absorption from the gut. Arch. Environ. Health, 34, 280-285

Batschelet, E., Brand, L. and Steiner, A., 1979. On the kinetics of lead in human body. J. Math. Biol., 8, 15-23.

Bell, R.R. and Spickett, J.T., 1981. The influence of milk in the diet on the toxicity of orally ingested lead in rats. Fd. Cosmet. Toxicol., 19, 429-436.

Bernard, S.R., 1977. Dosimetric data and metabolic model for lead. Health Phys., 32, 44-46.

Bjorklund, H., Lind, B., Picator, M., Heffer, B. and Olson, L., 1981. Lead, zinc and copper levels in intraocular brain tissue grafts, brain and blood of lead-exposed rats. Toxicol. Appl. Pharmacol., 60, 424-430.

Bogen, D.C., Welford, G.A. and Morse, R., 1975. General population exposure of stable lead and ^{210}Pb to residents of New York city. Health and Safety Laboratory Report HASL-299, December 1975. W.S. Energy Research and Development Administration, New York.

Bowen, H.J.M., 1979. Environmental Chemistry of the Elements. Academic Press, London.

Boyland, E., Dukes, C.E., Groves, P.L. and Mitclley, B.C.V., 1962. The induction of renal tumours by feeding lead acetate to rats. Br. J. Cancer, 16, 283-288.

Bruenger, F.W., Stevens, W. and Stover, B.J., 1973. The association of ^{210}Pb with constituents of erythrocytes. Health Phys., 25, 34-42.

Bushnell, P.J. and Deluca, H.F., 1981. Lactose facilitates the intestinal absorption of lead in weanling rats. Science, 211, 61-63.

Cantarow, A. and Trumper, M., 1944. Lead Poisoning. Williams and Wilkins, Baltimore, Maryland.

Cawse, P.A., 1975. A survey of atmospheric trace elements in the UK: results for 1974. Environmental and Medical Sciences Division, Atomic Energy Research Establishment Report. Harwell, UK.

Chang, L.W., Wade, P.R., Reuhl, K.R. and Olson, J., 1980. Ultrastructural changes in renal proximal tubules after tetraethyl lead intoxication. Environ. Res., 23, 208-223.

Chisolm, J.J. 1971. Treatment of lead poisoning. Modern Treatment, 8, 593-611.

Clausen, J. and Rastogi, S.C., 1977. Heavy metal pollution among auto-workers. I. Lead. Br. J. Ind. Med., 34, 208-215.

Cohen, N., 1970. The retention and distribution of lead-210 in the adult baboon. Annual Progress Report, 1st Sept. 1969 - 31st August 1970. NYO-3086-10, Vol. 1. Institute of Environmental Medicine, New York University, New York.

Conradi, S., Ronnevi, L-O and Vesterberg, O., 1978. Lead concentration in skeletal muscle in amyotrophic lateral scheloris patients and control subjects. J. Neurol. Neurosurg. Psychiat., 41, 1001-1004.

Constant, P., Marcus, M. and Maxwell, W., 1977. Sample fugitive lead emissions from two primary lead smelters. Report No. EPA-450/3-77-031. National Technical Information Service, Midwest Research Institute, US Environmental Protection Agency, Springfield, VA., USA, pp.92-98.

Coogan, P., Stein, L., Hsu, G. and Hass, G. 1972. The tumorigenic action of lead in rats. Lab. Invest., 26, p.473.

Cooper, W.C. and Gaffey, W.R., 1975. Mortality of lead workers. J. occup. Med., 17, 100-107.

Cotton, F.A. and Wilkinson, G., 1972. Advanced Inorganic Chemistry: A Comprehensive Text. 3rd edit. Wiley-Interscience, New York.

Damstra, T., 1977. Toxicological properties of lead. Environ. Health Perspect., 19, 297-307.

Davies, B.E., 1978. Plant-available lead and other metals in British garden soils. Sci. Tot. Environ., 9, 243-262.

Davies B.E., 1983. A graphical estimation of the normal lead content of some British soils. Geoderma, 29, 67-75.

Domanski, T. and Trojanowska, B., 1980. Studies on metabolic kinetics of lead and alkaline earth elements (Ca, Ba). Acta Physiol. Pol., 31, 439-447.

Edens, F.W., Benton, E., Barsien, S.J. and Morgan, G.W., 1976. Effect of dietary lead on reproductive performance in Japanese quail, Coturnix coturnix japonica. Toxicol. Appl. Pharmacol., 38, 307-314.

EEC, 1975a. Proposal for a Council Directive relating to the quality of water for human consumption. Off. J. Eur. Comm., C214, 2-17.

EEC, 1975b. Council Directive of 16 June 1975 concerning the quality required of surface water intended for the abstraction of drinking water in the member states. Off. J. Eur. Comm., L194, 26-31.

Engelhardt, E., Schaller, K.-H. Schiele, R. and Valentin, H., 1976. The human placenta's lead level as a parameter of the ecological lead exposure: its validity in comparison to the lead level in blood, the activity of the delta-aminolevulinic acid dehydratase and the concentration of the free erythrocyte porphyrins of newborns and their mothers. Zbl. Bakt. Hyg. I. Abt. Orig. B, 162, 528-543.

Environmental Protection Agency, 1978. Environmental Protection Agency regulations on national primary and secondary ambient air quality standards, 40 CFR 50. In: US Environment Reporter Reference File. Bureau of National Affairs Inc., Washington DC, pp.121:0101-121:0102, 121:0117-121:0122.

Fairhall, L.T. and Miller, J.W., 1941. A study of the relative toxicity of the molecular components of lead arsenate. Publ. Health Rep. (Wash.), 56, 1610-1625.

Faoro, R.B. and McMullen, T.B., 1977. National trends in trace metals in ambient air, 1965-1974. US Environmental Protection Agency, Washington Printing Office, Washington DC. EPA-450/1-77-003.

Fishbein, L., 1976. Environmental metallic carcinogens: an overview of exposure levels. J. Toxicol. Environ. Health, 2, 77-109.

Fleming, A.J., 1964. Industrial Hygiene and Medical Control Procedures. Arch. Environ. Health, 8, 266-277.

Forbes, W.F., Finch, A., Esterby, S.R. and Cherry, W.H., 1977. Studies of trace metal lead levels in human tissues - III. The investigation of lead levels in rib and vertebrae samples from Canadian residents. In: Hemphill, D.D. (Ed.) Trace Substances in Environmental Health X, University of Missouri Press, Columbia, Mo., 41-51.

Fouts, P.J. and Page, E.H., 1942. The effect of chronic lead poisoning on arterial blood pressure in dogs. Am. Heart J., 24, 329-351.

Furst, A., 1977. An overview of metal carcinogenesis. In: Schrauzer, G.N. (Ed.) Inorganic and Nutritional Aspects of Cancer. Plenum Press, New York, pp.1-12.

Furst, A., Schlauder, M. and Sasmore, D.P., 1976. Tumorigenic activity of lead chromate. Cancer Res., 36, 1779-1783.

Gerber, G.B., Léonard, A. and Jacquet, P., 1980. Toxicity, mutagenicity and teratogenicity of lead. Mutat. Res., 76, 115-141.

Gilfillan, S.C., 1965. J. occup. Med., 7, 53.

Goldberg, E.D., Bowen, V.T., Farrington, J.W., Harvey, G., Martin, J.H., Parker P.L., Risebrough, R.W., Robertson, W., Schneider, E. and Gamble, E., 1978. The mussel watch. Environ. Conserv., 5, 101-125.

Goyer, R.A. and Mushak, P., 1977. Lead toxicity laboratory aspects. In: Goyer, R.A. and Mehlman, M.A. (Eds.) Toxicology of Trace Elements. Advances in Modern Toxicology, Vol.2, Hemisphere Publishing Corp., Washington, D.C., pp.41-77.

Grant, L.D., Kimmel, C.A., West, G.L., Martinez-Vargas, C.M. and Howard, J.L., 1980. Chronic low-level lead toxicity in the rat II. Effects on postnatal physical and behavioural development. Toxicol. Appl. Pharmacol., 56, 42-58.

Greathouse, D.G. and Craun, G.F., 1977. Epidemiologic study of the relationship between lead in drinking water and blood lead levels. In: Hemphill, D.D. (Ed.) Trace Substances in Environmental Health, X. University of Missouri Press, Columbia, Mo., pp.9-24.

Green, V.A. Wise, G.W. and Callenback, J.C., 1978. Lead poisoning. In: Oehme, F.W. (Ed.) Toxicity of Heavy Metals in the Environment. Part 1. Marcel Dekker, New York, pp.123-141.

Gross, S.B. and Pfitzer, E.A., 1974. Influence of pathological change on lead in human tissues. In: Hamphill, D.D. (Ed.) Trace Substances in Environmental Health, VIII. University of Missouri Press, Columbia, Mo., pp.335-340

Hackett, P.L., Hess, J.O. and Sikov, M.R., 1982a. Effect of dose level and pregnancy on the distribution and toxicity of intravenous lead in rats. J. Toxicol. Environ. Health, 9, 1007-1020.

Hackett, P.L., Hess, J.O. and Sikov, M.R., 1982b. Distribution and effects of intravenous lead in the fetoplacental unit of the rat. J. Toxicol. Environ. Health, 9, 1021-1032.

Haley, T.J., 1977. Pediatric plumbism sources, symptoms and therapy. In: Brown, S.S. (Ed.) Clinical Chemistry and Chemical Toxicology of Metals. Elsevier/North-Holland Biomedical Press, pp.179-182.

Hamilton, D.L. 1978. Interrelationships of lead and iron retention in iron-deficient mice. Toxicol. Appl. Pharmacol., 46, 651-661.

Hamilton, E.I. and Minski, M.J., 1972/1973. Abundance of the chemical elements in man's diet and possible relations with its environmental factors. Sci. Tot. Environ., 1, 375-395.

Hammond, P.B., 1978. Metabolism and metabolic action of lead and other heavy metals. In: Oehme, F.W. (Ed.) Toxicity of Heavy Metals in the Environment, Part 1. Marcel Dekker, New York, pp.87-99.

Hammond, P.B., Clark, C.S., Gartside, P.S., Berger, O., Walker, A. and Michael, L.W., 1980. Fecal lead excretion in young children as related to sources of lead in their environment. Int. Arch. Occup. Environ. Health, 46, 191-202.

Hardy, H.L., Bishop, R.C. and Maloof, C.C., 1951. Treatment of lead poisoning with sodium citrate. AMA Arch. Ind. Hyg. Occup. Med., 3, 267-278.

Harrison, R.M. and Perry, R., 1977. The analysis of tetraalkyl lead compounds and their significance as urban air pollutants. Atmos. Environ., 11, 847-852.

Hart, M.H. and Smith, J.L., 1981. Effect of vitamin D and low dietary calcium on lead uptake and retention in rats. J. Nutr., 111, 694-698.

Henderson, D.A. and Inglis, J.A., 1957. The lead content of bone in chronic Bright's disease. Aust. Ann. Med., 6, 145-154.

Hicks, R.M., 1972. Chem.-Biol. Interact., 5, 361.

Hill, C.H., 1980, Interactions of vitamin C with lead and mercury. Ann. N.Y. Acad. Sci., 355, 262-266.

Hislop, J.S., Morton, A.G. and Haynes, J.W., 1977. An assessment of certain analytical factors affecting use of toe nails as monitors of human exposure to potentially toxic metals. In: Brown, S.S. (Ed.) Clinical Chemistry and Chemical Toxicology of Metals. Elsevier/Morth Holland Biomedical Press, Amsterdam, pp.323-326.

Horiuchi, K., 1965. Osaka City Med. J., 11, 265.

IARC, 1979. IARC Monographs on the Evalution of the Carcinogenic Risk of Chemicals to Humans. Volumes 1 to 20. Chemicals and Industrial Processes Associated with Cancer in Humans. Supplement 1.

IARC, 1980. IARC Monographs on the Evaluation of the Carcinogenic Risk of Chemicals to Humans. Volume 23. Some Metals and Metallic Compounds.

ICRP Task Group on Lung Dynamics, 1966. Deposition and retention models for internal dosimetry of the human respiratory tract. Health Phys., 12, 173-207.

ICRP Publication 23, 1975. Report of the Task Group on Reference Man. Pergamon Press, Oxford.

ICRP Publication 30, 1980. Limits for Intakes of Radionuclides by Workers. Part 2. Annals of the ICRP, Vol.4, No. 3/4.

Iyengar, G.V., Kollmer, W.E. and Bowen, H.J.M., 1978. The Elemental Composition of Human Tissues and Body Fluids. Verlag Chemie, Weinheim.

Jugo, S., 1977. Metabolism of toxic heavy metals in growing organisms: a review. Environ. Res., 13, 36-46.

Jugo, S., 1980, Chelatable fraction of [203]Pb in blood of young and adult rats. Environ. Res., 21, 336-342.

Karpatkin, S., 1961. Lead poisoning after taking lead acetate with suicidal intent. Report of a case with a discussion of the mechanism of anemia. AMA Arch. Environ. Health, 2, 679-684.

Kehoe, R.A., 1967. Industrial Lead Poisoning, Industrial Hygiene and Toxicity. Volume II. 2nd Revised Edition. Wiley Interscience, New York.

Keller, C.A. and Doherty, R.A., 1980a. Distribution and excretion of lead in young and adult female mice. Environ. Res., 21, 217-228.

Keller, C.A. and Doherty, R.A., 1980b. Effect of dose on lead retention and distribution in suckling and adult female mice. Toxicol. Appl. Pharmacol., 52, 285-293.

Kelman, B.J. and Walter, B.K., 1980. Transplacental movements of inorganic lead from mother to foetus. Proc. Soc. Exp. Biol. Med., 163, 278-282.

Khan, D.H., 1980. Lead in the soil environment. MARC Report No. 21. Monitoring and Assessment Research Centre, London.

Kimmel, C.A., Grant, L.D., Skan, C.S. and Gladen, B.C., 1980. Chronic low-level lead toxicity in the rat 1. Maternal toxicity and perinatal effects. Toxicol. Appl. Pharmacol., 56, 28-41.

Kostial, K. and Momcilovic, B., 1974. Arch. Environ. Health, 29, 28.

Kuhnert, P.M., Kuhnert, B.R. and Erhard, P., 1977. Effect of lead on delta-aminolevulinic acid dehydratase activity in maternal and fetal erythrocytes. In: Hemphill, D.D. (Ed.) Trace Substances in Environmental Health, X. University of Missouri Press, Columbia, Mo., pp.373-381.

Lauer, D.J., 1955. Clinical lead intoxication from brass-foundry operations. Ind. Health, 107-112.

Lepow, M.L., Bruckman, L., Gillette, M., Markowitz, S., Robino, R. and Kapish, J., 1975. Investigations into sources of lead in the environment of urban children. Environ. Res., 10, 415-426.

Levander, O.A., Welsh, S.O. and Morris, V.C., 1980. Erythrocyte deformability as affected by vitamin E deficiency and lead toxicity. Ann. N.Y. Acad. Sci., 355, 227-239.

Lilis, R., Fischbein, A., Eisinger, V., Blumberg, W.E., Diamond, S., Anderson, H.A., Rom, W., Rice, C., Sarkozi, L., Kon, S. and Selikoff, I.J., 1977. Prevalence of lead disease among secondary lead smelter workers and biological indicators of lead exposure. Environ. Res., 14, 255-285.

Lloyd, R.D., Mays, C.W., Atherton, D.R. and Bruenger, F.W., 1975. [210]Pb studies in beagles. Health Phys., 28, 575-583.

McCabe, L.J., Symons, J.M. and Lee, R.D. et al., 1970. Survey of community water supply systems. J. Amer. Water Works Assoc., 62, 670-687.

McClain, R.M. and Becker, B.A., 1975. Teratogenicity, fetal toxicity and placental transfer of lead nitrate in rats. Toxicol. Appl. Pharmacol., 31, 72-82.

Mackie, A.C., Stephens, R., Townshand, A. and Waldron, H.A., 1977. Tooth lead levels in Birmingham children. Arch. Environ. Health, pp.178-185.

MAFF, 1975. Survey of Lead in Food: First Supplementary Report. Working Party on the Monitoring of Foodstuffs for Heavy Metals. Fifth Report. Ministry of Agriculture, Fisheries and Food, HMSO, London.

Mahaffey, K.R. and Rader, J.I., 1980. Metabolic interactions: lead, calcium and iron. Ann. N.Y. Acad. Sci., 355, 285-308.

Malcolm, D. and Barnett, H.A.R., 1982. A mortality study of lead workers 1925-76. Br. J. Ind. Med., 39, 404-410.

Manton, W.I. and Malloy, C.R., 1983. Distribution of lead in body fluids after ingestion of soft solder. Br. J. Ind. Med., 40, 51-57.

Martin, M.H. and Coughtrey, P.J., 1983. Biological Monitoring of Heavy Metal Pollution: Land and Air. Applied Science Publishers, London.

Matthews, J.J. and Walpole, A.C., 1958. Brit. J. Cancer, 12, 234.

Metallgesellschaft, 1978. Metal Statistics 1976-1977. 65th Edition. Metallgesellschaft AG, Frankfurt am Main.

Miller, G.D., Massaro, T.F., Granlund, R.W. and Massaro, E.J., 1983. Tissue distribution of lead in the neonatal rat exposed to multiple doses of lead acetate. J. Toxicol. Env. Health, 11, 121-128.

Ministry of Health and Welfare, 1978. Drinking Water Standards, Tokyo.

Mitchell, D.G. and Aldous, K.M., 1974. Lead content of foodstuffs. Environ. Health Perspect. Exp., 7, 59.

Momcilovic, B., 1979. Lead metabolism in lactation. Experientia, 35, 517-518.

Momcilovic, B. and Kostial, K., 1974. Kinetics of lead retention and distribution in suckling and adult rats. Environ. Res., 8, 214-220.

Monier-Williams, G.W., 1949. Trace Elements in Food. Chapman and Hall, London.

Moore, M.R. and Meredith, P.A., 1979. The carcinogenicity of lead. Arch. Toxicol., 42, 87-94.

Morrow, P., Beiter, H., Amato, F. and Gibb, F.R., 1980. Pulmonary retention of lead: an experimental study in man. Environ. Res., 21, 373-384.

Murthy, G.K., Rhea, U.S. and Peeler, J.T., 1967. J. Dairy Sci., 50, 651.

NAS, 1972. Biologic Effects of Atmospheric Pollutants. Lead. Airborne Lead in Perspective. US National Academy of Sciences, Division of Medical Sciences and National Research Council, Washington D.C., pp.5-84, 131-144, 178-191, 226-248.

Nriagu, J.O. (Ed.), 1978. The Biogeochemistry of Lead in the Environment. Part A. Elsevier/North-Holland Biomedical Press, Amsterdam.

Nriagu, J.O., 1979. Global inventory of natural and anthropogenic emissions of trace metals to the atmosphere. Nature (Lond.)., 279, 409-411.

O'Brien, B.J., Smith, S. and Coleman, D.O., 1980. Lead pollution of the global environment. In: Progress Reports in Environmental Monitoring and Assessment-1. Lead. MARC Report No. 17, Monitoring and Assessment Research Centre, London.

Occupational Safety and Health Administration, 1979. Occupational safety and health standards, subpart Z - toxic and hazardous substances, 29 CFR 1910. In: US Occupational Safety and Health Reporter Reference File. Bureau of National Affairs Inc., Washington, DC, pp.31:8301-31, 31:8421-31:8429.

Oehme, F.W., 1978. Mechanisms of heavy metal inorganic toxicities. In: Oehme, F.W.(Ed.) Toxicity of Heavy Metals in the Environment, Part 1. Marcel Dekker, New York, pp.69-85.

Osheroff, M.R., Uno, H. and Bowman, R.E., 1982. Lead inclusion bodies in the anterior horn cells and neurons of the substantia nigra in the adult rhesus monkey. Toxicol. Appl. Pharmacol., 64, 570-576.

Oskarsson, A., Squibb, K.S. and Fowler, B.A., 1982. Intracellular binding of lead in the kidney: the partial isolation and characterisation of the postmitochondrial lead binding component. Biochem. Biophys. Res. Comm., 104, 290-298.

P'an, A.Y.S., 1981. Lead levels in saliva and in blood. J. Toxicol. Environ. Health, 7, 273-280.

Patterson, C.C., 1965. Contaminated and natural lead environments of man. Arch. Environ. Health, 11, 344.

Patterson, C., 1971. Lead. In: Hood, D.W. (Ed.) Impingement of Man on the Oceans. Wiley-Interscience, New York.

Pfaender, F.K., Shuman, M.S., Dempsey, H. and Harden, C.W., 1977. Monitoring Heavy Metals and Pesticides in the Cape Fear River Basin of North Carolina. Water Resources Institute of the University of North Carolina, Raleigh NC, pp.8-17.

Piotrowski, J.K. and Coleman, D.O., 1980. Environmental hazards of heavy metals: summary evaluation of lead, cadmium and mercury. MARC Report No. 20, Monitoring and Assessment Research Centre, London.

Piotrowski, J.K. and O'Brien, B.D., 1980. Analysis of the effects of lead in tissues upon human health using dose-response relationships. In: Progress Reports in Environmental Monitoring and Assessment-1. Lead. MARC Report No. 17, Monitoring and Assessment Research Centre, London.

Posner, A.S., 1961. Mineralised tissues. In: Van Wazar, J.R. (Ed.) Phosphorus and its Compounds, Vol.2. Wiley Interscience, New York, pp.1429-1459.

Quarterman, J., Humphries, W.R., Morrison, J.N. and Morrison, E., 1980. The influence of dietary amino acids on lead absorption. Environ. Res., 23, 54-67.

Rabinowitz, M.B., Kopple, J.D. and Wetherhill G.W., 1980. Effect of food intake and fasting on gastrointestinal lead absorption in humans. Am. J. Clin. Nutr., 33, 1784-1788.

Rabinowitz, M.B., Wetherhill, G.W. and Kopple, J.D., 1973. Lead metabolism in the normal human: stable isotope studies. Science, 182, 725-727.

Raghavan, S.R.V., Culver, B.D. and Gonick, H.C., 1980. Erythrocyte lead-binding protein after occupational exposure. 1. Relationship to lead toxicity. Environ. Res., 22, 264-270.

Reith, J.F., Engelsma, J. and Ditmarsch, M., 1974. Z. Lebensm.-Unters.-Forsch., 156, 271.

Rica, C.C. and Kirkbright, G.F., 1982. Determination of trace concentrations of lead and nickel in human milk by electrothermal atomisation atomic absorption spectrophotometry and inductively coupled plasma emission spectroscopy. Sci. Total Environ., 22, 193-201.

Robinson, R.O., 1978. Tetraethyl lead poisoning from gasoline sniffing. J. Amer. Med. Assoc., 240, 1373-1374.

Robinson, T.R., 1976. The health of long service tetraethyl lead workers. J. occup. Med., 18, 31-40.

Roels, H.A., Buchet J.-P., Lauwerys, R.R., Bruauz, P., Claeys-Thoreau, F., Lafontaine, A. and Verduyn, G., 1980. Exposure to lead by the oral and pulmonary routes of children living in the vinicity of a primary lead smelter. Environ. Res., 22, 81-94.

Roels, H., Lauwerys, R., Buchet, J.-P. and Hubermont, G., 1977. Effects of lead on lactating rats and their sucklings. Toxicology, 8, 107-113.

Rosen, J.F., Kraner, H.W. and Jones, K.W., 1982. Effects of CaNa$_2$ EDTA on lead and trace metal metabolism in bone organ culture. Toxicol. Appl. Pharmacol., 64, 230-235.

Rosen, J.F., Sorrell, M. and Roginsky, M., 1977. Interactions of lead, calcium, vitamin D, and nutrition in lead-burdened children. In: Brown, S.S. (Ed.) Clincial Chemistry and Chemical Toxicology of Metals. Elsevier/ North Holland Biomedical Press, Amsterdam, pp.27-31.

Roskill Information Services Limited, 1977. The Economics of Lead. 2nd edit. Roskill Information Service, London.

Russell, J.C., Griffin, T.B., McChesney, E.W. and Coulston, F. 1978. Metabolism of airborne particulate lead in continuously exposed rats: effect of penicillamine on mobilization. Ecotoxicol. Environ. Safety, 2, 49-53.

Safe Drinking Water Committee, 1977. Drinking Water and Health. Advisory Center on Toxicology, Assembly of Life Sciences, National Research Council, National Academy of Sciences. Washington, DC, pp.254-261.

Sanders, L.W., 1964. Tetraethyl lead intoxication. Arch. Environ. Health, 8, 270-277.

Schroeder, H.A. and Tipton, I.H., 1968. The human body burden of lead. Arch. Environ. Health, 17, 965-978.

Schroeder, H.A., Mitchener, M. and Hanover, N.H., 1971. Arch. Environ. Health, 23, 102.

Senatskommission, 1977. Maximale Arbeitsplatzkonzentrationen, 1977, Part 13. Deutsche Forschungsgemeinschaft, Bonn, p.16.

Shapiro, I.M., Needleman, H.L., Tuncay, O.C., 1972. The lead content of human deciduous and permanent teeth. Environ. Res., 5, 467-470.

Sharrett, A.R., Carter, A.P., Orheim, R.M. and Feinleib, M., 1982. Daily intake of lead, cadmium, copper, and zinc from drinking water: the Seattle study of trace metal exposure. Environ. Res., 28, 456-475.

Sirover, M.A. and Loeb, L.A., 1976. Infidelity of DNA synthesis in vitro: screening for potential metal mutagens or carcinogens. Science, 194, 1434-1436.

Smith, J.L., 1976. Metabolism and toxicity of lead. In: Prasad, A.S. and Oberleas, D. (Eds.) Trace Elements in Human Health and Disease, Volume II. Essential and Toxic Elements. Academic Press, New York, pp.443-452.

Sorrel, M., Roginsky, M. and Rosen, J.F., 1977. Interactions of lead, calcium, vitamin D, and nutrition in lead-burdened children. Arch. Environ. Health, 160-164.

Stankovic, M., Milic, S., Djuric, D. and Stankovic, B., 1977. Cadmium, lead and mercury content of human scalp hair in relation to exposure. In: Brown, S.S. (Ed.) Clinical Chemistry and Chemical Toxicology of Metals. Elsevier/North Holland Biomedical Press, Amsterdam, 327-331.

Thomas, B., Edmunds, J.W. and Curry, S.J., 1975. Lead content of canned fruit. J. Sci. Food Agric., 26, 1-4.

Tokudome, S. and Kuratsune, M., 1976. A cohort study on mortality from cancer and other causes among workers at a metal refinery. Int. J. Cancer, 17, 310-317.

Tola, S. and Nordman, C.H., 1977. Smoking and blood lead concentrations in lead-exposed workers and an unexposed population. Environ. Res., 13, 250-255.

Underwood, E.J., 1977. Trace Elements in Human and Animal Nutrition. 4th edit. Academic Press, New York.

UNEP, 1978. Lead: Evaluation Techniques for one of the Priority Pollutants. UNEP/GC/INFORMATION/8. United Nations Environmental Programme, Nairobi.

UNEP/WHO, 1977. Lead (Environmental Health Criteria 3). United Nations Environmental Programme/World Health Organisation, Geneva, pp.21-27, 30-41, 44-68, 80-86.

van Esch, G.J., van Genderen, H. and Vink, H.H., 1962. The induction of renal tumours by feeding of basic lead acetate to rats. Br. J. Cancer, 16, 289-297.

van Esch, G.J. and Kroes, R., 1969. The induction of renal tumours by feeding basic lead acetate to mice and hamsters. Br. J. Cancer, 23, 765-771.

Warren, H.V. and Delavault, R.E., 1971. Mem. Geol. Soc. Am., 123.

Watkins, D., Corbyons, T., Bradshaw, J. and Winefordner, J., 1976. Determination of lead in confection wrappers by atomic spectrometry. Anal. Chim. Acta., 85, 403-406.

Watson, W.S., Hume, R. and Moore, M.R., 1980. Oral absorption of lead and iron. Lancet, 2, 236-237.

Wells, A.C., Venn, J.B. and Heard, M.J. (1977). Deposition in the lung and uptake to blood of motor exhaust labelled with ^{203}Pb. In: Walton, W.H. (Ed.) Inhaled Particles IV. Pergamon Press, Oxford, pp.175-189.

WHO, 1970. European Standards for Drinking-Water, 2nd edit. World Health Organisation, Geneva, p.32.

WHO, 1971. International Standards for Drinking-Water, 3rd edit. World Health Organisation, Geneva, p.32.

WHO, 1973a. Trace Elements in Human Nutrition. World Health Organisation Technical Report Series No. 532. WHO, Geneva.

WHO, 1973b. The Hazards to Health and Ecological Effects of Persistent Substances in the Environment, Sources, Turnover in the Environment and Ecological Effects of Arsenic, Cadmium, Lead, Manganese and Mercury. Report on a Working Group, Stockholm, 29 October - 2 November.

WHO, 1977. Environmental Health Criteria 3: Lead. World Health Organisation, Geneva.

Williams, B., Dring. L.G. and Williams, R.T., 1978. The fate of triphenyllead acetate in the rat. Toxicol. Appl. Pharmacol., 46, 567-578.

Winell, M., 1975. An international comparison of hygenic standards for chemicals in the work environment. Ambio, 4, 34-36.

Ziegfeld, R.L., 1964. Importance and uses of lead. Arch. Environ. Health, 8, 202-212.

Zollinger, H.U., 1953. Durch chronische Bleivergiftung erzeugte Nierenadenome and Carcinome bei Ratten und ihre Beiziehungen zu den entresprechenden Neubildungen des Menschen. Virchows Arch. Pathol. Anat. Physiol., 323, 694-710.

Zook, E.G., Green, F.E. and Morris, E.R., 1970. Nutrient composition of selected wheats and wheat products. VI. Distribution of manganese, copper, nickel, zinc, magnesium, lead, tin, cadmium, chromium, and selenium as determined by atomic absorption spectroscopy and colorimetry. Cereal Chem., 47, 720-731.

Appendix 5
Nickel

5.1 INTRODUCTION

The chemical properties of nickel are related closely to those of iron and cobalt. In particular the properties of nickel metal are much like those of cobalt, except that nickel is less ferromagnetic and more inert to chemical oxidation. The chemistry of nickel compounds is essentially that of the 2+ state and in aqueous solution it usually exists either as the green nickelous ion, Ni^{2+}, or as a complex ion (Sienko and Plane, 1971). However, other oxidation states are possible including Ni^{1-} [as in $H_2Ni_2(CO)_6$], Ni^0 [as in $Ni(CO)_4$)], Ni^{1+} [as in $K_2Ni(CN)_3$], Ni^{3+} [as in NiF_6^{3-}] and Ni^{4+} [as in NiF_6^{2-}]. The properties of various common compounds of nickel were summarised by IARC (1976), while a useful brief history of the occurrence and utilisation of nickel, and a summary of its chemical properties, were given by Nriagu (1980a). Analysis of the element in biological materials and natural waters was discussed by Stoeppler (1980) and Sunderman (1980a). Production and uses of nickel have been summarised by Duke (1980). The primary nickel industry encompasses mining, milling, smelting and refining processes. In the non-communist world these processes are generally undertaken by a single company, although not necessarily in a single location. The two main ore types processed are sulphide and laterite ores and both may be smelted to matte (nickel-rich sulphide). About 20% of matte production is roasted to drive off the sulphur as sulphur dioxide, leaving marketable nickel oxide sinter. However, most of the matte undergoes electro-, vapo-, or hydrometallurgical refining to remove minor amounts of copper, iron, cobalt and other metals, and produce nearly pure nickel metal (Duke, 1980).

More than 75% of nickel production is consumed in the synthesis of alloys. The element is used to increase the strength and toughness of steel and cast iron at extreme temperatures and to provide resistance to corrosion in a variety of environments. A nickel-copper alloy is widely used in coinage and "nickel silver", which contains zinc in addition to nickel and copper, is commonly used as a base for electroplated articles. Pure nickel is principally used for electroplating and electroforming, with the largest proportion of this use being for consumer products, including plumbing fixtures. Nickel metal is used as a catalyst in various applications including the preparation of edible oils. Various nickel compounds are used in electroplating, storage batteries and in bonding ceramics to metal (Duke, 1980).

There are a large number of reviews concerning the distribution, metabolism and toxicity of nickel. Of particular note are the comprehensive study by the US National Academy of Sciences (NAS, 1975), the reviews by IARC (1976) and by Norseth and Piscator (1979), the review of occupational health aspects by Mastromatteo (1967), the review of uses of Ni-63 in biological research by Kasprzak and Sunderman (1979), the review of toxicity by Nielsen (1977), recent reviews on metabolism and carcinogenicity by Sunderman (1976a, 1977a, 1977b, 1981a), a review on carcinogenesis by Furst and Radding (1980), a review on mechanisms of metal carcinogenesis by Sunderman (1979a), a discussion of the treatment of nickel-induced air sinus carcinomas (Barton, 1977), a review on nickel carcinogenicity, mutagenicity and teratogenicity by Leonard et al. (1981) and the recent collections of articles on nickel in the environment (Nriagu, 1980b) and on nickel toxicology (Brown and Sunderman, 1980).

Oral toxicity of nickel is low and data reviewed by Nielsen (1977) indicate that dietary levels in excess of 100 µg g^{-1} are required to give significant depression of feed intake and growth in various species. With respect to low dietary levels, various studies [reviewed by Sunderman (1977a), discussed by Kasprzak and Sunderman (1979) and more recently reviewed by Nielsen (1980)] have demonstrated that nickel is an essential trace element in various mammalian species. Nickel deficiency is associated with retarded growth and reduction in blood haemoglobin concentrations, haematocrit values and erythrocyte counts. In particular, nickel deprivation impairs intestinal absorption of iron and thus causes anaemia. However, in a study on the F_1 and F_2 offspring of nickel deprived or nickel-supplemented rats, Nielsen et al. (1979) reported that severe iron deficiency appeared to be more detrimental to nickel-supplemented rats than to deficient rats, even though nickel supplementation increases haematocrit and haemoglobin levels in severely iron-deficient rats (Nielsen, 1980). In contrast, at marginally deficient or adequate iron levels, nickel-deprived rats did not perform as well as nickel supplemented controls (Nielsen et al., 1979). In conditions of zinc deficiency, nickel acts to reduce haemoglobin concentrations in erythrocytes as well as erythrocyte counts (Spears et al., 1978a). Overall, nickel-iron-zinc interactions with respect to gastrointestinal absorption and effects on blood is a subject requiring further investigation to elucidate the mechanisms involved. Independently of these results, nickel is demonstrated to be an essential element by its functional occurrence in the enzyme urease (Kasprzak and Sunderman, 1979).

Nickel salts administered intravenously or subcutaneously are highly toxic. LD_{50} values range from 6 mg nickel oxide per kg given intravenously to dogs to 600 mg nickel disodium EDTA per kg administered intraperitoneally to mice. Gross signs of nickel toxicity as a result of parenterally administered nickel salts include gastroenteritis, tremor, convulsions, paralysis, coma, anaphylactoid oedema and death (Nielsen, 1977). In hypersensitive individuals, skin contact with nickel, or solutions of nickel salts, can result in dermatitis (Nielsen, 1977).

With respect to inhalation, nickel carbonyl [$Ni(CO)_4$] is the main substance of concern. Nickel carbonyl is a colourless volatile liquid which boils at 43°C. Chronic exposure to nickel carbonyl can cause cancer, while acute exposure can give rise to dyspnoea, fatigue, nausea, vertigo, headache, odour of 'soot' in exhaled breath, vomiting, insomnia and irritability; in the longer term, respiratory distress and convulsions are seen in severe cases, but fever is not a prominent symptom. A detailed description of the symptoms, clinical course and therapy for nickel carbonyl poisoning has been given by Sunderman and Kincaid (1954) and by Nielsen (1977), who also discussed the limited data available relevant to the inhalation toxicity of other compounds of nickel.

Evidence for the carcinogenic action of nickel compounds has been summarised by the IARC (1976) and Sunderman (1977a, 1981a). Increased incidences of cancers of the lung and nasal cavities have been documented by epidemiological investigations of nickel refinery workers in Wales, Canada, Norway and Russia. A wide range of animal studies have been conducted and these have demonstrated that compounds of nickel can cause cancer after inhalation, intratracheal instillation, intramuscular injection, intraperitoneal injection, intrarenal injection, intratesticular injection and intraocular injection (Sunderman, 1981a). It is important to note that the tumourigenic effectiveness of nickel is related to the compound administered, with crystalline forms (e.g. α-Ni$_3$S$_2$ and β-NiS) being more effective than amorphous forms (Sunderman and Maenza, 1976; Sunderman et al., 1979a). This difference in effectiveness is almost undoubtedly related to distinctions in the phagocytosis of these various compounds (Costa and Mollenhauer, 1980a; 1980b; Costa el al., 1981).

Nickel has also been demonstrated to exhibit embryotoxic and terato-genic effects in various species (e.g. Schroeder and Mitchener, 1971; Sunderman et al., 1978a; Lu et al., 1979; Nadeenko et al., 1979; Gilani and Marano, 1980; Sunderman et al., 1980a; Storeng and Jonsen, 1981; and the review by Leonard et al., 1981).

5.2   INTAKE RATES

5.2.1   Typical dietary intakes

Typical dietary intakes of nickel have been discussed by several authors. Schroeder et al. (1961) measured nickel concentrations in a wide variety of foodstuffs and estimated average daily intakes as 300 to 600 μg; calculations for four laboratory workers came to 305, 340 360 and 480 μg, and an institutional diet contained 472 μg. Clements et al. (1980) measured the concentration of nickel in various foodstuffs in Italy and reviewed data for other countries. They concluded that daily intakes by adult man were typically 100-700 μg in Italy, 500 μg in Canada and 150-800 μg in the United States. For comparison, Myron et al. (1978) gave a typical dietary intake of 400 μg, while Solomons et al. (1982), in reviewing Swedish and American data, quoted 200 to 4460 μg d^{-1} ($\bar{x}$ = 750 μg d^{-1}) in Swedish diets and 168 ± 11 μg d^{-1} for nine institutional diets in North Dakota. On the basis of some of the data reveiwed above, Bennett (1982) estimated the normal dietary intake of nickel to be 170 μg d^{-1}, with a range of 165 to 500 μg d^{-1}. The ICRP (1975) considered a variety of data and concluded that a typical dietary intake is 400 μg d^{-1}, that a typical range is 200 to 600 μg d^{-1} and that selected diets might contain 700 to 900 μg d^{-1}. However, they included an estimate of 1120 ± 320 μg d^{-1} for a group of children. This is in contrast to the range of 30-300 μg d^{-1} given by Clemente et al. (1980) for Italian infants.

Concentrations of nickel in various foodstuffs have recently been reviewed by Coughtrey and Thorne (1983) who concluded that, in uncontaminated conditions, a concentration of 3 μg g^{-1} (d.w.) is representative of natural vegetation and the majority of agricultural vegetation; that a concentration of 0.3 μg g^{-1} (d.w.) is more representative for tuber crops and cereal grains; that typical concentrations in mammalian tissues are 0.1 to 0.5 μg g^{-1} (w.w.); that concentrations in milk are ~0.04 μg g^{-1}; and that typical concentrations in fish muscle and aquatic animals in general are 0.1 μg g^{-1} (w.w.) and 0.5 μg g^{-1} (w.w.) respectively. On the basis of these concentrations and using dietary data given by the ICRP (1975), the daily dietary intake of nickel can be estimated as follows.

Food type	European consumption (g d^{-1})	Assumed nickel concentration* (µg g^{-1})	Daily intake (µg)
Cereals	375	0.15	56
Starchy roots	377	0.06	23
Sugar	79	-	-
Pulses and nuts	15	1.5	23
Vegetables and fruits	316	0.6	190
Meat	111	0.3	33
Eggs	23	0.3	7
Fish	38	0.1	4
Milk	494	0.04	20
Fats and oils	44	0.6	26
Total	-	-	382

Note: * Converted to a wet weight basis throughout.

On the basis of the above discussion, it is probably appropriate to assume that the normal daily dietary intake of nickel is ∿400 µg.

5.2.2   Intakes in drinking water

Data on nickel concentrations in waters and the behaviour of the element in aquatic environments have been reviewed by Snodgrass (1980). In the United States, average nickel concentrations at the consumer's tap were 4.8 µg l^{-1} and 78% of samples exhibited a concentration above the detection limit (1 µg l^{-1}). Analysis of residues from public water supplies in 100 major cities of the United States gave nickel levels corresponding to water concentrations of 0.7 to 59 µg l^{-1} with a mean of 5.1 µg l^{-1}. For comparison, data for major US river basins gave an overall mean nickel concentration of 19 µg l^{-1} for samples in which nickel was detected.

Leonard et al. (1981) commented that the nickel content of drinking water has been reported to range from 0.3 µg l^{-1} in Finland to 4.8 µg l^{-1} in the USA, but that nickel concentrations in surface waters can reach 960 µg l^{-1}. Similarly, Bennett (1982) has commented that drinking water generally contains nickel at concentrations less than 10 µg l^{-1}, but that, in exceptional cases, values up to 75 µg l^{-1} are found and as much as 200 µg l^{-1} near mining areas. Coughtrey and Thorne (1983) summarised data on nickel in seawater and freshwater and concluded that, in uncontaminated conditions, concentrations of 1 and 5 µg l^{-1} are representative of the sea and of freshwaters respectively.

Assuming that a typical individual has a daily consumption of 1.65 l of water (ICRP, 1975), the concentrations listed above indicate that a typical intake rate via this route would be ∿10 µg d^{-1}, but that rates ∿300 µg d^{-1} could occur in restricted areas. For comparison, the ICRP (1975) quoted an estimated average US intake rate of 14 µg d^{-1}. Thus, in general, intakes of nickel in drinking water will be small in comparison with intakes in foodstuffs, but, in exceptional circumstances, the two routes could give rise to intakes of comparable magnitude.

5.2.3   Intakes by inhalation

The occurrence of nickel in air and its atmospheric chemistry has been reviewed by Schmidt and Andren (1980). Potentially significant natural sources include volcanos, exudation from vegetation, forest fires and meteoric dust. However, more nickel probably enters the atmosphere as a result of human activities including combustion of fossil fuels, mining and refining of nickel ores, waste incineration and steel production. Overall, Schmidt and Andren (1980) suggest that total global nickel emissions to the atmosphere are 5.1×10^7 kg y^{-1}, with 4.3×10^7 kg y^{-1} deriving from human related sources.

Atmospheric nickel concentrations for environments considered relatively free from man-made aerosol contamination are in the range 0.13 to 2.7 ng m^{-3} at remote continental sites, but vary from 0.023 to 10 ng m^{-3} at remote marine sites (Schmidt and Andren, 1980). At rural and suburban locations, air concentrations are generally in the range 3.5 to 9.5 ng m^{-3}, whereas in urban and industrial conditions air concentrations range from rural levels up to 250 ng m^{-3}, depending upon the extent and type of industrial activity, and also upon climatic conditions (Schmidt and Andren, 1980).

On the basis of the data reviewed above, it is probably appropriate to assume that average nickel concentrations in air are ~1 ng m^{-3} in remote continental locations, ~5 ng m^{-3} in rural and suburban locations and ~100 ng m^{-3} in large cities in temperate climates. Taking a typical inhalation rate to be 23 m^3 d^{-1} (ICRP, 1975), the following nickel intake rates are implied:

Location	Nickel intake (μg d^{-1})
remote continental	0.023
rural and suburban	0.12
urban	2.3

Although these values are low compared with the dietary intake (~400 μg d^{-1}), it must be remembered that the fractional gastrointestinal absorption of nickel is typically <0.05 (see Section 4.1).

Data on the chemical form of nickel in ambient air are virtually non-existent, but oxide, subsulphide, sulphate and carbonyl are all of possible significance (Schmidt and Andren, 1980).

Inhalation of nickel as a result of tobacco smoking can be a significant route of exposure. Sunderman and Sunderman (1961) measured the amount of nickel in six brands of American cigarettes and reported values of 1.59, 1.75, 1.85, 2.30 and 2.48 μg per cigarette in unfiltered brands, but 3.07 μg per cigarette in a filtered brand. They also studied the nickel partition in smoked tobacco and recorded the following results:

Nickel per gram of tobacco (μg)

Component	Unfiltered cigarette	Filtered cigarette	Cigar	Pipe
Total nickel	1.84	3.07	3.19	2.72
Ash + butt	1.31	2.34	2.01	2.20
Mainstream smoke	0.37	0.58	0.85	0.34
Sidestream smoke	0.16	0.11	0.33	0.18
Filter	-	0.04	-	-

These data indicate that 10 to 30% of nickel is found in the mainstream smoke and that a typical value is 20%.

In a more recent study, Menden et al. (1972) have reported on the nickel content of two brands of cigarettes. For the whole cigarette, the total nickel contents per cigarette were 4.25 ± 0.18 µg and 7.55 ± 0.50 µg for the two brands. The breakdown of these contents was as shown below.

	Nickel per cigarette (µg)	
Component	Brand 1	Brand 2
Smoked portion	3.10	5.51
Smoked butt	1.33±0.07	2.64±0.17
Tobacco smoke condensate	0.08	0.02±0.01
Ash	0.16	4.27±0.20
Sidestream	1.03	0.62

These data indicate that <0.02 of nickel in cigarettes is inhaled in particulates in mainstream smoke, but that 10 to 30% may be present in the local atmosphere due to loss in sidestream smoke. The reason for the difference between these results and those of Sunderman and Sunderman (1961) is almost undoubtedly because the technique used by Menden et al. (1972) would have failed to detect nickel carbonyl in the mainstream smoke and nickel in this form would have been attributed to the sidestream smoke, since the nickel content of this was estimated by difference.

Confirmation of the results of Sunderman and Sunderman (1961) is given by the work of Stahly (1973) in which four brands of cigarettes and eight samples of pipe tobacco were used. Nickel contents of the 12 tobaccos were reported to be in the range 0.5 to 10 ppm, and in the filters and papers of the cigarettes were from 5 to 10 and 10 to 20 ppm respectively. Nickel contents of one of the brands of cigarettes are summarised below:

State	Component	Nickel content per cigarette (µg)
Before smoking	Tobacco	2.9
	Filter	0.75
	Paper	0.75
After smoking	Ashes	2.0
	Butts	0.8
	Smoke	0.45
	Filter	1.1
	Not accounted for	0.05

In this study, which was designed to assay total nickel, including that present as nickel carbonyl, ∿10% of the nickel in the cigarettes was present in the mainstream smoke.

On the basis of the data reviewed above, it is probably appropriate to assume that the total nickel content of cigarettes is typically ∿5 µg per cigarette and that on smoking ∿15% of this will be inhaled in the mainstream smoke, almost entirely as nickel carbonyl. On this basis, an individual smoking 20 cigarettes per day would inhale ∿15 µg of nickel per day. Thus, nickel intakes due to cigarette smoking are likely to dominate over those due to inhalation of ambient air, except in industrial areas where nickel processing or steelmaking are being undertaken.

With respect to industrial exposure, nickel concentrations in air are substantially higher than the general levels recorded for industrialised urban areas. At the Falconbridge nickel refinery, Høgetveit and Barton (1977) reported that most sections of the plant have environmental levels below 400 µg m^{-3}, while Høgetveit et al. (1978) have given the following results, based on personal air sampling:

Department	Mean concentration in air (µg m^{-3})±s.d.
Roasting and smelting	0.86±1.20
Electrolytic	0.23±0.42
Other process	0.42±0.49

For the Clydach, South Wales, refinery, Morgan and Rouge (1979) have given the following personal air sampler results:

Department	Measured concentration of Ni in dust in air (mg m^{-3})			
	Mean	Max.	Min.	s.d.
Research	0.02	0.10	<0.01	0.02
Chemical products (a)	0.50	20.00	0.01	2.47
Chemical products (b)	0.45	12.07	<0.01	1.74
Calciners	0.28	0.70	<0.01	0.22
Nickel plant	0.25	2.26	0.02	0.45
Nickel powder	3.71	13.25	0.05	3.90
All plants	0.87	20.00	<0.01	1.47

In the above, the two results for chemical products derived from two separate examinations of the same department.

With respect to other industrial operations, Bernacki et al. (1978a) reported that the most highly exposed groups of workers in an aircraft engine factory worked in conditions where concentrations of nickel in air were <300 µg m^{-3}. Clausen and Rastogi (1977) measured nickel concentrations in air in automobile repair shops and reported values ranging from 0.02 to 0.49 µg m^{-3}. In electroplating shops, Bernacki et al. (1980) studied nickel in air using personal air samplers and reported a mean value (±s.d.) of 9.3±4.4 µg m^{-3}. In comparison, Tola et al. (1979) reported values of between ∿50 µg m^{-3} and 150 µg m^{-3}.

Thus, in modern working conditions, workers are unlikely to be exposed to nickel concentrations in air in excess of a few hundred micrograms per cubic metre, and even at these levels inhalation will generally be limited by the wearing of face masks or other apparatus.

5.2.4   Summary

On the basis of data reviewed in this section, estimated intake rates for nickel are as given below.

TABLE 1

DISTRIBUTION OF STABLE NICKEL IN HUMAN TISSUES [1]

Organ, tissue or fluid	Concentration in $\mu g\ g^{-1}$ (number of samples)	Weighted mean[2] ($\mu g\ g^{-1}$)	Unweighted mean[2] ($\mu g\ g^{-1}$)	Number of samples[2]
Adrenal	0.429(13), 0.26(16)	0.336	0.345	29
Aorta	<0.07(104), 0.084(16), 0.238(15), 0.140(65), 0.182(5), 0.2(4), 0.9(1)	0.157	0.14-0.15	106
Blood (total)	0.027(63), 0.0048(17), 0.022(76), 0.054(61), 0.032(153), 0.079(140), 0.061(38), 0.076(20), 0.18(70), 0.041(8), 0.022(23)	0.063	0.054	849
Blood (erythrocytes)	0.050(16), 0.048(61), 0.106(25), 0.072(2), 0.094(200)	0.083	0.074	304
Blood (plasma)	0.021(26), 0.059(61), 0.01(17), 0.066(25), 0.06(?), 0.0595(200), 0.012(1)	0.054	0.041	330
Blood (serum)	0.0026(40), 0.029(17), 0.039(12), 0.058(48), 0.0078(69), 0.04(105), 0.055(3), 0.03(1)	0.030	0.033	295
Bone	59.4(341)	59.4	59.4	341
Brain	<0.075(129), <0.075(17), <0.075(18), <0.075(51), <0.075(8), 0.034(61), 0.14(2), ND(1), 0.4(?)	0.037		
Breast	ND(?)		0.07-0.12	63
Diaphragm[6]	<0.06(91)			

TABLE 1   (Contd.)

Organ, tissue or fluid	Concentration in µg g⁻¹ (number of samples)	Weighted mean (2) ($\mu g\ g^{-1}$)	Unweighted mean (2) ($\mu g\ g^{-1}$)	Number of samples (2)
G.I. tract:				
Small intestine	0.33(21)	0.33	0.33	21
Caecum	0.17(31)	0.17	0.17	31
Colon	0.096(108), ND(?)	0.096	0.096	108
Duodenum	0.04(67)	0.04	0.04	67
Ileum	0.072(84)	0.072	0.072	84
Jejunum	<0.04(102)	-	-	-
Rectum	0.128(42)	0.128	0.128	42
Stomach	0.04(130), 0.49(9), 0.18(10)	0.077	0.237	149
Hair	1.8(184), 2.7(40), 0.6(?), 1.1(90), <5(776), 2.2(121), 3.6(1), 1.9(2), 6.5(?)	1.85	2.3-2.8	438
Heart	0.0063(4), 0.006(4), <0.055(140), <0.055(43), <0.055(20), <0.055(62), 0.142(8), 0.044(66), 0.23(20)	0.085	0.05-0.07	102
Kidney	0.055(144), <0.055(48), 0.132(31), 0.077(66), 0.11(9), 0.41(116), 0.036(64), 0.135(6), 0.22(20), 6.0(?)	0.161	0.71(?)	456
Liver	0.0089(4), 1.28(43)(3), 0.189(11), 0.009(4), <0.064(148), <0.064(45), <0.064(33), 0.064(67), 0.090(9), 0.044(67), 0.195(5), 0.514(116), 0.32(13), 0.2(?), 0.11(10)	0.376	0.20-0.21	349

TABLE 1 (Contd.)

Organ, tissue or fluid	Concentration in μg g^{-1} (number of samples)	Weighted mean(2) (μg g^{-1})	Unweighted mean(2) (μg g^{-1})	Number of samples(2)
Lung	0.0019(4), 0.061(4), <0.055(141), 0.066(44), 0.264(34), 0.11(69), 0.22(7), 0.088(68), 0.06(10), 0.47(23), 0.2(11), 0.15(10)	0.149	0.14	284
Lymph node	0.3(6)	0.3	0.3	6
Mature milk	0.020-0.083(60)	–	0.052	60
Muscle (skeletal)	0.4(15), 0.2(?), <0.18(8)	0.4	0.2-0.26	15
Nails	11.9(17), 0.033(1)	11.2	6.0	18
Oesophagus (6)	<0.06(66)	–	–	–
Omentum (6)	0.27(75)	0.27	0.27	75
Ovary	<0.049(16), <0.049(2), <0.049(11)	–	–	–
Pancreas	<0.061(139), <0.061(6), <0.061(26), 0.061(58), 0.133(4), 0.067(64), 0.32(16)	0.095	0.08-0.11	142
Prostate	<0.063(50), 0.48(4)	0.48	0.24-0.27	4
Skin	0.32(22), 0.05(1)	0.31	0.19	23
Spleen	<0.070(143), <0.070(40), <0.070(34), <0.70(62), 0.209(8), 0.051(67), 0.178(3), 0.382(116), 0.72(14)	0.289	0.17-0.20	208
Sweat	0.063(14), 0.079(30), 0.163(30), 0.052(33), 0.132(15)	0.097	0.098	122

TABLE 1   (Contd.)

Organ, tissue or fluid	Concentration in μg g^{-1} (number of samples)	Weighted mean (2) (μg g^{-1})	Unweighted mean (2) (μg g^{-1})	Number of samples (2)
Sweat (24h collection) (4)	0.128(6)	0.128	0.128	6
Testis	<0.055(72), <0.055(2), <0.055(18), <0.055(39), 0.089(4), 0.67(5), 0.4(?)	0.412	0.17-0.20	9
Thyroid	<0.055(21), 0.22(7)	0.22	0.11-0.14	7
Tooth (dentine)	0.96(?)	0.96	0.96	?
Trachea	0.08(60)	0.08	0.08	60
Urinary bladder	0.04(110), 0.28(4)	0.048	0.16	114
Urine (8)	0.0046(39), 0.0023(26), 0.018(17), 0.085(?), 0.0101(154), 0.040(?), 0.085(?), 0.040(?)	0.0089	0.036	236
Urine (24h) (5) (8)	0.0037(39), 0.0017(26), 0.0143(17), 0.0179(?), 0.0936(2), 0.0144(24), 0.407(20), 0.079(2), 0.0086(3), 0.665(2), 0.0079(11)	0.073	0.119	146
Uterus	<0.061(32)	-	-	-

Notes:

(1)   Data are from Iyengar et al. (1978), but are converted to fresh weight using the dry and ash weight fractions given in that review

(2)   Weighted means are based on all studies where the number of subjects is specified, unweighted means are based on all studies, giving equal weight to each, and number of samples is the sum over all studies used in the weighted mean calculation

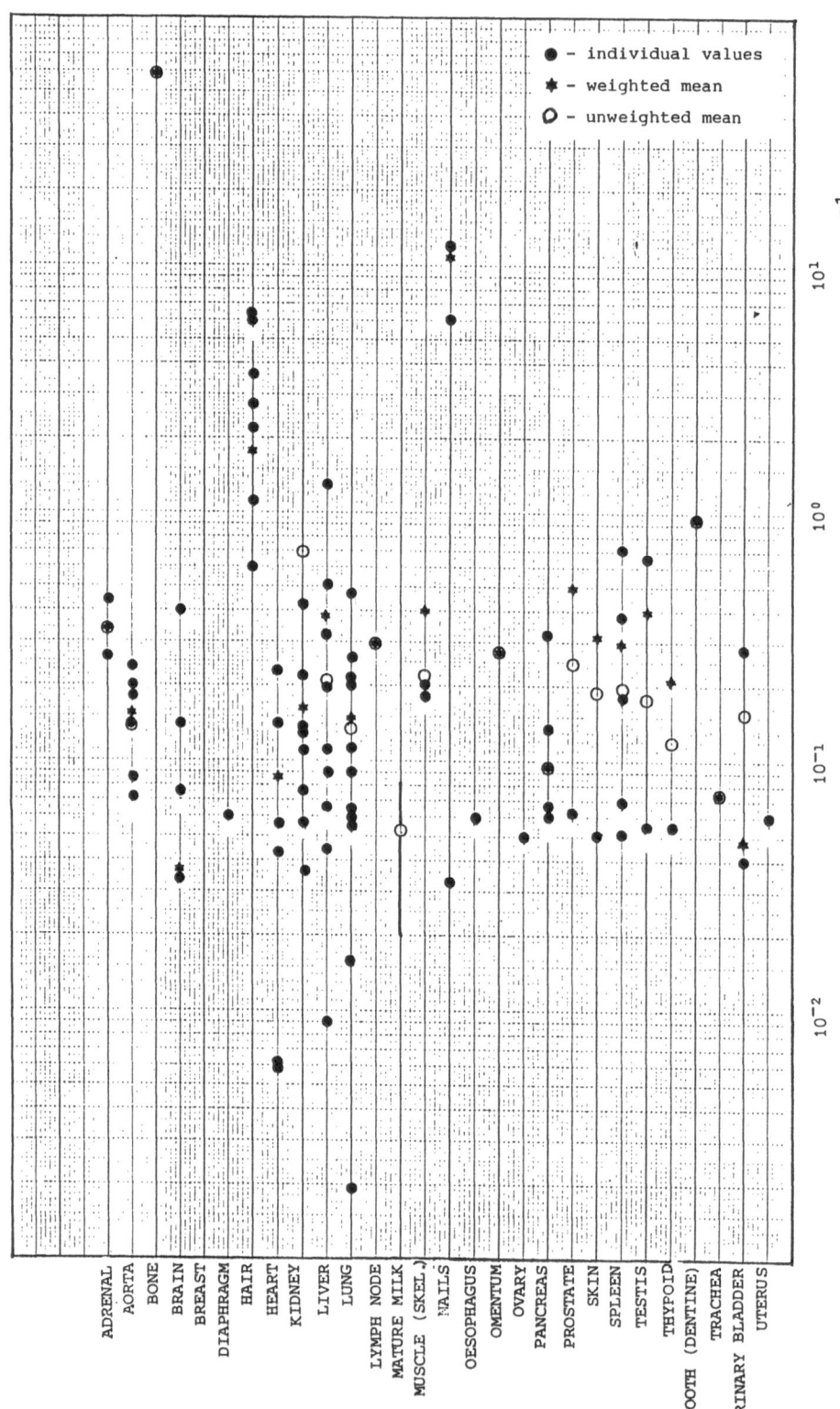

FIGURE 1   DISTRIBUTION OF STABLE NICKEL IN HUMAN TISSUES

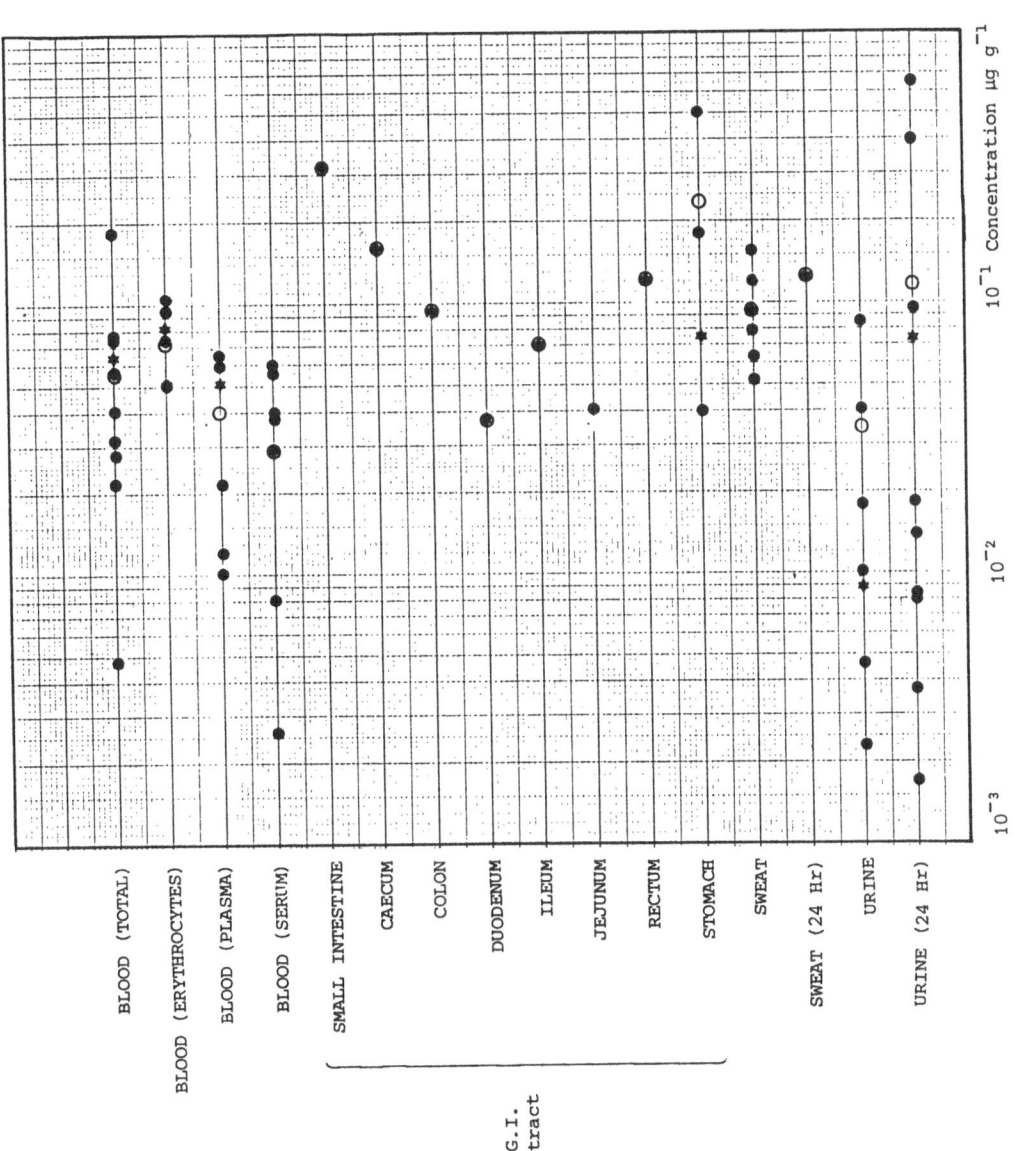

FIGURE 1 Cont.

Route of intake	Typical intake rate ($\mu g\ d^{-1}$)	Comments
Diet	400	Typical range 100 to 800 $\mu g\ d^{-1}$.
Drinking water	∿10	Rates of up to 300 $\mu g\ d^{-1}$ could occur in restricted areas.
Ambient air	0.12	Value for rural and suburban conditions. In urban conditions 2.3 $\mu g\ d^{-1}$ would be more representative.
Smoking	∿15	Based on 20 cigarettes per day. This nickel is likely to be almost entirely in the form of nickel carbonyl.
Occupational exposure	7-2100	Based on atmospheric concentrations of 1 to 300 μg m^{-3} and a 40 h working week.

5.3   DISTRIBUTION OF NICKEL IN HUMAN TISSUES

Data on the distribution of stable nickel in human tissues have been collated by Iyengar et al. (1978). Data from this review have been converted to concentrations in wet tissue. The results of these calculations are summarised in Table 1 and illustrated in Fig. 1. On the basis of these data, it is reasonable to conclude that nickel is probably concentrated in bone, and to some extent in hair and nails, but that it is relatively uniformly distributed throughout all other organs and tissues of the body.

With respect to tissue fluids, reported nickel concentrations have decreased throughout the years, probably due to improvements in analytical methods (Norseth and Piscator, 1979). Some additional values for concentrations in human organs, tissues and, more particularly, fluids are summarised in Table 2.

On the basis of data given in Tables 1 and 2, the following conclusions can be drawn:

- nickel concentrations in serum and urine are typically 2.5 $\mu g\ l^{-1}$;
- plasma concentrations are probably similar to serum concentrations, but whole-blood concentrations may be ∿5 $\mu g\ l^{-1}$;
- faecal concentrations are ∿3.3 $\mu g\ g^{-1}$ w.w., corresponding to faecal excretion rates ∿260 $\mu g\ d^{-1}$;
- hair concentrations are typically ∿1 $\mu g\ g^{-1}$;
- bone concentrations are not well known, with values of 0.33 and 54 $\mu g\ g^{-1}$ having been recorded;
- general levels in tissues are probably not higher than 0.2 $\mu g\ g^{-1}$ (w.w.), but they could be more than an order of magnitude lower than this.

Taking a nickel concentration in urine of 2.5 $\mu g\ l^{-1}$ and a daily urinary excretion of 1.4 l (ICRP, 1975), the daily excretion of nickel in urine is estimated as 3.5 μg. Thus, total urinary plus faecal nickel excretion is estimated as ∿260 $\mu g\ d^{-1}$, somewhat lower, but comparable with, an average dietary + water intake ∿410 $\mu g\ d^{-1}$ (Section 2.4).

TABLE 2

REPORTED CONCENTRATIONS OF NICKEL IN HUMAN
ORGANS, TISSUES AND TISSUE FLUIDS FOR
NON-OCCUPATIONALLY EXPOSED INDIVIDUALS

Organ, tissue or tissue fluid	Concentration	Reference	Comments
Serum	2.6 ± 0.9 µg l^{-1}	Horak and Sunderman, 1973	Corresponds to 258 ± 126 µg d^{-1}
Urine	2.2 ± 1.2 µg l^{-1}		
Faeces	3.3 ± 0.8 µg g^{-1} (w.w.)		
Sweat	49 ± 18 µg l^{-1}		
Hair	0.22 ± 0.08 µg g^{-1} (d.w.)		
Serum	4.6 ± 1.4 µg l^{-1}	McNeely et al., 1972	Sudbury values only. Hartford values reported in Horak and Sunderman, (1973)
Urine	7.2 ± 3.9 µg l^{-1}		
Serum	2.6 ± 0.8 µg l^{-1}	McNeely et al. 1971	Male controls
	2.7 ± 0.8 µg l^{-1}		Female controls
	4.0 ± 1.8 µg l^{-1}		Acute myocardial infarction 1-12h
	5.4 ± 2.8 µg l^{-1}		13-24h
	4.9 ± 2.7 µg l^{-1}		25-36h
	3.0 ± 1.7 µg l^{-1}		37-48h
	2.8 ± 1.9 µg l^{-1}		49-72h
	2.6 ± 1.3 µg l^{-1}		73-96h
	2.7 ± 3.1 µg l^{-1}		97-120h
	2.7 ± 1.2 µg l^{-1}		Acute myocardial ischemia 1-12h
	3.4 ± 1.4 µg l^{-1}		13-24h
	3.0 ± 1.8 µg l^{-1}		25-36h
	2.9 ± 1.2 µg l^{-1}		37-48h
	2.6 ± 1.0 µg l^{-1}		49-72h
	2.6 ± 0.6 µg l^{-1}		73-96h
	2.0 ± 0.6 µg l^{-1}		97-120h

TABLE 2 (Contd.)

Organ, tissue or tissue fluid	Concentration	Reference	Comments
Serum	3.5 ± 1.1 µg l⁻¹	McNeely et al., 1971	Acute stroke 13-36h
	4.5 ± 2.0 µg l⁻¹		37-72h
	7.2 µg l⁻¹		Burns 37-72h
	2.7 ± 0.9 µg l⁻¹		Trauma with fracture 13-36h
	3.0 ± 1.1 µg l⁻¹		37-72h
	1.7 ± 0.7 µg l⁻¹		Chronic Uremia
	1.6 ± 0.8 µg l⁻¹		Hepatic cirrhosis
	2.3 ± 0.9 µg l⁻¹		Alcoholic delirium tremens
	2.3 ± 1.4 µg l⁻¹		Muscular dystrophy
	3.0 ± 1.2 µg l⁻¹		Postpartum mothers
	3.0 ± 1.2 µg l⁻¹		Newborn infants (cord blood)
Whole blood	6.0 ± 1.0 µg l⁻¹	Zachariasen et al., 1975	8 healthy persons living at
Plasma	4.7 ± 1.0 µg l⁻¹		Kristiansand South, Norway
Urine	24 ± 4 µg l⁻¹		
Hair	0.51 (0.20-1.30)	Creason et al., 1975	Children⎫ Values are geometric mean.
	0.74 (0.27-2.07)		Adults ⎬ Range in parentheses is ± 1 geom. s.d. All values are in µg g⁻¹
Serum or Plasma	2.1 ± 1.1 µg l⁻¹	Sunderman, 1980a	Review
	2.5 ± 0.5 µg l⁻¹		Matsumoto, Japan
	1.9 ± 1.4 µg l⁻¹		Santiago, Spain
Urine	2.6 ± 1.2 µg l⁻¹		Kristiansand, Norway
	2.7 ± 1.1 µg l⁻¹		Julich, W. Germany
	4.9 ± 4.2 µg l⁻¹		Matsumoto, Japan
			Kristiansand, Norway

TABLE 2   (Contd.)

Organ, tissue or tissue fluid	Concentration	Reference	Comments
Whole blood	4.8±1.3 µg l⁻¹	Sunderman, 1980a	Review values, some of these are also included elsewhere in this table
Serum	2.6±0.9 µg l⁻¹		
Urine	2.2±1.2 µg l⁻¹		
Faeces	14.2±2.7 µg g⁻¹		
Scalp hair	0.22±0.08 µg g⁻¹		
Arm sweat	52±36 µg l⁻¹		
Parotid saliva	2.2±1.2 µg l⁻¹		
Palatine tonsils	0.14±0.07 µg g⁻¹ (w.w.)		Autopsy specimens. All values µg g⁻¹ (w.w.)
Nasal mucosa	0.13±0.20 µg g⁻¹ (w.w.)		
Bone	0.333±0.147		
Lung	0.085±0.065		
Kidney	0.0105±0.0041		
Liver	0.0082±0.0023		
Heart	0.0064±0.0016		
Serum	2.6 µg l⁻¹	Howard, 1980	Healthy controls
	1.8 µg l⁻¹		Hepatic disease
	2.7 µg l⁻¹		Hospital controls
	5.6 µg l⁻¹		Acute myocardial infarction, 0-6h
	6.2 µg l⁻¹		6-12h
	6.9 µg l⁻¹		12-24h
	6.9 µg l⁻¹		24-36h
	6.7 µg l⁻¹		36-48h
	6.5 µg l⁻¹		48-72h
	6.2 µg l⁻¹		72-96h
	5.7 µg l⁻¹		96-120h
	5.2 µg l⁻¹		120-216h
	3.2 µg l⁻¹		Myocardial ischemia, no infarction

TABLE 2 (Contd.)

Organ, tissue or tissue fluid	Concentration	Reference	Comments
Lung Lymph nodes	0.23 ± 0.06 µg g^{-1} (w.w.) 0.81 ± 0.41 µg g^{-1} (w.w.)	Bernstein et al., 1974	New York City residents
Scalp hair Plasma Urine	0.6 µg g^{-1} 1.0 µg g^{-1} 1.6 µg l^{-1} 2.0 µg l^{-1} 0.6 µg l^{-1}	Spruit and Bongaarts, 1977a, 1977b	Men Women Men Women Men No difference between hypersensitive and non-hypersensitive subjects
Teeth	16 µg g^{-1} 16 µg g^{-1}	Stack et al., 1976	Foetal enamel } 4 foetuses Foetal dentine
Scalp hair Pubic hair Whole blood Cord blood Placenta	1.7 µg g^{-1} 0.7 µg g^{-1} 0.85 µg l^{-1} 0.81 µg l^{-1} 0.034 µg g^{-1} (w.w.)	Creason et al., 1977	Maternal Maternal Maternal
Liver Brain Heart Lung Skel. muscle Bone Kidney	0.15±0.12 0.038±0.026 0.14±0.13 0.068±0.049 0.048±0.032 0.14±0.09 0.03-0.32	Casey and Robinson, 1978	Foetal tissues. Values ± s.d. given on a wet weight basis Range of values on 21 foetuses

Notes (Cont.):

(3) Defatted

(4) Based on excretion of 650 ml d^{-1} (ICRP, 1975)

(5) Based on excretion of 1400 ml d^{-1} (ICRP), 1975)

(6) Ash to wet weight conversion based on muscle

(7) Heavily biased to a single study giving 6 $\mu g\ g^{-1}$ on an unspecified number of individuals

(8) Values of weighted and unweighted means for all urine studies are 0.034 and 0.084 $\mu g\ g^{-1}$ respectively

5.4   METABOLISM

5.4.1   Gastrointestinal absorption

The fractional absorption of nickel from the gastrointestinal tract is generally thought to be low, both for dietary nickel and for inorganic compounds of the element. Underwood (1977) estimated fractional absorption at 0.01 to 0.10, even at high intakes. In setting standards for limiting exposure of workers to radioactive nickel, the ICRP (1981) used a value of 0.05 for the fractional gastrointestinal absorption of all inorganic compounds of the element, though they noted that fractional absorption values of as much as 0.5 have sometimes been quoted for dietary nickel (see also ICRP, 1975 and Veterans Administration Hospital, 1975). Data reviewed by Norseth and Piscator (1979) indicate a fractional absorption of no more than 0.1 in man, while, for domestic animals, Coughtrey and Thorne (1983) concluded that it is probably conservative to take the fractional absorption of dietary nickel and inorganic compounds of the element as 0.05. Data reviewed by Mushak (1980) indicate that the fractional absorption of nickel in dietary or liquid form is typically between 0.01 and 0.06. In discussing the toxicity of nickel, Nielsen (1977) concluded that nickel or nickel salts are relatively non-toxic when taken orally and that abnormally high levels of dietary nickel are required to overcome homeostatic mechanisms that control nickel metabolism. He stated that nickel toxicity in humans via the oral route occurs only in extreme and unusual circumstances.

In mice, Oskarrson and Tjalve (1979a) reported that, at five days after oral administration of $^{63}NiCl_2$, the highest content of radioactivity was present in the intestinal contents. They commented that only a small fraction of the administered radioactivity was absorbed from the gastrointestinal tract, but did not quantify this statement.

In rats, Ho and Furst (1973) showed that, regardless of the amount of nickel administered orally as the chloride, from 3 to 6% of the metal occurred in the urine and the rest in the faeces. In similar animals injected intraperitoneally, only 1 to 2% of nickel was excreted in the faeces. From these two results, it can be concluded that the fractional gastrointestinal absorption of nickel in the orally dosed rats was 0.03 to 0.06.

In a study in which rats were maintained on a diet containing 25 mg Ni per 100g of diet, Phatak and Patwardhan (1952) recorded urinary and faecal nickel excretion after various periods of feeding. Results were as listed below.

Period of feeding (mo)	Nickel content (mg)		
	Urine*	Faeces*	Retained
4	0.14	12.3	0.66
8	0.20	12.9	0.80
12	0.11	14.9	0.29
16	0.14	15.3	0.36

*   Excretion measured over 4 days.

Because retained material would have been mainly in gut contents, the fractional absorption implied by these results is ~0.01.

In Syrian golden hamsters, Wehner and Craig (1972) reported that they were unable to detect any increase in the nickel content of lungs, liver, kidneys and carcass following an oral intake of 5 mg of the element. This is indicative of limited gastrointestinal absorption, but the results are not quantifiable.

In experiments on rabbits (Decsy and Sunderman, 1974) the serum nickel concentration was reported to be 1.5 μg l^{-1} at 2.5 h after oral dosing at a level of 240 μg kg^{-1}. In contrast, at 2 h after intravenous dosing at the same level, the serum concentration was reported to be 720 μg l^{-1}. These results are suggestive of a fractional gastrointestinal absorption of 0.01, but, in the absence of data on the time dependence of serum concentrations in these studies, this cannot be confirmed.

In calves, O'Dell et al. (1971) have reported urinary and faecal levels of nickel for different levels of dietary supplementation. Assuming that most systemic nickel is excreted in the urine, these data can be converted to fractional gastrointestinal absorption. Results of this calculation are summarised below.

Level of supplementation (ppm)	Urinary nickel (mg d^{-1})	Faecal nickel (mg d^{-1})	Fractional absorption
0	0.47	9.83	0.046
62.5	7.16	260.56	0.027
250	24.75	1285.30	0.019
1000	45.31	1020.90	0.042

Fractional gastrointestinal absorption was remarkably constant in this study, even at dietary nickel levels which were high enough to cause gross depression of feed consumption and weight gain.

Spears et al. (1978b) studied the retention of an oral dose of ^{63}NiCl$_2$ in lambs on a low nickel or on a nickel-supplemented diet. On the low nickel diet, 74.4% of the Ni-63 was excreted in the faeces in the first 72 h after administration and 0.8±0.2% in the urine. Corresponding figures for the nickel-supplemented diet were 64.7±3.3% and 2.0±1.0%. In each case, tissue levels at 72 h post-administration were ≤0.02% dose kg^{-1}, corresponding to a total systemic burden ≤0.4% of the administered dose. These data indicate a fractional gastrointestinal absorption ∿0.01 to 0.03, but considerable retention in the gastrointestinal tract at three days after ingestion.

For man, the data on urinary and faecal contents reviewed in Section 3 are indicative of a fractional gastrointestinal absorption ∿0.01 for dietary nickel. In a study of nickel feeding to nickel-sensitive patients with hand eczema, Jordan and King (1979) reported that following a dose of 0.5 mg of nickel as nickel sulphate hexahydrate the highest increase in urinary nickel was from 10.5 μg/24 h to 32.16 μg/24 h. Bearing in mind the rapid excretion of nickel (Section 4.3), this is indicative of a fractional gastrointestinal absorption ∿0.05.

In a similar study, Christensen and Lagesson (1980) reported urinary excretion of nickel following oral dosing of eight subjects with 5.6 mg of nickel as the sulphate. The results of this study can be interpreted as representing a fractional gastrointestinal absorption of 0.05. Also, Cronin et al. (1980) reported that in the 24 h following oral doses of

0.6, 1.25 and 2.5 mg of nickel the total urinary excretion in female patients was 48-89, 62-253 and 95-206 µg respectively. These excretion rates are consistent with a fractional gastrointestinal absorption of ∿0.1 to 0.2.

In balance studies, Nodiya (1972) recorded urinary and faecal nickel values in ten students of an occupational technical school. Average urinary and faecal excretion rates were 29 µg d^{-1} and 258 µg d^{-1} respectively, indicating a fractional gastrointestinal absorption ∿0.1.

Solomons et al. (1982) studied the relative availability of orally administered nickel to man by monitoring changes in blood plasma levels after oral dosing with the sulphate. Their data demonstrate that simultaneous ingestion of nickel sulphate and cows' milk, orange juice, tea or coffee depresses absorption, whereas coca cola has little effect. These authors also reported that 1 g of ascorbic acid depressed absorption, but that phytic acid did not significantly affect plasma nickel.

On the basis of the data reviewed above, a best estimate for the fractional absorption of nickel from the gastrointestinal tract of man is 0.05, but a range of 0.01 to 0.20 is not unusual, depending upon chemical form administered, nature of the diet, nickel status, and state of health. Absorption does not seem to be modified substantially by the amount of nickel present in the diet.

5.4.2   Retention in the respiratory system

Carcinogenesis of the respiratory tract due to nickel exposure has been identified as a significant problem in occupationally exposed individuals (Section 5.1). The metabolism of compounds of nickel following inhalation exposure has been discussed in several publications (ICRP, 1981; Coughtrey and Thorne, 1983; Sunderman, 1977a; Mushak, 1980; Norseth and Piscator, 1979). For convenience of discussion it is appropriate to distinguish between the behaviour of nickel carbonyl and other forms of nickel.

5.4.2.1   Nickel carbonyl

Nickel carbonyl, $Ni(CO)_4$, is a volatile colourless liquid which is highly toxic when inhaled (Section 5.1). As Sunderman (1977a) has stated "the pulmonary parenchyma has consistently been found to be the prinicpal target tissue of $Ni(CO)_4$ toxicity, regardless of the route of administration. Type I alveolar cells (membranous pneumocytes) are primarily damaged by $Ni(CO)_4$, but type II alveolar cells (granular pneumocytes) are also affected." On the basis of a review of animal data, Sunderman (1977a) has also concluded that "$Ni(CO)_4$ can cross the alveolar membranes in either direction without metabolic alteration. During the first 2 to 4 hours after exposure of rats or rabbits to $Ni(CO)_4$, the lung is a major excretory organ for $Ni(CO)_4$. Thereafter, $Ni(CO)_4$ is progressively oxidized within erythrocytes and other cells to liberate $Ni(II)$, which is excreted in the urine, and carbon monoxide which is eliminated in the expired breath." These comments on nickel carbonyl are consistent with those of the ICRP (1981) who noted that, following inhalation, nickel carbonyl is almost completely absorbed from the lungs, but that the compound is briefly retained on parenchymal lung surfaces before its entry into the systemic circulation. The ICRP (1981) also stated that "nickel entering the systemic circulation as nickel carbonyl is broken down in the red cells, and other tissues, to Ni° and CO. The Ni° is oxidised intracellularly to Ni^{2+} and released to the blood serum, where it behaves similarly to intravenously injected nickel compounds." For the purpose of estimating dose to man the ICRP (1981) assumed that all nickel entering the respiratory system as nickel carbonyl is deposited there and that it is then translocated to the systemic circulation with a biological half-life of 0.1 days. After entry into the systemic circulation the metabolic model for other inorganic compounds of nickel was assumed to apply.

Experimental studies on the metabolism of nickel carbonyl in various mammalian species are discussed below.

Armit (1908) studied the metabolism of inhaled $Ni(CO)_4$ in rabbits and cats and drew the following conclusions:

- in the lungs nickel carbonyl is dissociated and a nickel compound is deposited on the respiratory surface;

- some of the nickel finds its way directly through the lymphatic channels into the bronchial [lymph] glands.

However, these conclusions were based on a variety of histochemical staining techniques, the validity of which it is difficult to assess.

Dissociation of nickel carbonyl in the lungs is substantiated by an autoradiographic study in which $^{63}Ni(CO)_4$ or $Ni(^{14}CO)_4$ was administered to mice intravenously or by inhalation (Oskarsson and Tjalve, 1977). In mice given $^{63}Ni(CO)_4$ by either route, a high radioactivity was present in the lung at all survival intervals, whereas in mice given $Ni(^{14}CO)_4$ the radioactivity was restricted mainly to the blood, presumably due to the formation of ^{14}C-labelled carboxyhaemoglobin.

Quantitative data on the distribution of nickel carbonyl in mice and rabbits following inhalation were given by West and Sunderman (1958) who reported the following tissue concentrations in animals exposed to the vapour for 30 minutes. Animals treated with EDTA were injected with the chelate immediately after exposure.

Animal	Treatment	Tissue concentration ($\mu g\ g^{-1}$)			
		Lung	Liver	Kidney	Brain
Mouse	Control	9.12±2.89	2.06±0.41	10.03±2.55	-
	$CaNa_2$-EDTA	8.23±1.78	5.09±2.11	11.01±2.74	-
Rabbit-1	Control	10.87	1.78	12.12	-
-2	$CaNa_2$-EDTA	12.01	3.68	4.94	-
-5	Control	12.73	6.08	5.15	3.14
-6	$CaNa_2$-EDTA	13.07	3.87	6.20	3.85

The mice were exposed to air concentrations of 60 mg m^{-3} and the results given above are from mice that died within 3 days as a result of this exposure. Rabbits 1 and 2 were exposed to 2 g m^{-3} and rabbits 5 and 6 to 1.75 g m^{-3}. The time of assay for these animals was not recorded. In two other rabbits exposed to 1.75 g m^{-3}, average nickel concentrations in urine in the first 24 h post-exposure were ~15 $\mu g\ ml^{-1}$.

In studies on dogs, Tedeschi and Sunderman (1957) reported that following inhalation exposure to nickel carbonyl there was a striking increase in excretion of nickel in urine in the first three days after exposure, but that in days 4 to 6 the amount of nickel in urine tended to return to pre-exposure levels. From detailed balance studies on one dog it was concluded that approximately 99% of the ingested and inhaled nickel was eliminated in the urine and faeces within six days.

In studies on rats, Ghiringhelli and Agamennone (1957) reported high concentrations of nickel in the lungs after 30 minute exposures to air containing 0.4 g m^{-3} of nickel carbonyl. At this time, concentrations in brain, liver, kidneys and blood were also high. All tissues appeared to decrease in content at a similar rate, with a biological half-life of ~1d. Excretion data were presented for five rats exposed to 30 ppm $Ni(CO)_4$, but this level was not sufficient to give significantly enhanced excretion rates.

More recently, Sunderman and Selin (1968) reported on the tissue distribution and excretion of nickel in rats following intravenous injection and inhalation of nickel carbonyl. They commented that the tissue distribution of ^{63}Ni 24 hours after inhalation of $^{63}Ni(CO)_4$ differed from the distribution found after intravenous injection. A comparison of their data is given below:

Tissue	Percent of dose		Percent of body burden	
	Intravenous	Inhalation	Intravenous	Inhalation
Muscle + fat	7.3±1.4	9.8±1.7	41.2±2.5	30.4±5.4
Bone + connective tissue	5.5±0.7	5.0±2.8	31.1±3.7	15.6±8.6
Viscera + blood	4.7±1.4	16.0±2.9	26.6±6.7	49.7±9.2
Brain + spinal cord	0.20±0.06	1.4±0.4	1.1±0.6	4.4±1.1
Total (excluding pelt)	17.7±2.3	32.2±2.0	100	100

The main absolute difference between routes of exposure is an enhanced retention in viscera and blood following inhalation. Excretion was also compared between the two routes and the results are listed below.

Day	Percent of dose excreted						
	Injection				Inhalation		
	Urine	Faeces	Breath	Total	Urine	Faeces	Total
1	27.0±6.1	0.8±0.2	38.4±7.2	66.2	17.2±1.4	17.7±4.1	34.9
2	2.0±1.7	0.5±0.2	-	2.5	7.5±1.9	3.1±1.9	10.6
3	1.6±0.8	0.6±0.4	-	2.2	6.0±0.7	4.7±2.6	10.7
4	0.6±0.5	0.5±0.3	-	1.1	3.8±1.5	4.5±2.6	8.3
1 to 4	31.2±10.1	2.4±0.8	38.4±7.2	72.0	34.4±3.6	29.7±8.9	64.1

The significance of the exhalation route is clear from the injection studies, but was not investigated in the inhalation exposure mode. The other main point of interest is the enhanced faecal excretion in the inhalation case. Sunderman and Selin (1968) attributed this to ingestion of nickel present on contaminated fur and this seems likely to have been the case.

Data on the retention and excretion of nickel in man, following acute exposure to nickel carbonyl, have been reported (Sunderman and Kincaid, 1954; Sunderman and Sunderman, 1958; Sunderman, 1964; Jones, 1973; Adams, 1980). Interpretation of these data is complicated by the high levels of intake and by the use of dithiocarb (sodium

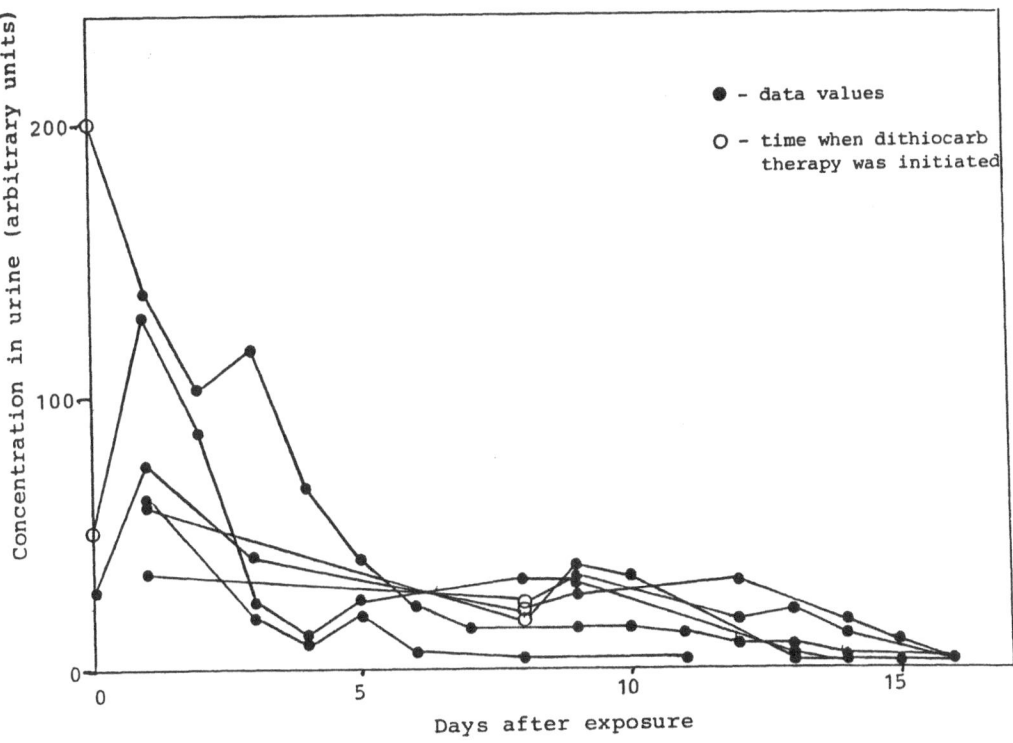

Note:
(1) Data from Sunderman and Sunderman (1958)

FIGURE 2   CONCENTRATION OF NICKEL IN THE URINE OF
WORKERS ACCIDENTALLY EXPOSED TO NICKEL
CARBONYL.

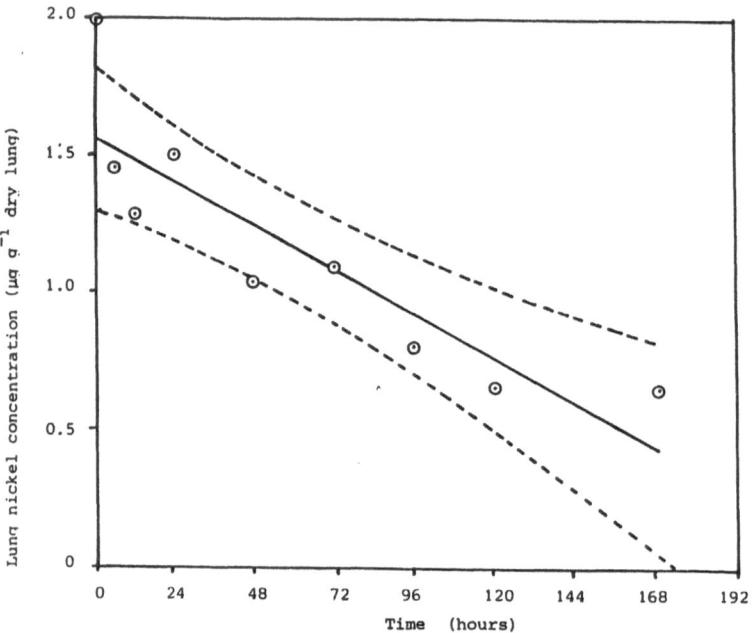

Notes:

(1)   Data from Adkins et al. (1979).

(2)   Broken lines are 95% confidence limits.

FIGURE 3.   CLEARANCE OF NICKEL FROM MICE LUNGS AFTER
            INHALATION OF A NiCl$_2$ ATMOSPHERE FOR 2 Hrs.

diethyldithiocarbamate) in treatment. Representative urinary excretion data from some of the reported exposures are plotted in Fig. 2, which illustrates that rapid early urinary excretion of nickel is not universally associated with acute inhalation exposure to the carbonyl.

On the basis of the data reviewed above, it is concluded that the ICRP (1981) model provides the best currently available representation of the initial uptake of nickel carbonyl, but that further work on nickel carbonyl metabolism is required before any detailed model can be developed. In particular, dissociation and nickel retention on respiratory surfaces needs considerably more investigation.

5.4.2.2 Other compounds of nickel

With respect to compounds of nickel other than nickel carbonyl, it is important to note the observation that the potential of such compounds for inducing cell transformation is related to the degree to which they are phagocytosed (Costa and Mollenhauer, 1980a; 1980b; 1980c; Costa et al., 1981). Thus, interactions of inhaled nickel particles with lung macrophages and other phagocytic cells may be of significance with respect to neoplastic transformation. It is noted that, as a result of studies on rabbits exposed by inhalation to metallic nickel dust, Johannson et al. (1980) commented that while after a short time of nickel exposure lung macrophages seem to retain, or even increase, their functional capacity (see also Jarstrand et al., 1978 and Bingham et al., 1972), they probably have a decreased function after longer exposure. Johannsen et al. noted that, in long-term experiments nickel particles were occasionally seen within macrophages. These particles were small and were located in secondary lysosomes and residual bodies. Particles outside macrophages were surrounded by lamellar bodies, which may have a role in preventing cells in the lungs from coming into close contact with foreign material. The intracellular location of nickel entering cells in soluble form, or solubilised within the cell, is discussed in Section 4.3.

Data on the gross distribution and retention of compounds of nickel in the lung are rather limited. On the basis of the recommendations of the ICRP Task Group on Lung Dynamics (ICRP, 1966) and the results of experiments on hamsters (Wehner and Craig, 1972) and rats (Ziemer and Carvalho, 1980), the ICRP (1981) assigned oxides, hydroxides and carbides of nickel to inhalation class W and all other commonly occurring compounds of the element to inhalation class D.

Adkins et al. (1979) studied the deposition and retention of $NiCl_2$ in mice following a 2 h exposure. Deposition was studied for aerosol concentrations ranging from zero to 1000 μg Ni m^{-3} and retention was studied at an exposure of 583.73±10.89 μg Ni m^{-3}. It is noted that exposure at the 500 μg Ni m^{-3} level was sufficient to reduce the resistance of these mice to streptococcal infection; in particular, nickel-exposed mice demonstrated a reduced capacity to clear inhaled streptococci. Thus, some impairment of lung function is indicated at these levels of exposure. Results of the study demonstrated that nickel deposition in the lungs was directly proportional to the concentration in air. Lung concentrations fell relatively rapidly in the first week post-exposure. This can either be interpreted as a linear (Fig. 3) or an exponential (Fig. 4) decrease. On the exponential interpretation, the half-life for lung retention was ~110 h.

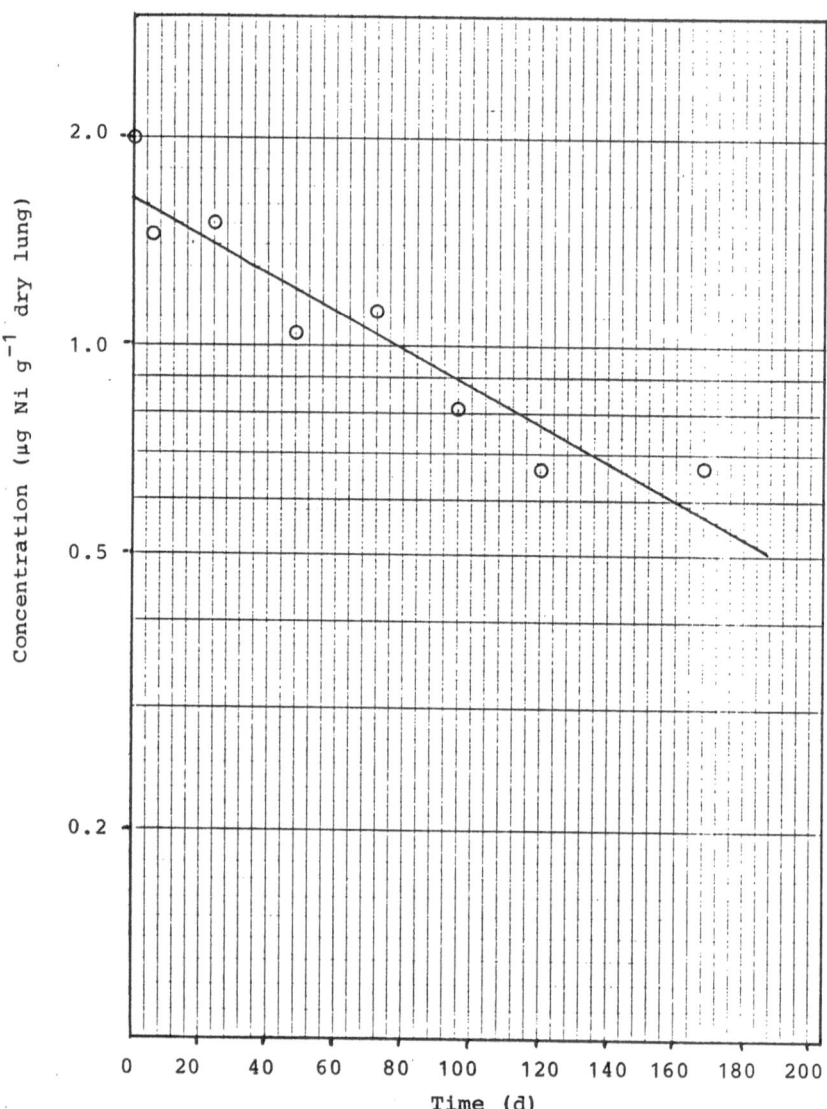

Note:

(1) Data from Fig.3 replotted on a semi-log plot

FIGURE 4.   CLEARANCE OF NICKEL FROM MICE LUNGS

Clary (1975) studied the distribution of Ni-63 in the rat following intratracheal instillation of ^{63}NiCl$_2$ and reported the following data on tissue concentration (decays per minute per gram).

Tissue	Time after injection		
	6h	24h	72h
Kidney	(1.96 ± 0.30)x10^5	(1.09 ± 0.19)x10^5	(9.01 ± 1.19)x10^3
Lung	(1.11 ± 0.20)x10^5	(5.61 ± 1.31)x10^4	(2.98 ± 1.86)x10^4
Adrenal	(1.59 ± 0.37)x10^4	(8.55 ± 1.66)x10^3	(4.99 ± 0.27)x10
Liver	(1.14 ± 0.36)x10^4	(3.01 ± 1.06)x10^3	(5.15 ± 0.84)x10^2
Pancreas	(9.83 ± 2.51)x10^3	(3.70 ± 1.09)x10^3	(5.52 ± 0.79)x10^2
Spleen	(9.50 ± 3.14)x10^3	(4.61 ± 1.97)x10^3	(1.12 ± 0.13)x10^3
Heart	(9.19 ± 1.10)x10^3	(2.94 ± 0.43)x10^3	(1.57 ± 0.17)x10^2
Testis	(4.67 ± 0.53)x10^3	(2.28 ± 0.52)x10^3	(5.57 ± 1.31)x10^2

These data are consistent with an early phase of rapid lung clearance followed by a slower phase with a biological half-life of ~50 h.

The retention of NiCl$_2$ and NiO in rat lung and associated lymph nodes following intratracheal instillation has been studied by English et al. (1981). Results of their study, summarised in Fig. 5, indicate that NiO is retained in the lung with a biological half-life of ~60 d and that significant translocation to lymph nodes occurs. In contrast, NiCl$_2$ is cleared rapidly from both lung and lymph nodes, with more than 90% of the nickel being lost in the first day. The longer-term components of lung retention observed with the chloride are likely to represent redeposition of systemic nickel in that tissue (Section 5.4.3). In the case of NiO, concentrations of nickel in all tissues other than lung and lymph nodes were typically two or three orders of magnitude lower than the concentration in lung at all times after intratracheal instillation. In the case of NiCl$_2$, concentrations in other tissues were comparable with concentrations in lung at all times greater than one day post-instillation. Urinary excretion dominated over faecal excretion in the case of NiCl$_2$, but in the case of NiO, the contributions of the two routes were similar (Fig. 5). This indicates that, notwithstanding its slow removal from the lung, a substantial fraction of the NiO which is removed is translocated to the systemic circulation rather than to the gut.

Williams et al. (1980) studied the removal of Ni^{2+} from the airways of the isolated perfused rat lung following intratracheal instillation of the chloride in isotonic solution. They reported a biological half-life for removal which increased as the amount instilled decreased, ranging from 4.58 ± 0.34 h at 127 nmol per lung to 19.7 ± 6.49 h at 1 nmol per lung. In a corresponding in vivo study, they reported that the rate of removal was independent of the amount instilled. The clearance half-life in this case was ~8 h. Williams et al. (1980) concluded that Ni^{2+} is removed from the airways of the rat lung by a process of diffusion. Very similar data are reported in a second paper from this group (Menzel et al., 1980).

With respect to the half-life of nickel in the rat lung, Oberdoerster and Hochrainer (1980) demonstrated that continuous long-term exposure to NiO may lead to impaired lung clearance. Thus, in these circumstances more nickel might be expected to be accumulated in the lung than would be estimated by extrapolation from the results of short-term exposures.

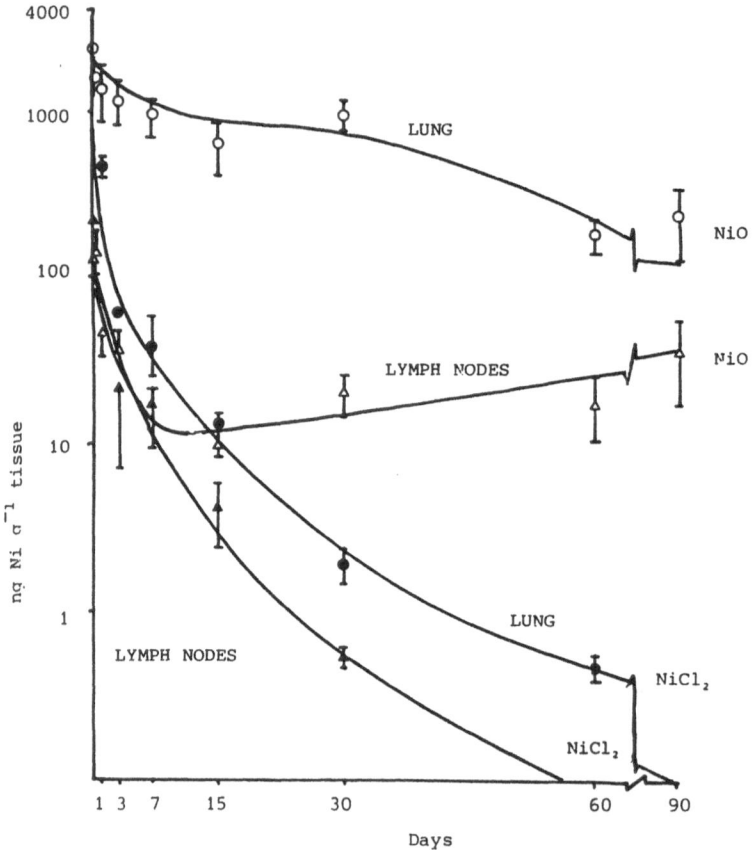

Note:

(1)   Data from English et al. (1981).

FIGURE 5.   CHANGE IN NICKEL CONCENTRATION IN RAT LUNG
            AND ASSOCIATED LYMPH NODES FOLLOWING AN
            INTRATRACHEAL INJECTION OF $NiCl_2$ OR NiO.

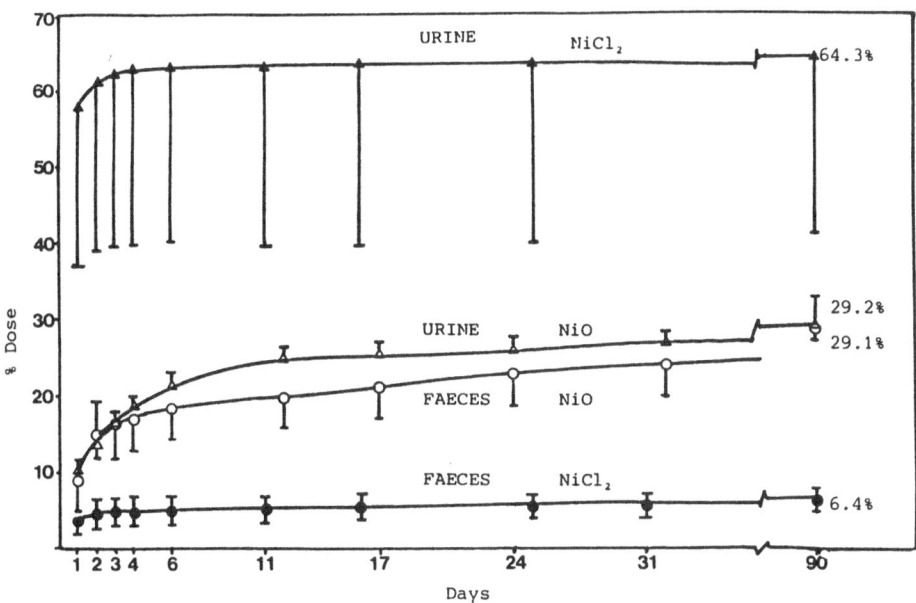

Notes:

(1)   Data from English et al. (1981)

FIGURE 6.   ACCUMULATED EXCRETION OF NICKEL VIA URINE AND
FAECES FOLLOWING INTRATRACHEAL INJECTION OF
$NiCl_2$ OR NiO.

Wehner and Craig (1972) studied the retention of NiO in Syrian golden hamsters following inhalation. The data presented indicated that the NiO, was cleared from the lungs with a biological half-life of ~60 d. It is notable that Wehner and Craig failed to find significant quantities of nickel in the livers and kidneys at any post-exposure time. More recently, Wehner et al. (1975) have reported results from three month sub-acute toxicity studies with NiO and cigarette smoke in Syrian golden hamsters. During a 61 d exposure, the animals were estimated to have inhaled 50.9 mg of the aerosol (mass median diameter 2.1 μm). The distribution of the retained material was as listed below.

Exposure	Quantity retained (mg)	Distribution (% of retained)		
		Lung	Liver	Kidneys
NiO	10.27	99.75	0.21	0.04
NiO + smoke	9.79	99.73	0.22	0.05

Taking a 60d half-life in the lungs, these results imply that ~40% of inhaled nickel was deposited in the lungs, consistent with the calculated value for an aerosol of this diameter (ICRP, 1966). The results confirm the limited uptake and retention of nickel in tissues other than the lung. Whether this is due to limited translocation, or to rapid excretion of the translocated material, cannot be determined from the results reported.

For man, Bernstein et al. (1974) have set up a single compartment model to represent clearance from the lung and have used this to estimate the biological half-lives of various metals in the lungs of New York City residents. Results from this study indicate a biological half-life of 330 d for the pulmonary clearance of nickel, but the chemical form inhaled is not known.

Other data on nickel in man following inhalation relate primarily to biological monitoring. Thus, Høgetveit et al. (1978) illustrated the rapid fall in plasma nickel concentration (biological half-life ~2 d) after insistence on the use of a protective mask. These authors noted the generally poor correlation between atmospheric levels and both plasma and urine nickel concentrations. Limited correlation between atmospheric and urinary nickel was also a feature of the results presented by Morgan and Ronge (1979). In contrast, Tola et al. (1979) concluded that both urine and plasma nickel concentrations may be used as biological indicators of exposure to soluble nickel compounds in an electroplating shop, while Bernacki et al. (1978b) found a correlation between mean air concentration and mean urine concentration for groups of workers, but not for individual workers within the groups. However, Bernacki et al. (1980) have pointed out that while end-shift urine concentrations are correlated with air concentrations, no correlation is observed for beginning or mid-shift urine samples. It is noted that general levels of materials in workplace air are seldom a good measure of intake.

Finally, with respect to longer-term monitoring, Torjussen and Andersen (1979) have estimated that nickel is released from the nasal mucosa with a half-life of ~3.5 y. However, as Bernacki et al. (1980) have noted, although nasal mucosal biopsy under local anaesthesia is a relatively safe procedure, the technique would probably be applied only in workers who have definite risks of developing respiratory cancers.

On the basis of the data reviewed above, it seems that NiCl$_2$ is properly assigned to inhalation class D of the ICRP lung model and NiO to inhalation class W. The absence of relevant data on α-Ni$_3$S$_2$ (crystalline nickel subsulphide) and β-NiS (crystalline nickel sulphide) is disturbing, in view of their industrial significance and potential carcinogenic activity (see Section 1). In the absence of further data, it is recommended that the ICRP lung model be used for all inorganic compounds of nickel and that the following classification of those compounds be used:

Inhalation class	Compounds
W	oxides, hydroxides, carbides, Ni$_3$S$_2$ (amorphous and crystalline) NiS (amorphous and crystalline)
D	all other commonly occuring compounds

This classification is likely to over-estimate, rather than under-estimate, the mobility of the nickel sulphides.

5.4.3 Systemic metabolism

The metabolism of various compounds of nickel following administration to experimental animals and man by various routes has been studied extensively and it is convenient to discuss the subject under the following headings:
- binding of nickel to constituents of blood, serum and urine;
- uptake by cells and intracellular binding;
- distribution and retention in tissues, and transfer to the foetus.

5.4.3.1 Binding of nickel to constituents of blood, and urine

The binding of nickel to the various constituents of blood has been discussed widely. Data reviewed in Section 3 indicate that concentrations in erythrocytes and plasma are similar, and this is in agreement with results from comparative studies by Herring et al. (1960). However, in rats, Smith and Hackley (1968) found that plasma concentrations were about twice whole blood concentrations at all times after intravenous injection of the chloride. Similar results have been reported for human blood following oral intake of nickel sulphate (Christensen and Lagesson, 1980) and for rat blood following chronic dietary intake (Whanger, 1973). In contrast, after the intravenous injection of ^{63}Ni(CO)$_4$ into rats, Kasprzak and Sunderman (1969) found that the proportion of blood ^{63}Ni in erythrocytes diminished from 48±4.5% at 1 h post-injection to 8±0.3% at 6h. In the same experiment, but using ^{63}Ni(^{14}CO)$_4$, Kasprzak and Sunderman found that during the entire period from 1 to 24 h post-injection 95.4% of C-14 in blood was associated with erythrocytes. These data are indicative of the hypothesis that a substantial proportion of intravenously injected Ni(CO)$_4$ is taken up by erythrocytes in unmodified form before being broken down into carbon monoxide, which binds to haemoglobin, and free nickel, which is released to the extracellular environment.

Recently, Barton et al. (1980) have reported that in blood samples from refinery workers the distribution of nickel in blood was 24% in

TABLE 3

BINDING OF NICKEL TO CONSTITUENTS OF SERUM

Reference	Results
Sunderman et al., 1972	Fractionation of serum nickel ($\mu g \ l^{-1}$). Component Rabbit Human Starting serum 9.0 2.6 Ultrafilterable 1.4 1.0 Albumin-bound 3.6 0.9 Nickeloplasmin 4.0 0.7
Hendel and Sunderman, 1972	Percent ultrafilterable nickel in various species. Man 41 (36-45) Dog >85 (>78->95) Rat 27 Rabbit 16 (15-17) Lobster 38 (31-45)
Nomoto et al., 1973	After up to 21 days of repeated injections of $^{63}Ni \ Cl_2$ Only 1.2% of total serum ^{63}Ni was present in nickeloplasmin. In contrast 44% of stable nickel was in nickeloplasmin, indicating a long equilibration time for this component of serum.
Callan and Sunderman, 1973	Species variations in the affinity of albumin for Ni(II) are responsible, at least in part, for species differences in the proportions of serum ultrafilterable and protein-bound nickel.
Decsy and Sunderman, 1974	Demonstration of the difficulty of labelling rabbit nickeloplasmin with ^{63}Ni in vivo and in vitro. Comparison of the in vivo and in vitro results suggested that ^{63}Ni-nickeloplasmin might be a ternary complex of serum α_1-macroglobulin with an ultrafilterable ^{63}Ni-constituent if serum.

TABLE 3 (Contd.)

Reference	Results
Asato et al., 1975	Different complexes in rabbit serum assayed by thin layer chromatography. Time-dependence of total serum nickel and ultrafilterable nickel after intravenous injection. | Time after injection (h)	Total serum nickel ($\mu mol\ l^{-1}$)	Percent ultrafilterable
---	---	---
0.25	23	29
0.5	18	27
1.0	15	21
2.0	12	17	
Lucassen and Sarkar, 1979, see also Sarker, 1980	^{63}Ni Cl$_2$ added to human blood serum in vitro. Of total ^{63}Ni, 95.7% was associated with albumin, 4.2% was bound to low-molecular-weight components and ≤0.1% was associated with a high-molecular-weight protein. L-histidine was identified as the main low-molecular-weight binding component.
Gitlitz et al., 1975	Observation of histidinuria in nickel-intoxicated rats led to the suggestion that a nickel-histidine chelate might be involved in the renal excretion of Ni(II).
Nomoto, 1980	43% of human serum nickel was found to be bound to α_2-macroglobulin.
Sunderman et al., 1981	Identification of five macromolecular nickel binding constituents in the renal cytosol of rats. The rest of the nickel in the cytosol was associated with low molecular weight (<2000) components.

plasma, 13% in erythrocytes and 63% in a composite fraction representing white blood cells, fibrin and platelets.

In summary, it appears that nickel has no particular affinity for erythrocytes, which substantiates the comment of Mushak (1980) that, although the exact partitioning of nickel between erythrocytes and plasma or serum has not been determined, it appears that serum levels reliably reflect blood burdens and exposure status.

Serum albumin is the main carrier protein for nickel in human, bovine, rabbit and rat sera. A second macromolecular carrier in the sera of rabbit and man is a nickel-rich metalloprotein identified as an α-macroglobulin in rabbits (nickeloplasmin) and a 9.5S α-glycoprotein in man (Mushak, 1980). In addition to protein-bound nickel, several ultrafilterable complexes have been isolated in rabbit and human sera and in rabbit urine (Asato et al., 1975; Lucassen and Sarkar, 1979; Van Soestbergen and Sunderman, 1972). Various individual studies on nickel-binding in serum are summarised in Table 3; the chemistry of nickel-albumin interactions was discussed by Rao (1962) and Cotton (1964); the dissolution of nickel subsulphide in rat serum was studied by Kasprzak and Sunderman (1977) and the dissolution of various compounds of nickel in whole blood was studied by Andersen et al. (1980).

Data on chemical forms of nickel in urine are more limited than for serum. Van Soestbergen and Sunderman (1972) observed five distinct ultra-filterable nickel complexes in serum and three in urine. Free Ni^{2+} was not identified in either fluid, in agreement with the observation of Verma et al. (1980) that, following intraperitoneal injection of $NiCl_2$ into rats, the element is excreted in urine as complexes and not as the free metal.

With respect to saliva, Hofsøy et al. (1979) reported that 40 to 60% of salivary nickel in rabbits is ultrafilterable and that excretion of nickel in saliva is low, whether or not stimulation of salivation is carried out.

5.4.3.2   Uptake by cells and intracellular binding

Distinctions in the uptake of compounds of nickel have already been discussed in the context of inhalation (Section 4.2.2). Briefly, crystal-line forms are more readily phagocytosed than amorphous forms and this is reflected in the differences in carcinogenic effectiveness between the two. This section includes a brief review of phagocytosis and a discussion of the distribution of dissolved nickel between intracellular consitituents.

The subject of nickel phagocytosis was well summarised by Costa and Mollenhauer (1980b), who made the following suggestions and observations;
- the biological effects of Ni_3S_2 and NiS, including cytotoxicity, in vitro cell transformation and in-vivo production of tumours are preceded by phagocytosis of particles;
- particles of >10 μm diameter can be phagocytosed, but particles of this size have limited carcinogenic potential due to the loss of integrity of the transforming cell;
- phagocytosed particles are found in the cytoplasm, in particular, close to the nuclear membrane, but essentially no large particles (>0.1 μm) are found in the nucleus;

TABLE 4

DATA ON THE INTRACELLULAR BINDING OF COMPOUNDS OF NICKEL

Reference	Results
Heath and Webb, 1967	Distribution of nickel in cells of primary rhabdomyosarcomas of rats induced by powdered metallic nickel.
Webb et al., 1972	Intranuclear distribution of nickel in primary rhabdomyosarcomas of rats induced by powdered metallic nickel.
Webb and Weinzierl, 1972	Distribution of ^{63}Ni in mouse dermal fibroblasts after growth in $^{63}Ni^{2+}$ labelled serum and muscle diffusate.
Whanger, 1973	Intracellular distribution of nickel in the kidneys of rats after chronic exposure to excess dietary nickel. Nickel found mainly in the soluble fraction, with rather less in nuclei plus debris and very small amounts in mitochondria and microsomes.

Heath and Webb, 1967:

	% of total	
Component	Rat 1	Rat 2
Nuclear	0.84	0.94
Mitochondrial	0.11	0.01
Microsomal	0.01	}0.05
Soluble	0.04	

Webb et al., 1972:

Fraction	% of total	$\mu g\ Ni^{2+}/$ mg nucleic acid P
Nuclei	–	29.2
Nuclear sap	14.3	39.6
Chromatin	16.3	24.2
Crude nucleoli	62.8	41.7
Purified nucleoli	–	58.6

Webb and Weinzierl, 1972:

Component	% total recovered
Mitochondrial	22.7
Microsomal	10.7
Cell sap	30.1
Nucleus: total	36.5
nucleoli	17.2
sap + DNA	7.2

TABLE 4   (Contd.)

Reference	Results
Jasmin and Solymoss, 1977	Distribution of nickel in subcellular fractions from kidney homogenates after intrarenal injection of Ni_3S_2 in rats. Times are months post-injection.

Fraction		% of total		
	Control	+1	+2	+4
Nuclear	0.88	0.973	0.935	0.790
Mitochondrial	-	0.013	0.028	0.171
Microsomal	-	0.008	0.000	0.038
Cytosol	0.12	0.006	0.037	0

Reference	Results
Mathur et al., 1978	Distribution of nickel (μg/fraction obtained from 1g of fresh tissue) in subcellular fractions of the myocardium of rats injected intra-peritoneally with 3 and 6 mg kg^{-1} of nickel as nickel sulphate.

Fraction	Control	3mg		6mg	
	-	7d	14d	7d	14d
Nuclear	0.62	1.00	1.11	1.30	1.68
Mitochondrial	0.59	0.83	1.60	1.30	1.69
Microsomal	0.56	0.68	0.78	1.10	1.33
Cytosolic	0.47	0.63	0.76	0.81	0.97

Reference	Results
Oskarsson and Tjalve, 1979b	One and 24 hours after the administration of [63]Ni Cl_2 and [63]Ni $(CO)_4$ to mice, [63]Ni was present in association with both particulate and soluble cellular constituents in the lung, liver and kidney. After disruption of organelles by sonication a considerable part of the [63]Ni was still bound to cellular fragments. Distributions following [63]Ni Cl_2 and [63]Ni $(CO)_4$ exhibited considerable similarities.
Costa et al., 1981	Nickel derived from α-Ni_3S_2 , α-NiS and amorphous $Ni\ S$ is strongly concentrated in the nuclear fraction of Chinese hamster ovary cells exposed in solution culture.

- benzopyrene enhances phagocytosis, possibly by rendering the particles more lipophilic or by stimulating absorption-enhancing enzymes;
- there is a good correlation in vitro between the number of cells containing particles and the number of particles per cell;
- Ni_3S_2, but not NiS, can be treated with poly-L-lysine to enhance its uptake; this may be due to a differential coating action on the two compounds.

It is noted that particles of Ni_3S_2 that are present in the body are subject to chemical modification and dissolution. Thus, following intramuscular injection of nickel subsulphide into mice, and on the basis of a review of other data, Oskarsson et al. (1979) commented that there is a gradual solubilisation of Ni_3S_2 from the site of injection during tumourigenesis and that x-ray diffraction studies of the crystalline residues in the tumours indicated that the administered α-Ni_3S_2 had been converted to α-Ni_7S_6, β-NiS and small amounts of additional unidentified products. Transformation from α-Ni_3S_2 to β-NiS has also been reported for solid intramuscular implants in rats, but other chemical forms were not detected in these studies (Dewally and Hildebrand, 1980).

Finally, with respect to phagocytosis, it is interesting to note that in studies in which $^{63}Ni_3S_2$ and $Ni_3{}^{35}S_2$ dusts were administered to rats by intramuscular injection, Kasprzak (1974) found that neither ^{63}Ni nor ^{35}S was detected within rhabdomyocytes at the site of injection or within rhabdomyoblasts in the induced tumours. However, Kasprzak speculated that the neutral formalin used as a tissue fixative may have eluted intracellular ^{63}Ni-complexes, without dissolving the highly insoluble extracellular particles of Ni_3S_2.

Data on the intracellular distribution of nickel are summarised in Table 4. In general, nickel is mainly associated with the nuclear fraction. Within the nucleus, the nickel is mainly associated with the nucleoli.

5.4.3.3   Distribution and retention in tissues and transfer to the foetus

There have been a large number of studies on the distribution and retention of nickel in mammals. However, the bulk of the data are for mice and rats, rather than for larger animals and man.

Major features of nickel metabolism have been discussed briefly by the ICRP (1981) who noted the following points.

- In mice, rats and rabbits, nickel is deposited preferentially in the kidneys. However, in man the concentration of stable nickel in the kidneys is similar to the average concentration in all soft tissues and it is probably appropriate to attribute the high concentration in the kidneys at early times after intravenous or intraperitoneal injection to the rapid excretion of nickel in the urine.
- In rats there is an early phase of rapid urinary excretion which is essentially complete in the first twelve hours after injection; the residual body burden of nickel is excreted considerably less rapidly.
- The concentration of stable nickel in human tissues seems to imply a component of retention with a very long biological half-life ($\sim$1000 d).

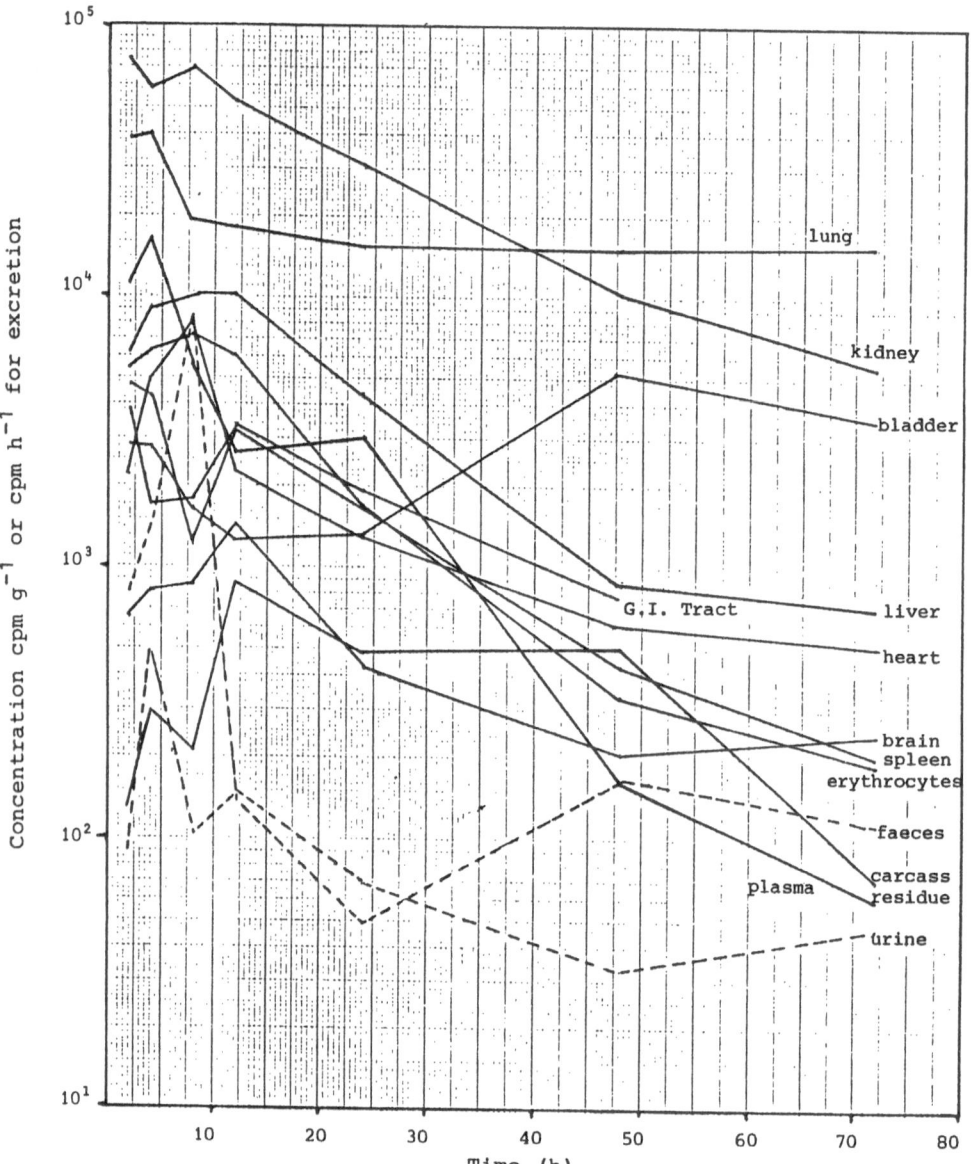

Note:

(1)   Data from Wase et al. (1954)

FIGURE 7.   DISTRIBUTION OF NICKEL IN MOUSE TISSUES FOLLOWING
             INTRAPERITONEAL INJECTION

- Nickel has not been found to have any affinity for mineralised tissues.

The data reviewed in this section are discussed in the context of these various points.

Data on the distribution and retention of nickel in mice are contained in the papers of Wase et al. (1954), Schroeder et al. (1964), Oskarsson and Tjalve (1977; 1979a; 1980), Bergman et al. (1980) and Jacobsen et al. (1978).

Wase et al. (1954) studied tissue distribution and excretion following intraperitoneal injection of the chloride. Results, shown in Fig. 7, demonstrate high concentrations in lung and kidney; rapid loss from all tissues, except lung; and limited accumulation in erythrocytes. In contrast to most other studies, faecal excretion appeared to be more important than urinary excretion, but the high, and rapidly changing, kidney concentration indicates an important role for kidney uptake and loss.

Schroeder et al. (1964) studied the distribution of nickel in mice after lifetime exposure to nickel in drinking water. The following results were presented.

| Tissue | Concentration ($\mu g \ g^{-1}$ w.w.) | | | |
| | Exposed | | Controls | |
	Male	Female	Male	Female
Kidney	0.93	1.07	0.52	0.46
Liver	0.78	0.75	0.62	0.20
Heart	1.05	0.72	0.43	0.0
Lung	1.13	0.53	0.32	0.61
Spleen	2.76	4.16	0.42	0.33

Oskarsson and Tjalve (1977) used whole-body autoradiography to study the distribution of intravenously injected $^{63}NiCl_2$ and $^{63}Ni(CO)_4$, and inhaled $^{63}Ni(CO)_4$. In mice given $^{63}NiCl_2$ there was a high initial radioactivity in the connective tissues and cartilage. A high radioactivity was also seen in the kidney, reflecting the main excretory pathway. At later survival intervals, the distribution was characterised by retention of radioactivity in the lungs. With $^{63}Ni(CO)_4$, injected by either route, a high level of radioactivity was present in the lung parenchyma at all survival intervals. A considerable amount of radioactivity was also present in the brain, the adrenal cortex, adipose tissues, the heart, the diaphragm and the kidneys. Similar autoradiographic studies on mice given $^{63}NiCl_2$, by intravenous or intraperitoneal injection or oral administration, were reported by Oskarsson and Tjalve (1979a). This study also included gross tissue assays on mice injected intravenously with 1.2 µCi of $^{63}NiCl_2$ per kg body weight. Major findings of this study can be summarised as follows.

- Five minutes after intravenous injection of $^{63}NiCl_2$, the distribution of ^{63}Ni was characterised by high activity concentrations in connective tissues and cartilages. In addition, activity was high in blood, kidneys and urinary bladder. The distribution was similar until 7 h post-administration, except that there was a relative increase in the radioactivity of the cartilages and a decrease in the radioactivity of the connective tissues. At 24 h, the activity level in blood was low, but levels were high in lungs,

TABLE 5

DISTRIBUTION OF ^{63}Ni IN THE TISSUES OF MICE
FOLLOWING INTRAVENOUS INJECTION OF ^{63}Ni Cl_2

Organ or tissue	Count rate (Cpm per 100µg or per 100µl for serum)			
	1h	24h	5d	10d
Lung	13800(13100–14600)	5990(5210–6840)	3594(2840–4700)	1347(1310–1400)
Liver	4920(4120–6600)	1770(1270–2050)	1060(985–1170)	345(270–330)
Kidney	117000(79600–141000)	15400(13500–18400)	3330(2530–4740)	1371(863–1680)
Pancreas	4870(3840–5570)	1100(1040–1200)	417(339–485)	480(195–890)
Sternal cartilage	8390(7160–10000)	37100(14300–68400)	1620(1110–2550)	487(251–908)
Serum	25800(21900–29700)	628(556–666)	n.d.	n.d.

Note:

From Oskarsson and Tjalve (1979a), 3 mice were used at each interval and ranges of results are given in parenthesis

TABLE 6

EFFECTS OF COMPLEXING AGENTS ON THE DISTRIBUTION OF INTRAVENOUSLY INJECTED ^{63}Ni Cl$_2$ IN MICE AT 4 HOURS AFTER INJECTION[1]

	Tissue concentration (dpm per 100µg w.w.)					
	Lung	Liver	Kidney	Brain	Erythrocytes	Serum[2]
Control (^{63}Ni Cl$_2$ only)	73400 ±1850	16900 ±440	544000 ±61700	2240 ±105	13600 ±1250	103000 ±5890
Dithiocarb 10 min. before ^{63}Ni Cl$_2$	161000 ±15100	264000 ±22800	326000 ±20000	127000 ±11400	68800 ±16900	106000 ±11900
Dithiocarb 10 min. after ^{63}Ni Cl$_2$	124000 ±6790	257000 ±71100	266000 ±22500	86500 ±11000	61500 ±9040	101000 ±2070
Dithiocarb 3h 50 min. after ^{63}Ni Cl$_2$	55600 ±4680	57800 ±10500	149000 ±24400	14500 ±7400	32300 ±1270	90400 ±12200
DL-penicillamine 10 min. before ^{63}Ni Cl$_2$	2920 ±753	2250 ±47	4150 ±596	491 ±154	646 ±52	2150 ±689

Notes:

(1) From Oskarsson and Tjalve (1980)

(2) dpm per 100µl

cartilage, kidneys and the squamous epithelium of the forestomach. At longer times (to 3 weeks) relative levels of activity in cartilage declined, but labelling of the central nervous system increased.

- Following intravenous injection of $^{63}NiCl_2$, the ^{63}Ni was localised in small areas of the cortex of the kidney, though up to 24 h post-injection some was also present in the cortico-medullary zone. Microautoradiography indicated that the activity was probably localised in the distal convoluted tubuli, but was low in the glomeruli and proximal convoluted tubuli.

- In the lung, the activity was limited to the parenchyma, with little in the bronchial epithelium. In the forestomach, the tissue of accumulation was the keratinised stratified squamous epithelium.

- In the skin, considerable radioactivity was present in the connective tissues of the dermis at 5 minutes and in the epidermis up to 10d.

- After intraperitoneal injection, the peritoneal coat of the liver attained a high degree of labelling.

- After oral administration much of the activity was found in the gut contents, but the distribution of the remainder was similar to that obtaining after intravenous injection.

- Results of the radiochemical assay of various tissues (Table 5) were consistent with the results of the autoradiographic study.

With respect to their data, and on the basis of in vitro incubation studies, Oskarson and Tjalve (1979a) commented that the chondroitin sulphate of cartilage and the keratin of skin have cation binding properties which may explain the binding of $^{63}Ni(II)$ in these tissues.

In a further study, Oskarsson and Tjalve (1980) reported on the distribution of ^{63}Ni in mice following intravenous injection of $^{63}NiCl_2$, with or without treatment with sodium diethyldithiocarbamate (dithiocarb) or DL-penicillamine. Results of these studies are given in Table 6. On the basis of this experiment, the authors proposed that Ni^{2+} forms a lipophilic complex with dithiocarb and a hydrophilic complex with penicillamine. The lipophilic complex would penetrate readily through cell membranes and be retained in tissues, while the hydrophilic complex would be excreted rapidly. In contrast, West and Sunderman (1958) found that $CaNa_2$-EDTA was ineffective in modifying the distribution of nickel in mice following inhalation of nickel carbonyl (see Section 4.2.1).

Results from an autoradiographic study by Bergman et al. (1980) were similar to those reviewed above. In mice, intravenously injected with $^{63}NiCl_2$, high concentrations of activity were found in the urogenital, circulatory and respiratory organs in the first 24 h after injection. At later times, the lungs, kidneys, central nervous system and skin were the main organs and tissues of accumulation. In pregnant mice, Bergman et al. (1980) reported that autoradiographs demonstrated penetration of nickel through the placenta and into the foetus, but no quantitative data were given. Transplacental transfer of nickel in mice, after administration of toxic levels of the stable element, was also demonstrated by Lu et al. (1979). Jacobsen et al. (1978) studied the distribution and retention of ^{63}Ni in adult mice and embryos after intraperitoneal injection of $^{63}NiCl_2$. These authors also included data on transfers from mother to suckling in the milk. Detailed data from this study are summarised in Tables 7 to 10.

TABLE 7

RETENTION OF ^{63}Ni IN MOUSE TISSUES AFTER
INTRAPERITONEAL INJECTION OF ^{63}Ni Cl$_2$

Tissue	cpm per mg (w.w.)					
	15 min.	1h	2h	1d	5d	22d
Liver	758	380	504	49	14	10
Kidney	4335	437	449	797	77	4
Heart	788	342	571	43	6	trace
Brain	96	54	96	23	8	0
Calvaria	1026	274	262	68	13	16
Long bones	635	343	335	59	15	8
Incisors	161	124	199	120	31	13
Blood	2084	1144	1402	39	7	0

Note:
From Jacobsen et al. (1978)

TABLE 8

CONCENTRATION OF ^{63}Ni IN PREGNANT MICE AND FOETUSES
AFTER INTRAPERITONEAL INJECTION OF ^{63}Ni Cl$_2$

Tissue	cpm per mg (w.w.)	
	Mouse	Foetus
Liver	20 (19-21)	70 (14-188)
Kidney	217 (182-227)	189 (50-438)
Heart	10 (6-12)	57 (26-128)
Brain	7 (5-8)	172 (53-474)
Calvaria	10 (9-12)	195 (172-207)
Long bones	33 (13-62)	134 (33-289)
Blood	5 (3-6)	—

Note:
From Jacobsen et al. (1978), injected day 18
of gestation, killed day 20

TABLE 9

CONCENTRATIONS OF ^{63}Ni IN TISSUES OF LACTATING
MICE AND 5-DAY-OLD SUCKLINGS AFTER
INTRAPERITONEAL INJECTION OF ^{63}Ni Cl$_2$

Tissue	cpm per mg (w.w.)	
	Mouse	Suckling
Liver	55 (33-100)	10 (5-23)
Kidney	259 (100-459)	14 (6-17)
Heart	66 (23-150)	18 (7-45)
Brain	28 (19-42)	17 (5-42)
Calvaria	42 (33-56)	32 (12-47)
Long bones	56 (53-60)	16 (5-29)
Blood	8 (8-9)	-

Note:
From Jacobsen et al. (1978); injected day
3 after delivery, killed day 5

TABLE 10

RETENTION OF ^{63}Ni IN MOUSE SUCKLINGS
AFTER UPTAKE FROM MILK

Tissue	cpm per mg (w.w.)					
	Suckling					Mother
	1d	2d	3d	4d	5d	5d
Liver	421	45	45	35	7	12
Kidney	333	76	48	23	7	17
Heart	650	269	170	45	15	9
Brain	46	35	60	30	8	10
Calvaria	397	156	116	75	21	9
Long bones	224	97	69	39	20	21
Incisors	359	201	96	78	28	50
Blood	-	-	-	-	-	1

Note:
From Jacobsen et al. (1978), mothers injected immediately
after delivery

Data on the distribution of nickel in rats following various routes of administration are numerous (Phatak and Patwardham, 1952; Sunderman et al., 1957; 1978a; Sunderman and Selin, 1968; Smith and Hackley, 1968; Kasprzak and Sunderman, 1969; Mikheev, 1971; Ho and Furst, 1973; Whanger, 1973; Schroeder et al., 1974; Clary, 1975; Ambrose et al., 1976; Sunderman et al., 1976a; 1976b; Mathur et al., 1978; Shen et al., 1979; Sarkar, 1980; English et al., 1981) and some of these data have been used in the development of compartmental models of nickel metabolism (Onkelinx et al., 1973; Chausmer, 1976; Onkelinx, 1977; Onkelinx and Sunderman, 1980). For convenience, models and associated data are discussed together, and this discussion is followed by a brief summary of other data which have not been used in model derivation.

Chausmer (1976) applied a compartmental analysis to the data of Smith and Hackley (1968). These data were obtained from experiments in which rats were injected intravenously with $^{63}NiCl_2$, and organ, tissue and excreta assays were performed to 72 h post-injection. In these studies, over 50% of the injected activity was excreted in the urine in the first 8 h after injection, while, in the first 72 h after injection, ∿60% was excreted in urine and 5% in faeces. Data on tissue distributions obtained in this study are summarised in Tables 11 and 12. On the basis of these data, Chausmer (1976) gave the following retention functions $C(t)$, expressed as % ^{63}Ni retention per g of tissue.

$$C_{PLASMA}(t) = 1.472 \exp(-2.0852t) + 1.117 \exp(-0.1032t)$$

$$C_{KIDNEY}(t) = 5.890 \exp(-0.3356t) + 1.232 \exp(-0.0192t)$$

$$C_{LUNG}(t) = 0.805 \exp(-0.8148t) + 0.317 \exp(-0.0575t)$$

$$C_{LIVER}(t) = 0.290 \exp(-1.1062t) + 0.149 \exp(-0.0938t)$$

$$C_{SPLEEN}(t) = 0.407 \exp(-1.0679t) + 0.087 \exp(-0.0351t)$$

$$C_{BONE}(t) = 1.4229 \exp(-1.8175t)$$

where t is in hours.

The recent modelling paper by Onkelinx and Sunderman (1980) used data from several studies on both rats and rabbits (Onkelinx et al., 1973; Sunderman et al., 1976b; Shen et al., 1979; Van Soestbergen and Sunderman, 1972) and analysed these data in terms of a two compartment model (Fig. 8). Using the nomenclature given in Fig. 8, the equations governing this model are:

$$dS_1/dt = -(f_e/V_1 + f_t/V_1) S_1 + f_e S_2/V_2$$

$$dS_2/dt = f_e(S_1 - S_2)/V_2$$

where S_1 and S_2 are the concentrations of ^{63}Ni in the two compartments. Values of the various model parameters are summarised below.

TABLE 11

DISTRIBUTION OF ^{63}Ni IN RATS FOLLOWING INTRAVENOUS
INJECTION OF ^{63}Ni Cl$_2$

Time after dose	Kidney	Lung	Spleen	Liver	Femur
Hours	% dose/g fresh tissue				
0.25	6.54±0.50	0.97±0.06	0.40±0.30	0.36±0.03	0.24±0.02
1	5.47±0.38	0.66±0.03	0.22±0.01	0.24±0.01	0.16±0.01
2	4.46±0.36	0.42±0.03	0.14±0.01	0.14±0.01	0.08±0.01
4	2.36±0.16	0.32±0.01	0.10±0.00	0.12±0.01	0.04±0.00
8	1.57±0.16	0.18±0.01	0.05±0.00	0.06±0.01	0.01±0.00
16	0.95±0.06	0.11±0.01	0.03±0.00	0.03±0.00	n.d.
24	0.92±0.11	0.11±0.01	0.07±0.01	0.02±0.00	n.d.
48	0.52±0.04	0.03±0.00	0.01±0.00	n.d.	0.01±0.00
72	0.27±0.02	0.02±0.00	0.01±0.00	n.d.	0.01±0.00

Note:
From Smith and Hackley (1968)

TABLE 12

DISTRIBUTION OF ^{63}Ni IN RATS FOLLOWING INTRAVENOUS
INJECTION OF ^{63}Ni Cl$_2$

	Hours after dose				
	0.25	2	6	16	72
	% dose/g fresh tissue				
Kidney	2.49±0.54	2.57±1.24	0.59±0.23	0.20±0.06	0.11±0.06
Adrenal	0.92±0.14	0.28±0.03	0.15±0.01	0.12±0.02	0.03±0.01
Ovary	0.90±0.33	0.23±0.06	0.11±0.02	0.09±0.01	n.d.
Lung	0.81±0.04	0.29±0.04	0.14±0.03	0.09±0.01	0.01±0.00
Heart	0.64±0.04	0.21±0.02	0.11±0.01	0.07±0.01	n.d.
Eye	0.56±0.06	0.19±0.03	0.13±0.04	0.08±0.03	0.01±0.00
Thymus	0.55±0.03	0.15±0.02	0.12±0.02	0.04±0.01	n.d.
Pancreas	0.54±0.05	0.16±0.03	0.12±0.03	0.08±0.01	n.d.
Spleen	0.48±0.03	0.13±0.01	0.11±0.01	0.09±0.01	0.01±0.00
Liver	0.40±0.03	0.13±0.02	0.08±0.01	0.05±0.01	n.d.
Skin	0.38±0.08	0.20±0.05	0.07±0.01	0.04±0.01	n.d.
G.I. tract	0.33±0.04	0.21±0.04	0.11±0.03	0.10±0.01	n.d.
Muscle	0.29±0.07	0.11±0.05	0.04±0.01	0.03±0.05	n.d.
Teeth	0.21±0.04	0.08±0.02	0.04±0.01	0.03±0.01	0.01±0.00
Femur	0.15±0.02	0.05±0.01	0.03±0.01	0.01±0.00	n.d.
Brain	0.15±0.02	0.04±0.01	0.04±0.01	0.05±0.02	n.d.
Adipose	0.14±0.04	0.04±0.01	0.02±0.00	0.01±0.01	n.d.
Carcass	–	–	–	–	n.d.

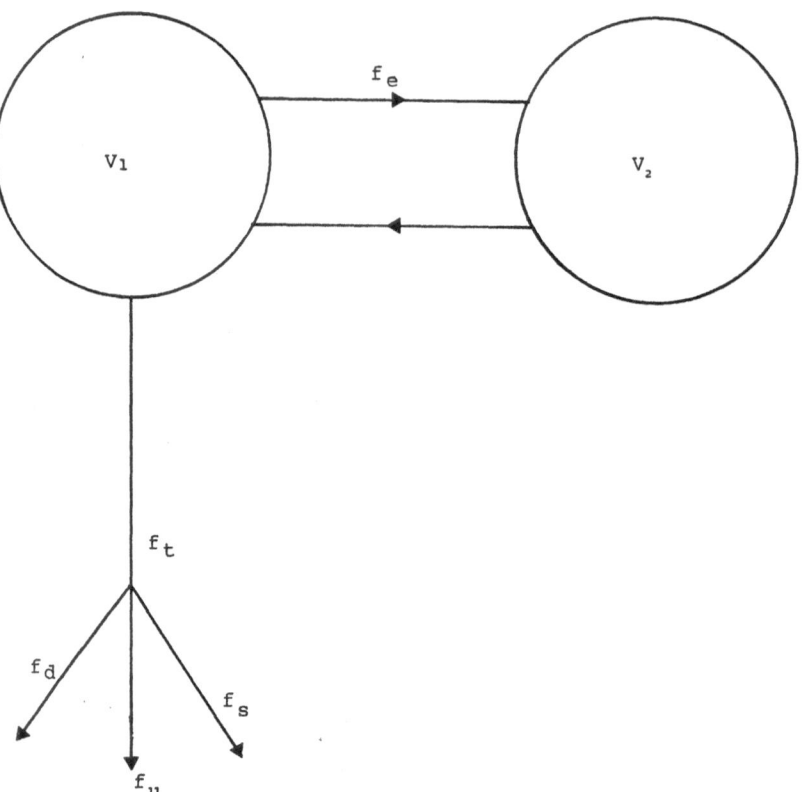

Notes:

(1)   From Onkelinx and Sunderman (1980).

(2) f_e = exchange rate (ml h^{-1}).

      f_t = total excretory clearance (ml h^{-1}).

      f_d = clearance to digestive tract (ml h^{-1}).

      f_u = clearance to urine (ml h^{-1}).

      f_s = deposition in non-exchangable, or very slowly exchangable body resevoirs (ml h^{-1}).

  V_1, V_2 = compartment volumes (ml)

FIGURE 8.   TWO-COMPARTMENT MODEL FOR Ni (II) METABOLISM IN RATS AND RABBITS

Parameter	Units	Wistar rat	Fischer rat	Rabbit
V_1	ml	75.1	59.2	697
V_2	ml	8.3	31.6	265
f_e	ml h^{-1}	0.12	0.92	2.31
f_t	ml h^{-1}	8.14	7.73	61.2
f_u	ml h^{-1}	6.39	6.70	54.1
f_d	ml h^{-1}	1.28	0.75	-
f_s	ml h^{-1}	0.47	0.28	-
body weight	g	208	165	3400

In the case of rabbits, measurements of faecal nickel could not be performed, hence f_d and f_s could not be calculated.

An important point to note with this model is that f_s/f_t is $\sim$0.05 in
rats, implying that $\sim$5% of nickel is eventually transferred to a
long-term body store. It is this long-term component of retention that
determines nickel accumulation in the body.

Onkelinx and Sunderman (1980) also discussed the effect of the
chelate triethylenetetramine (TETA) upon Ni(II) metabolism in rats.
Plasma clearance curves with and without TETA treatment are summarised
below.

Control: $C_{PLASMA}(t) = 35600 \exp(-0.15t) + 1110 \exp(-0.025t)$

TETA treated: $C_{PLASMA}(t) = 14560 \exp(-1.93t) + 5401 \exp(-0.12t)$
$$+ 430 \exp(-0.027t)$$

In each case, the injected dose was 2173 µg per rat and 0.75 mmol kg^{-1} of
TETA was injected intramuscularly 1 minute before intraperitoneal injection of $^{63}NiCl_2$. From the form of the clearance curves, Onkelinx and
Sunderman (1980) argued that nickel chelation by TETA is rapid and that
the first component of loss in the TETA-treated rats represented rapid
urinary excretion of the chelated complex. The other two components of
loss are very similar, in relative magnitude and biological half-life, to
those observed after injection of $^{63}NiCl_2$. For this reason, they can be
interpreted as clearance of uncomplexed Ni(II). The urinary excretion
observed in control and TETA-treated rats supports this hypothesis, with
36±23% and 70±7% of the injected activity excreted in the urine of
control and TETA-treated rats respectively during the first 6 h after
$^{63}NiCl_2$ injection.

The following data were given for the distribution of ^{63}Ni in the
body 6 h after injection of $^{63}NiCl_2$:

TABLE 13

THE DISTRIBUTION OF NICKEL IN RATS FED A
NICKEL-CONTAINING DIET

Concentration ($\mu g\ g^{-1}$ w.w.)

Tissue	4 mo feeding	8 mo feeding	12 mo feeding	16 mo feeding	4 mo feeding low protein diet	4 mo feeding normal diet	8 mo feeding low protein diet	8 mo feeding normal diet
Bone	75	84	86.3	73	41.5	66	64	79
Liver	2.8	3.6	1.7	1.3	2.8	3.1	2.4	4.1
Kidney	5.5	28.2	20	23	4.3	6.9	16.8	22
Spleen	27	53.6	27.7	19	16.6	26.5	29.0	42.3
Heart	21	25.7	30	20	6.2	21.3	19.0	23.5
Intestine	6.1	7.1	5.2	4.6	9.2	5.7	5.8	6.1
Testes	4.3	11	6.4	5.2	2.8	6.6	6.6	8.6
Blood	7.6	9.1	5.0	4.5	5.7	5.9	5.8	6.1
Skin	0.7	0.9	-	-	-	0.1	0.2	0.4

Note: From Phatak and Patwardhan (1952).

TABLE 14

DISTRIBUTION OF NICKEL IN TISSUES OF RATS GIVEN REPEATED
DAILY INTRAPERITONEAL INJECTIONS OF THE SULPHATE

Tissue	Concentration $\mu g\ g^{-1}$ (w.w.)				
	Control	3 mg Ni $kg^{-1}\ d^{-1}$		6 mg Ni $kg^{-1}\ d^{-1}$	
	–	7d	14d	7d	14d
Kidney	0.51±0.007	0.62±0.05	1.20±0.06	1.03±0.12	1.33±0.08
Liver	0.17±0.009	0.26±0.02	0.42±0.04	0.63±0.06	0.95±0.11
Myocardium	2.23±0.06	3.13±0.24	4.19±0.41	4.49±0.37	5.67±0.16
Spleen	0.60±0.04	0.87±0.11	1.81±0.05	1.27±0.09	2.05±0.27
Testis	0.32±0.01	0.49±0.01	0.75±0.03	0.67±0.06	1.03±0.02
Bone	0.15±0.01	0.37±0.009	0.72±0.07	0.60±0.05	1.12±0.05

Note:
From Mathur et al. (1978)

TABLE 15

DISTRIBUTION OF NICKEL IN RATS AT VARIOUS LEVELS
OF NICKEL IN THE DIET

Tissue	Diet (ppm Ni added)			
	0	100	500	1000
Heart	0.9	1.3	0.9	2.1
Kidney	5.0	8.1	25.4	40.7
Liver	0.7	0.9	2.4	4.0
Testes	1.6	2.3	3.8	7.2

Note:
From Whanger (1973), concentrations are
ppm (d.w.), mean values for 6 rats

TABLE 16

DISTRIBUTION OF NICKEL IN CONTROL RATS AND RATS FED 5 ppm
NICKEL IN THEIR DIET OVER THEIR LIFE SPAN

Tissue	Concentration ($\mu g\ g^{-1}$)	
	Control	Nickel fed
Liver	1.3±0.12	1.20±0.20
Lung	2.4±0.53	2.7±0.52
Heart	3.0±0.94	3.2±0.39
Kidney	1.7±0.46	3.0±0.70
Spleen	6.2±1.83	4.9±0.87

Note:
From Schroeder et al. (1974)

TABLE 17

TISSUE CONCENTRATION OF NICKEL IN RATS RECEIVING NICKEL
SULPHATE IN THEIR DIET FOR TWO YEARS

Sex	Diet conc. (ppm)	Tissue conc. (ppm w.w.)			
		Bone	Liver	Kidney	Fat
Female	0	0.53	0.094	0.14	0.51
	2500	0.82	0.64	3.4	1.0
Male	0	<0.096	0.055	<0.14	<0.055
	2500	0.64	0.68	4.9	1.4

Note:
From Ambrose et al. (1976)

Organ	Concentration ($\mu g\ g^{-1}$ w.w.)	
	Control	TETA treated
Kidney	16.6±3.8	12.0±1.2
Liver	2.3±0.3	7.7±2.5
Lung	3.7±0.5	0.80±0.11
Heart	1.76±0.24	0.24±0.06
Spleen	1.59±0.70	0.43±0.22

These data were not used by Onkelinx and Sunderman (1980).

Onkelinx and Sunderman (1980) also considered the clearance of ^{63}Ni from the body of Fischer rats following intramuscular injection of a dust of ^{63}Ni$_3$S$_2$ alone or combined with manganese. This experiment was originally described by Sunderman et al. (1976a) who gave whole body retention functions of the form:

$$R(t) = A_1\ exp(-\lambda_1 t) + A_2\ exp(-\lambda_2 t) + A_3\ exp(-\lambda_3 t)$$

Values of A_i and $T_{\frac{1}{2}}^i$ ($=ln2/\lambda_i$) were as summarised below:

	A_1(%)	$T_{\frac{1}{2}}^1$(d)	A_2(%)	$T_{\frac{1}{2}}^2$(d)	A_3(%)	$T_{\frac{1}{2}}^3$(d)
Control	63±8	14±1	27±6	60±24	11±2	$\cong\infty$
+ Mn	55±12	15±1	30±6	55±18	15±8	$\cong\infty$

With respect to other data concerning nickel in rats, Phatak and Patwardhan (1952) presented data on the distribution of nickel in rats fed a diet containing 250 $\mu g\ g^{-1}$ of nickel. Results from this study are summarised in Table 13. Sunderman et al. (1957) reported that kidney concentrations of nickel were factors of 3.3, 6.1 and 2.0 higher than concentrations in the livers of control animals, animals chronically exposed to nickel carbonyl and animals acutely exposed to toxic levels of nickel carbonyl respectively. Data on the distribution of nickel in the body of rats, following inhalation of nickel carbonyl and other compounds of nickel, are discussed in Section 4.2. Data for chronically exposed animals are summarised in Tables 14 to 17, and data on the distribution of ^{63}Ni following single intraperitoneal or intratracheal administration of ^{63}NiCl$_2$ are summarised in Tables 18 to 20. In addition, Sunderman et al. (1978a) gave data on the distribution of ^{63}Ni in non-pregnant and pregnant rats following intramuscular injection 24 h before death. These data are summarised in Table 21.

One other study on rats is relevant. Kasprzak and Sunderman (1969) reported data on the exhalation of ^{14}C and ^{63}Ni following intravenous injection of labelled nickel carbonyl. On the basis of this and previous studies, the authors proposed that after intravenous injection of Ni(CO)$_4$ in LD$_{50}$ dosage, approximately 36% of the dose is exhaled without metabolic alteration, while the remainder undergoes intracellular decomposition. In erythrocytes, decomposition is accelerated, with haemoglobin acting as an acceptor for the released carbon monoxide.

With respect to species other than rats and mice, data are very limited. Some data on rabbits have already been discussed, in the context of the modelling studies of Onkelinx and Sunderman (1980). In addition, Parker and Sunderman (1974) studied the distribution of ^{63}Ni in rabbit tissue following intravenous injection of ^{63}NiCl$_2$. Results from these

TABLE 18

DISTRIBUTION OF ^{63}Ni IN RATS FOLLOWING
INTRAPERITONEAL INJECTION OF ^{63}Ni Cl$_2$

Tissue	% dose g^{-1} (w.w.)		
	6h	18h	24h
Heart	0.135	0.04	0.07
Kidney	3.55	1.42	1.54
Liver	0.06	0.02	0.04
Lung	0.20	0.09	0.09
Spleen	0.32	0.14	0.07
Muscle	0.045	0.03	0.02
Serum	0.76	0.24	0.29
Urine	5.57	4.31	-

Note:
From Sarkar (1980)

TABLE 19

TISSUE CONCENTRATIONS OF NICKEL IN THE RAT FOLLOWING
INTRATRACHEAL INJECTION OF NICKEL CHLORIDE

Tissue	Concentration (% I.A. g^{-1})								
	2h	8h	24h	3d	7d	15d	30d	60d	90d
Heart	0.72 ±0.30	0.18 ±0.03	0.15 ±0.10	0.0031 ±0.0003	0.0019 ±0.0002	0.0176 ±0.0007	0.0019 ±0.0002	n.d.	n.d.
Spleen	0.19 ±0.01	0.07 ±0.02	0.11 ±0.02	0.0068 ±0.0024	0.0081 ±0.0044	0.0095 ±0.0019	0.0022 ±0.0002	0.0012 ±0.0002	0.0034 ±0.0019
Duodenum	0.18 ±0.06	0.15 ±0.04	0.07 ±0.01	0.0034 ±0.0003	0.0039 ±0.0015	0.0053 ±0.0015	0.0025 ±0.0	n.d.	0.0008 ±0.0003
Pancreas	0.12 ±0.01	0.12 ±0.03	0.07 ±0.01	0.0039 ±0.0005	0.0032 ±0.0014	0.0081 ±0.0027	0.0027 ±0.0002	0.0014 ±0.0003	0.0010 ±0.0003
Pituitary	0.11 ±0.02	0.18 ±0.06	0.16 ±0.03	0.0272 ±0.0061	0.0166 ±0.0025	0.0136 ±0.0020	0.0127 ±0.0025	0.0053 ±0.0008	0.0117 ±0.0020
Ovaries	0.24 ±0.04	0.21 ±0.06	0.09 ±0.01	0.0053 ±0.0014	0.0053 ±0.0020	0.0068 ±0.0019	0.0024 ±0.0003	0.0005 ±0.0002	0.0012 ±0.0003
Adrenals	0.17 ±0.02	0.15 ±0.04	0.16 ±0.02	0.019 ±0.0059	0.0144 ±0.0046	0.0178 ±0.0049	0.0053 ±0.0011	0.0014 ±0.0002	0.0019 ±0.0002
Bone	0.52 ±0.12	0.22 ±0.04	0.06 ±0.01	0.0142 ±0.0039	0.0064 ±0.0005	0.0061 ±0.0003	0.0044 ±0.0015	0.0022 ±0.0003	0.0029 ±0.0002
Skin	0.17 ±0.05	0.12 ±0.02	0.05 ±0.01	0.0076 ±0.0019	0.0073 ±0.0025	0.0154 ±0.0025	0.0022 ±0.0010	0.0024 ±0.0008	n.d.

Note: From English et al. (1981); mean ± standard error of mean

TABLE 20

TISSUE CONCENTRATIONS OF NICKEL IN THE RAT FOLLOWING
INTRACTRACHEAL INJECTION OF NICKEL OXIDE

Tissue	\multicolumn{9}{c}{Concentration (% I.A. g^{-1})}
	2h	8h	24h	3d	7d	15d	30d	60d	90d
Heart	0.0781 ±0.0134	0.603 ±0.169	0.0210 ±0.0080	0.0453 ±0.0158	0.0127 ±0.0008	0.0064 ±0.0027	0.0176 ±0.0032	0.0032 ±0.0010	0.0005 ±0.0002
Spleen	0.0215 ±0.0015	0.213 ±0.049	0.0429 ±0.0168	0.0186 ±0.0061	0.0456 ±0.0069	0.0307 ±0.0037	0.0037 ±0.0010	0.0027 ±0.0012	0.0071 ±0.0012
Duodenum	0.0424 ±0.0129	0.0636 ±0.0244	0.0403 ±0.0195	0.0090 ±0.0015	0.0092 ±0.0010	0.0034 ±0.0003	0.0086 ±0.0015	0.0014 ±0.0003	0.0010 ±0.0003
Pancreas	0.0275 ±0.0029	0.0264 ±0.0063	0.0146 ±0.0029	0.0069 ±0.0012	0.0054 ±0.0005	0.0042 ±0.0005	0.0105 ±0.0029	0.0014 ±0.0003	0.0015 ±0.0002
Pituitary	0.0280 ±0.0019	0.0371 ±0.0012	0.0827 ±0.0020	0.0058 ±0.0010	0.0083 ±0.0010	0.0146 ±0.0034	0.0127 ±0.0014	0.0176 ±0.0061	0.0261 ±0.0080
Ovaries	0.0624 ±0.0236	0.225 ±0.164	0.0108 ±0.0025	0.0100 ±0.0017	0.0356 ±0.0110	0.0041 ±0.0012	0.0095 ±0.0029	0.0017 ±0.0003	0.0008 ±0.0003
Adrenal	0.0341 ±0.0039	0.0185 ±0.0044	0.0134 ±0.0056	0.0092 ±0.0008	0.0471 ±0.0183	0.0054 ±0.0002	0.0078 ±0.0012	0.0020 ±0.0002	0.0010 ±0.0003
Bone	0.592 ±0.234	0.278 ±0.080	0.0195 ±0.0041	0.0451 ±0.0225	0.0186 ±0.0088	0.0032 ±0.0003	0.0066 ±0.0008	0.0019 ±0.0002	0.0034 ±0.0008
Skin	0.0603 ±0.0051	0.0325 ±0.0073	0.0166 ±0.0022	0.0129 ±0.0027	0.0119 ±0.0025	0.0037 ±0.0008	0.0025 ±0.0005	0.0014 ±0.0002	0.0014 ±0.0003

Note:
From English et al. (1981), mean ± standard error of mean

TABLE 21

DISTRIBUTION OF ^{63}Ni IN RATS 24h AFTER
INTRAMUSCULAR INJECTION OF ^{63}Ni Cl_2

Organ, tissue or fluid	Concentration µg g^{-1} (w.w.)		
	Non-pregnant	Pregnant: day 9	Pregnant: day 19
Kidney	16.35±3.13	12.22±2.65	9.64±1.71
Serum	3.67±0.48	3.17±0.61	1.79±0.10
Adrenal	2.92±0.47	1.89±0.39	1.49±0.27
Lung	2.32±0.70	1.95±0.30	2.04±0.27
Ovary	2.24±1.07	1.97±0.59	0.91±0.25
Uterus	2.07±0.26	–	–
Spleen	0.78±0.20	0.62±0.26	0.70±0.19
Heart	0.71±0.12	0.46±0.10	0.61±0.19
Liver	0.57±0.30	0.62±0.19	0.44±0.06
Skeletal muscle	0.19±0.03	0.16±0.03	0.13±0.02
Pituitary	0.13±0.05	1.09±0.25	0.91±0.24
Foetuses and membranes	–	2.00±0.38	–
Placenta	–	–	2.61±0.65
Foetuses	–	–	1.18±0.43
Amniotic fluid	–	–	0.62±0.21

Note:
From Sunderman et al. (1978a): mean ± std deviation

TABLE 22

DISTRIBUTION OF ^{63}Ni IN RABBITS AFTER
INTRAVENOUS INJECTION OF ^{63}Ni Cl$_2$ (1)

Tissue or fluid	Concentration (cpm mg^{-1} (w.w.))	
	(2)	(3)
Body fluids:		
Urine	20000(16000-30000)	720(270-930)
Serum	3000(2200-4100)	14(8.2-20)
Whole blood	2300(1400-3200)	8.6(4.7-12)
Viscera:		
Kidney	8800(8100-9200)	810(360-1700)
Lung	1100(960-1300)	17(9.5-32)
Heart	920(750-1100)	6.8(4.8-8.9)
Pancreas	750(680-810)	14(3.0-29)
Duodenum	640(480-790)	8.8(7.6-10)
Spleen	450(390-530)	38(22-51)
Liver	390(300-460)	8.8(5.8-13)
Endocrine glands:		
Pituitary	3200(3100-3300)	45(34-60)
Testis	870(530-1200)	15(10-31)
Adrenal	670(520-810)	14(11-19)
Skin and connective tissues:		
Skin	1250(1200-1300)	16(12-30)
Bone	500(460-550)	4.5(2.5-12)
Muscle	300(280-320)	3.1(2.0-3.9)
Central nervous system:		
Spinal cord	73(63-83)	2.4(1.5-3.9)
Cerebellum	62(59-66)	3.0(1.5-4.3)
Medulla oblongata	44(42-47)	2.8(2.0-3.5)
Hypothalamus	37(34-46)	3.0(1.7-4.8)
Eye:		
Sclerae		9.1(5.6-12)
Iris and ciliary		3.6(3.2-4.3)
Cornea		3.0(2.2-4.3)
Retina		1.9(1.5-2.1)
Lens		1.0(0.7-1.7)
Vitreous humor		0.4(0.2-0.5)

Notes:

(1)   From Parker and Sunderman (1974)

(2)   Single injection killed 2h later

(3)   Daily injections for 34-38d and killed 24h after the
      last injection

studies are summarised in Table 22. Anke et al. (1980) studied the distribution of nickel in kids of nickel deficient and normal goats and concluded that nickel is effectively conserved by the foetus, even under conditions of dietary nickel deficiency. Spears et al. (1978b) reported on the distribution of ^{63}Ni in lambs fed low nickel and nickel supplemented diets; results from this study are given in Table 23.

With respect to man, Christensen and Lagesson (1980) used data from oral uptake studies to estimate that the biological half-life of nickel in serum is 11 h. However, these studies extended to only 32h post-ingestion and would not, therefore, have bbserved any long-term components of serum retention.

The data discussed in this sub-section allow the following conclusions to be drawn.

- Data on plasma levels and the early excretion of nickel in rats and rabbits can be fitted by a two compartment model in which some nickel is transferred from one of the compartments to a non-exchanging or slowly exchanging body 'pool'.
- Data on tissue concentrations at early times after exposure are suggestive of the hypothesis that the kidney acts as a temporary 'sink' for circulatory nickel prior to urinary excretion.
- Data on the relative concentrations of nickel in organs and tissues other than the kidneys are not self-consistent within or between species. In the absence of more detailed data on man, it is probably appropriate to assume that nickel is uniformly distributed throughout all organs and tissues other than the kidneys. However, hair and nail concentrations may be about an order of magnitude higher than tissue concentrations.
- The initial biological half-life of nickel in human plasma is ~11h.
- Concentrations of nickel in foetal organs or tissues are typically comparable to, or higher than, those in the corresponding organs and tissues of the mother.
- Chelation therapy for nickel poisoning probably operates by complexing a fraction of the inter-cellular nickel, though some chelates may also interact, to some extent, with intra-cellular nickel. In either case, the metabolism of the unchelated nickel is not thought to be modified substantially. Chelated nickel may be excreted in this form, or the chelates may be broken down and the nickel recirculated (see also Tandon and Srivastava, 1980).

On the basis of these conclusions, a relatively simple compartmental model of nickel metabolism is probably appropriate in assessing and interpreting human exposure. This model is shown in Fig. 9. With respect to coefficients for use in this model the following assumptions are made:

i) $\lambda_1 + \lambda_2 = 1.5$ d^{-1}, corresponding to a half-life in the blood of 11 h;
ii) $\lambda_1 = 1.05$ d^{-1}, corresponding to 70% of nickel going to early excretion (ICRP, 1981);
iii) $\lambda_3 = 6$ d^{-1} (Table 12);
iv) $\lambda_4 = 5.78 \times 10^{-4}$ d^{-1}.

The value of λ_4 is defined so as to give an equilibrium concentration of nickel in tissues ~0.2 μg g^{-1} for the typical intake rates defined in Section 2.4. With respect to λ_4, it can be assumed that ~90% of excretion will be via urine. Details of the combination of these compartments to give total tissue contents are shown in Fig. 9. The fraction of 'all

TABLE 23

^{63}Ni DISTRIBUTION IN LAMBS FED LOW NICKEL
OR NICKEL SUPPLEMENTED DIETS

Tissue	Concentration (% I.A. kg^{-1} (w.w.))	
	Low Ni	5 ppm Ni
Kidney	0.1282±0.0362	0.3223±0.0552
Lung	0.0095±0.0014	0.0204±0.0028
Spleen	0.0094±0.0013	0.0208±0.0133
Heart	0.0073±0.0020	0.0078±0.0006
Testis	0.0049±0.0009	0.0104±0.0036
Liver	0.0070±0.0002	0.0136±0.0033
Brain	0.0068±0.0010	0.0069±0.0006

Note:
From Spears et al. (1978b), distribution at 72h
post-injection, mean ± standard error on mean

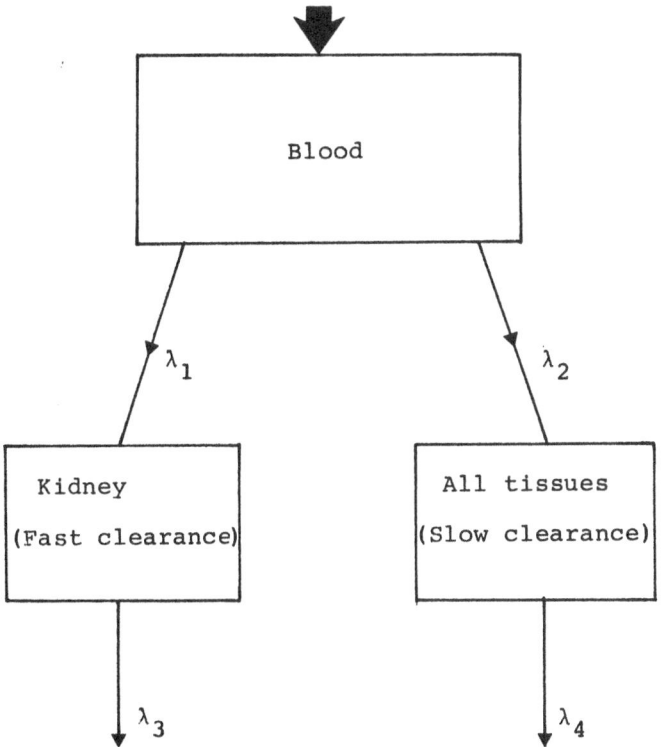

Note:

    (1)   Kidney content = [Kidney(Fast clearance)]

                                              + 0.005 [All tissues(slow clearance)]

        Blood content = [Blood] + 0.002 [All tissues(slow clearance)]

        Other tissues = 0.993 [All tissues(slow clearance)]

FIGURE 9.   SIMPLE MODEL FOR THE METABOLISM OF NICKEL IN MAN
                 AFTER ENTRY OF THE ELEMENT INTO THE SYSTEMIC
                 CIRCULATION

tissues (slow clearance)' assigned to blood is determined by the requirement to give an equilibrium whole-blood concentration of 5 µg l^{-1}.

It is noted that this model does not apply to nickel entering the
body by intramuscular injection or implantation (e.g. via puncture
wounds). Clearance from the site of intramuscular injection will be very
dependent upon the type of material injected and the location of the
site.

With respect to chelation therapy, the above model can be used, but,
at the time of injection of the chelate, nickel in blood should be
partitioned into two fractions. One fraction can be assumed to be Ni^{2+}
and will continue to behave according to the model proposed above. The
second fraction will be the nickel-chelate complex and will behave
metabolically as does the chelate; providing that the nickel-chelate
complex is sufficiently strongly bound to preclude significant
dissociation in vivo. The fractional binding to specific chelates and the
post-binding metabolism of those chelates will need to be investigated
separately for each individual case. For TETA, the reader is referred to
data discussed in this section.

5.4.4   Other metabolic data

5.4.4.1   Transfer to the foetus

Data on transfer to the foetus and to the suckling animal are
discussed in Section 4.3.2. In the absence of specific data for man, it
is probably appropriate to assume that the nickel concentration in the
foetus is not substantially different from the nickel concentration in
the mother at any time.

5.4.4.2   Transcutaneous absorption

On the basis of experiments on corpses, Kolpakov (1963) concluded
that the corneal epidermis prevented nickel sulphate penetration through
the skin, but that Malpigian layer, dermis and hypodermis were easily
permeable. More recently, Lloyd (1980) has reported that, in experiments
on guinea pigs, ^{63}Ni accumulated within one hour in the highly
keratinized areas, the stratum corneum and hair shafts. He noted that an
early route of entry into the skin may be via the skin appendages and
observed that after 24 h exposure 0.51, 0.05 and 5.33% of the applied
activity was found in urine, plasma and excised skin respectively.

The data reviewed above indicate that significant absorption through
the intact skin may occur, but that this is a relatively slow process.
The data available are not sufficient to define a quantitative model, but
it may be prudent to assume that, when a nickel salt in solution is
applied to the skin, a total of about 1% of the nickel is absorbed and
enters the systemic circulation in the first 24 hours post-application.

5.5   EFFECTS OF STATE OF HEALTH, ADMINISTRATION OF TOXIC LEVELS
        AND THERAPEUTIC PROCEDURES

5.5.1   State of health

No data appear to be available concerning the metabolism of nickel in different states of health. However, the implication of the kidneys in early and late excretion indicates that renal dysfunction is likely to have a profound modifying effect on nickel retention. The observed concentration of nickel in the distal convoluted tubuli suggests that failures of resorption could increase early excretion of nickel, but reduced circulatory flow to the kidneys would limit early excretion.

5.5.2   Administration of toxic levels

The data available are not sufficient to justify any modifications to the models for different levels of exposure.

5.5.3   Therapeutic procedures

The use of chelates to modify the whole-body retention of nickel is discussed in Section 4.3 where recommendations are given concerning appropriate changes to the proposed model.

5.6.   MODEL SUMMARY

The following model is recommended for nickel, on the basis of data reviewed in previous sections of this Chapter.

5.6.1   Gastrointestinal absorption

A best estimate of fractional absorption from the gastrointestinal tract is 0.05, but a range of 0.01 to 0.20 is not unusual, depending on chemical form administered, nature of the diet, nickel status and state of health. Absorption does not seem to be modified substantially by the amount of nickel present in the diet.

5.6.2   Retention in the respiratory system

It is assumed that all nickel entering the respiratory system as nickel carbonyl is deposited there and that it is then translocated to the systemic circulation with a biological half-life of 0.1 d. After entry into the systemic circulation, the metabolic model for other inorganic compounds of nickel is assumed to apply. However, it is emphasised that further work on nickel carbonyl metabolism is required before a detailed model can be developed.

For other compounds of nickel, the ICRP lung model is taken to apply, using the following classification:

Inhalation class	Compounds
W	oxides, hydroxides, carbides, Ni_3S_2 (amorphous and crystalline) NiS (amorphous and crystalline)
D	all other commonly occuring compounds

This classification is likely to ·over-estimate, rather than under-estimate, the mobility of the nickel sulphides.

5.6.3   Systemic metabolism

The model illustrated in Fig. 9 should be used, in conjunction with the following rate coefficients:

$\lambda_1 = 1.05\ d^{-1}$.
$\lambda_2 = 0.45\ d^{-1}$.
$\lambda_3 = 6.0\ d^{-1}$.
$\lambda_4 = 5.78 \times 10^{-4}\ d^{-1}$.

In estimating urinary and faecal excretion it can be assumed that 90% of material leaving the 'all tissues (slow clearance)' compartment goes to urinary excretion and that the remainder goes to faecal excretion.

The model does not apply to nickel entering the body by intramuscular injection or implantation. Clearance from the site of intramuscular injection will be very dependent upon the type of material injected and the location of the site.

The same model can be used when chelation therapy is employed. However, at the time of injection of the chelate, nickel in blood should be partitioned into two fractions. One fraction can be assumed to be Ni^{2+} and will continue to behave in the same fashion as before. The second fraction will be the nickel-chelate complex and will behave metabolically as the chelate.

5.6.4   Transfer to the foetus

In the absence of specific data for man, nickel concentrations in the foetus cannot be specified, but are likely to be of the same order as those in the mother at any time.

5.6.5   Transcutaneous absorption

The data available are not sufficient to define a quantitative model, but it may be prudent to assume that, when a nickel salt in solution is applied to the skin, a total of about 1% of the nickel is absorbed and enters the systemic circulation in the first 24 hours post-application.

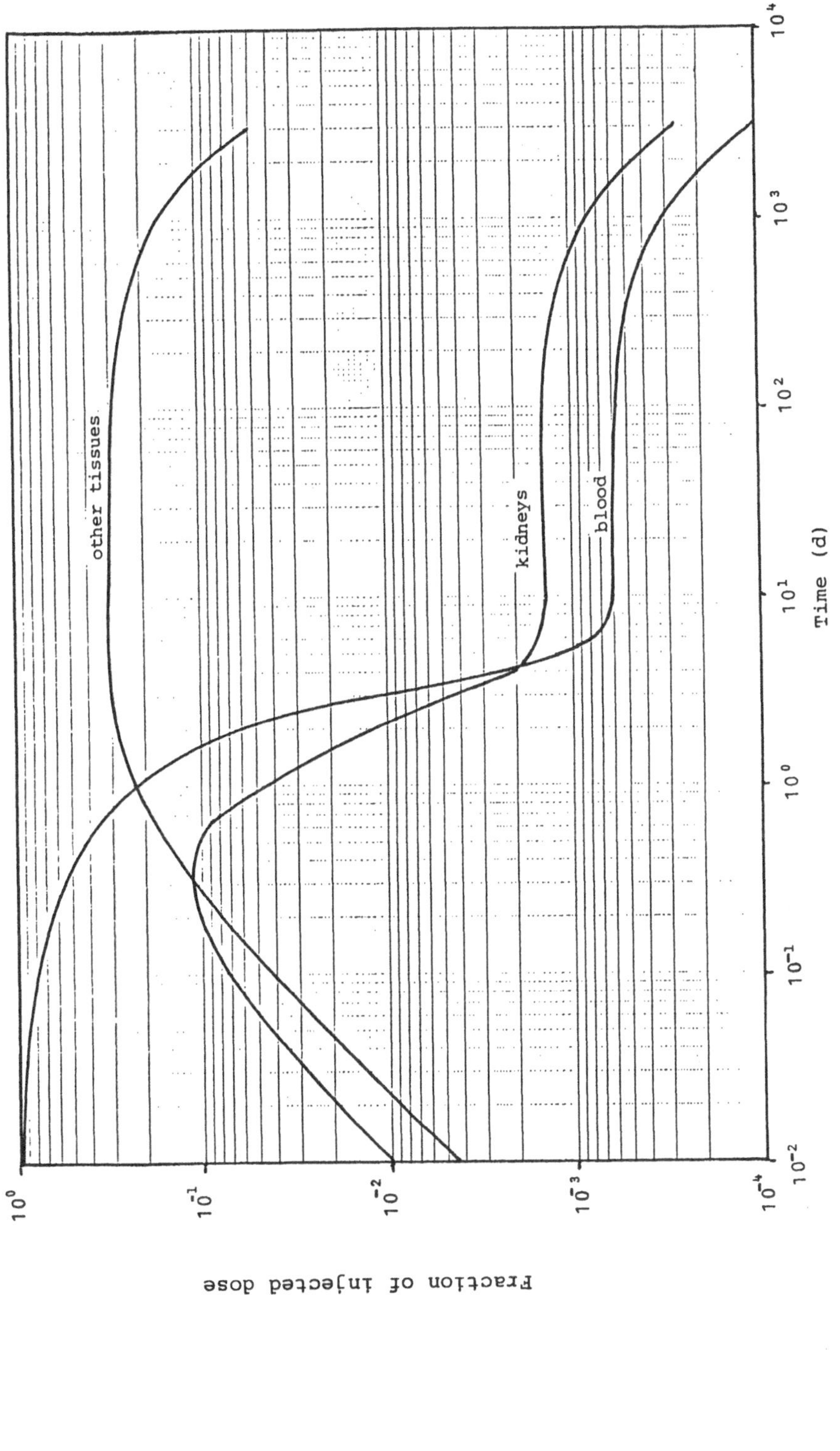

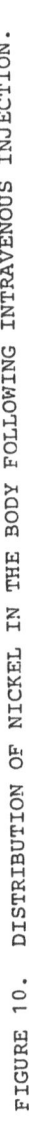

FIGURE 10. DISTRIBUTION OF NICKEL IN THE BODY FOLLOWING INTRAVENOUS INJECTION.

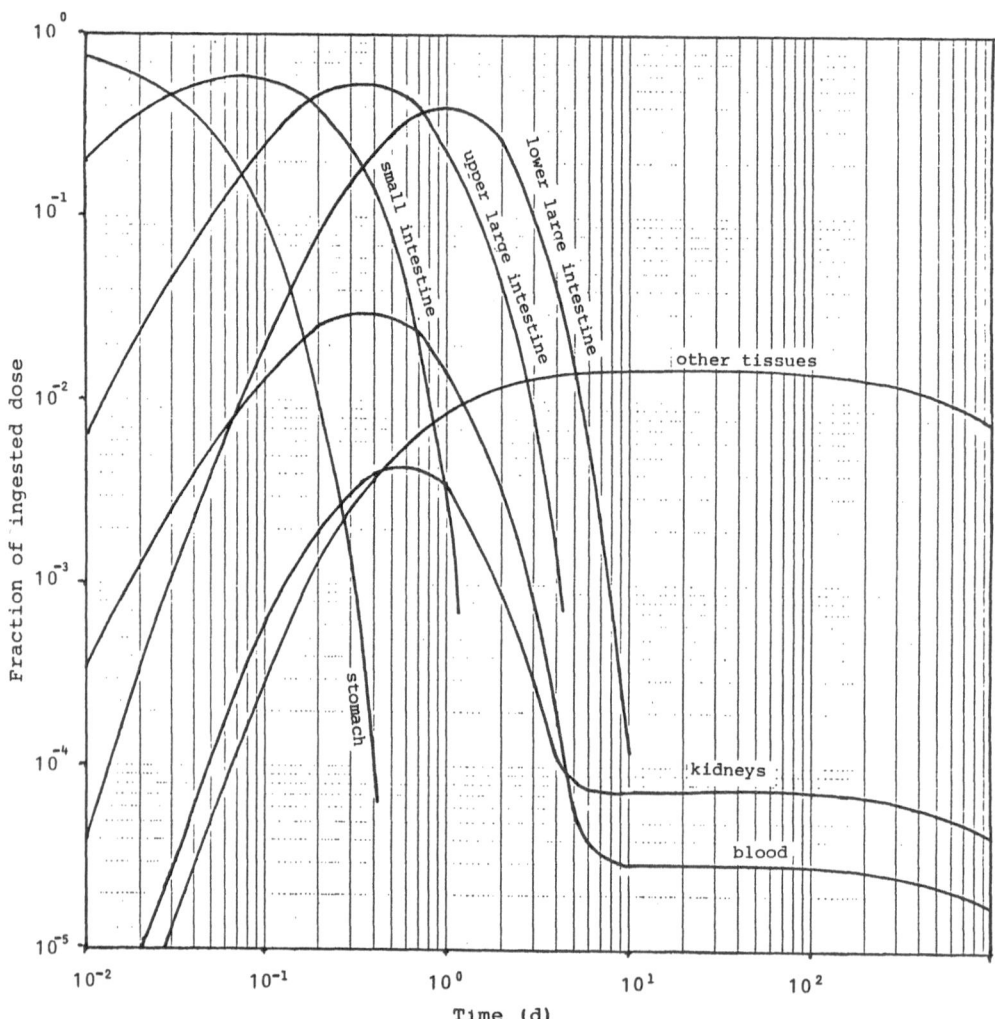

FIGURE 11.   DISTRIBUTION OF NICKEL IN THE BODY AFTER INGESTION.

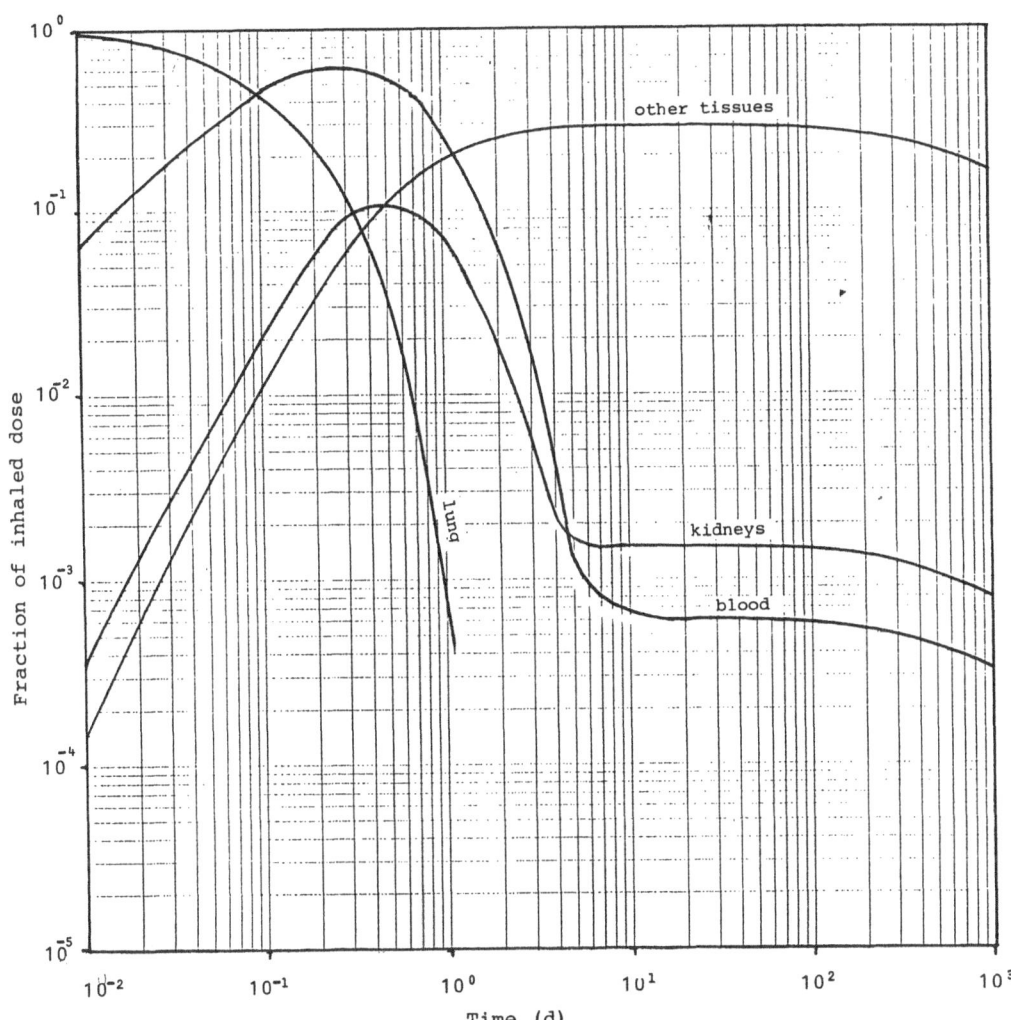

FIGURE 12.   DISTRIBUTION OF NICKEL IN THE BODY AFTER INHALATION
OF NICKEL CARBONYL.

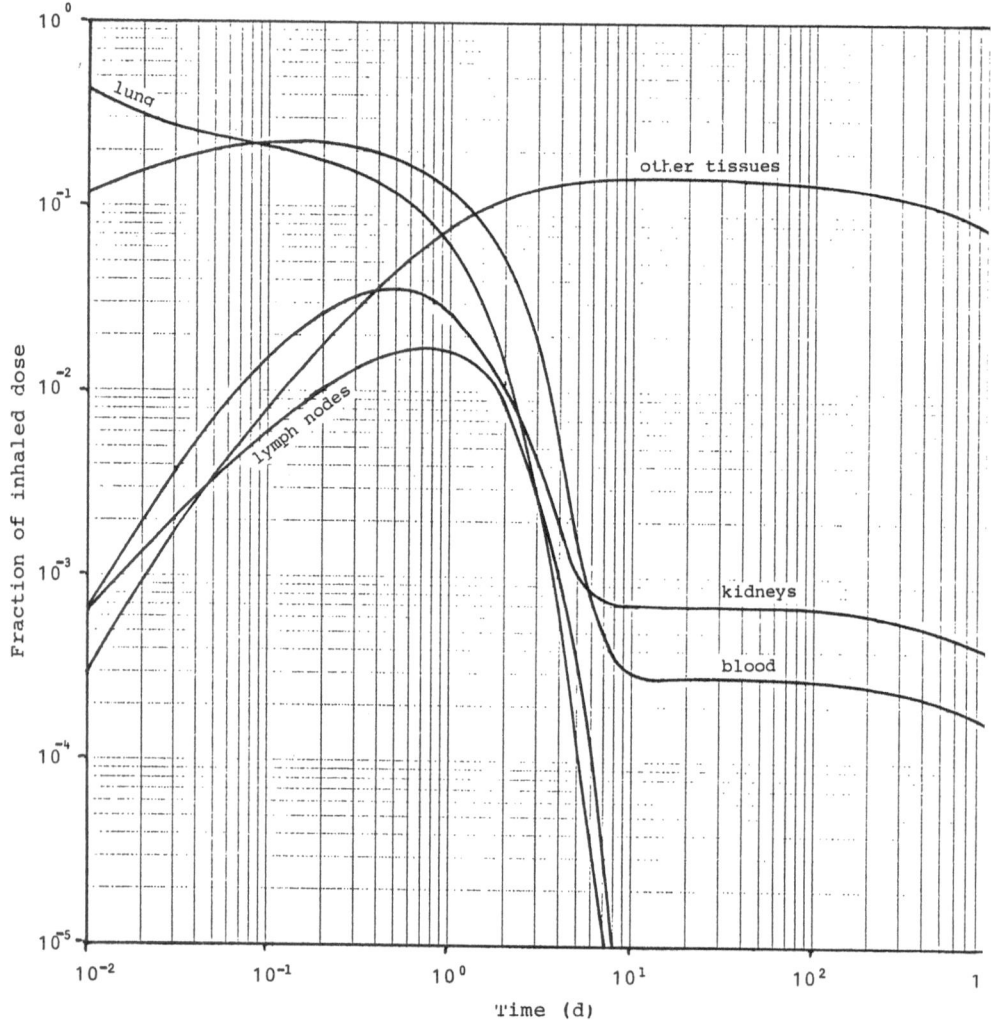

FIGURE 13.   DISTRIBUTION OF NICKEL IN THE BODY FOLLOWING
INHALATION OF A CLASS D COMPOUND.

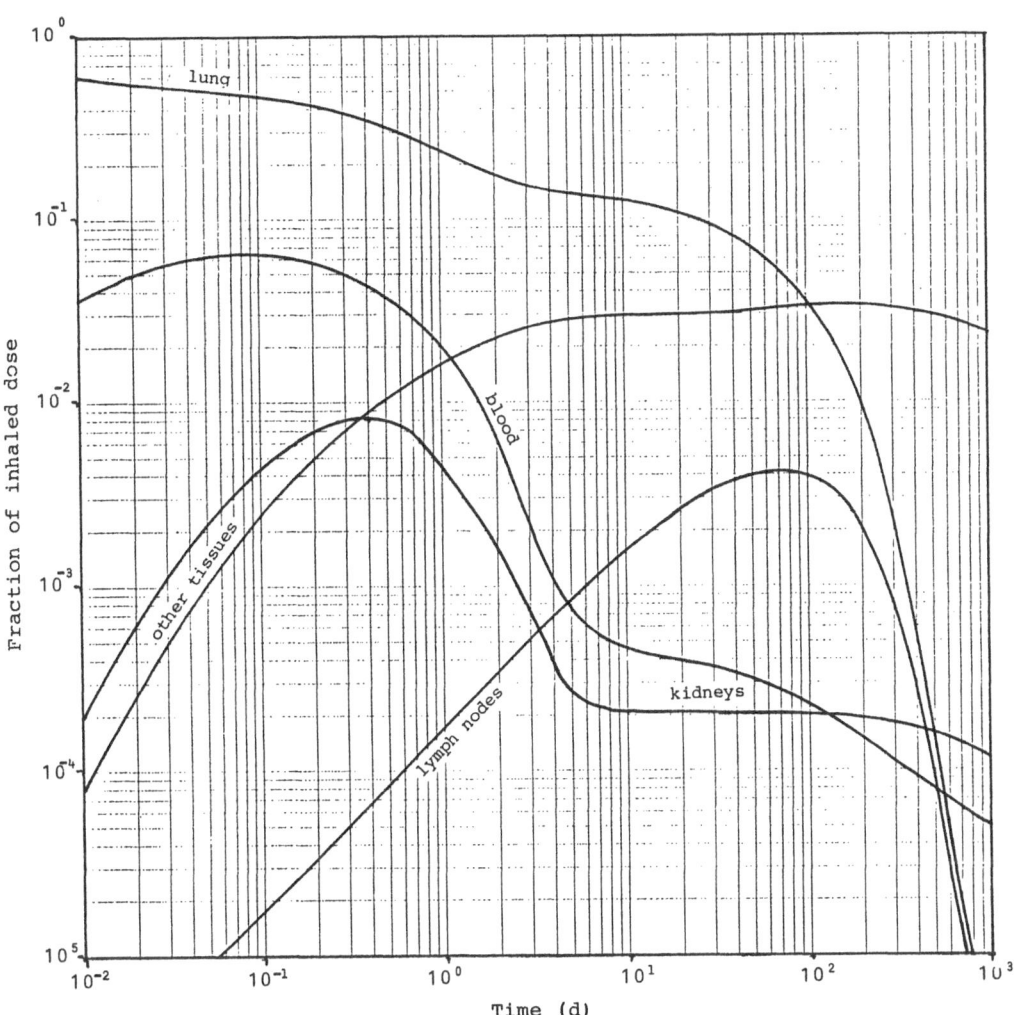

FIGURE 14.   DISTRIBUTION OF NICKEL IN THE BODY FOLLOWING
INHALATION OF A CLASS W COMPOUND.

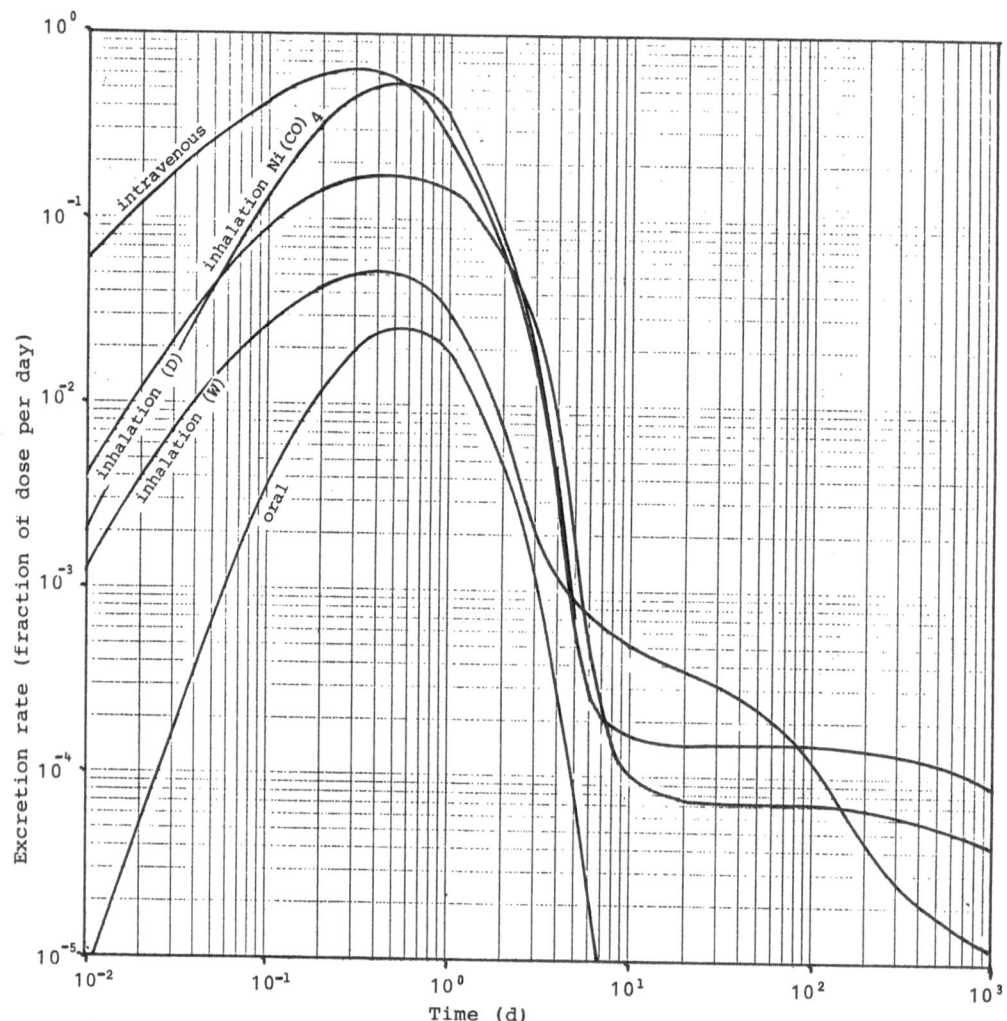

FIGURE 15.   URINARY EXCRETION OF NICKEL FOLLOWING INTAKE
VIA DIFFERENT ROUTES.

5.6.6   Effects of state of health

Renal dysfunction is likely to have a profound modifying effect on the retention of nickel in the body, but has not been studied and cannot currently be quantified.

5.6.7   Administration of toxic levels

The data available are not sufficient to justify any modifications to the models for different levels of exposure.

5.7   ILLUSTRATIVE CALCULATIONS

For the purpose of illustration of the proposed model, five sets of results are presented. These are time-dependent distributions of nickel in the body following instantaneous entry of a unit quantity by the following routes and in the following chemical forms:

- intravenous injection (all compounds);
- oral (all compounds);
- inhalation (nickel carbonyl);
- inhalation (class D compound);
- inhalation (class W compound).

Results of these calculations are shown in Figs. 10 to 14. The fractional gastrointestinal absorption was taken as 0.05 throughout. Also for comparison, the urinary excretion rates for each of these routes of intake are shown in Fig. 15.

5.8   REFERENCES

Adams, D.B., 1980. The routine determination of nickel and creatinine in urine. In: Brown, S.S. and Sunderman, F.W. Jr. (Eds.). Nickel Toxicology, Academic Press, New York, pp. 98-102.

Adkins, B. Jr., Richards, J.H. and Gardner, D.E., 1979. Enhancement of experimental respiratory infection following nickel inhalation. Environ. Res., 20, 33-42.

Ambrose, A.M., Larson, P.S., Borzelleca, J.F. and Hennigar, G.R. Jr., 1976. Long-term toxicologic assessment of nickel in rats and dogs. J. Food Sci. Technol., 13, 181-187.

Andersen, I., Høgetveit, A.C., Barton, R.T. and Glad, W.R., 1980. Rates of solubilization of nickel compounds in aqueous solutions and biological fluids. In: Brown, S.S. and Sunderman, F.W. Jr. (Eds.). Nickel Toxicology, Academic Press, New York, pp.77-80.

Anke, M., Grun, M. and Kronemann, H., 1980. Distribution of nickel in nickel-deficient goats and their offspring. In: Brown, S.S. and Sunderman, F.W. Jr. (Eds.). Nickel Toxicology, Academic Press, New York, pp.69-72.

Armit, H.W., 1908. The toxicology of nickel carbonyl. Part II. J. Hyg., VIII, 565-600.

Asato, N., Van Soestbergen, M. and Sunderman, F.W. Jr., 1975. Binding of ^{63}Ni(II) to ultrafilterable constituents of rabbit serum in vivo and in vitro. Clin. Chem., 21, 521-527.

Barton, R.T., 1977. Nickel carcinogenesis of the respiratory tract. J. Otolaryngol., 6, 412-422.

Barton, R.T., Andersen, I. and Høgetveit, A.C., 1980. Distribution of nickel in blood fractions. In: Brown, S.S. and Sunderman, F.W. Jr. (Eds.). Nickel Toxicology, Academic Press, New York, pp.85-88.

Bennett, B.G., 1982. Exposure of man to environmental nickel - an exposure commitment assessment. Sci. Total Environ., 22, 203-212.

Bergman, B., Bergman, M., Magnusson, B. and Soremark, R., 1980. The distribution of nickel in mice. An autoradiographic study. J. Oral Rehabil., 7, 319-324.

Bernacki, E.J., Parsons, G.E. and Sunderman, F.W. Jr., 1978a. Investigation of exposure to nickel and lung cancer mortality. Case control study at aircraft engine factory. Ann. Clin. Lab. Sci., 8, 190-194.

Bernacki, E.J., Parsons, G.E., Roy, B.R. Mikac-Devic, M., Kennedy, C.D. and Sunderman, F.W. Jr., 1978b. Urine nickel concentrations in nickel-exposed workers. Ann. Clin. Lab. Sci., 8, 184-189.

Bernacki, E.J., Zygowicz, E. and Sunderman, F.W. Jr., 1980. Fluctuations of nickel concentrations in urine of electroplating workers. Ann. Clin. Lab. Sci., 10, 33-39.

Bernstein, D.M., Kneip, T.J., Kleinman, M.T., Riddick, R. and Eisenbud, M., 1974. Uptake and distribution of airborne trace metals in man. In: Hemphill, D.D. (Ed.). Trace Substances in Environmental Health, 8th Annual Conference, University of Missouri, pp.329-334.

Bingham, E., Barkley, W., Zerwas, M., Stemmer, K. and Taylor, P., 1972. Response of alveolar macrophages to metals I. Inhalation of lead and nickel. Arch. Environ. Health, 25, 406-414.

Brown, S.S. and Sunderman, F.W. Jr. (Eds.). 1980. Nickel Toxicology, Academic Press, London.

Callan, W.M. and Sunderman, F.W. Jr., 1973. Species variation in binding of ^{63}Ni(II) by serum albumin. Res. Comm. Chem. Pathol. Pharmacol., 5, 459-472.

Casey, C.E. and Robinson, M.F., 1978. Copper, managanese, zinc, nickel, cadmium and lead in human foetal tissues. Br. J. Nutr., 39, 639-646.

Chausmer, A.B., 1976. Measurement of exchangable nickel in the rat. Nutr. Rep. Int., 14, 323-326.

Christensen, O.B. and Lagesson, V., 1980. Concentrations of nickel in blood and urine after oral administration. In: Brown, S.S. and Sunderman, F.W. Jr. (Eds.). Nickel Toxicology, Academic Press, New York, pp.95-98.

Clary, J.J., 1975. Nickel chloride-induced metabolic changes in the rat and guinea pig. Toxicol. Appl. Pharmacol., 31, 55-65.

Clausen, J. and Rastogi, S.C., 1977. Heavy metal pollution among auto-workers II. Cadmium, chromium, copper, manganese and nickel. Br. J. Ind. Med., 34, 216-220.

Clemente, G.F., Rossi, L.C. and Santaroni, G.P., 1980. Nickel in foods and dietary intake of nickel. In: Nriagu, J.O. (Ed.). Nickel in the Environment, John Wiley and Sons, New York, pp.493-498.

Costa, M. and Mollenhauer, H.H., 1980a. Carcinogenic activity of partic-ulate nickel compounds is proportional to their cellular uptake. Science, 209, 515-517.

Costa, M. and Mollenhauer, H.H., 1980b. Phagocytosis of nickel subsulfide particles during the early stages of neoplastic transformation in tissue culture. Cancer Res., 40, 2688-2694.

Costa, M. and Mollenhauer, H.H., 1980c. Phagocytosis of particulate nickel compounds is related to their carcinogenic activity. In: Brown, S.S. and Sunderman, F.W. Jr. (Eds.). Nickel Toxicology, Academic Press, New York, pp.43-46.

Costa, M., Simmons-Hansen, J., Bedrossian, C.W.M., Bonura, J. and Caprioli, R.M., 1981. Phagocytosis, cellular distribution and carcino-genic activity of particulate nickel compounds in tissue culture. Cancer Res., 41, 2868-2876.

Cotton, D.W.K., 1964. Studies on the binding of protein by nickel. With special reference to its role in nickel sensitivity. Brit. J. Dermatol., 76, 99-109.

Creason, J.P., Hinners, T.A., Bumgarner, J.E. and Pinkerton, C., 1975. Trace elements in hair, as related to exposure in Metropolitan New York. Clin. Chem., 21, 603-612.

Creason, J.P., Svendsgaard, D., Bumgarner, J., Pinkerton, C. and Hinners, T., 1977. Maternal-fetal tissue levels of 16 trace elements in 8 selected Continental United States communities. In: Hemphill, D.D. (Ed.). Trace substances in Environmental Health, Vol. 10, University of Missouri, pp.53-62.

Cronin, E., Di Michiel, D. and Brown, S.S., 1980. Oral challenge in nickel-sensitive women with hand eczema. In: Brown, S.S. and Sunderman, F.W. Jr. (Eds.). Nickel Toxicology, Academic Press, New York, pp.149-152.

Coughtrey, P.J. and Thorne, M.C., 1983. Radionuclide Distribution and Transport in Terrestrial and Aquatic Ecosystems. A Critical Review of Data, Vol. 2, A.A. Balkema, Rotterdam.

Decsy, M.I. and Sunderman, F.W. Jr., 1974. Binding of ^{63}Ni to rabbit serum α_1-macroglobulin in vivo and vitro. Bioinorg. Chem., 3, 95-105.

Dewally, D. and Hildebrand, H.F., 1980. The fate of nickel subsulfide implants during carcinogensis. In: Brown, S.S. and Sunderman, F.W. Jr. (Eds.). Nickel Toxicology, Academic Press, New York, pp.51-54.

Duke, J.M., 1980. Production and uses of nickel. In: Nriagu, J.O. (Ed.). Nickel in the Environment, John Wiley and Sons, New York, pp.51-65.

English, J.C., Parker, R.D.R., Sharma, R.P. and Oberg, S.G., 1981. Toxicokinetics of nickel in rats after intratracheal administration of a soluble and insoluble form. Am. Ind. Hyg. Assoc. J., 42, 486- 492.

Furst, A. and Radding, S.B., 1980. An update on nickel carcinogenesis. In: Nriagu, J.O. (Ed.). Nickel in the Environment, John Wiley and Sons, New York, pp.585-600.

Ghiringhelli, L. and Agamennone, M., 1957. Il metabolismo del nichel in animali sperementalmente avvelenati con nichelcarbonile. Med. Lavoro, 48, 187-194.

Gilani, S.H. and Marano, M., 1980. Congenital abnormalities in nickel poisoning in chick embryos. Arch. Environ. Contam. Toxicol., 9, 17-22, 1980.

Gitlitz, P.H., Sunderman, F.W. Jr. and Goldblatt, P.J., 1975. Aminoaciduria and proteinuria in rats after a single intraperitoneal injection of Ni(II). Toxicol. Appl. Pharmacol., 34, 430-440.

Heath, J.C. and Webb, M., 1967. Content and intracellular distribution of the inducing metal in the primary rhabdomyosarcomata induced in the rat by cobalt, nickel and cadmium. Br. J. Cancer, 21, 768-779.

Hendel, R.C. and Sunderman, F.W. Jr., 1972. Species variations in the proportions of ultrafilterable and protein-bound serum nickel. Res. Comm. Chem. Pathol. Pharmacol., 4, 141-146.

Herring, W.B., Leavell, B.S., Paixao, L.M. and Yoe, J.H., 1960. Trace metals in human plasma and red blood cells. Am. J. Clin. Nutr., 8, 846-854.

Ho, W. and Furst, A., 1973. Nickel excretion by rats following a single treatment. Proc. West. Pharmacol. Soc., 16, 245-248.

Hofsøy, H., Paulsen, G. and Jonsen, J., 1979. Secretion of nickel in rabbit saliva. Ann. Clin. Lab. Sci., 9, 479-486.

Høgetveit, A.C. and Barton, R. Th., 1977. Monitoring nickel exposure in refinery workers. In: Brown, S.S. (Ed.). Clinical Chemistry and Chemical Toxicology of Metals, Elsevier/North-Holland Biomedical Press, pp. 265-268.

Høgetveit, A. Ch., Barton, R. Th. and Kostøl, C.O., 1978. Plasma nickel as a primary index of exposure in nickel refining. Ann. occup. Hyg., 21, 113-120.

Horak, E. and Sunderman, F.W. Jr., 1973. Faecal nickel excretion by healthy adults. Clin. Chem., 19, 429-430.

Howard, J.M.H., 1980. Serum nickel in myocardial infarction. Clin. Chem., 26, p.1515.

IARC, 1976. Nickel and nickel compounds. IARC Monographs on the Evaluation of Carcinogenic Risk of Chemicals to Man. 11, 75-112.

ICRP, 1966. Report of the Task Group on Lung Dynamics. Deposition and retention models for the internal dosimetry of the human respiratory tract. Health Phys., 12, 173-207.

ICRP, 1975. Report of the Task Group on Reference Man, Pergamon Press, Oxford.

ICRP, 1981. Limits for Intakes of Radionuclides by Workers, ICRP Publication 30, Part 3. Annals of the ICRP, 6, No. 2/3.

Iyengar, G.V., Kollmer, W.E. and Bowen, H.J.M., 1978. The Elemental Composition of Human Tissues and Body Fluids. Verlag Chemie, Weinheim.

Jacobsen, N., Alfheim, I. and Jonsen, J., 1978. Nickel and strontium distribution in some mouse tissues passage through placenta and mammary glands. Res. Comm. Chem. Pathol. Pharmacol., 20, 571-584.

Jarstrand, C., Lundborg, M., Wiernik, A. and Camner, P., 1978. Alveolar macrophage function in nickel dust exposed rabbits. Toxicology, 11, 353-359.

Jasmin, G. and Solymoss, B., 1977. The topical effects of nickel subsulfide on renal parenchyma. In: Schrauzer, G.N. (Ed.). Inorganic and Nutritional Aspects of Cancer. Plenum Press, New York, pp.69-83.

Johannson, A., Camner, P., Jarstrand, C. and Wiernik, A., 1980. Morphology and function of alveolar macrophages after long-term nickel exposure. Environ. Res., 23, 170-180.

Jones, C.C., 1973. Nickel carbonyl poisoning. Report of a fatal case. Arch. Environ. Health, 26, 245-248.

Jordan, W.P. and King, S.E., 1979. Nickel feeding in nickel-sensitive patients with hand eczema. Am. Acad. Dermatol., 1, 506-508.

Kasprzak, K.S., 1974. An autoradiographic study of nickel carcinogenesis in rats following injection of $^{63}Ni_3S_2$ and $Ni_3{}^{35}S_2$. Res. Comm. Chem. Pathol. Pharmacol., 8, 141-150.

Kasprzak, K.S. and Sunderman, F.W. Jr., 1969. The metabolism of nickel carbonyl-^{14}C. Toxicol. Appl. Pharmacol., 15, 295-303.

Kasprzak, K.S. and Sunderman, F.W. Jr., 1977. Mechanisms of the dissolution of nickel subsulphide in rat serum. Res. Comm. Chem. Pathol. Pharmacol., 16, 95-108.

Kasprzak, K.S. and Sunderman, F.W. Jr., 1979. Radioactive ^{63}Ni in biological research. Pure & Appl. Chem., 51, 1375-1389.

Kolpakov, F.I., 1963. Skin permeability for nickel compounds. Arkh. Patol., 25, 38-45.

Leonard, A., Gerber, G.B. and Jacquet, P., 1981. Carcinogenicity, mutagenicity and teratogenicity of nickel. Mutat. Res., 87, 1-15.

Lloyd, G.K., 1980. Dermal absorption and conjugation of nickel in relation to the induction of allergic contact dermatitis - preliminary results. In: Brown, S.S. and Sunderman, F.W. Jr. (Eds.). Nickel Toxicology, Academic Press, New York, pp.145-148.

Lu, C.-C., Matsumoto, N. and Iijima, S., 1979. Teratogenic effects of nickel chloride on embryonic mice and its transfer to embryonic mice. Teratology, 19, 137-142.

Lucassen, M. and Sarkar, B., 1979. Nickel(II)-binding constituents of human blood serum. J. Toxicol. Environ. Health, 5, 897-905.

Mastromatteo, E., 1967. Nickel: A review of its occupational health aspects. J. occup. Med., 9, 127-136.

Mathur, A.K., Dikshith, T.S.S., Lal, M.M. and Tandon, S.K., 1978. Distribution of nickel and cytogenetic changes in poisoned rats. Toxicology, 10, 105-113.

McNeely, M.D., Sunderman, F.W. Jr., Nechay, M.W. and Levine, H., 1971. Abnormal concentrations of nickel in serum in cases of myocardial infarction, stroke, burns, hepatic cirrhosis, and uremia. Clin. Chem., 17, 1123-1128.

McNeely, M.D., Nechay, M.W. and Sunderman, F.W. Jr., 1972. Measurements of nickel in serum and urine as indices of environmental exposure to nickel. Clin. Chem., 18, 992-995.

Menden, E.E., Elia, V.J., Michael, L.W. and Petering, H.G., 1972. Distribution of cadmium and nickel of tobacco during cigarette smoking. Environ. Sci. Technol., 6, 830-832.

Menzel, D.B., Williams, S.J., Graham, J.A., Miller, F.J. and Gardiner, D.H., 1980. Permeability of the lung to inhaled heavy metals. In: Holmstedt, B., Lauwerys, R., Mercier, M. and Roberfroid, M. (Eds). Mechanisms of Toxicity and Hazard Evaluation. Elsevier/North-Holland Biomedical Press, pp.551-554.

Mikheev, M.I., 1971. Distribution and elimination of the nickel carbonyl. Gig. Tr. Prof. Zabol., 15, 35-38.

Morgan, L.G. and Rouge, P.J.C., 1979. A study into the correlation between atmospheric and biological monitoring of nickel in nickel refinery workers. Ann. occup. Hyg., 22, 311-317.

Mushak, P., 1980. Metabolism and systemic toxicity of nickel. In: Nriagu, J.O. (Ed.). Nickel in the Environment. John Wiley and Sons, New York, pp.499-523.

Myron, D.R., Zimmerman, T.J., Shuler, T.R., Klevay, L.M., Lee, D.E. and Nielsen, F.H., 1978. Intake of nickel and vanadium by humans: a survey of selected diets. Am. J. Clin. Nutr., 31, 527-531.

Nadeenko, V.G., Lenchenko, V.G., Azkhipenko, T.A. Saichenko, S.P. and Petrova, N.N., 1979. Embryotoxic effect of nickel ingested with drinking water. Gig. Sanit., 6, 86-88.

NAS, 1975. Nickel. A Report of the Committee on Medical and Biologic Effects of Environmental Pollutants. National Academy of Sciences, Washington, D.C.

Nielsen, F.H., 1977. Nickel toxicity. In: Goyer, R.A. and Mehlman, M.A. (Eds.). Advances in Modern Toxicology, Vol. 2, Hemisphere Publishing Corp., Washington, D.C.

Nielsen, F.H., 1980. Evidence of the essentiality of arsenic, nickel and vanadium and their possible nutritional significance. In: Draper, H.H. (Ed.). Advances in Nutritional Research, Vol. 3, Plenum Press, New York, pp.157-172.

Nielsen, F.H., Zimmerman, T.J., Collings, M.E. and Myron, D.R., 1979. Nickel deprivation in rats: nickel-iron interactions. J. Nutr., 109, 1623-1632.

Nodiya, P.I., 1972. Cobalt and nickel balances in students of an occupational technical school. Gig. Sanit., 37, 108-109.

Nomoto, S., 1980. Fractionation and quantitative determination of alpha-2 macroglobulin-combined nickel in serum by affinity column chromatography. In: Brown, S.S. and Sunderman, F.W. Jr. (Eds.). Nickel Toxicology, Academic Press, New York, pp.89-90.

Nomoto, S., Decsy, M.I., Murphy, J.R. and Sunderman, F.W. Jr., 1973. Isolation of [63]Ni-labeled nickeloplasmin from rabbit serum. Biochem. Med., 8, 171-181.

Norseth, T. and Piscator, M., 1979. Nickel. In: Friberg, L., Nordberg, G.F. and Vouk, V.B. (Eds.). Handbook on the Toxicology of Metals, Elsevier/ North-Holland Biomedical Press, pp.541-553.

Nriagu, J.O., 1980a. Global cycle and properties of nickel. In: Nriagu, J.O. (Ed.). Nickel in the Environment. John Wiley and Sons, New York, pp.1-26.

Nriagu, J.O. (Ed.), 1980b. Nickel in the Environment. John Wiley and Sons, New York.

Oberdoerster, G. and Hochrainer, D., 1980. Effect of continuous nickel oxide exposure on lung clearance. In: Brown, S.S. and Sunderman, F.W. Jr. (Eds.). Nickel Toxicology, Academic Press, London, pp.125-128.

O'Dell, G.D., Miller, W.J., Moore, S.L., King, W.A., Ellers, J.C. and Jurecek, H., 1971. Effect of dietary nickel level on excretion and nickel content of tissues in male calves. J. Anim. Sci., 32, 769-773.

Oskarsson, A. and Tjalve, H., 1977. Autoradiography of nickel chloride and nickel carbonyl in mice. Acta Pharmacol. Toxicol., 41, Suppl. 1, pp.158-159.

Oskarsson, A. and Tjalve, H., 1979a. An autoradiographic study on the distribution of $^{63}NiCl_2$ in mice. Ann. Clin. Lab. Sci., 9, 47-59.

Oskarsson, A. and Tjalve, 1979b. Binding of ^{63}Ni by cellular constituents in some tissues of mice after the administration of $^{63}NiCl_2$ and $^{63}Ni(CO)_4$. Acta pharmacol. et toxicol., 45, 306-314.

Oskarsson, A. and Tjalve, H., 1980. Effects of diethyldithiocarbamate and penicillamine on the tissue distribution of $^{63}NiCl_2$ in mice. Arch. Toxicol., 45, 45-52.

Oskarsson, A., Andersson, Y. and Tjalve, H., 1979. Fate of nickel subsulfide during carcinogenesis studied by autoradiography and x-ray powder diffraction. Cancer Res., 39, 4175-4182.

Onkelinx, C., 1977. Whole-body kinetics of metal salts in rats. In: Brown, S.S. (Ed.). Clinical Chemistry and Chemical Toxicology of Metals. Elsevier/North-Holland Biomedical Press, pp.37-40.

Onkelinx, C., Becker, J. and Sunderman, F.W. Jr., 1973. Compartmental analysis of the metabolism of $^{63}Ni(II)$ in rats and rabbits. Res. Comm. Chem. Pathol. Pharmacol., 6, 663-676.

Onkelinx, C. and Sunderman, F.W. Jr., 1980. Modelling of nickel metabolism. In: Nriagu, J.O. (Ed.). Nickel in the Environment, John Wiley and Sons, New York, pp.525-545.

Parker, K. and Sunderman, F.W. Jr., 1974. Distribution of ^{63}Ni in rabbit tissues following intravenous injection of $^{63}NiCl_2$. Res. Comm. Chem. Pathol. Pharmacol., 7, 755-762.

Phatak, S.S. and Patwardhan, V.N., 1952. Toxicity of nickel-accumulation of nickel in rats fed on nickel-containing diets and its elimination. J. Sci. Ind. Res., IIB, 173-176.

Rao, M.S.N., 1962. A study on the interaction of nickel (II) with bovine serum albumin. J. Amer. Chem. Soc., 84, 1788-1790.

Sarkar, B., 1980. Nickel in blood and kidney. In: Brown, S.S. and Sunderman, F.W. Jr. (Eds.). Nickel Toxicology, Academic Press, New York, pp.81-84.

Schmidt, J.A. and Andren, A.W., 1980. The atmospheric chemistry of nickel. In: Nriagu, J.O. (Ed). Nickel in the Environment. John Wiley and Sons, New York, pp.93-135.

Schroeder, H.A. and Mitchener, M., 1971. Toxic effects of trace elements on the reproduction of mice and rats. Arch. Environ. Health, 23, 102-106.

Schroeder, H.A., Balassa, J.J. and Tipton, I.H., 1961. Abnormal trace metals in man-nickel. J. chron. Dis., 15, 51-65.

Schroeder, H.A., Mitchener, M. and Nason, A.P., 1974. Life-term effects of nickel in rats: survival, tumors, interactions with trace elements and tissue levels. J. Nutr., 104, 239-243.

Shen, S.K., Williams, S., Onkelinx, C. and Sunderman, F.W. Jr., 1979. Use of implanted minipumps to study the effects of chelating drugs on renal ^{63}Ni clearance in rats. Toxicol. Appl. Pharmacol., 51, 209-217.

Sienko, M.J. and Plane, R.A., 1971. Chemistry, 4th edit., McGraw-Hill, New York.

Smith, J.C. and Hackley, B., 1968. Distribution and excretion of nickel-63 administered intravenously to rats. J. Nutr., 95, 541-546.

Snodgrass, W.J., 1980. Distribution and behaviour of nickel in the aquatic environment. In: Nriagu, J.O. (Ed.) Nickel in the Environment, John Wiley and Sons, New York, pp.203-274.

Solomons, N.W., Viteri, F., Shuler, T.R. and Nielsen, F.H., 1982. Bioavailability of nickel in man: effects of foods and chemically - defined dietary constituents on the absorption of inorganic nickel. J. Nutr., 112, 39-50.

Spears, J.W., Hatfield, E.E. and Forbes, R.M., 1978a. Interrelationship between nickel and zinc in the rat. J. Nutr., 108, 307-312.

Spears, J.W., Hatfield, E.E., Forbes, R.M. and Koenig, S.E., 1978b. Studies on the role of nickel in the ruminant. J. Nutr., 108, 313-320.

Spruit, D. and Bongaarts, P.J.M., 1977a. Nickel content of plasma, urine and hair in contact dermatitis. In: Brown, S.S. (Ed.). Clinical Chemistry and Chemical Toxicology of Metals, Elsevier/North-Holland Biomedical Press, pp.261-264.

Spruit, D. and Bongaarts, P.J.M., 1977b. Nickel content of plasma, urine and hair in contact dermatitis. Dermatologica, 154, 291-300.

Stack, M.V., Burkitt, A.J. and Nickless, G., 1976. Trace metals in teeth at birth (1957-1963 and 1972-1973). Bull. Environ. Contam. Toxicol., 16, 764-766.

Stahly, E.E., 1973. Some considerations of metal carbonyls in tobacco smoke. Chem. Ind., 13, 620-623.

Stoeppler, M., 1980. Analysis of nickel in biological materials and natural waters. In: Nriagu, J.O. (Ed.). Nickel in the Environment, John Wiley and Sons, New York, pp.661-821.

Storeng, R. and Jonsen, J., 1981. Nickel toxicity in early embryogenesis in mice. Toxicology, 20, 45-51.

Sunderman, F.W., 1964. Nickel and copper mobilization by sodium diethyl-dithiocarbamate. J. New Drugs, 4, 154-161.

Sunderman, F.W. Jr., 1976a. A review of the carcinogenicities of nickel, chromium and arsenic compounds in man and animals. Prevent. Med., 5, 279-294.

Sunderman, F.W. Jr., 1977a. The metabolism and toxicology of nickel. In: Brown, S.S. (Ed.). Clinical Chemistry and Chemical Toxicology of Metals, Elsevier/North-Holland Biomedical Press, pp.231-259. See also: Sunderman F.W. Jr., A review of the metabolism and toxicology of nickel. Ann. Clin. Lab. Sci., 7, 377-398, 1977, which is essentially an identical article.

Sunderman, F.W. Jr., 1977b. Metal carcinogenesis. In: Goyer, R.A. and Mehlman, M.A. (Eds.). Toxicology of Trace Elements. Advances in Modern Toxicology, Vol. 2, Hemisphere Publishing Corp., Washington, D.C., 1977.

Sunderman, F.W. Jr., 1979a. Mechanisms of metal carcinogenesis. Biol. Trace Element Res., 1, 63-86, 1979.

Sunderman, F.W. Jr., 1980a. Analytical biochemistry of nickel. Pure & Appl. Chem., 52, 527-544, 1980.

Sunderman, F.W. Jr., 1981a. Recent research on nickel carcinogenesis. Environ. Health Perspect., 40, 131-141.

Sunderman, F.W. and Kincaid, J.F., 1954. Nickel poisoning II. Studies on patients suffering from actue exposure to vapours of nickel carbonyl. J. Am. Med. Assoc., 155, 889-894.

Sunderman, F.W. Jr. and Maenza, R.M., 1976. Comparisons of carcinogen-icities of nickel compounds in rats. Res. Comm. Chem. Pathol. Pharmacol., 14, 319-330.

Sunderman, F.W. Jr. and Selin, C.E., 1968. The metabolism of nickel-63 carbonyl. Toxicol. Appl. Pharmacol., 12, 207-218.

Sunderman, F.W. and Sunderman, F.W. Jr., 1958. Nickel poisoning VIII. Dithiocarb: a new therapeutic agent for persons exposed to nickel carbonyl. Am. J. Med. Sci., 236, 26-31.

Sunderman, F.W. and Sunderman, F.W. Jr., 1961. Nickel poisoning XI. Implication of nickel as a pulmonary carcinogen in tobacco smoke. Am. J. Clin. Pathol., 35, 203-209.

Sunderman, F.W., Kincaid, J.F., Donnelly, A.J. and West, B., 1957. Nickel poisoning IV. Chronic exposure of rats to nickel carbonyl; a report after one year of observation. Arch. Ind. Health, 16, 480-485.

Sunderman, F.W. Jr., Decsy, M.I. and McNeely, M.D., 1972. Nickel metabolism in health and disease. In: Hopps, H.C. and Cannon, H.L. (Eds.). Geochemical Environment in Relation to Health and Disease, New York Academy of Sciences, 199, 300-312.

Sunderman, F.W. Jr., Kasprzak, K.S., Lau, T.J., Minghetti, P.P., Maenza, R.M., Becker, N., Onkelinx, C. and Goldblatt, P.J., 1976a. Effects of manganese on carcinogenicity and metabolism of nickel subsulfide. Cancer Res., 36, 1790-1800.

Sunderman, F.W. Jr., Kasprzak, K., Horak, E., Gitlitz, P. and Onkelinx, C., 1976b. Effects of triethylenetetramine upon the metabolism and toxicity of $^{63}NiCl_2$ in rats. Toxicol. Appl. Pharmacol., 38, 177-188.

Sunderman, F.W. Jr., Shen, S.K., Mitchell, J.M., Allpass, P.R. and Damjanov, I., 1978a. Embryotoxicity and fetal toxicity of nickel in rats. Toxicol. Appl. Pharmacol., 43, 381-390.

Sunderman, F.W. Jr., Taubman, S.B. and Allpass, P.R., 1979. Comparisons of the carcinogenicities of nickel compounds following intramuscular administration to rats. Ann. Clin. Lab. Sci., 9, p.441.

Sunderman, F.W. Jr., Shen, S.K., Reid, M.C. and Allpass, P.R., 1980a. Teratogenicity and embryotoxicity of nickel carbonyl in Syrian Hamsters. In: Brown, S.S. and Sunderman, F.W. Jr. (Eds.). Nickel Toxicology, Academic Press, London, pp.133-116.

Sunderman, F.W. Jr., Costa, E.R., Fraser, C., Hui, G., Levine, J.J. and Tse, T.P.H., 1981. ^{63}Nickel - constituents in renal cytosol of rats after injection of ^{63}nickel chloride. Ann. Clin. Lab. Sci., 11, 488-496.

Tandon, S.K. and Srivastava, R.C., 1980. Amelioration of nickel intoxication by chelating agents. In: Nriagu, J.O. (Ed.) Nickel in the Environment, John Wiley and Sons, New York, pp.569-583.

Tedeschi, R.E. and Sunderman, F.W., 1957. Nickel poisoning V. The metabolism of nickel under normal conditions and after exposure to nickel carbonyl. AMA Arch. Ind. Health, 16, 486-488.

Tola, S., Kilpio, J. and Virtamo, M., 1979. Urinary and plasma concentrations of nickel as indicators of exposure to nickel in an electroplating shop. J. occup. Med., 21, 184-188.

Torjussen, W. and Andersen, I., 1979. Nickel concentrations in nasal mucosa, plasma and urine in active and retired nickel workers. Ann. Clin. Lab. Sci., 9, 289-298.

Underwood, E.J., 1977. Trace Elements in Human and Animal Nutrition (4th edit.), Academic Press, New York.

Van Soestbergen, M. and Sunderman, F.W. Jr., 1972. [63]Ni complexes in rabbit serum and urine after injection of [63]NiCl$_2$. Clin. Chem., 18, 1478-1484.

Verma, H.S., Rajbehari, J. and Tandon, S.K., 1980. Pattern of urinary [63]Ni excretion in rats. Toxicol. Lett., 5, 223-226.

Veterans Administration Hospital, Hines, Ill., 1975. Metabolism of ^{90}Sr and of other elements in man. 1 July 1974-30 June 1975. COO-1231-104.

Webb, M., Heath, J.C. and Hopkins, T., 1972. Intranuclear distribution of the inducing metal in primary rhabdomyosarcomata induced in the rat by nickel, cobalt and cadmium. Br. J. Cancer, 26, 274-278.

Webb, M. and Wienzierl, S.M., 1972. Uptake of [63]Ni^{2+} from its complexes with proteins and other ligands by mouse dermal fibroblasts in vitro. Br. J. Cancer, 26, 292-298.

Wehner, A.P. and Craig, D.K., 1972. Toxicology of inhaled NiO and CoO in Syrian Golden Hamsters. Am. Ind. Hyg. Assoc. J., 33, 140-155.

Wehner, A.P., Busch, R.H., Olson, R.J. and Craig, D.K., 1975. Chronic inhalation of nickel oxide and cigarette smoke by hamsters. Am. Ind. Hyg. Assoc. J., 36, 801-810.

West, B. and Sunderman, F.W., 1958. Nickel poisoning Vi. A note concerning the ineffectiveness of edathamil calcium-disodium (calcium disodium ethylenediaminetetraacetic acid). AMA Arch. Ind. Health, 18, 480-482.

Whanger, P.D., 1973. Effects of dietary nickel on enzyme activities and mineral contents in rats. Toxicol. Appl. Pharmacol, 25, 323-331.

Zachariasen, H., Andersen, I., Kostøl, C. and Barton, R., 1975. Technique for determining nickel in blood by flameless atomic absorption spectrophotometry. Clin. Chem., 21, 562-567.

Ziemer, P.L. and Carvalho, S.M., 1980. Distribution and clearance of inhaled [63]NiCl$_2$ by rats. In: Radiation Protection: A Systematic Approach to Safety. Proceedings of the 5th Congress of the International Radiation Protection Society. Jerusalem. March, 1980. Vol. 2, Pergamon Press, Oxford, pp.1075-1079.

Appendix 6
Chromium

CONTENTS

6.1 INTRODUCTION

Chromium is a group VIB metallic element, notable for the brilliant red, yellow or green colour of its salts. First discovered in 1797 by Nicholas-Louis Vaugelin, it was isolated in 1798 by reduction of chromium oxide, CrO_3, with charcoal at high temperature (NAS 1974). The only commercial source of the metal is chromite, an ore of varying composition, nominally composed of varying mixtures of iron and chromium oxides (Stern 1982). Chromium is now recognized as an essential trace element for man, the first conclusive evidence being obtained by Mertz and Schwarz (1954; discussed in Mertz 1969). Recent literature pertaining to the nutritional role of chromium in man and animals has been reviewed extensively by Guthrie (1982). Exploitation of chromium is relatively recent, its use in metallurgy started to become important around 1910 and chrome plating, in the modern form, dates from around 1926 (Rollinson 1973). Since 1950 the use of chromium has increased substantially and the element is now of considerable importance (NAS 1974). World production of chromite ore was estimated to be 8 million tonnes in 1980 (Leonard and Lauwerys 1980) with the major producers being USSR and the Union of South Africa (Stern 1982). Leonard and Lauwerys (1980) listed the major uses of chromium as follows:

- in metallurgy, chromium is used in the manufacture of chrome-steel or chrome-nickel-steel alloys;
- chromite ore is used as a refractory agent;
- chromium salts are used as pigments and mordants in the textile industry, in tanning, in hardening photographic emulsions, as catalysts for organic and inorganic reactions, in ceramics and in explosives;
- in medicine, sodium radiochromate has been used to evaluate the life-span of erythrocytes.

A detailed consideration of the production of chromium and its compounds, and the occupational exposure arising there from, is presented by Stern (1982).

Chromium has oxidation states from Cr^{2-} to Cr^{6+}, but most commonly occurs as Cr^0, Cr^{2+}, Cr^{3+} and Cr^{6+}. Divalent chromium is rapidly oxidised to trivalent, and only Cr^{3+} and Cr^{6+} occur in nature (NAS 1974). Of the chromium ions, trivalent chromium is the most stable and important oxidation state. Hexavalent chromium is relatively stable in fresh water, probably because of the low concentrations of reducing material (Cutshall et al. 1966; Fukai 1967). Trivalent chromium is associated mainly with particulate matter, suggesting that organic particles may reduce and bind the element, leaving the hexavelent form in solution (Curl et al. 1965). Bowen (1979) has noted that hexavalent chromium is mobile in soils and plants, but is rapidly reduced to the less toxic, immobile, trivalent chromium.

Over the past 20 to 30 years a considerable literature has emerged concerning many aspects of chromium in the environment, including distribution, toxicity and metabolism in man and animals. Much of the work concerning the retention, distribution and carcinogenicity of chromium was performed in the 1950's and 1960's (e.g. Baetjer 1950a,b; Baetjer 1956; Baetjer et al. 1955; Baetjer et al. 1959; Bourne and Yee 1950; Davis 1956; Gafafer 1953; Hueper 1966; Jett et al. 1968; Kleinfeld and

Rosso 1965; Nater 1962; Schroeder et al. 1962; 1964; 1965; Visek et al. 1953), but more recent work has also been conducted (e.g. Sanderson 1976; Sayato et al. 1980), particularly as analytic methods for determining chromium have become more refined, allowing more reliable and accurate estimates of chromium concentrations (NAS 1974). Also, a large number of reviews have been published covering environmental chemistry and trans- fer, as well as absorption, retention, distribution, metabolism, dietary requirements, toxicity and carcinogenesis of chromium in man and animals (e.g. Schroeder 1968; Levander 1975; Sunderman 1979; Leonard and Lauwerys 1980; Bowen 1979; Norseth 1981; Underwood 1977; Hayes 1982; Coughtrey and Thorne 1983). Where possible, the original literature has been referred to in this appendix, but considerable reference has also been made to previous reviews.

Chromium may be environmentally damaging (e.g. Breeze 1973) and chromium compounds have been recognized for a long time as industrial poisons to man (e.g. Samitz 1955; Leonard and Lauwerys 1980; Norseth 1981). Occupational exposure is reported to represent the main source of human contamination (Leonard and Lauwerys 1980).

In a discussion of chromium toxicity in the chrome-plating industry, it was noted by Royle (1975) that:

"The toxic effects of exposure to chromium and its
compounds have been well known since the early nineteenth century .... in the United Kingdom notification
of cases of chrome ulceration to H.M. Chief Inspector
of Factories has been a statutory obligation since 1919".

The International Agency for Research on Cancer (IARC 1979) concluded that there is 'sufficient' evidence of chromium carcinogenicity in experimental animals and man, although the "specific compound(s) which may be responsible for a carcinogenic effect in humans cannot be speci- fied precisely". Hayes (1982) reviewed the carcinogenicity of chromium and its compounds in man and animals. It was not possible to exclusively identify the responsible agents, but in several instances strong and positive associations could be demonstrated between occupational exposure and development of cancer. It is of note that some compounds of chromium are used in cancer therapy, for example, intraperitoneally injected P-32 labelled, chromic phosphate has been used in the therapy of confirmed Stage 1 ovarian adenocarcinoma (Piver et al. 1982). In an earlier review of literature relating to chromium toxicity, the US National Academy of Sciences (NAS 1974) noted the following points:

- Chromium as a metal is biologically inert and does not produce harmful or toxic effects in man or laboratory animals.
- Trivalent chromium compounds have no established toxicity, either from ingestion or inhalation. On skin, Cr(III) may bind to proteins in the superficial layers and may be linked to dermatitis, but does not cause ulceration.
- Hexavalent chromium compounds are both corrosive and irritant, and may be absorbed by ingestion, inhalation or through the skin. Acute poisoning is generally rare.
- Hexavalent chromium causes ulceration primarily of skin and nasal septum and, rarely, the throat.

- The only important long-term health effect of hexavalent chromium is an increased risk of lung cancer. Other respiratory effects include irritation of mucous membranes, causing sneezing, rhinorrhea, irritation and redness of the throat and generalised bronchospasm. Sensitization may develop.

With regard to the toxicity of trivalent chromium, Leonard and Lauwerys (1980) noted that:

"It can be considered as evident, however, that the ultimate mutagen which binds to the genetic material is the trivalent form produced intracellularly from hexavalent chromium, the apparent lack of activity of the trivalent form being due to its poor cellular uptake."

It was demonstrated by Gentile et al. (1981) that "several chelants, in proportion to concentration, reduce or eliminate the mutagenicity of $Cr_2O_3^{2}$". The chelating agents were stated to include EDTA, salicylate (SA) and Tiron (disodium 1,2-dihydroxybenzene-3,5-disulphonate). Cr(III) as chromic chloride was rendered slightly mutagenic by SA and citrate. Although acute poisoning by hexavalent chromium may be rare, it has been recorded. Leonard and Lauwerys (1980) described the symptoms as severe inflammation of the digestive tract from the oesophagus to the jejunum with necrosis and even perforation. Death by cardiovascular collapse may follow. Without treatment, the lethal dose is estimated at 1 to 3 g (Moeschlin 1972; Langard 1980; Leonard and Lauwerys 1980). Finally, it has been noted that in the past 'therapy of chromium ulcers, whether subcutaneous or nasal, has not been highly successful' (NAS 1974). However, since 1956 in Great Britain, a striking reduction in chromium ulcers of the skin has been achieved by the treating of all breaks in the skin with an ointment containing 10% sodium calcium edetate (EDTA, Versenate) and covering with an impervious dressing (NAS 1974).

Although of less concern than toxicity in the context of metabolism and industrial exposure, symptoms of chromium deficiency have been identified in man and laboratory animals (NAS 1974; Levander 1975; Leonard and Lauwerys 1980; Casey and Hawbidge 1980). Low chromium status may complicate a number of conditions including protein-calorie malnutrition and diabetes, and has been suggested as an aetiological factor in coronary heart disease (Casey and Hambidge 1980). Impairment of 'glucose-tolerance' is generally the first symptom of mild chromium deficiency in animals; glucose removal rates decline within a few weeks, but can be cured by a single dose of chromium (NAS 1974). More severe deficiency results in mild impairment of growth and longevity; fasting hyperglycemia and glycosuria; and diminished stress resistance (NAS 1974). Chromium deficiency in man is mainly detectable by the demonstration of a chromium-responsive impairment of physiological function, generally of glucose metabolism (NAS 1974; Levander 1975; Leonard and Lauwerys 1980).

TABLE 1

CHROMIUM CONCENTRATIONS IN ROCKS, SOILS AND
SEDIMENTS (μg g^{-1} d.w.)

Material	Concentration	Reference and comments
Rocks:		
Earth's crust	125	IARC (1980): R Overall mean value, based on Hartford (1979)
Earth's crust	200	Coughtrey and Thorne
Sedimentary rocks	100-500	(1983): R
Igneous rocks	100	Values presented are
Acid rocks	2	derived from both
Shales	90	primary sources and
Sandstones	35-40	review articles, and do
Basic rocks	2000	not necessarily repre-
Magmatic rocks of the	70	sent 'mean' values or
upper continental crust		'typical' ranges. [1]
Limestone	11	
Carbonates	10	
Coals	5-60	
Superphosphates	66-243	
Soils:		
General range	tr[2]-250	IARC (1980): R
Estimated typical value	50	Coughtrey and Thorne (1983) [3]
Sediments:		
Estimated typical value, marine and freshwater sediments	75	Coughtrey and Thorne (1983)

Notes:

(1)   Data presented are to illustrate the variability of chromium concentration in parent materials

(2)   tr, trace

(3)   Coughtrey and Thorne (1983) note that previous authors had adopted values of 100 to 200 μg g^{-1} d.w.

6.2 INTAKE RATES

6.2.1 Elemental abundance

Chromium is distributed widely in the geosphere, but is concentrated in basic rocks, where it may occur at levels of ~2000 µg g^{-1} (Table 1). Chromium is reported to have an overall mean crustal concentration of 125 µg g^{-1} (Hartford 1979; IARC 1980) and is the twentieth most abundant element (Hartford 1979), ranking with vanadium, zinc, copper and tungsten. Data presented by Coughtrey and Thorne (1983) demonstrate the extreme variability of chromium concentrations in soil, from trace levels to 3000 µg g^{-1} d.w. Chromium is particularly abundant in soils derived from basalt or serpentine (IARC 1980). On the basis of a review of available data, Coughtrey and Thorne (1983) estimated a mean concentration of chromium in soil to be ~50 µg g^{-1} d.w. However, Coughtrey and Thorne noted that previous authors had adopted values of 100 to 200 µg g^{-1} d.w. The US National Academy of Sciences (1974) commented that discrepancies in analytic data for chromium, due to unreliable and highly variable analytic methods used in the past, are such that any estimated mean value must be treated with caution. This is taken to be especially true for reported chromium concentrations in water, air and biological materials; data for geochemical materials may be somewhat more reliable (NAS 1974).

A similar variability in chromium concentrations is notable in sediments, compared with soils, and available data have been summarised by Coughtrey and Thorne (1983). On the basis of data reviewed, Coughtrey and Thorne (1983) commented that chromium concentrations in marine sediments may vary from 1 to 2000 µg g^{-1} d.w., with a similar range for estuarine sediments. In freshwater sediments the concentration of chromium is generally between 18 and 140 µg g^{-1} d.w. (Coughtrey and Thorne 1983), but up to 1240 µg g^{-1} d.w. has been reported for samples from the R. Rhine (DeGroot and Allersma 1975). Coughtrey and Thorne (1983) assigned a mean value of 75 µg g^{-1} d.w. for chromium in all sediments. Less variability has been reported for chromium concentrations in water. Data reviewed by IARC (1980), indicate that marine water generally contains less than 1 µg l^{-1}. Freshwater typically contains 1-10 µg l^{-1} (IARC 1980 and see Table 2), although concentrations of up to 2000 µg l^{-1} have been reported on metallurgical mine drainage sites.

Chromium and compounds of chromium have a wide variety of industrial uses, reviewed by IARC (1980), and approximately 2.5x10^9 kg of chromium are mined each year (Bowen 1979). As a result of mining activities and natural cycling of the element, it has been estimated that 6.7x10^6 kg of chromium are added to the oceans each year (Fishbein 1976; IARC 1980). In view of the above, a considerable amount of the variability of chromium concentrations reported for soil, sediment and water may be attributed to the activity of man.

Within the biosphere, chromium is apparently ubiquitous, although some plant species are known to accumulate chromium to a considerable extent, such as Leptospermum scoparium and Pimelia suteri (Bowen 1979). Average concentrations in potential foodstuffs are presented in Table 3. Reported values vary from 0.0013 µg g^{-1} d.w. for brocoli to 5.2 µg g^{-1} d.w. for lettuce, and 0.02 µg g^{-1} d.w. for crabs to 49 µg g^{-1} d.w. for mussel (reviewed in Coughtrey and Thorne 1983). Data

TABLE 2

CHROMIUM CONCENTRATION IN WATER ($\mu g \ l^{-1}$)

Type	Concentration	Reference and comments
Seawater:		
General	<<1.0	IARC (1980): R
Estimated typical value	0.25	Coughtrey and Thorne (1983): R
Freshwater	1-10	IARC (1980): R
US, mean value	9.7	IARC (1980): R
Estimated typical value	2.5	Coughtrey and Thorne (1983): R

TABLE 3

CHROMIUM CONCENTRATION IN FOODSTUFFS

Material	Concentration	Reference and comments
Aquatic: Plants Crustaceans Molluscs Fish: freshwater Fish: marine Other organisms	1.0 µg g^{-1} d.w. 0.6 µg g^{-1} w.w. 0.6 µg g^{-1} w.w. 0.1 µg g^{-1} whole body 0.05 µg g^{-1} muscle 0.2 µg g^{-1} w.w.	Coughtrey and Thorne (1983): R Estimated typical values
Terrestrial: Plants: natural and agricultural	1.0 µg g^{-1} d.w.	May be elevated near roadsides, areas of mineralisation, phosphate processing factories or power- plants
Meat	0.06 µg g^{-1} w.w.	Underwood (1977): R from Kirkpatrick and Coffin (1975a)
Milk	13 µg l^{-1} 8 µg l^{-1} 10 µg l^{-1}	Kirchgessner (1959) Hambidge (1971) Schroeder et al. (1962)
Tobacco: cigarettes Tobacco Tobacco: cured	0.24-14.6 µg g^{-1} d.w. 10.7 (1.9-15.4) µg g^{-1} d.w. 1.14-4.96 µg g^{-1} d.w.	IARC (1980): R Frank et al. (1977) Frank et al. (1977)
Drinking water:[1] USA General General	ND-36 [2] 3.8-6.2 [3] 2.5 [4]	IARC (1980): R ICRP (1975): R IARC (1980): R

Notes:

(1)   WHO, European and US standard for maximum permissable concentration of chromium in drinking water is 50 µg l^{-1} (IARC   1980).

(2)   ND, not detectable. Median value in this case reported to be 0.43 µg l^{-1} (from, Hartford 1979).

(3)   Estimated on the basis of a daily intake of 1.6 l water by Reference Man (ICRP 1975), and data reviewed by ICRP (1975) indicating that 6-10 µg of chromium is ingested by Reference Man, per day, in drinking water.

(4)   Estimated on the basis of a daily intake of 1.6 l water by Reference Man (ICRP 1975), and data reviewed by IARC (1980) indicating that 4 µg Cr d^{-1} is ingested from drinking water per day.

pertaining to the transport of chromium, and its radioisotopes, through
the terrestrial and aquatic environments, were also reviewed by Coughtrey
and Thorne (1983). In a review of the environmental chemistry of
chromium, Bowen (1979) noted the following mean or median concentrations:

Geosphere:

Granite	4	$\mu g\ g^{-1}$
Basalt	90	$\mu g\ g^{-1}$
Soil	70	$\mu g\ g^{-1}$
Shale	90	$\mu g\ g^{-1}$
Limestone	11	$\mu g\ g^{-1}$
Sandstone	35	$\mu g\ g^{-1}$
Seawater	0.3	$\mu g\ l^{-1}$
Freshwater	1	$\mu g\ l^{-1}$
Air (Europe)	0.025	$\mu g\ m^{-3}$

Biosphere:

Land plants	0.03 - 10	$\mu g\ g^{-1}$ d.w.
Edible vegetables	0.016 - 14	$\mu g\ g^{-1}$ d.w.
Mammalian muscle	<0.002 - 0.84	$\mu g\ g^{-1}$ d.w.
Mammalian bone	0.1 - 33	$\mu g\ g^{-1}$ d.w.
Marine algae	0.5 -13	$\mu g\ g^{-1}$ d.w.
Marine fish	0.03 - 2	$\mu g\ g^{-1}$ d.w.

6.2.2   Typical dietary

Data presented in Section 6.2.1 and Table 3 indicate that all plant
and animal tissues contain chromium in detectable amounts, although it
has been noted by the ICRP (1975) that 'spices appear to be the richest
source'. Guthrie (1975) reported concentrations of 3.9 $\mu g\ g^{-1}$ in thyme,
whereas Schroeder et al. (1962) obtained value of 3.7 $\mu g\ g^{-1}$ and
10.0 $\mu g\ g^{-1}$. Guthrie (1982) noted that extreme variability in values for
the chromium content of various foods can be found both between and
within laboratories. Values reported in Table 3 are intended to serve
only as guides. Dietary intakes can be expected to vary with local
dietary custom and personal preference. Appreciable losses of chromium
have been reported in normal processing and preparation of foods
(Underwood 1977). Masironi et al. (1973) analysed the chromium content of
molasses, unrefined, brown and highly refined sugar from several
countries, by flameless atomic absorption with low temperature ashing.
They obtained mean values of 0.266 ±0.058, 0.162 ± 0.038, 0.064 ±0.005
and 0.02 ±0.003 $\mu g\ Cr\ g^{-1}$ respectively. Glinsmann et al. (1966) noted
that the high intake of refined sugar in US diets, typically 120 $g\ d^{-1}$
per person contributes very little chromium and may lead to an overall
body loss due to the chromium-depleting action of glucose (see
Section 6.6). In a further study, Zook et al. (1970) reported mean levels
of 0.38 ± 0.06 $\mu g\ Cr\ g^{-1}$ and 0.37 ±0.06 $\mu g\ Cr\ g^{-1}$ for common hard wheat
and soft wheat respectively, compared with 0.22 ±0.08 and
0.29 ±0.15 $\mu g\ Cr\ g^{-1}$ in the respective flours. In contrast, Murakami
et al. (1965) noted that for three recommended 'well-balanced' Japanese
diets, higher levels of chromium were detected in cooked servings as
compared with the raw ingredients.

TABLE 4

ESTIMATED DAILY AVERAGE INTAKE OF CHROMIUM

Country or Area	Cr intake (μg d^{-1})	Method of Estimation	Reference
	30–3500	Review of information	ICRP (1975), from Gandolfo and Sampaolo (1963)
	30–200	Review of information [1]	ICRP (1975)
	73–740 (mean ∿200)	Review of information long term study of 4 individuals	ICRP (1975), from Schroeder (1968), Tipton and Stewart (1967), Tipton et al. (1966)
	150 10–400 (mean ∿80)	Review of information: Estimated typical value	ICRP (1975, 1980) IARC (1980), from Hartford (1979)
	280	Review of information [2]	IARC (1980), from Fishbein (1976)
Vermont, USA	80	Institutional diet	Underwood (1977), from Schroeder et al. (1962)
New York, USA	50	Institutional diet [4]	Underwood (1977), from Glinsmann and Mertz (1966), Levine et al. (1968)
USA	5 to >100		Underwood (1977), from WHO (1973)
Japan	130–253	Recommended diets [5]	Underwood (1977), from WHO (1973)
New York	5–115 (mean 65)	'Ad libitum'	Levine et al. (1968)
Italy	64	200 g dinner	Mertz (1969)
India	11–55	Vegetarian diet	Joseph et al. (1968)
W. Germany	62 (11–195)	Duplicated – food and beverages	Schelenz (1977)
Finland	29	Calculated representative intake	Varo and Koivistoinen (1980)

TABLE 4 (contd)

Country or Area	Cr intake ($\mu g \ d^{-1}$)	Method of Estimation	Reference
Finland	31 (14–45)	Self chosen diets of pregnant women	Kumpulainen et al. (1980)
Sweden	182 (44–588)	Self chosen diets of elderly men and women	Abdulla and Svenson (1979)
USA	50 (30–80)	Calculated representative intake	Schroeder et al. (1962)
USA	52	Typical institutional diet	Schlettwein-Gsell and Mommsen-Straub (1971)
USA	52 (5–115)	Institutional diets of elderly subjects	Levine et al. (1968)
USA	62±28 [3] (37–130)	Representative diets containing 43% fats	Kumpulainen et al. (1979)
USA	65	Representative diet	Schlettwein-Gsell and Mommsen-Straub (1971)
USA	77±23 (33–125)	Meals from 50 colleges	Walker and Page (1977)
USA	78	Typical institutional diet	Schroeder et al. (196:
USA	89±56 (25–224)	Representative diets containing 25% fat	Kumpulainen et al. (1979)
USA	123	Hospital diet	Schroeder (1971)
USA	200±30	Self chosen diets of 1 man	Tipton et al. (1969)
USA	200±40	Self chosen diets of 1 man	Tipton and Stewart (1969)
USA	290±60	Self chosen diets of 1 man	Tipton et al. (1969)
USA	330	Self chosen diets of 1 woman	Tipton et al. (1966)
USA	400	Self chosen diets of 1 man	Tipton et al. (1966)
USA	<455	Representative institutional summer diet	Gormican (1970)

TABLE 4 (contd)

Country or Area	Cr intake ($\mu g\ d^{-1}$)	Method of Estimation	Reference
USA	<887	Representative institutional winter diet	Gormican (1970)
USA	<860	Self chosen diets of 48 young women	White (1969)
USA	2,620	Self chosen diets of men and women	Chah et al. (1976)
India	76–189	Typical Indian diets	Rao and Rao (1980)
India	109 (90–127)	Rice-based diets	Rao et al. (1977)
India	150 (100–300)	Self chosen diets	Soman et al. (1969)
New Zealand	81±32 (39–190)	Self chosen diets of 14 women	Guthrie (1973)
New Zealand	229 (166–292)	Representative diets	Dick et al. (1978)
Japan	135	Representative diets	Murakami et al. (1965)
Canada	136 (136–152)	Representative diets	Kirkpatrick and Coffin (1974)
USSR	690–820	Representative diets	Schlettwein-Gsell and Mommsen-Straub (1971)

Notes:

(1)   Considered to be a 'more usual daily intake' (ICRP 1975), of which 6 to 10 µg may be contributed by drinking water (ICRP 1975, from Anderson, pers. comm. to Howells 1966; Hadjimarkos 1967; Schroeder et al. 1962)

(2)   A further 4 µg d^{-1} is estimated to be consumed in drinking water

(3)   Mean ± SE

(4)   Diabetics and old people, in whom some positive response to Cr supplementation was obtained

(5)   Higher values were obtained when cooked servings were analysed

Estimated daily average intakes of chromium are presented in Table 4, indicating a range of 5 to 3500 µg Cr d^{-1}. The ICRP (1975) considered a usual daily intake to be around 30 to 200 µg and, in defining a standard man for radiological protection purposes, assumed a mean value of 150 µg d^{-1} (ICRP 1975, 1980). On the basis of data presented by Schroeder (1970), the US National Academy of Sciences (1974) estimated a typical dietary intake of 280 µg Cr d^{-1} or ∿100 µg Cr d^{-1} for hospital diets. However, it is noted that 'estimates of the contribution of chromium from food, water and air vary significantly from author to author' (NAS 1974). Diets containing in excess of 500 µg Cr d^{-1} appear to be uncommon, unless local land contamination is present. In a review of daily intakes, Guthrie (1982) concluded that "many of the estimates are probably too high." Guthrie (1982) considered that most normal daily intakes are below 200 µg d^{-1} and intakes higher than this generally derive from earlier references using less sensitive instrumentation. The same limitations may also apply to many of the reported intakes in the 100-200 µg d^{-1} range. On the basis of data presented in Table 4 and with respect to the comment of Guthrie (1982), it is reasonable to assume that a typical dietary intake of chromium in Europe and N. America will not generally exceed 100 µg d^{-1} and that the ICRP estimate of 150 ug d^{-1} is a cautious upper limit for typical dietary intakes. Less confidence can be expressed with regard to estimating a typical lower limit to dietary intake, and a reasonable estimate of mean daily dietary intake is taken to be 75 µg d^{-1}.

Dietary information presented by ICRP (1975) in conjunction with chromium concentrations reported in Table 3, can be used to estimate daily intakes of chromium as presented in Table 5. Although many assumptions have been made to derive the daily dietary intake of >69 µg Cr, in Table 5 it is nonetheless in good agreement with the value of 75 µg Cr d^{-1} proposed above.

6.2.3   Chromium in drinking water

By comparison with data for concentrations of chromium in plant and animal foodstuffs, relatively little information is available for the concentration of chromium in drinking water. On the basis of data reviewed by IARC (1980) and ICRP (1975), as presented in Table 3, concentrations of chromium in drinking water are taken generally to be <10 µg l^{-1} and may be less than 1 µg l^{-1}. In a survey of chromium levels in public water supplies in the USA, Hartford (1979) recorded a median value of 0.43 µg l^{-1}. Extremely high levels of chromium (up to 2.0 mg l^{-1}) have been reported for waters from areas of metallurgical mining activity (Leland et al. 1978), but such waters should not be considered as public water supplies. If it is assumed that the chromium concentration in drinking water is generally between 0.5 to 5 µg l^{-1} and that the daily fluid intake of man is 1.6 litres (ICRP 1975), then a dietary intake from water of 0.8 to 8 µg Cr d^{-1} is calculated. This represents <1% to <10% of the estimated chromium intake in food. By comparison, Schroeder (1970) estimated a daily intake of 4 µg Cr in water for individuals on a 'self-selected diet' and 0-84 µg Cr d^{-1} (mean 1 µg Cr d^{-1}) for individuals on a hospital diet.

TABLE 5

ESTIMATED DIETARY INTAKE OF CHROMIUM ON BASIS
OF INDIVIDUAL DIETARY DATA

Food type	U.K. per caput consumption (1) g d^{-1}	Assumed chromium concentration in food (μg g^{-1}) (2)	Daily intake (μg)	Comments
Milk	382	0.01	3.8	From Table 3
Cheese	12	0.05	0.6	Assuming that cheese has 20% volume of milk and no chromium is lost in production
Meat and products	137	0.06	8.2	From Table 3
Fish and seafood	21	0.1	2.1	From Table 3
Eggs	34	0.01	0.3	Assumed to have a concentration equal to milk
Fats	44	?	?	No data available
Sugar and preserves	77	0.02	1.5	Value from Masironi et al. (1973) for refined sugar
Potatoes, other vegetables and fruit	428	0.1	42.8	From Table 3, assuming d.w. is equal to 10% w.w.

TABLE 5 Cont.

Food type	U.K. per caput consumption[1] g d^{-1}	Assumed chromium concentration in food (μg g^{-1}) [2]	Daily intake (μg)	Comments
Cereals	246	0.04	9.8	Value from Zook et al. (1970) for wheat, assuming d.w. is equal to 10% w.w.
Total	1381		>69.1	

Notes:

(1) Data from ICRP (1975) for period 1962 to 1965

(2) All values have been converted to fresh weight

6.2.4   Inhalation of chromium

Reported concentrations of chromium in ambient air have been collated and discussed by Bowen (1979) and IARC (1980) and available data are presented in Table 6. Burning of coal and smelting of metals are major sources of chromium release to the atmosphere (IARC 1980) and levels of 220 to 2200 μg Cr m^{-3} have been recorded in emitted gases of coal-fired power stations, in the absence of fly-ash collection (Fishbein 1976). Cement-producing plants have been identified by IARC (1980) as further sources of chromium in air. Portland cement contains 27.5 to 60 μg Cr g^{-1} and soluble chromium in cement averages 4.1 μg g^{-1} of which 2.9 μg g^{-1} is hexavalent chromium (IARC 1980). Asbestos contains approximately 1500 μg Cr g^{-1} (Fishbein 1976) and IARC (1980) noted that "wearing of brake linings thus represents a source of chromium [to atmosphere] since asbestos particles are emitted in this way".

Air samples analysed from 23 localities in northern England and Wales had chromium levels of 0.9 to 21.5 μg m^{-3} (IARC 1980). However, those samples were obtained during 1956-1958 and, Salmon et al. (1977) presented data indicating that, at one rural site in the UK, atmospheric chromium declined by 11.3% y^{-1} during the period 1957-1974. On the basis of a review of available literature, Bowen (1979) estimated a median air concentration of chromium as 0.025 μg m^{-3} in Europe. Values for North America and Japan are reported to be 0.06 and 0.02 to 0.07 μg m^{-3} respectively (Bowen 1979).

Within the working environment of factories producing or extensively utilising chromium, or compounds of chromium, high levels of chromium in air have been reported. Airborne concentrations of 'chromates' in the kilns and mills of 4 US plants processing chromium, over the period 1930 to 1947, ranged between 10 and 41600 μg m^{-3} (Machle and Gregorius 1948). More recently, Gomes (1972) reported a chromium in air concentration of >1000 μg m^{-3} in the electro-plating area of one Brazilian hard-chrome plant using solutions of Cr(VI). A further seven similar plants were surveyed and found to exhibit air concentrations of 100 to 400 μg m^{-3} (Gomes 1972). Guillemin and Berode (1978) found a higher exposure of workers to chromium in 'hard' chromium-plating plants, relative to 'bright' chromium-plating. The chromium- and nickel-plating area of a chromium-plating factory in the US was reported to exhibit a mean concentration of 3.24 μg Cr(VI) m^{-3} in air (and a range of <0.71 to 9.12 μg m^{-3} (National Institute for Occupational Safety and Health 1975). Data presented in Table 5 indicate that in European and North American factories, current mean levels of chromium in the working environment are unlikely to exceed 10 μg m^{-3}.

The amount of chromium inhaled by an occupationally exposed worker in Europe can be calculated, given the following assumptions:

- during light activity the respiration rate of Reference Man is 0.02 m^3 min^{-1}; when engaged in heavy work the rate of respiration increases to 0.043 m^3 min^{-1}; with minimal activity the basal rate of respiration is 0.0075 m^3 min^{-1} (ICRP 1975):
- a working day consists of 8 h occupational activity; 8 h non-occupational, or light, activity; 8 h rest:
- the air concentration of chromium in the working environment is 5-10 μg m^{-3}; in all other areas chromium is present at a concentration of 0.025 μg m^{-3}.

TABLE 6

CONCENTRATION OF CHROMIUM IN AIR SAMPLES (μg m^{-3})

Remarks	Concentration	Location and material	Reference
Maximum statutory concentrations	50	Sweden and Czechoslovakia, MPC(1). Chromic acid and chromates	IARC (1980)
	10	USSR, MPC. Chromic acid and chromates	IARC (1980)
	100	Japan, TC(2). Barium chromate, calcium chromate, lead chromate, potassium chromate, potassium dichromate, sodium chromate, sodium dichromate (estimated as CrO_3)	IARC (1980)
	500	Japan, TC. Strontium chromate, $CrCl_3$ (estimated as CrO_3)	IARC (1980)
	1000	Japan, TC. Chromium sulphate	IARC (1980)
	5000	Japan, TC. Zinc chromate hydroxide, zinc pottasium hydroxide (estimated as CrO_3)	IARC (1980)
Industry: 1930–1947	10–4600	US kilns and mills	IARC (1980)
1930–1947	200–21000	US kilns and mills, packing areas	IARC (1980)
1930–1947	3–2170	US kilns and mills, other areas	IARC (1980)
ca 1950–1953	110–150	Italy, chromate factory (Cr-VI)	IARC (1980)

TABLE 6 (Cont.)

Remarks	Concentration	Location and material	Reference
Industry cont.: pre 1943	210-600	Chromium platers (Cr-VI)	IARC (1980)
post 1943	45-50	Chromium platers, following installation of air vents (Cr-VI)	IARC (1980)
ca 1974	<0.71-9.12	US, chromium-nickel plating area (Cr-VI)	IARC (1980)
ca 1952	3	Finland, highest reported value (Cr-III)	IARC (1980)
pre 1960	180-1400	Chromium platers (Cr-VI)	IARC (1980)
post 1960	3-9	Chromium platers, after installation of air vents	
ca	~100->1000	Brazil, electroplaters (Cr-VI)	IARC (1980)
ca 1970	~100	Brazil, working environment in brilliant chrome eletro-plating industries (Cr-VI)	IARC (1980)
ca 1975	220-2200	Coal fired power station, emitted gas	IARC (1980)
ca 1975	1.8-500	As above, after fly-ash collection	IARC (1980)
	<0.002-0.2	UK, USA, contaminated areas of heavy metallurgical industries	ICRP (1975), from Schroeder et al. (1962), Stocks et al. (1961), Tabor and Warren (1958)

376 PHARMACODYNAMIC MODELS OF SELECTED TOXIC CHEMICALS IN MAN

TABLE 6 (Cont.)

Remarks	Concentration	Location and material	Reference
Urban and industrialised areas:			
ca 1975	0.016	6 US cities, with metallurgical chromium producers	IARC (1980)
ca 1975	0.012	3 US cities, with chromium chemical producers	IARC (1980)
ca 1975	0.016	8 US cities, with refractories	IARC (1980)
1956–1958	0.9–21.5	23 areas in Northern England and waters	IARC (1980
1972–1975	0.01–0.04	15 areas in Belgium	Kretzschmar et al. (1977)
Mean or median concentrations, rural areas or areas not known to be industrialised:			
	0.002–0.02	Typical value	IARC (1980)
1964–1965	0.015	Chromium as metal, US	IARC (1980)
1957–1974	0.01	Chilton, Oxfordshire	Salmon et al. (1977)
1976	0.0007	Shetland	Bowen (1979)
1974	0.0007	Northern Norway	Bowen (1979)
1971	0.0006	North West Canada	Bowen (1979)
1977	5×10^{-6}	South Pole	Bowen (1979)

TABLE 6 (Cont.)

Remarks	Concentration	Location and material	Reference
Mean or median concentrations, rural areas or areas not known to be industrialised, cont.	0.025 (0.001-0.14)	Europe, median (range)	Bowen (1979)
	0.06 (0.001-0.3)	North America, median (range)	Bowen (1979)
	0.02-0.07	Japan	Bowen (1979)
	0.045-0.067	Hawaii or Etna volcano	Bowen (1979)

Notes:

(1) MPC, Maximum permissible concentration

(2) TC, Tolerance concentration

(3) Based on a reported daily mean intake of 0.28 µg in air, and a volume of 22.8 m^3 reported per day (ICRP 1975)

Engaged in heavy work, an occupationally exposed worker not wearing any protective face-mask would thus be expected to inhale 103 to 206 µg Cr d^{-1} in a working day, compared with 48 to 96 µg Cr d^{-1} for an exposed worker engaged in light activity and 0.6 µg Cr d^{-1} for a worker not occupationally exposed to high levels of chromium, and engaged in light activity. Averaged over a 7 day week, the mean daily inhalation of chromium by each of these groups, assuming a 40 h working week, would be ~75 to 150 µg, 35 to 70 µg and 0.6 µg respectively. In view of the above, it is clear that for workers in the chromium industry intakes of chromium by inhalation could be as large as dietary intakes. For members of the public not occupationally exposed, inhalation of chromium is not likely to exceed a mean level of 1 µg d^{-1} in Europe, or 2 µg d^{-1} in North America and Japan. In a study of mean daily chromium intakes, Schroeder (1970) estimated that 0.28 µg d^{-1} was typically inhaled, but recorded a range of 0 to 0.8 µg d^{-1} in a hospital environment. Smoking of tobacco can be an additional source of chromium. Cigarettes typically contain between 1 to 15 µg Cr g^{-1}, depending upon source of tobacco used (IARC 1980). Frank et al. (1977) reported a mean concentration of 10.7 µg g^{-1} in tobacco, and 1.14 to 4.96 µg g^{-1} in the cured leaf (Table 3). From these data, a typical value of ~5 µg g^{-1} for tobacco in cigarettes appears reasonable. With respect to intakes via this route, it has been estimated, for arsenic, that 10% of the available chromium in cigarette tobacco is inhaled (Appendix 1, Sections 1.2.3 and 1.4.2). However, data presented in Chapter 5, indicate some variability for estimates in the percentage of nickel present in cigaratte tobacco detectable in mainstream smoke (<2% to 30%) and it was assumed in Appendix 5 that ~15% of nickel would be inhaled in the mainstream smoke. On the basis of the figures for arsenic and nickel, a smoker of 20 cigarettes per day, equivalent to 20 g tobacco, would inhale an additional 10 to 15 µg Cr d^{-1}.

6.2.5   Summary

Based on the information presented in this section, the following ranges for normal daily intakes of chromium can be estimated.

TABLE 7

THE DISTRIBUTION OF STABLE CHROMIUM IN HUMAN TISSUES (1)

Organ, tissue or tissue fluid	Concentration in $\mu g \ g^{-1}$ (number of samples)	Weighted mean(2) ($\mu g \ g^{-1}$)	Unweighted mean(2) ($\mu g \ g^{-1}$)	Number of samples
Adrenal	0.429(13) 0.28(17)	0.345	0.355	30
Aorta	0.028(103), 0.092(15), 0.14(10), 0.14(65), 0.42(5), <0.00014(5)	0.085	0.137	198
Blood (total)	0.038(10), 0.028(23), 0.023(61), 0.107(47), 0.038(33), 0.071(?), 0.028(102), 0.0065(8), 0.034(2), 0.053(1), 0.028(8), 0.047(?), 0.026(6), 0.028(154), 0.035(10)	0.036	0.039	>465
Blood (erythrocytes)	0.026(23), 0.019(61), 0.385(16), 0.0656(32), 0.022(6), 0.102(8)	0.075	0.103	146
Blood (plasma)	0.029(132), 0.026(61), 0.164(16), 0.038(29), 0.029(8)	0.038	0.057	246
Blood (serum)	0.02(12), 0.005(7), 0.022(17), 0.018(25), 0.016(48), 0.018(69), 0.006(20), 0.0098(5), 0.013(?), 0.014(1), 0.01(4), 0.0093(177), 0.0022(37), 0.01(39)	0.012	0.012	>461
Bone (3)	33(341), 0.1(?), 6(1)	32.9	13.0	>342
Brain	0.003(128), 0.033(17), 0.0315(18), 0.0405(51), 0.0525(8), 0.0118(61), 0.36(7), 0.139(8), 0.099(9), 0.182(4), 0.126(1), 0.01(10)	0.032	0.091	322
Breast(4)	0.052(8)	0.052	0.052	8
Diaphragm(4)	0.028(91)	0.028	0.028	91

TABLE 7 (Cont.)

Organ, tissue or tissue fluid	Concentration in µg g^{-1} (number of samples)	Weighted mean (2) (µg g^{-1})	Unweighted mean (2) (µg g^{-1})	Number of samples
Gastrointestinal tract				
Unspecified	0.1(20), 0.034(42)	0.055	0.067	62
Caecum	0.050(14)	0.050	0.050	14
Colon	0.0106(6), 0.031(108)	0.030	0.021	114
Duodenum	0.0184(67)	0.018	0.018	67
Ileum	0.032(84)	0.032	0.032	84
Jejunum	0.013(101)	0.013	0.013	101
Rectum	0.033(42)	0.033	0.033	42
Stomach	0.016(130), 0.28(8)	0.031	0.148	138
Hair	0.77(164), 0.85(33), 0.55(90), 0.13(54), 3.3(2), 3.25(116), 3.65(750), 3.1(14), 3.2(20), 1.3(23), 1.3(26), 2(?)	2.71	1.95	>1292
Heart	0.016(140), 0.023(43), 0.061(20), 0.052(62), 0.52(8), 0.019(66), 0.13(21), 0.011(11)	0.043	0.104	371
Kidney	0.011(142), 0.036(48), 0.143(31), 0.264(66), 0.187(9), 1.06(116), 0.025(64), 0.27(5), 0.03(8), 0.86(1), 0.03(8)	0.309	0.265	498
Larynx	0.003(48)	0.003	0.003	48
Liver	0.163(24), 0.079(43), 0.300(11), 0.009(146), 0.0128(45), 0.031(33), 0.059(67), 0.074(9), 0.033(67), 0.918(4), 0.603(116), 0.27(24), 0.0054(5), 0.08(11), 0.05(1)	0.167	0.179	606

TABLE 7 (Cont.)

Organ, tissue or tissue fluid	Concentration in μg g^{-1} (number of samples)	Weighted mean (2) (μg g^{-1})	Unweighted mean (2) (μg g^{-1})	Number of samples
Lung	0.22(139), 0.187(44), 0.297(34), 0.352(69), 2.86(7), 0.55(68), 2.9(2), 0.72(23), 0.24(10), 0.5(11), 2.3(2), 0.24(1), 1.36(1)	0.407	0.979	411
Lymph node	2.2(6)	2.2	2.2	6
Milk	0.010-0.029(78)	-	-	-
Muscle	<0.012(136), 0.18(16), 0.005(6), <0.91(8)	0.132	0.046-0.277	22
Nails	6.2(17)	6.2	6.2	17
Oesophagus	<0.027(66)	-	-	-
Omentum (5)	0.17(75)	0.17	0.17	75
Ovary	0.021(16), 0.021(2), 0.56(11), 0.03(5)	0.197	0.158	34
Pancreas	0.019(139), 0.024(6), 0.079(26), 0.073(58), 0.073(4), 0.058(64), 0.20(22)	0.055	0.075	319
Placenta	0.036(60), 0.09(3)(6)	0.039	0.063	63
Prostate	0.011(50), 0.28(8)	0.048	0.145	58
Skin	0.28(22), 0.46(2), 7.3(2), 0.17(1)	0.809	2.05	27

TABLE 7 (Cont.)

Organ, tissue or tissue fluid	Concentration in $\mu g\ g^{-1}$ (number of samples)	Weighted mean(2) ($\mu g\ g^{-1}$)	Unweighted mean(2) ($\mu g\ g^{-1}$)	Number of samples
Spleen	0.00695(143), 0.031(40), 0.076(34), 0.040(62), 0.278(8), 0.022(67), 0.267(4), 1.38(116), 0.63(23), 0.157(1)	0.375	0.289	498
Sweat (24h) (7)	0.091(6)	0.091	0.091	6
Testis	0.018(72), 0.047(2), 0.085(18), 0.144(39), 0.322(4), 0.39(13), 0.06(6)	0.099	0.152	154
Thyroid	0.017(21), 0.0046(9)	0.013	0.022	30
Tooth (dentine)	0.005(15), 2(8)	0.699	1.00	23
Tooth (enamel)	0.005(15), 1.02(6), 3.2(28)	1.96	1.41	49
Trachea	0.054(60)	0.054	0.054	60
Urinary bladder	0.027(110), 0.42(4)	0.041	0.224	114
Urine (9)	0.0049(10), 0.01(?), 0.0094(9), 0.012(20), 0.0052(12), 0.00072(2), 0.004(154), 0.0007(1), 0.0051(10)	0.0051	0.0058	>218
Urine (24h) (8) (9)	0.0051(9), 0.0129(3), 0.0821(2), 0.0064(10), 0.107(2), 0.00043(1), 0.0193(1), 0.00043(?), 0.0057(?),	0.0197	0.0266	>28
Uterus (4)	0.019(32)	0.019	0.019	32

TABLE 7 (Cont.)

Notes:

(1) Data are from Iyengar et al. (1978), but are all converted to fresh weight using the dry and ash weight fractions given in that publication

(2) Weighted means are based on all studies where the number of subjects is specified and a mean value is given. Unweighted means are based on all studies

(3) Concentrations are not specified as ash, dry or fresh. This could make a difference of a factor of decrease of two, since fresh weight has been assumed

(4) Ash and dry to fresh conversion factors based on muscle

(5) Ash to fresh conversion factor based on muscle

(6) Dry to fresh conversion factor based on spleen

(7) Assuming a daily excretion of 650 ml (Reference Man, ICRP 1975)

(8) Assuming a daily excretion of 1.6 l (Reference Man, ICRP 1975)

(9) Weighted and unweighted means for all urine studies are 0.0067 and 0.0162 $\mu g \ g^{-1}$ respectively

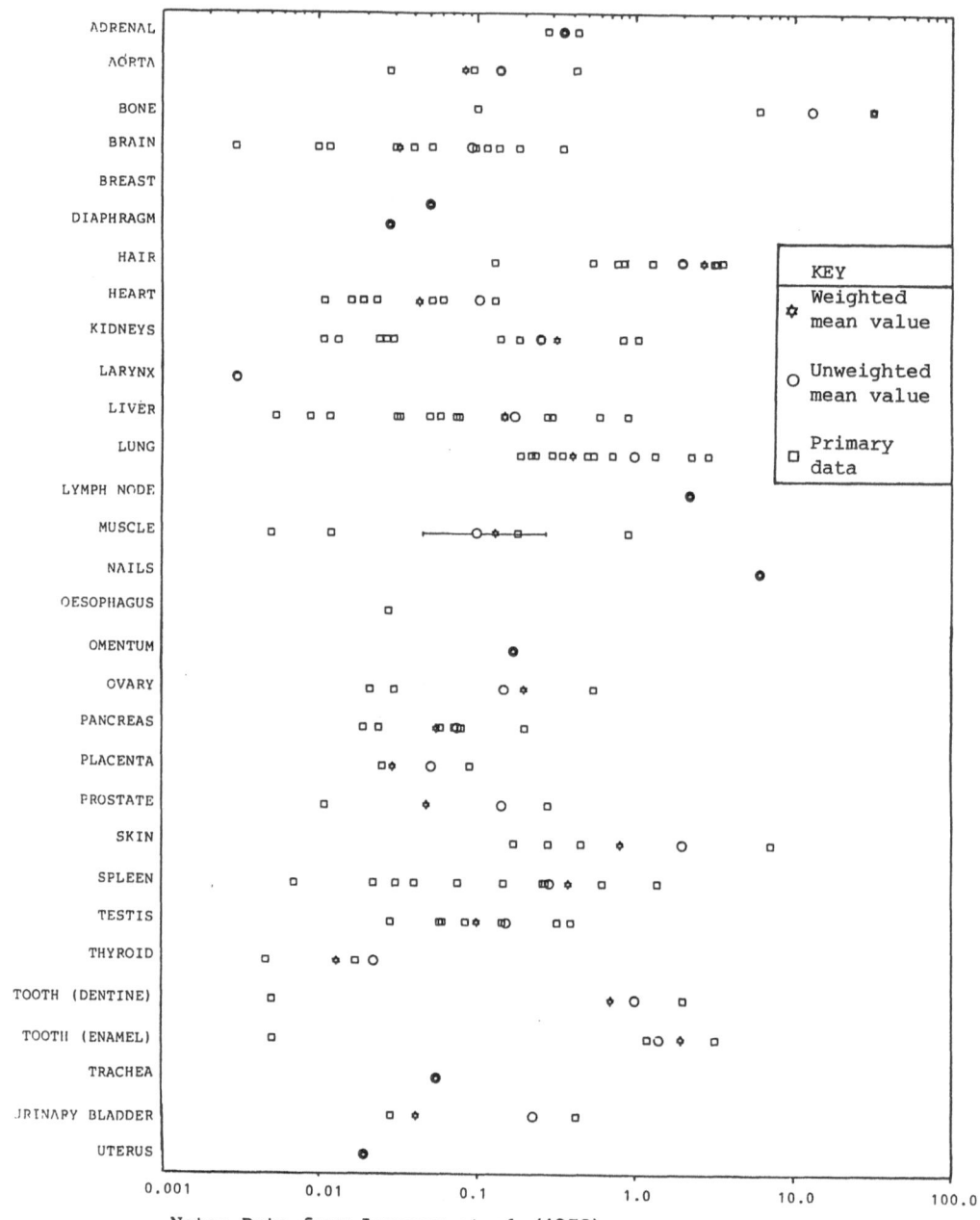

Note: Data from Iyengar et al.(1978)

FIGURE 1. DISTRIBUTION OF STABLE CHROMIUM IN TISSUES
ORGANS AND FLUIDS OF MAN. (1)

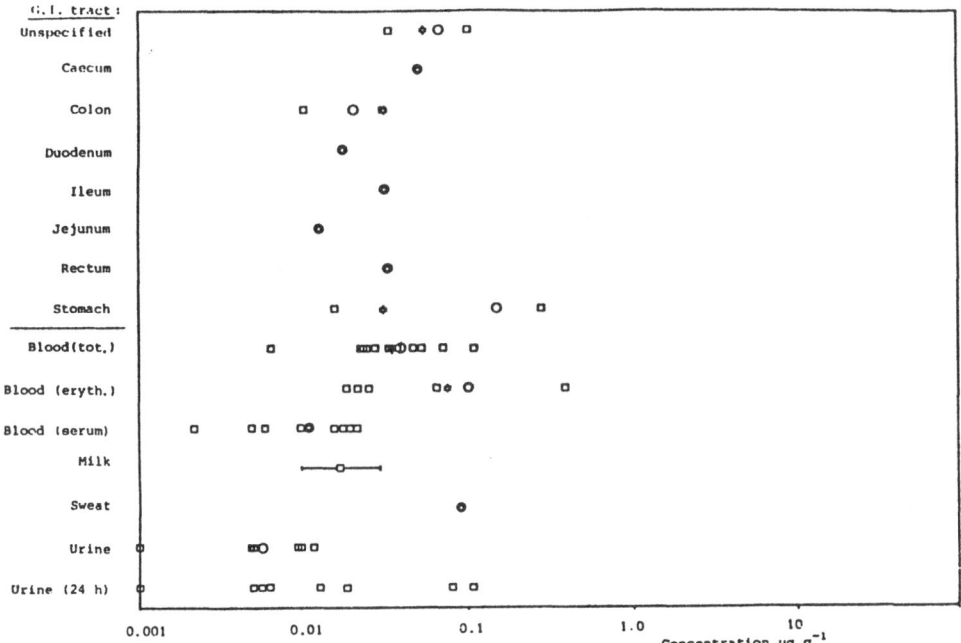

FIGURE 1. contd.

Route of intake	Typical intake (μg Cr d^{-1})	Comments
Diet	30 - 200	The ICRP (1975, 1980) estimated a mean intake of 150 μg d^{-1}, but in this study a typical intake is assumed to be 75 μg d^{-1}. Diets containing in excess 500 μg d^{-1} are uncommon, but have been reported.
Drinking water	0.8 - 8	Best estimate on the basis of relatively limited data.
Air	$\sim$1 - 2	Based on median air concentrations in Europe, N. America and Japan. Occupational exposure may result in inhalation of >200 μg in a working day, based on estimates for a European worker engaged in heavy activity.
Smoking	$\sim$10	Based on a daily consumption of 20 cigarettes ($\sim$20 g tobacco) and 10 to 15% volatilisation of chromium in tobacco.

6.3   DISTRIBUTION OF CHROMIUM IN HUMAN TISSUES AND FLUIDS

Iyengar et al. (1978) reviewed the chromium content of a wide range of human tissues and body fluids. Data presented in Table 7 are derived from the review of Iyengar .et al. (1978), but, for convenience of comparison, all concentrations have been converted to μg chromium per gram fresh tissue. Dry weight and ash weight fractions for each organ, listed by Iyengar et al. (1978) have been used to derive fresh weight equivalents. Data presented in Table 7 are also displayed in graphical form in Fig. 1.

Several other, less extensive, reviews of chromium distribution in man are also available, (e.g. Baetjer 1956; IARC 1980; ICRP 1975) and data presented in Tables 8 and 9 summarise the available information. Additional data, for the concentration of chromium in hair from human infants (Hambidge and Baum 1972) and chromium distribution in animals following subcutaneous injection, intravenous injection and intratracheal injection (Visek et al. 1953; Baetjer et al. 1959; Onkelinx 1977; Yoshirawa and Hara 1980) are presented in Tables 10 to 14. On the basis of information listed in Tables 7 to 14, the following conclusions may be drawn.

- Chromium apparently concentrates in hair, nails, tooth (enamel) and bone of man, where it is typically found at levels in excess of 1 μg g^{-1} w.w.
- Considerable variability of chromium concentrations in human tissues and fluids is notable, both within and between reviews of the literature.

TABLE 8

REPORTED MEAN VALUES, OR RANGES, OF CHROMIUM CONCENTRATION IN TISSUES AND BODY FLUIDS OF PERSONS WITHOUT AND WITH KNOWN EXPOSURE TO CHROMIUM

μg Cr g^{-1} w.w.

Organ, tissue or tissue fluid	Iyengar et al.[1]	Baetjer[2] Normal tissues	Baetjer[2] Chromate workers	ICRP[3]
Adrenal	0.345	0-0.41	0.05-0.76	0.05
Aorta	0.085		0.03	0.023
Blood (total)	0.036			0.025
Blood (erythrocytes)	0.075			0.018
Blood (plasma)	0.038			0.049
Blood (serum)	0.012			
Bone	32.9	0.05	0-2.92[4]	1.76[6]
Brain	0.032	0-0.04	0-0.05	0.003
Breast	0.052			
Diaphragm	0.028			
Gastrointestinal tract:				
unspecified	0.055	0.01[5]	0.04-0.8[5]	0.057
caecum	0.050			0.071
colon	0.030			0.017
duodenum	0.018			0.025
ileum	0.032	0.1	0.04-0.05	0.014
jejunum	0.013			0.027
rectum	0.033			
stomach	0.031	0-0.05	0.04-0.11	0.014

TABLE 8 (Cont.)

µg Cr g^{-1} w.w.

Organ, tissue or tissue fluid	Iyengar et al.[1]	Baetjer[2] Normal tissues	Baetjer[2] Chromate workers	ICRP[3]
Hair	2.71		0.31	3.8
Heart	0.043		0-0.2	0.016
Kidney	0.309	0-0.096	0-2.11	0.01
Larynx	0.003		0.21	0.0005
Liver	0.0167	0.01-0.11	0-1.59	0.009
Lung	0.407	0-0.33	1.3-98.9	0.092
Lymph node	2.2	0-0.01	0.12-75.9	0.1
Milk	0.010-0.029			
Muscle	0.132	0-0.08	0-0.19	0.12
Nails	6.2			
Oesophagus	<0.027			0.033
Omentum	0.17			
Ovary	0.197			
Pancreas	0.055	0.210	0.08-0.36	0.018
Placenta	0.039			
Prostate	0.048			
Skin	0.809		0.05	0.01
Spleen	0.375	0-0.98	0-0.91	1.31
Sweat (24 hours)	0.091			0.007
Testis	0.099			
Thyroid	0.013	0.43	0.24-0.53	0.017
Tooth (dentine)	0.699			0.014

TABLE 8 (Cont.)

Organ, tissue or tissue fluid	Iyengar et al.(1)	Baetjer(2) μg Cr g^{-1} w.w.		ICRP(3)
		Normal tissues	Chromate workers	
Tooth (enamel)	1.96			0.048
Trachea	0.054		0-0.32	0.022
Urinary bladder	0.041		0-2.26	
Urine	0.0051			
Urine (24 hours)	0.0196			0.087
Uterus	0.019			

Notes:

(1)   Iyengar et al. (1978), data from Table 7, weighted mean

(2)   Baetjer (1956), also reported in IARC (1980)

(3)   ICRP (1975)

(4)   Additional values reviewed in this study were (μg g^{-1} w.w.):

Tissue or fluid	Normal tissues	Chromate workers
Lung tumour	-	0-16.6
Metastatic tumour	-	0.02-1.0
Nasal septum	-	2.87
Cartilage	-	0.06
Bile	-	0.01

(5)   Reported to be, abdominal lymph node

(6)   Cortical bone

TABLE 9

CONCENTRATION OF CHROMIUM IN BLOOD AND URINE FROM PERSONS
WITH VARYING DEGREES OF EXPOSURE TO CHROMIUM[1]

Degree of exposure to chromium	Blood concentration $\mu g\ ml^{-1}$	Urine concentration $\mu g\ ml^{-1}$
No exposure	0-0.2	0-0.16
Slight exposure	-	0-0.18
Chromate workers	0-5.8	0-0.78
Chromium platers	-	0-2.8
Chromite workers	0-0.02	0

Notes:

Data from various literature sources, reported by Baetjer
(1956), and presented in summary by IARC (1980)

TABLE 10

MEAN HAIR CHROMIUM CONCENTRATIONS OF HUMAN
SUBJECTS AGED 0 TO 35 MONTHS [1]

Age of subjects	No. of subjects	Hair chromium concentration ($\mu g \ g^{-1}$) [1]
0-7 days	25	0.910±0.139
3-6 months	6	1.493±0.386
8 months	8	0.850±0.106
10-12 months	11	0.631±0.062
1-2 years	23	0.525±0.059
2-3 years	20	0.412±0.047

Notes:

(1)   Data from Hambidge and Baum (1972)

(2)   Mean ± 1 s.e.

TABLE 11

DISTRIBUTION OF CHROMIUM IN ORGANS OF GUINEA-PIG INTRATRACHEALLY
INJECTED WITH CHROMATE OR CHROMIC CHLORIDE (1)

% of dose, normalised to 200 µg Cr per guinea-pig
remaining in tissues at times after administration

Material	Time after injection	Lungs	RBC(2)	Plasma	Liver	Kidney	Spleen	Urine(3)
Na₂CrO₄ and K₂Cr₂O₄	10 min.	14.5	14.0	5.0	2.0	3.0	0.5	13.5
	1 day	11.0	8.5	1.0	3.5	3.0	<0.5	26.5
	2 days	5.0	7.5	1.0	4.5	3.0	0.5	17.0
	4 days	6.0	9.5	0.5	3.0	2.0	0.5	
	15 days	4.0	5.0	0.5	1.0	0.5	1.0	
	30 days	2.5	6.0	1.0	3.0	0.5	1.0	
	80 days	1.5	1.0	0.5	0.5	<0.5	0.5	
	90 days	1.0	<0.5 (4)	<0.5	0	<0.5	0.5	
	120 days	1.5	0.5	0.5	<0.5	0.5	1.0	
	140 days	0.5	0	0	0.5	0	0.5	
CrCl₃	10 min.	69.0	1.5	2.5	0	0.5	<0.5	6.0
	1 day	45.0	1.0	1.0	0	0.5	<0.5	8.5
	2 days	62.5	0	0.5	0	0.5	<0.5	11.5
	4 days	43.0	0.5	0.5	0	<0.5	<0.5	
	15 days	33.5	0.5	<0.5	0	0.5	<0.5	
	30 days	30.0	0	0	0	<0.5	<0.5	
	60 days	13.0	0	0	0	<0.5	0	

Notes:

(1) Data revised from Baetjer et al. (1959)

(2) RBC: red blood cells

(3) Cumulative excretion

(4) All values greater than 0 but less than 0.5 are recorded as <0.5

TABLE 12

DISTRIBUTION OF CHROMIUM IN MICE INJECTED SUBCUTANEOUSLY
WITH TRIVALENT AND HEXAVALENT CHROMIUM[1]

μg Cr g^{-1} w.w.

Organ	Cr (III)				Cr (VI)			
	days post-injection				days post-injection			
	5	12	19	33	5	12	19	33
Heart	2.7±0.9	3.4±0.9	4.1±0.9	4.4±1.2	5.4±0.6	11.4±3.2	11.0±2.3	14.1±2.9
Lung	2.3±0.3	2.8±0.6	3.5±1.0	3.4±1.1	10.9±1.9	18.9±1.8	22.6±2.3	32.5±9.2
Liver	1.3±0.1	2.7±1.6	4.6±0.6	6.7±0.6	18.3±3.7	34.3±7.6	83.4±15.1	126.2±37.4
Spleen	5.1±0.8	7.0±0.7	10.5±1.3	5.4±1.9	18.8±3.0	54.3±10.6	123.7±33.5	247.5±32.5
Kidney	1.9±0.5	3.2±0.4	9.3±3.2	4.8±2.8	27.1±3.6	35.2±3.4	49.5±12.6	72.4±20.1

Note:

Data from Yoshikawa and Hara (1980). All results are presented as mean ± 1 s.d. 5 replicates were taken of each sample

TABLE 13

SUMMARY OF Cr-51 DISTRIBUTION AND RETENTION IN RATS FOLLOWING
INTRAVENOUS INJECTION IN DIFFERENT CHEMICAL FORMS

a) 4 days post-administration
b) 42 days post-administration (1)

a)

% of injected Cr-51 remaining in various organs following administration as:

Organ	Na_3CrO_2 (2)	$CrCl_3$	NO_2CrO_4	$CrCl_3$ acetate	Buffered by: citrate
Liver	87.0	51.0	4.8	1.5	2.9
Spleen	8.5	1.6	0.46	0.15	0.38
Bone marrow (3)	16.0	3.8	1.4	0.4	1.9
Whole bone (4)	<26.0	<19.0	<6.7	<18.0	<3.5
Lungs	2.9	0.4	0.7	0.2	0.38
Kidneys	0.12	0.88	4.2	1.2	0.26
Blood	<0.14	0.34	3.5	0.2	<0.14
Cumulative: urine	0.6	15	35	56	75
% excretion: faeces	1.6	20	17	8	17
Total	127	108	72	85	100

TABLE 13 (Cont.)

b)

% of injected Cr-51 remaining in various organs following administration as:

Organ	Na_3CrO_2	$CrCl_3$ (5)	NO_2CrO_4	$CrCl_3$ acetate	Buffered by: citrate
Liver	59.0	24.0	0.64	1.7	1.6
Spleen	4.1	2.1	2.4	0.21	0.11
Bone marrow	2.4	3.8	0.4	<0.05	<0.05
Whole bone	<3.9	<11.0	<0.4	<17.0	<6.2
Lungs	0.27	0.2	0.09	0.14	<0.04
Kidneys	0.08	0.52	0.48	0.50	0.14
Blood	<0.14	<0.14	0.27	<0.14	<0.14
Chemical behaviour	Colloidal	Colloidal under these conditions	Probably ionic under these conditions	Complex	Complex
Electropharetic patter	Colloidal in serum	Protein bound	Ionic in serum bound by haemoglobin in cells	Complex	–
pH of administered solution	11	3 to 4	7	5.5	4.0

TABLE 13 (Cont.)

Notes:

(1) Data adapted from original presentation of Visek et al. (1953), making the following assumptions:

- average body weight of rats used, male and female, 250g

Organ	% of total body weight	Actual weight (g w.w.)
Liver	3.7	9.2
Spleen	0.2	0.5
Bone marrow	1.0	2.5
whole bone	7.1	17.7
Lungs	0.7	1.8
Kidneys	0.8	2.0
Blood	2.7	6.8

(2) All values represent the mean from 4 rats, results presented to 2 significant figures only

(3) Not included in total body content as it is already a factor of whole bone

(4) Values for whole bone are estimated from reported concentrations in the tibial epiphysia, which represented the bone with the highest concentration

(5) Rats at 45 days, not 42 days

TABLE 14

DISTRIBUTION OF Cr-51 IN SHEEP FOLLOWING
INTRAVENOUS INJECTION OF Cr-51 Cl$_3$ [1]

Tissue	% of dose (g^{-1} fresh tissue)	
	A[2]	B[3]
Blood	0.00166	0.00075
Lung	0.0114	0.0727
Liver	0.00788	0.00284
Spleen	0.00739	0.00332
Bone marrow	0.0042	0.00256
Kidney	0.00557	0.00434
Lymph node	0.00408	0.00209
Pancreas	0.00067	0.00033
Loin muscle	0.00026	0.00061
Gastrocnemius muscle	0.00011	0.00004
Vertebra	0.00276	0.00294
Metatarsus shaft	0.00043	0.00052
Metatarsus epiphysis	0.00092	0.00095
Incisors	0.00081	0.00094
Angle mandible	0.00333	0.00325
White bone marrow	0.00038	0.00017
Urinary excretion[4]	0.00327	0.00603
Faecal excretion[4]	0.00033	0.00022

Notes:

(1) Data from Visek et al. (1953). Sheep were killed
     7 days after administration of chromium. All values
     are expressed as relative concentrations at time of
     death

(2) Sheep 107, received 4 mg of chromium

(3) Sheep 68, received 8 mg of chromium

(4) Cumulative excretion to 7 days

- Chromium concentrations in human newborn have been reported to be higher than concentrations in adults (Schroeder et al. 1962; Hambidge and Baum 1972); data recorded in Table 10, for concentrations of chromium in hair of newborn humans, are in accord with the above statement but some variability is also apparent.
- Data from experiments on animals indicate that the initial distribution and subsequent retention of chromium is dependent upon the chemical form administered.
- Chromium is concentrated in the bone of rats and, depending on chemical form of chromium administered, there is limited evidence for concentration in lung. Organs of the reticulo-endothelial system apparently concentrate hexavalent forms of chromium.
- The total body content of chromium in man is ~20 mg of which 15 mg is concentrated in the bone (assuming a typical value for the concentration in bone of 3 $\mu g\ g^{-1}$, on the basis of data presented in Tables 7 and 8).

It has been noted by Schroeder et al. (1962) and Coughtrey and Thorne (1983) that more data are available for the distribution of chromium in man than animals. However, considerably more chemical form related and time-dependent data for the distribution of chromium, are available for animals than man. Data presented by Baetjer et al. (1959) and summarised in Table 11 indicate that trivalent chromic chloride, intratracheally injected into guinea-pig, is more tenaciously retained in the lung than hexavalent potassium chromate or sodium chromate. Correspondingly, less excretion of chromic chloride was recorded compared with chromate. These results are in accord with those of Yoshikawa and Hara (1980), presented in Table 12, demonstrating that hexavalent chromium is more mobile in mouse body-tissues and fluids than trivalent chromium, and also indicating an accumulation of hexavalent chromium by organs of the reticulo-endothelial system. Visek et al. (1953) obtained data on the distribution of chromium-51 in rats following intravenous injection of several chemical forms. these data are summarised in Table 13. Trivalent chromium, whether administered as sodium chromite or chromic chloride was rapidly concentrated in organs of the reticulo-endothelial system, primarily liver. Hexavalent chromium, administered as sodium chromate was also concentrated, to a limited extent, in organs of the reticulo-endothelial system, but a substantially higher rate of excretion was recorded. Chromic chloride isotonically buffered in acetate or citrate showed a limited accumulation in the liver, but excretion was rapid and within 4 days 75% of the initially administered dose had been excreted in urine, with an additional 17% excreted in faeces.

In view of the above comments, it is concluded that, in man, chromium is deposited primarily in the bone with limited deposition and accumulation in the liver, spleen and kidneys. Coughtrey and Thorne (1983), in a review of chromium in domestic animals and man, suggested that the elevated concentration of chromium which may be observed in lung and lymph nodes, probably derives from inhalation of chromium containing dusts, which is in accord with data reviewed by Baetjer (1956), and summarised in Table 8.

Finally, it is noted that Mertz et al. (1974) commented that chromium is difficult to analyse in biological systems and that 'no one analytical value for chromium in biological materials can be considered absolute'. Consequently, the data discussed above should not be considered as definitives

6.4   METABOLISM

6.4.1   Gastrointestinal absorption

The gastrointestinal absorption of chromium has not been studied extensively in man or animals, although several reviews of available data have discussed this matter, principally with respect to man (e.g. ICRP 1975: Underwood 1977; IARC 1980; ICRP 1980; Guthrie 1982; Langara 1982; Coughtrey and Thorne 1983). The site and mechanism of chromium absorption is not known, although, as discussed by Underwood (1977), the mid-section of small intestine in rats is most permeable to the passage of chromium by diffusion and there is evidence to suggest a common pathway for the absorption of zinc and chromium. Experimental data and estimated values for fractional gastrointenstinal absorption (f_1) are presented in Table 15, from which it is readily apparent that there exists considerable variability in values.

Inorganic trivalent compounds of chromium, such as chromic chloride, are generally little absorbed, with f_1 values typically around 0.005 to 0.02 in rats and 0.004 in man (Table 15). Hexavalent compounds, such as sodium chromate, typically exhibit f_1 values of 0.02 to 0.06 in rats and 0.1 in man. For the purpose of dosimetric calculations in man, the ICRP (1975; 1980) assigned f_1 values of ~0.01 and 0.1 to trivalent and hexavalent compounds of chromium respectively. However, the data of Donaldson and Barreras (1966) indicate that, in rats, the gastrointestinal absorption of trivalent or hexavalent chromium is similar following gastric administration, with f_1 values of 0.02 (Cr-III) and 0.023 (Cr-VI). Following jejunal administration, differences in f_1 were more marked, 0.084 (Cr-III) and 0.24 (Cr-VI), suggesting that, in the highly acidic environment of the stomach, reduction of Cr (VI) to Cr (III) may occur. This is in accord with the comment of Coughtrey and Thorne (1983), .in their review of the literature, that "some Cr-VI compounds will be reduced to Cr-III on their passage through the stomach". Underwood (1977) did not distinguish between trivalent and hexavalent compounds, but assigned an f_1 value of 0.01 to 0.03 to all inorganic compounds in man and animals. In view of the above comments, it is thought appropriate to assign a single value of f_1 to all inorganic compounds of chromium in man, and data presented in Table 15 suggest a mean f_1 value of ~0.05.

The fractional gastrointestinal absorption of organic or biologically incorporated forms of chromium may be substantially higher than for inorganic compounds, although data are extremely variable (Table 15). Information considered in several reviews (e.g. ICRP 1975; Underwood 1977; IARC 1980; Coughtrey and Thorne 1983) has suggested that up to 0.5 of dietary chromium may be absorbed and, on this basis an f_1 value of 0.25 is taken to be appropriate for man. This value is in accord with the proposal of Coughtrey and Thorne (1983) for man and domestic animals.

TABLE 15

FRACTIONAL GASTROINTESTINAL ABSORPTION OF DIETARY CHROMIUM

Compound	Species	Age of animal (1)	Amount administered	Fractional absorption	Reference	Comments
Chromium lactate (in milk)	Rat	25-35 d	23.7 mg Cr 34.5 mg Cr 132.0 mg Cr	3×10^{-4} 6×10^{-3} 3×10^{-3}	Conn et al. (1932)	0.79 mg Cr d^{-1} for 30 d 1.15 mg Cr d^{-1} for 30 d 4.4 mg Cr d^{-1} for 30 d
51-CrCl$_3$	Rat		1 ng	2×10^{-2} (?)	Donaldson and Barreras (1966)	Gastric administration, absorption estimated as Cr not excreted in faeces over 7 days jejunal administration, absorption estimated as above. Gastric administration, absorption estimated as above. Jejunal administration absorption estimated as above
51-CrCl$_3$	Rat		1 ng	8.4×10^{-2}		
Na$_2$ 51-CrO$_4$	Rat		1 ng	2.3×10^{-2}		
Na$_2$ 51-CrO$_4$	Rat		1 ng	2.4×10^{-1}		
51-CrCl$_3$	Man	21-68 yrs	20 ng	4.0×10^{-3}		Oral administration. Absorption estimated as Cr-51 not excreted in faeces over 6 days. Duodenal administration, absorption estimated as above. Oral administration, absorption estimated as above. Duodenal administration absorption estimated as above
51-CrCl$_3$	Man	21-68 yrs	20 ng	6.3×10^{-3}		
Na$_2$ 51-CrO$_4$	Man	21-68 yrs	20 ng	1.06×10^{-1}		
Na$_2$ 51-CrO$_4$	Man	21-68 yrs	20 ng	4.35×10^{-1}		
51-Cr-EDTA	Chickens	6-9 weeks	5 μCi	5.0×10^{-3}	Sklan et al. (1975)	Estimated in tests conducted on Cr-51 as a non-absorbed reference marker
51-CrCl$_3$	Rat		0.5 to 2 μCi	$<5.0\times10^{-3}$	Visek et al. (1953)	From tissue distribution studies
Na$_2$ 51-CrO$_4$	Rat		57 μg Cr	6×10^{-2}	Mackenzie et al. (1959)	Fasted rats 24 hours prior to oral dose
Na$_2$ 51-CrO$_4$	Rat		57 μg Cr	3×10^{-2}		Non-fasted rats
Cr$_2$O$_3$	Rat		1.7g	1.6×10^{-1}	Ivankovic and Preussmann (1975)	
Cr(III)	Man			0.01	ICRP (1980)	Review
Cr (VI)	Man			0.1		
Inorganic Cr	Man and animals			0.01 to 0.03	Underwood (1977)	Review
Cr biologically incorporated in brewers yeast	Rat			0.1 0.25		

TABLE 15 (Cont.)

Compound	Species	Age of animal	Amount administered	Fractional absorption	Reference	Comments
Cr (III) salts	Man			<0.005	ICRP (1975)	Review
Cr (IV) salts	Man			<0.1		
Dietary Cr	Man			up to 0.5		Review, based on ICRP (1975)
Dietary Cr	Man and domestic animals			0.25	Coughtrey and Thorne	
Cr (VI)	Man			0.02 to 0.5	IARC (1980)	Review, based on Donaldson and Barreras (1966)

Notes:

(1)   Age at beginning of study period

(2)   Absorbed chromium is excreted in urine and bile, hence faecal excretion represents unabsorbed dietary chromium together with some biliary excretion (ICRP 1975). Consequently, where absorption has been estimated on the basis of material ingested, but not excreted in faeces, this represents a lower estimation of absorption

6.4.2   Retention in the respiratory system

There have been many studies on the toxicity and carcinogenicity of chromium in the respiratory tract and other sites, following occupational exposure to chromium in air (e.g. Zvaifler 1944; Pokrovskaya and Shabynina 1973; Waterhouse 1975; Davies 1978) and experimental work has been performed on laboratory animals to establish the aeteological factor(s) in chromate induced cancer (e.g. Grogan 1957; Lane and Mass 1977). By comparison there have been relatively few studies concerning the retention and distribution of chromium following inhalation in various chemical states, by man or animals.

It can be inferred from the clinical studies that hexavalent chromium is the main carcinogen of concern (e.g. Langard and Norseth 1975; Lane and Mass 1977; Davies 1978). Oshaki et al. (1978) reported that 'smoking [of tobacco] is probably an accelerating factor on chromium hazard'. On the basis of experimental studies involving tracheal grafts in rats, Lane and Mass (1977) concluded that chromium carbonyl is a carcinogen which can act synergistically with benzo(a)pyrene. The carcinogenicity of inhaled chromium is not confined to the lungs. In a study of cancer among chromium ferro-alloy workers, Pokrovskaya and Shabynina (1973) reported that mortality from malignant tumours in lungs, stomach, oesophagus and 'all locations' [presumably all other locations] was significantly higher in workers compared to controls (p = 0.001 for workers aged 50 years or more). It should be noted that, in that study, the chromium-containing dusts also contained 3-4-benzopyrene, which as noted above (Lane and Mass 1977) apparently acts synergistically with chromium.

On the basis of extremely limited data, the ICRP Task Group on Lung Dynamics (ICRP 1966) assigned oxides and hydroxides of chromium to inhalation class Y, halides and nitrates to inhalation class W and all other compounds to inhalation class D. These recommendations are in accord with experimental data obtained for dogs by Morrow et al. (1968). Aerosolized suspensions of $^{51}CrO_3$ were inhaled by dogs in a 'nose only' apparatus. The effective half-life of retention was calculated to be approximately 26 days in two dogs. This is very close to the physical half-life for chromium-51, and Morrow et al. (1968) concluded that the biological half-life of retention "cannot be stated more definitely than a 200-day minimum." They further concluded that the lung clearance of chromium, and other poorly soluble materials tested, can be described as a single exponential process. Following inhalation of $^{51}CrCl_3$ by dogs, Morrow et al. (1968) reported a biological half-life of 25 days after the first 24 h in lung. This is in agreement with a further set of experiments, in the same study, by Morrow et al. (1968). Intramuscular injection of $^{51}CrCl_3$ in rats indicated a biological half-life $T_{0.5}B$ in excess of 150 days at the site of injection, but at all other sites (representing absorbed chromium) the biological half-life was around 25 days. Thus, absorbed chromic chloride is rapidly excreted, but an important degree of tissue fixation occurs, possibly indicative of chemical changes within the tissues.

Two recent reviews of data relating to the retention of chromium following inhalation (ICRP 1980; Coughtrey and Thorne 1983) have not noted any additional data to the above, and for the purposes of this study the ICRP (1966) recommendations are adopted. The ICRP (1980) also argued that it would be prudent to assume, for the purposes of radiological protection, that when chromium enters the gastrointestinal tract after inhalation it will be in the hexavalent state. However, data presented by Mertz (1969) suggest that chromium will be predominantly in the trivalent state in biological materials. Furthermore, no distinction is made in the present review between the fractional gastrointestinal absorption of trivalent or hexavalent chromium, where either is present in an inorganic form, and a single f_1 value of 0.05 is assigned (Section 6.4.1).

Langard et al. (1978) noted that chromium as zinc chromate (Zn_2CrO_4) was rapidly absorbed by rats following inhalation. The fraction of chromium absorbed was not reported, although the concentration of chromium in faeces was noted to be elevated from a pre-inhalation value of 0.007 mg g^{-1} w.w to ~0.5 mg g^{-1} w.w. within 24 hours, declining to ~0.1 mg g^{-1} within 6 days. Chromium blood-levels were elevated five-fold within 100 minutes of inhaling zinc chromate and continued to show a similar rate of increase for the next 150 minutes. Chromium thus taken up by the blood was eliminated slowly; 9% of the initial peak concentration was found after 37 days. Langard et al. (1978) noted that this result was commensurate with chromium entering the bloodstream in hexavalent form and binding with the erythrocytes. This hypothesis remains to be confirmed, but tends to support the argument of the ICRP (1980) that inhaled chromium may remain in the hexavalent form, at least for a limited period.

6.4.3   Systemic metabolism

Chromium-51, in the hexavalent or trivalent state, has found several uses in medicine, such as determining blood volume and red blood cell survival (e.g. Ebaugh et al. 1953; Korst 1968; Gray and Sterling 1950). Chromium-51 has also been used in measurements of platelet survival (e.g. Aas and Gardner 1958) and in autoradiography (e.g. Christian et al. 1977). Other isotopes of chromium, principally chromium-48 and the non-radioactive chromium-50, have also been found of use in medicine (Sanderson 1982). Consequently, the metabolism of chromium, has been studied in some detail, both in man and animals and data have been reviewed by NAS (1974), ICRP (1975; 1980), Mertz (1969) and Coughtrey and Thorne (1983). A review of the applications of chromium-51 in cell biology and medicine was presented by Sanderson (1982).

6.4.3.1   Uptake and binding of chromium by constituents of blood, serum and other tissues.

The uptake and binding of chromium in blood and serum is dependant on the chemical form administered, particularly with regard to the valence state. Gray and Sterling (1950) used chromium-51 as sodium chromate to label dog erythrocytes and as chromic chloride to label plasma. Gray and Sterling reported that of trivalent chromium taken up by whole blood 'in vitro' essentially all was in the plasma. It is also notable that of Cr (III) administered by stomach tube to rats at a dose of 0.1 µg per kg body weight (Hopkins and Schwarz 1964), more than 99% of the absorbed chromium was in the non-cellular component of blood, where it was attached to transferrin in a distribution similar to that observed for Fe-55. When the transferrin was precipitated, 80% of the chromium-51 was in the precipitate. Applying excessive amounts of chromium resulted in binding to other proteins at the expense of β-globulin (Hopkins and Schwarz 1964, and reported in the reviews of Mertz 1969; NAS 1974). In man, the bulk of chromium is in the albumin fraction, and only 30% to 40% is in globulins, of which transferrin (siderophilin) is one (NAS 1974).

Labelling red blood cells with chromium-51 as chromate does not result in uniform distribution (Korst 1968), since younger red blood cells and reticulocytes accumulate roughly three times the average chromium concentration. Although leucocytes and platelets are also labelled by hexavalent chromium "the difference in size of populations nullifies most of this artifact in studies of erythrocytes" (Korst 1968). The rate of binding to red blood cells was reported by Korst (1968) to be dependent upon temperature and pH. Chromium released as a result of erythrocyte death does not label other red blood cells. This is consistent with the suggestion of Mertz (1969) that once inside the erythrocyte, chromate is reduced to the trivalent form and bound to haemoglobin. After subsequent release, the chromium, as with Cr(III) injected directly into the bloodstream, firmly attaches to plasma proteins without penetrating the erythrocyte cell membrane. Hexavalent chromium must rapidly penetrate the erythrocyte cell membrane, since the transport process is in competition with the reducing capacity of the plasma (Mertz 1969). Reported data indicate that red blood cells reach 50% chromium saturation within 15 minutes 'in vitro' (Gray and Sterling 1950; Gabrieli et al. 1963; Ingrand 1964). The dynamics of 'in vitro' uptake of chromate-51 by human leucocytes was studied by Lilien et al. (1970), who reported a unidirectional uptake of chromate over a 1 hour incubation with extracellular chromate concentrations of up to 200 μmoles 1^{-1}. Under these conditions, intracellular chromium-51 is in a form which is non-exchangeable and influx is temperature sensitive, with a Q_{10} (that is, the change in rate of influx over a temperature inverval of 10°C) over the temperature range of 17°C to 37°C of approximately 2. Influx may be energy dependent since a variety of metabolic poisons strongly inhibit uptake. Lilien et al. (1970) summarised the uptake dynamics of chromate as follows.

"The unidirectional influx of chromate follows Michaelis-Menten kinetics; the maximum velocity is 52 mμmoles/g dry weight of cells per min. and the chromate concentration at which influx velocity is half maximal is 87 μmoles/liter. This transport mechanism is highly specific for chromate; other divalent tetrahedral anions only slightly inhibit influx at concentrations up to 10 times that of chromate. Metavanadate, however, competitively inhibits chromate influx at equimolar concentrations. Exposure of cells to unlabelled chromate leads to inhibition of subsequent influx of 51-chromate. It is suggested that this is due to a primary inhibitory effect of chromate on cellular energy metabolism."

Of chromate which enters the erythrocytes, a small fraction is bound to constituents of the cell other than haemoglobin (e.g. Gabrieli et al. 1963; Mertz 1969).

Prins (1962) investigated three explanations for the finding that chromium-51 in labelled erythrocytes is mainly in the Hb-A_3 fraction, which contains 10% of total cell haemoglobin:

-      after reacting with chromate the haemoglobin is so altered as
       to be chromatographically inseperable from Hb-A$_3$;
-      Hb-A$_3$ has a strong affinity to chromate;
-      in the chromatograph Hb-A$_3$ and the fraction taking up chromate
       coincide.

Whilst the above suggestions are not mutually incompatible, Prins (1962) concluded, on the basis of experimental data, that not all the chromate is attached to haemoglobin and some at least is complexed with a low molecular weight protein, possibly glutathione. On the basis of a review of the literature, Mertz (1969) noted that most of the chromate entering erythrocytes is bound to the globin fraction of haemoglobin, but some is bound to the haem and some to another substance of low molecular weight. Unpublished experimental determinations by Mertz and Thurman (summarised by Mertz 1969) indicate that the low molecular weight chromium complex can be easily separated from the haemoglobin-bound chromium by ion-exchange chromatography, since the low molecular weight complex passes through an Amberlite IRC-50 column unadsorbed. It was stated that "the chromium-containing complex isolated by this method from chromate-treated, lysed erythrocytes exhibited no more biological activity in the fat-pad assay than simple, inorganic chromium compounds." These conclusions are in accord with the earlier experimental studies of Gabrieli et al. (1963). When passing 51-chromate labelled haemolysate through a small Sephadex column, Gabriel et al. (1963) recorded two peaks in radioactivity, the first of which (Fraction I) paralleled the increase and decrease of the haemoglobin content of the effluent. The second peak (Fraction II) was not associated with haemogolobin. Full recovery of radioactivity was realised. Further studies, mixing Fraction II with untagged haemoglobin, did not result in labelling the haemoglobin. Similarly, Fraction II did not label whole erythrocytes; although in 2 separate experiments small amounts (1.2% and 1.8%) did enter the cells during incubation, Sephadex fractionation after lysis of these erythrocytes showed that intra-erythrocyte 51-chromium was not bound to haemoglobin.

Although data presented by Langárd et al. (1978) indicate that inhaled chromate may enter the bloodstream in the hexavalent form (Section 6.4.2), it is likely that the majority of chromium in biological tissues will be in trivalent form (Mertz 1969; ICRP 1980; Coughtrey and Thorne 1983) and the remainder of this section considers the uptake, distribution and retention of trivalent chromium.

Uptake of chromium by tissues is dependent on chemical form (Mertz 1969) but, with the exception of chromates, all chemical forms are cleared rapidly from the blood (Mertz 1969; NAS 1974) and are taken up by tissues. On the basis of a study in which tracer quantities of chromium-51 as the chloride (CrCl$_3$) were injected into healthy subjects direct, or following incubation with the subjects' own plasma, Sargent et al. (1979) proposed the following function for the percentage retention of chromium in blood.

$$R_{BLOOD}(t) = 5.06e^{-76.4t} + 7.91e^{-2.62t} + 3.35e^{-0.372t} + 3.14e^{-0.084t}$$

where t is in days.

Data presented by Sargent et al. (1979) do not suggest any longer term components of retention, but further components of short-term retention are not excluded.

NAS (1974) reported that other tissues and organs concentrate chromium by 10 to 100 times relative to the concentration in blood and, "this indicates that the blood ordinarily is not a usable indicator of chromium nutritional status." This remark was made also by Mertz (1969). Although data presented in Table 7 and Section 3 do not necessarily support the statement that chromium is concentrated 10 to 100 times in all tissues compared with blood, it is clear nonetheless that certain tissues, notably bone, do accumulate chromium to a considerable degree.

Mertz (1969) reported, on the basis of an extensive review of available literature, that organs of the reticulo-endothelial system (e.g. liver, spleen and bone marrow) have a high affinity for chromium. This probably largely represents phagocytosis of colloidal particles, though chromic chloride is also concentrated in the liver. Injected chromium-51 (in the trivalent form) is predominantly taken up by bone, particularly the bone marrow. However, this chromium is not associated with cellular elements of marrow, but with a tricholoroacetic acid precipitable protein fraction (Mertz 1969).

In mice, tissue uptake of chromium appears to decline with age. Vittorio et al. (1962) intraperitoneally injected young and old mice with chromate, and measured the chromium concentrations in liver, stomach, epididymal fat pad, thymus, kidney and testes. Concentrations in older mice were reported to be about half of those found in the younger mice. Schroeder et al. (1962) commented that, "these observations may offer one explanation for the declining tissue chromium levels with age, detected in a survey of the US population." In a review of the literature, the US National Academy of Sciences (1974) noted that, in healthy young people, a challenge with a glucose load or insulin results in the plasma chromium concentration rising rapidly to twice the concentration in the fasting state. The site of the 'pool' from which this chromium is derived is not defined and, as with observations on chromium uptake in mice (above), the response declines with increasing age or impairment of glucose-tolerance. The response is improved by chromium supplementation.

Edwards et al. (1961) studied the subcellular distribution of naturally occurring chromium in rats fed a commercially obtained diet. They found that 49% of the chromium was concentrated in the nuclear fraction (distinguishing it from zinc, iron, copper, molybdenum and manganese, which have far less affinity for the nuclear fraction) and 23% was in the supernatant. The remainder was evenly divided between mitochondria and microsomes. Following an acute dose of chromium, Vittorio and Wight (1963) recovered only 3% of the injected dose from the nucleic acid fraction of liver, compared with 30% in the proteins.

A recent review of the mechanisms of uptake of chromium (Langárd 1982) noted that the pathways are better elucidated for hexavalent chromium than for trivalent chromium. The following simplified account of chromate uptake by red blood cells following inhalation or ingestion, is largely based upon the above review.

In the airways and gastrointestinal tract, it is likely that chromates are taken up by epithelial cells by means of simple diffusion through the plasma membrane, where reduction of the chromate is facilitated by enzymatically mobilised electrons (available from electron donors such as GSH, NADPH and NADH). Details of the mechanisms of

BRONCHIAL   EPITHELIAL CELL   BLOOD
LUMEN

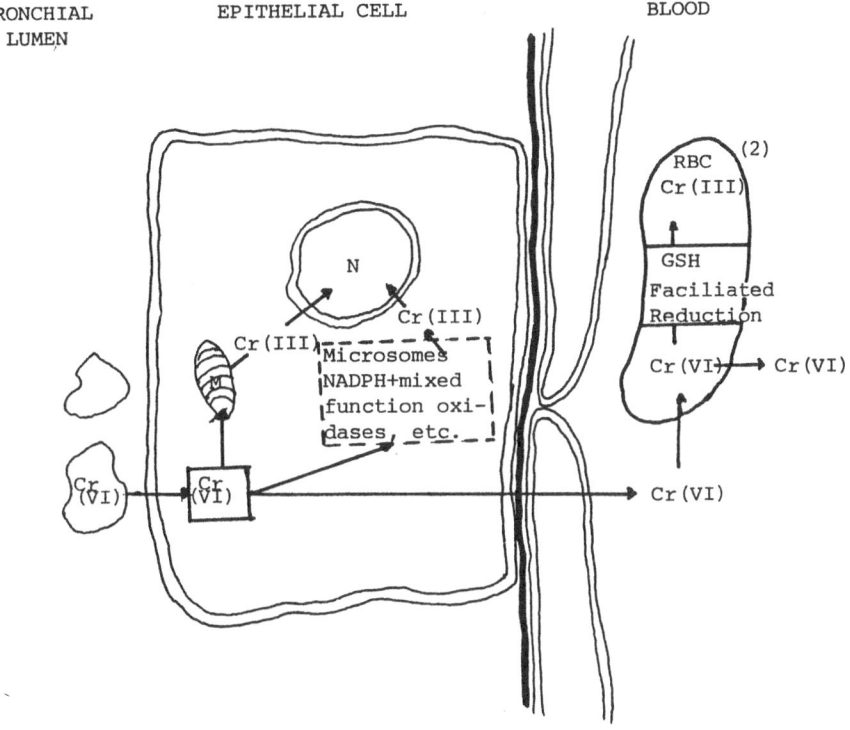

Note: (1) Redrawn from Langard (1982)
       (2) GSH: Glutathione
           RBC: Red blood cell
             M: Mitochondrion
             N: Nucleus

FIGURE 2. SUGGESTED MODEL OF CHROMATE UPTAKE IN THE
           LUNGS AND IN THE GASTROINTESTINAL TRACT (1)

intracellular reduction have been recently discussed by several authors (e.g. De Flora 1978; Löfroth 1978; Langård 1979; Jenette 1979; Langård and Hensten-Pettersen 1981; Garcia and Jenette 1981; cited in Langård 1982). The reducing capacity inside the cell is limited, hence both hexavalent and trivalent chromium can co-exist in cytoplasm. Hexavalent chromium is released from the cell by simple diffusion into the bloodstream and taken up by the blood cells. Within the erythrocytes a surplus of glutathione (GSH) reduces the chromium to the trivalent form. Recent data presented by Alexander et al. (1982) generally support the above account, and the pathways are illustrated schematically in Fig. 2.

It is clear from the above discussion that the uptake and distribution of chromium within and between tissues is dependent on a number of variables, which may be summarised as follows:

-    physical and chemical form of chromium administered or absorbed;
-    temperature and pH of bathing solutions in 'in vitro' experiments;
-    presence of metabolic inhibitors, such as 'metavanadate';
-    quantity of chromium administered or previously present in the bloodstream;
-    age of the animal.

Competition between chromium and other, similar, anions does not appear to be of significance.

6.4.3.2   Retention in tissues

A simple descriptional model of the metabolism of trivalent chromium in man is presented in Fig. 3. Chromium, which is cleared rapidly from the blood, is retained for much longer in various organs of the body and it is likely that there is no equilibrium between tissue stores and chromium circulating in the bloodstream (Mertz 1969). Tissue retention of chromium is highly dependent upon chemical form. Mertz (1969) cited one study in which 64% and 92% of chromium acetate and citrate respectively were excreted within 4 days, whereas chromic chloride was much more effectively retained. Unfortunately, no further details of that experiment, the animals involved or the amounts and method of administration, were supplied.

A common failing in early experiments was the use of non-physiological amounts of chromium, in order to facilitate subsequent detection. Hopkins (1965) studied much lower levels of chromium, administering 0.1 µg and 1 µg per kg body weight to rats. Both doses were handled similarly, and organ retention was only slightly higher for the 0.1 µg kg^{-1} dose. As with previous experiments (employing higher dose levels of chromium), brain, heart, lungs and pancreas retained little of the dose, whereas bone, spleen, testes and epididymis accumulated chromium with time. Testicular chromium increased rapidly two to four-fold over initial values.

The ICRP (1980) noted that hexavalently administered chromium incorporated into erythrocytes has a biological half-life of retention of approximately 30 days in normal persons, whereas of chromium administered as trivalent chromic chloride roughly 25% is excreted within 24 hours.

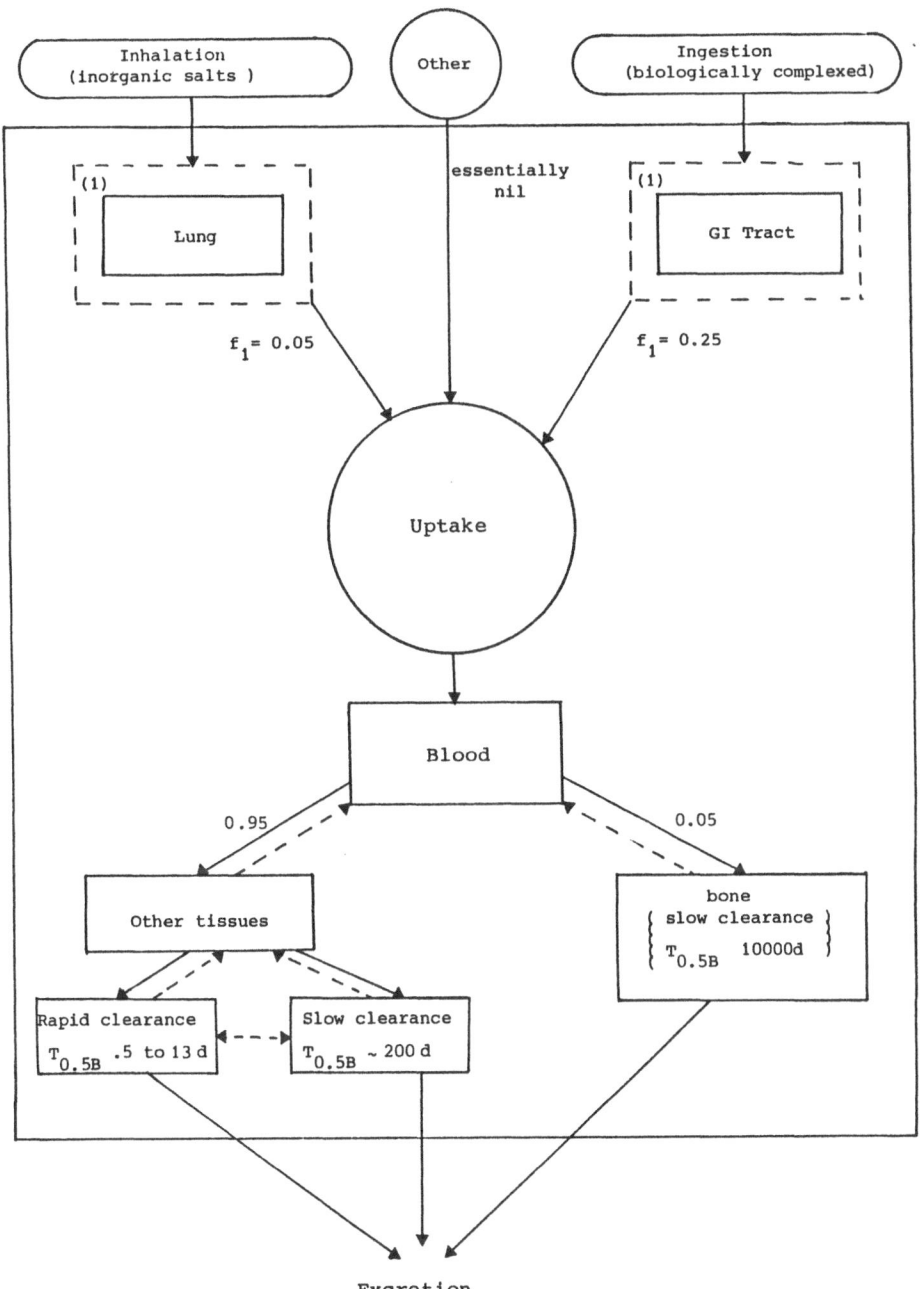

FIGURE 3   SIMPLE MODEL FOR THE METABOLISM OF TRIVALENT
CHROMIUM.

Note:

Chromium is cleared rapidly from the blood and is probably not in equilibrium with other tissues. Dotted lines represent possible metabolic pathways for chromium, levels of which are known to rise in blood when challenged with a glucose or insulin load.

Of chromium leaving the blood, a fraction of 0.05 is assigned to the bone. Of the remainder 0.2, 0.02, 0.04, 0.02 and 0.72 are assigned to the liver, lungs, kidneys, spleen and all other tissues respectively. The lung and GI tract as organs of input are based on the ICRP (1980) model.

At least 80% of the absorbed chromium is excreted in urine.

FIGURE 3   Cont.

This latter value is in approximate agreement with the blood retention function proposed by Sargent et al. (1979) and presented in Section 6.4.3.1. Furthermore, as noted in Sections 6.4.2 and 6.4.3.1, it is likely that by the time chromium has been absorbed, following ingestion or inhalation, it will be in the trivalent form and will not bind appreciably to red blood cells. Thus, data relating to Cr(III) is taken to be pertinent to developing a model for chromium retention in man. In rats (Mertz et al. 1965; reviewed in ICRP 1980) the whole body retention of chromium-51 intraveneously injected as $^{51}CrCl_3.6H_2O$ was well described by a function of the form:

$$R(t) = 0.43e^{-0.693t/0.5} + 0.32e^{-0.693t/5.0} + 0.25\ e^{-0.693t/83.4}$$

where t is in days.

Results from a more recent experiment on rats (Sayato et al. 1980) agree very closely with the above, although a biological half-life for the term of longest retention is given as 91.8 days following peroral administration.

Data for Reference Man (ICRP 1975) and subsequent reviews of the literature (e.g. Iyengar et al. 1978; IARC 1980; see also Tables 7 and 8 and Section 3) indicate that chromium is preferentially concentrated in bone. The ICRP (1980) assumed that of chromium leaving the transfer compartment of the metabolic model for man, 0.05 goes to bone where it is retained with a biological half-life of 1000 days. A further fraction of 0.3 was assumed to go directly to excretion, with a half-life of 0.5 days. The remainder was assumed to be uniformly distributed throughout all other organs and tissues with two components of retention, with half-lives of 6 and 80 days.

In a recent review of the literature, Coughtrey and Thorne (1983) noted that the distribution of chromium in man reported by Iyengar et al. (1978) suggested that chromium is retained in bone with a half-life of 10000 days rather than 1000 days. They further suggested that, of chromium present in all other tissues, fractions of 0.43, 0.32 and 0.2 are retained with half-lives of ~0.5 days (representing rapid excretion), 6 days and 80 days respectively. A non-uniform distribution of chromium was assumed and fractions of 0.1, 0.1, 0.02, 0.01 and 0.77 were assigned to lung, liver, kidneys, spleen and all other tissues respectively. Available data for the distribution of chromium in man display considerable variability, but on the basis of values presented in Tables 7 and 8 the above assignment may require some modification. It is of significance that data presented in Tables 7 and 8 indicate a much greater body content of chromium than previously noted by the ICRP (1975; 1980), and that 3.6 to 6.4 mg of this body content is in the soft tissue compared with the ICRP (1975; 1980) estimate of 1.8 mg. On the basis of a total soft tissue content of 5 mg, a long-term component of retention in soft tissue of biological half-life of around 200 days appears reasonable. Baetjer et al. (1959) concluded, on the basis of autopsy samples from men who had worked in chromate plants, that acid soluble and insoluble chromium are firmly bound to lung tissue and apparently retained for several years. This is compatible with data presented by Sargent et al. (1979) indicating a long-term component of biological retention of chromium in healthy individuals of around 192 days. Short and medium-term values for retention were found to be 0.59 days and

12.7 days, which are comparable with the retention function proposed for rats by Mertz et al. (1965). Fractions of 0.35, 0.26 and 0.39 were assigned respectively to short, medium and long-term components of retention in the whole-body. On the basis of these various data, the whole-body retention function of chromium in man is given by:

$$R(t) = 0.95 \ [0.35e^{-0.693t/0.6} + 0.26e^{-0.693t/13} + 0.39e^{-0.693t/200}]$$
$$+ 0.05e^{-0.693t/10000}$$

where t is in days.

The distribution of chromium within the body is given by resolving the above function into its component parts as follows:

$$R_{bone}(t) = 0.05e^{-0.693t/10000}$$

$$R_{other}(t) = 0.95a \ [0.35e^{-0.693t/0.5} + 0.26e^{-0.693t/13} + 0.39e^{-0.693t/200}]$$

where t is in days and

a takes the value of 0.2, 0.02, 0.04, 0.02 and 0.7 for lung, liver, kidneys, spleen and all other tissues respectively.

The value assigned to a above differ somewhat from the recommendations of Coughtrey and Thorne (1983), based on a retention function for chromium in rats, and the reported distribution of chromium in man. In particular, a greater fraction is assigned above to the lung, and rather less to the liver. The ICRP (1980) assigned uniform distribution to chromium in soft tissues, which is reasonable agreement with the above, although a substantially greater fraction is assigned to spleen in this new model. Although hexavalent chromium concentrates in all organs of the reticulo-endothelial system (Section 6.3), this does not apply to such a marked extent to trivalent forms of chromium (Tables 12 and 13). The above model has been developed specifically with regard to trivalent chromium, since this probably reflects the normal form in dietary intake and in biological samples (Section 6.4.3.1).

If the above functions are integrated over all time, f_1 is assumed to be 0.25 (Section 6.3) and a typical total daily dietary intake of chromium is assumed to be 80 µg (Section 6.2) then the following amounts of chromium in tissues of man can be calculated, and compared with data summarised from Table 7:

Organ tissue or fluid	Chromium content (µg) Observed	Calculated
Bone[1]	15000	14428
Kidney	95.8	88.8
Liver	30.1	44.4
Lung	407	444
Spleen	67.5	44.4
All others[2]	3086-6171	1594.4

Notes: (1) assuming a 'representative' bone concentration of 3 µg g^{-1}.

(2) assuming a concentration of 0.05 to 0.1 µg^{-1}.

It can be seen from the above that the observed and calculated chromium content of bone is in good agreement. Soft tissue contents of chromium àre generally in close agreement for organs identified above, but the calculated whole-body content is lower than that observed. The concentration of chromium in liver calculated from the compilation of Iyengar et al. (1978) is at the lower end of the range of values reported by Baetjer (1956; and see Table 8),and a higher value may be 'typical' of liver, but insufficient data are available to resolve this.

In view of the uncertainties regarding the metabolism of chromium in man by comparison with rats, and uncertainties previously noted with regard to values for f_1 and total dietary intake (Sections 2 and 3), the above agreement between observed and calculated chromium content in tissue is taken to be reasonable. Insufficient data are available at present to justify altering the proposed retention function for high levels of dietary intake. Moreover, results obtained by Hopkins (1965) indicate that over a ten-fold variation in dietary intake by rats, organ retention of chromium was little affected.

6.4.4   Other metabolic information

6.4.4.1   Skin absorption

Chrome ulcers are exclusively caused by occupational contact and were first reported in 1827 (Pederson 1982). Allergic contact dermatitis to chromium compounds is much more common than the irritant reaction (Pederson 1982). Although not exclusively of occupational origin, it was noted by Polak et al. (1973) that "[contact] chromium eczema is one of the most important occupational dermatoses and is becoming more wide-spread with the increasing use of chromium in different industries." A large proportion of such eczemas are due to contact with cement, caused by hypersensitivity to the hexavalent chromium salt content (see also Section 6.2.4). As a point of interest, Polak et al. (1973) noted that "chromium eczema occurs less often in people who come into contact with high concentrations of chromium salts .... than in those who work with material containing mere traces of chromium salts." In addition to the sensitising properties of hexavalent chromium, skin eczema can also be induced by divalent chromium [e.g. $Cr(CH_3COO)_2$] or trivalent chromium [e.g. $KCr(SO_4)_2$ and $Cr(NO_2)_2$] (Polak et al. 1973). Metallic chromium is not known to be immunogenic (Walsh 1955; Pederson 1982).

Chromium compounds, like all low molecular weight substances, are immunogenic only when bound to proteins. Numerous experiments have been performed, both 'in vivo' and 'in vitro', demonstrating the ability of chromium to conjugate with proteins, and the literature was briefly reviewed by Polak et al. (1973). On the basis of this review, Polak et al. (1973) concluded that "only trivalent chromium is able to conjugate with proteins of the skin and other organs and of the blood whereas hexavalent chromium is taken up by cells, i.e. penetrates through the cell membranes". Thus, whereas trivalent chromium may be the main valence state responsible for contact skin eczema, it is clear that hexavalent chromium will be more readily absorbed. After absorption it may be reduced to the immunologically active trivalent form, and bound to the relevant protein forming the full antigen (Pederson 1982).

Several 'in vivo' and 'in vitro' studies have been conducted, both on experimental animals and man, confirming the ability of certain chromate compounds (e.g. potassium dicromate and sodium chromate) to penetrate the skin and subsequently be detectable in blood, urine and various inner organs. Literature available up to 1980 was reviewed by Pederson (1982), from which the following conclusions or suggestions have been drawn.

- Percutaneous absorption of Cr-51 labelled compounds in guinea pigs, presented as disappearance of activity (%) during a 5 hour period, is maximal at 4% with a 0.261 M chromate solution. At higher and lower concentrations the relative disappearance rates approached the limits of detection. There is a maximum plateau value for absorption (Wahlberg 1965).
- The absolute maximum plateau value of absorption for chromic trichloride is 315-330 nM l^{-1} cm^{-2}, for sodium chromate the value is 690-725 nM l^{-1} cm^{-2} (Wahlbergand Skeg 1965).
- Percutaneous absorption of sodium chromate is relatively greater at PH 6.5 or higher, compared with pH 5.6 or lower (Wahlberg 1968a).
- Sodium lauryl sulphate as a skin pretreatment or as a test substance additive increases the percutaneous absorption (Wahlberg 1968b).
- Use of petrolatum as a vehicle increases absorption by 2 to 7 times, compared with use of water (Lidén and Lundberg 1979).
- Diffusion rates of chloride, nitrate and sulphate salts of chromium through epidermis removed from skin at autopsy are greater at pH 5 or pH 9 relative to pH 7 (Samitz et al. 1967).
- Chromium compounds which have penetrated into human skin may be retained for considerable period, depending upon allergic responses of the individual and chromium solution applied. After 2 months 3-5% of sodium chromate may remain at the injection site; for chromic trichloride a disappearance half-life from the site may be in excess of 380 days (Pederson et al. 1969; Pederson et al. 1970; Pederson and Naversten 1973; Fregert 1979).

More recently Kelly et al. (1982) reported on a case of accidental immersion in a solution of trivalent chromium, indicating considerable percutaneous absorption. The solution was of acidic chromium (III) sulphate ($Cr_2(SO_4)_3$ 40% w/w) and Na_2SO_4 (8% w/w) and H_2SO_4 at pH 2.83 and 80°C. The patient (a 56 year old white male) sustained 70% burns of variable thickness to skin of the limbs, thorax and abdomen. His face and neck did not come into contact with the solution and none was swallowed. Five and a half hours after exposure his blood load of chromium indicated that at least 176 mg had been absorbed. At death, 47 hours after the accident, his total body burden of chromium was 155 mg, exchange transfusion had removed 15 mg, urinary excretion 12 mg and faecal excretion 3 mg. In view of the extreme conditions, little can be inferred regarding the rate of percutaneous absorption or the subsequent toxic effects, but clearly substantial uptake occurred.

Baranowska-Dutkiewicz (1981) applied solutions of hexavalent chromium (as Na_2CrO_4) at 0.01, 0.1 and 0.2 molar, to the forearms of 27 volunteers. Results obtained indicated that:

- the absolute absorption increased with increasing chromium concentration in applied solution;

TABLE 16

CHROMIUM-51 CONCENTRATION IN MATERNAL
AND NEW BORN TISSUES OF RAT

cpm g^{-1} tissue	
Liver, maternal	48.0
Liver, foetal	187.0
Heart, maternal	29.7
Heart, foetal	45.8
Kidney, maternal	39.0
Kidney, foetal	44.5

Note:

Data from Mertz and Roginski (1971). A pregnant rat received
3 doses of Cr-51 labelled yeast extract by stomach tube. Counts
of radioactivity were taken from pooled tissue samples from new
born and corresponding samples from the mother

- the rate of absorption decreased as time of exposure increased;
- the amount of Cr(VI) absorbed, expressed as a percentage of the applied dose was highest with a 0.01 molar solution (7.7 to 23%) and lowest with a 0.2 molar solution (3.4 to 10.6%).

The absorption rate, over one hour, was 1.1, 6.5 and 10 μg cm^{-2} h^{-1} for the increasing strengths of solution respectively. These results are similar to those previously reported for rats (Dutkiewicz and Konczalik 1966). On the basis of findings reported (with n equal to 27 and an area of absorption of 20.4cm^2), Baranowska-Dutkiewicz (1981) proposed a function to model skin absorption, of the form:

$$y = m^{0.7447} t^{0.6407} e^{-2.9785+\mu}; \quad r = 0.996$$

where   y is the amount of chromium absorbed,
          m is the molar concentration of sodium chromate,
          t is the time of exposure in minutes and
          μ is a residual.

In view of the above, it is reasonable to assume that if a solution of hexavalent chromium comes into contact with the skin, a fraction of 0.1 will be absorbed. Insufficient data are available to propose a function for the absorption of trivalent chromium through skin, but the fractional absorption of this form of chromium is not likely to be significant by comparison with that of hexavalent chromium.

6.4.4.2   Cross placental transfer of chromium

Chromium is often reported to be present in higher concentrations in newborn animals and man than in adults (e.g. Schroeder et al. 1962). Although data presented in Table 10 for the concentration of chromium in the hair of newborn infants do not support the above statement, it is clear from Table 16 that chromium levels in foetal rats may be substantially higher than in maternal tissue. Data presented by Pribulada (1963) indicate a progressive increase in the chromium concentrations in hollow bones of human foetus with gestational age (12 to 40 weeks). Consequently, one might assume that cross-placental transfer of chromium, from mother to foetus,would be readily observable. However, in an extensive review of available literature the US National Academy of Sciences (1974) commented as follows:

"In spite of considerable efforts by several investigators, no transfer of chromium from mother to fetus, regardless of valence state or chemical form has been demonstrated ......
The chromium concentration in the newborn rat cannot be increased by feeding the mother chromium chloride, even at very high concentrations in drinking water. It is, however, influenced by natural sources of chromium in the diet .....
On the basis of these findings, it appears that chromium must be present in a special organic complex if it is to be available to the fetus."

Visek et al. (1953) had previously summarised their findings on rats as follows:

"Insignificant amounts of Cr^{51} were found to cross the placenta of rats in the 24 hours following intravenous injection regardless of the chemical form of the isotope, its valence state, the gestational stage (15 to 20 days), the animal or the number of fetuses per litter. In no case did the recovery of Cr^{51} per litter exceed 0.13% of the injected dose."

Data presented by Mertz et al. (1970) and Mertz and Roginski (1971) demonstrated that when chromium-51 was incorporated into glucose-tolerance factor by brewer's yeast and administered to pregnant rats by stomach tube, considerable transfer to the litter occurred. Using preparations of varying specific activity, Mertz et al. (1970) obtained the following net counts per ten minutes in mother (body weight ~300 g) and litters (total wight ~60-70 g) at birth, after 3 to 5 stomach tubed doses of chromium-51 as yeast extract to mothers.

	Net counts (10 min.)	
Rat Number[1]	In Mother	In total litter
32	900	150
34	988	240
35	1096	183
42	283	0
44	1006	350
Mean ± SE	911 ± 132	203 ± 50
71	321 600	172 400
72	209 400	132 400
73	34 700	14 200

Note: Rats 32 to 44 low specific activity, 71 to 73 high specific activity.

Davidson and Burt (1973) compared plasma chromium concentrations in healthy pregnant and non-pregnant women of similar ages. Plasma chromium was found to be significantly lower in the fasting pregnant subjects (2.97 ± 0.11 µg l^{-1}) compared with fasting non-pregnant subjects (4.70 ± 0.15 µg l^{-1}). A challenge with glucose, administered intravenously or orally, resulted in a fall in plasma chromium levels in non-pregnant women, but did not provoke such a response in pregnant subjects.

On the basis of an investigation on changes in the urinary excretion of chromium during pregnancy, and the effect of intravenous glucose tolerance tests on urinary excretion of chromium in late pregnancy, Saner (1981) concluded that "habitual dietary intake [of chromium] does not meet the increased chromium requirement and that prophylaxis may be of benefit and appears to be advisable in pregnancy." Although Knopp (1982) argued that chromium supplementation during pregnancy is probably unwarranted, it is clear nonetheless that pregnancy does have a significant modifying effect on the metabolism of chromium. However, in the absence of more time and/or dose related metabolic data, no alteration to the presently proposed metabolic model (Section 6.4.3.2) can be justified.

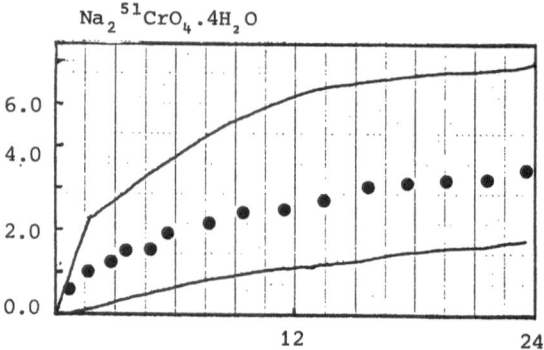

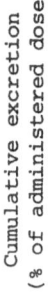

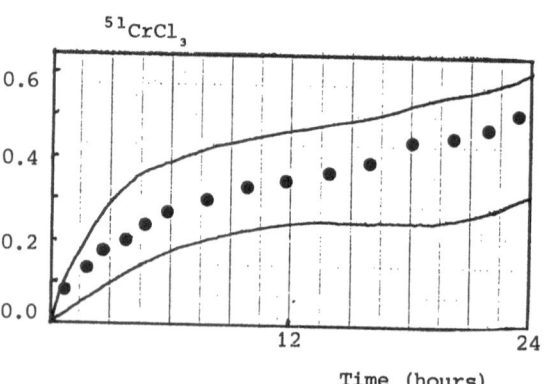

Note: Data from Cikrt and Bencko (1979). Amount
        administered was 31.4 µg of Cr, labelled with
        Cr-51, per 200g of body weight for both com-
        pounds.

FIGURE 4   CUMULATIVE BILIARY EXCRETION OF
             Cr-51 IN RATS DURING 24 HOURS
             AFTER INTRAVENOUS ADMINISTRATION.

An early study by Conn et al. (1932) indicated that no more than 0.03% of chromium administered in milk as chromium lactate was absorbed by young rats. Although data presented in Section 6.4.1 indicate that a higher rate of absorption can be expected in general for biologically complexed chromium, there is no evidence that fractional uptake is appreciably higher in infants on a milk diet compared with dietary uptake in adults. In view of the reported decline in chromium tissue levels with age (Section 6.3), it is likely that the major fraction of chromium in newborn infants will have been derived from cross-placental transfer of specific organic complexes of chromium.

6.4.4.3   Loss of chromium in milk

In a recent review of literature pertaining to chromium distribution and metabolism in man and domestic animals, Coughtrey and Thorne (1983) stated that "there do not appear to be any relevant data available concerning the transfer of radioactive chromium to milk." Limited data are available for the concentrations of stable chromium in human and cow's milk (Medvedeva 1966; Underwood 1977; see also Table 7). On the basis of these very limited data, Coughtrey and Thorne (1983) proposed a function for the loss of chromium in the milk of cows. Integrating their function over all time, Coughtrey and Thorne (1983) noted that "the total fraction of chromium which is lost in the milk of a lactating cow is estimated to be 0.43 and hence the loss of chromium in milk could significantly modify the retention function for a non-lactating animal. Since there are no relevant data it is not possible to make an allowance for this." A similar situation pertains also for man.

6.5   URINARY AND FAECAL EXCRETION OF CHROMIUM

In a review of the literature, the US National Academy of Sciences (NAS 1974) reported values for the concentration of chromium in human urine ranging from non-detectable to 860 µg l^{-1}. Two carefully controlled studies gave values of 5 and 4 µg l^{-1} respectively (Imbus et al. 1963; Pierce and Cholak 1966) and a further study of 20 young adults gave a 24 hour urinary excretion of 8.4 µg, with a range of 1.6 to 21 µg (Hambidge 1971). At least 80% of chromium excretion is estimated to be in urine with 0.5 to 20% of an intravenous dose to animals excreted in faeces (NAS 1974). Cirkt and Bencko (1979) reported that 0.6% and 6.0% of trivalent and hexavalent chromium respectively were excreted in the bile of rats within 24 hours following intravenous injection, (see Fig. 4). Similar results were obtained also by Norseth et al. (1982), with 0.1% and 6-8% of injected doses of Cr-III (as $CrCl_3.6H_2O$) and Cr-VI (as Na_2CrO_4) respectively excreted in bile during the first five hours after treatment.

The data sited above are commensurate with a total 24 hour urinary excretion of chromium by man in the order of 10 µg, which is somewhat lower than the 70 µg d^{-1} urinary loss estimated by ICRP (1975). If it is assumed that a further 2 µg d^{-1} of absorbed chromium is excreted in the faeces (see above), that chromium in man is in balance, and that f_1 for dietary intakes of chromium is 0.25, then a daily dietary intake of 48 µg

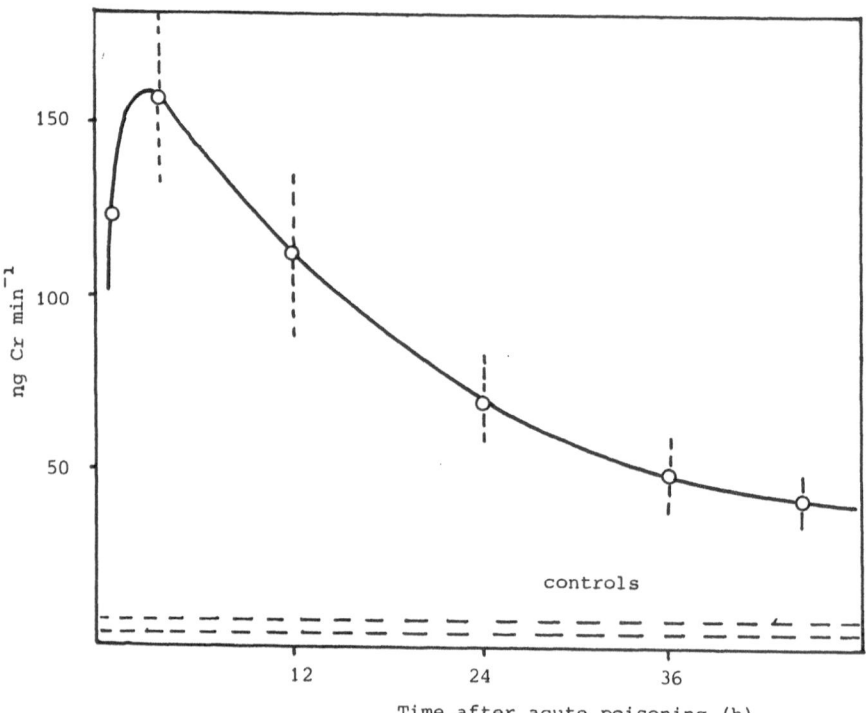

Note: (1) Data from Mutti et al. (1979)
            1.5 mg $K_2Cr_2O_7$ 100 g^{-1} body weight administered.

FIGURE 5.   URINARY EXCRETION OF CHROMIUM AFTER SUBCUTANEOUS
            INJECTION OF A SINGLE DOSE OF POTASSIUM DICHROMATE
            IN RATS [1].

is indicated. This is somewhat lower than the total intake of around 80 $\mu g\ d^{-1}$ (including food, water and air) estimated in Section 6.2, but given the uncertainties attached to each value, the agreement is reasonable. Furthermore, f_1 will be lower if chromium is ingested in the form of a simple salt, which concomittantly implies a higher rate of intake. However, it should be noted that Guthrie (1982) has reviewed data for the urinary excretion of chromium and concluded that, since 1978, "most investigators have agreed that normal urinary chromium concentrations are in the order of 1 ng / ml which corresponds to daily excretions of approximately 0.3-2.0 ug." This in agreement with recent data presented by Anderson et al. (1982) and if this is appropriate to normal rates of intake it may imply a substantially lower value for f_1, and serves to illustrate the uncertainties present in determining a 'typical' value. Additionally, it may be noted that since urine and blood are, from a practical point of view, the only biological materials available for measurement of chromium exposure in workers (Langård 1982), it is clearly desirable to establish with certainty a normal base line concentration of chromium in urine.

Collins et al. (1961) noted that in dogs renal clearance of chromium decreases exponentially with time (up to 8 hours) after a single intravenous injection of $^{51}CrCl_3$. A similar result was demonstrated by Mutti et al. (1979a) following a single subcutaneous injection of potassium dichromate to rats. Urinary levels of chromium were highly elevated during the first hour after injection and results to 48 hours indicate that early clearance exhibited a biological half-life of ∿0.5 days, with a second component exhibiting a half-life in the order of a few days, as shown in Fig. 5. On the basis of a literature review, the NAS (1974) reported 3 components for urinary excretion in rats. these components exhibited biological half-lives of 0.5, 5.9 and 83.4 days (see also the whole-body retention function for rats given in Section 4.3.2). The NAS noted that data on man are more limited. Therapeutic trials on the turnover of chromium, in glucose tolerance testing, indicate a slow turnover rate. On termination of chromium supplementation the glucose tolerance remains normal for approximately 30 days, slowly returning to pre-treatment levels. Gylseth et al. (1977) demonstrated that, for shift workers in a chromium welding factory, urinary excretion is highly correlated with the concentration of chromium in air during the shift, as illustrated in Fig. 6. Given that the 3 component model of retention applies also to man (as detailed in Section 4.3.2), the first component ($T_{0.5} \cong 0.5$ days) is considered by NAS (1974) probably to represent an effective means of eliminating excessive chromium. However, no data are available to suggest that this component of loss is dose-dependent, hence it cannot be considered as a mechanism of regulation.

Glomerular filtration and tubular reabsorption are involved in renal excretion of chromium, but tubular excretion is probably of minor importance (Collins et al. 1961; Matti et al. 1979b; Langård 1982). Nearly all chromium in urine is in low molecular weight complexes, protein-bound chromium is excreted only to a very small degree (NAS 1974).

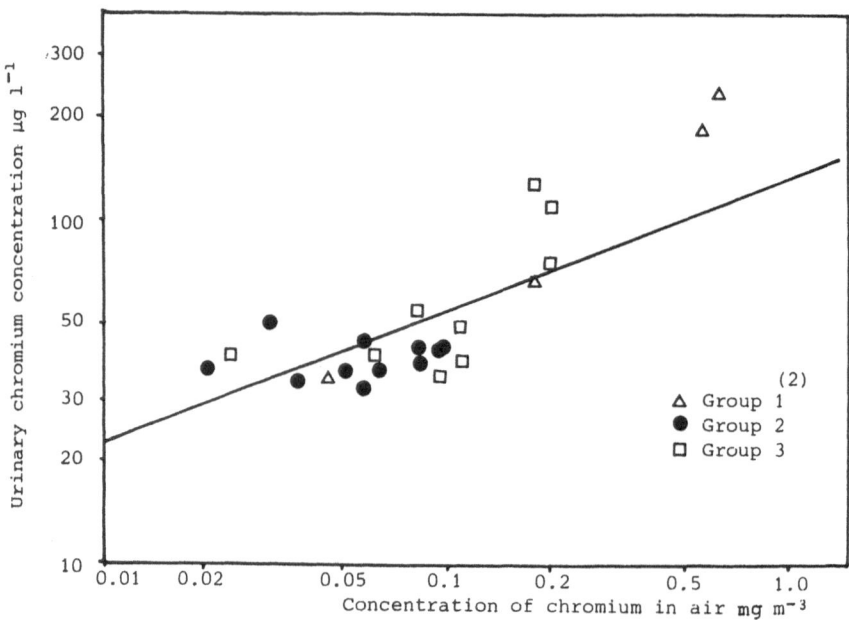

Note: (1) Data from Gylseth et al. (1977)

(2) Groups represent different work areas within
the factory

Group 1 - steel tank 26% chromium
Group 2 - steel tank 18% chromium
Group 3 - Cylindric milk tanks 18% chromium
              and nickel-steel alloy 9% chromium

FIGURE 6.   RELATION BETWEEN URINARY CHROMIUM CONCENTRATION
OF WELDERS AND THE CONCENTRATION OF CHROMIUM
IN AIR DURING A WORK SHIFT [1].

TABLE 17

DISTRIBUTION OF CHROMIUM IN ORGANS
AND BLOOD OF RATS INJECTED WITH
1, 2 or 3 mg Cr kg^{-1} (1)

Dose of Cr (mg/kg)	1		2		3	
Days of exposure	30	60	30	60	30	60
Liver	15.1±0.76 (2)	14.1±1.12	31.7±1.25	36.2±1.26[b]	38.1±1.50	43.3±2.71
Kidneys	5.6±0.37	8.1±0.98[b]	14.2±0.86	18.5±1.77[b]	12.9±0.91	25.8±1.18[a]
Testes	1.8±0.31	3.2±0.22[a]	3.2±0.24	7.2±0.81[a]	5.7±0.39	19.2±1.40[a]
Brain	2.1±0.42	2.8±0.26	2.7±0.17	7.1±1.30[a]	9.2±0.96	11.0±1.52
Blood (3)	ND (4)	ND	5.6±0.75	8.2±0.45[a]	8.5±0.69	12.0±0.55[a]

Notes: (1) Data from Tandon et al. (1979)
(2) Each value represents mean ± S.E. of 6 rats. In 12 control animals the concentration
of chromium was below the detection limit (1 µg g^{-1}). Significant difference indicatec
by a and b are at the $p<0.01$ level and $p<0.05$ respectively, when compared to the value at
30 days as evaluated by the student's t-test.
(3) Blood chromium concentration is given as µg ml^{-1}
(4) ND, not detectable (<1 µg g^{-1}).

TABLE 18

THE RELATIVE DISTRIBUTION OF CHROMIUM IN SUB-CELLULAR FRACTIONS OF RAT LIVER AT DOSE LEVELS OF 1, 2 AND 3 mg kg^{-1} (1)

% of liver Cr (mean ± S.E.) (2)

Fraction	Dose of Cr (mg kg^{-1})					
	1		2		3	
	Days of exposure					
	30	60	30	60	30	60
Nuclear	64.9±3.18	72.7±3.30(3)	47.2±2.63	44.9±2.50	45.0±3.85	51.7±3.17
Mitochondrial	28.0±3.14	20.4±3.89	39.1±1.93[a]	41.3±1.84[a]	43.2±3.46[a]	43.8±2.67[a]
Post mitochondrial supernatant	7.1±1.16	6.9±1.32	13.7±1.21	13.6±1.26	11.8±1.31	4.7±0.69

Notes: (1) Data from Tandon et al. (1979)

(2) Total liver chromium is the sum of chromium found in all 3 fractions.

(3) Each value is the mean of 6 rats; in 12 control animals the concentration was below the detection limit (1 ugg^{-1}). Significant difference indicated by a, is at the p<0.01, when compared to the corresponding value at 1 mg Cr μg^{-1} dose level as evaluated by the student's t-test.

TABLE 19

PLASMA CHROMIUM-51 CONCENTRATION IN
NORMAL, ELDERLY AND DIABETIC SUBJECTS (1)

Percent of original dose

Subject	1 hour	Time after administration 2 hours	4 hours	24 hours	48 hours	72 hours
Normal subjects age 21-69 $\bar{x}$	0.099(11) (2)	0.082(23) (3)	0.073(20)	0.080(11)	0.181(9)	0.139(9)
SEM ±	0.031	0.021	0.015	0.028	0.104	0.067
Normal subjects age 70 and over $\bar{x}$	0.025(5)	0.060(16)	0.042(10)	0.030(10)	0.021(9)	0.017(7)
SEM ±	0.009	0.010	0.009	0.005	0.005	0.006
Insulin-dependent diabetics $\bar{x}$	0.389(16)	0.398(18)	0.269(16)	0.185(14)	0.52(15)	0.125(11)
SEM ±	0.160	0.183	0.128	0.112	0.016	0.044
Diabetics controlled by oral agent or diet values $\bar{x}$	no values	0.038(9)	0.040(9)	0.024(7)	0.022(7)	0.014(4)
SEM ±		0.009	0.008	0.005	0.004	0.003

Notes: (1) Data from Doisy et al. (1971).
        (2) Numbers in parentheses indicate numbers of patients studied.
        (3) In initial studies, plasma samples were obtained at 2 and 4 hours only.

TABLE 20

MEAN URINE CHROMIUM-51 OUTPUT
IN NORMAL, ELDERLY AND DIABETIC SUBJECTS (1)

Subject	Output (% of original dose) (2)			
	Time after administration			
	0-24 hours	24-48 hours	48-72 hours	Total
Normal subjects $\bar{x}$ age 21-69	0.466(24) (3)	0.158(24)	0.064(21)	0.695(21)
SEM ±	0.052	0.032	0.008	0.066
Normal subjects $\bar{x}$ age 70 and over	0.364(17)	0.162(17)	0.097(17)	0.623(17)
SEM ±	0.064	0.029	0.039	0.099
Insulin dependent $\bar{x}$ diabetics	0.893(22)	0.316(22)	0.210(18)	1.383(18)
SEM ±	0.131	0.080	0.063	0.169
Diabetics controlled $\bar{x}$ by oral agent or diet	0.453(10)	0.107(10)	0.038(9)	0.636(9)
SEM ±	0.104	0.016	0.005	0.121

Notes: (1) Data from Doisy et al. (1971).

(2) Mean values which are significantly different (p<0.05) from means in normals under 70 years are underlined.

(3) Numbers in parentheses indicate numbers of patients studied.

TABLE 21

PARAMETERS A_i AND r_j FOR BEST-FIT TO WHOLE-BODY RETENTION CURVES (1) (2)

Patient	Diagnosis	Method of injection (3)	Whole Body Retention Parameters						Blood Retention Parameters							
			A_1	r_1	A_2	r_2	A_3	r_3	A_4	r_4	A_5	r_5	A_6	r_6	A_7	r_7
A	Normal	hom	.367	1.12	.257	.0376	.342	.00334	9.60	248	13.5	4.11	7.50	.313	2.42	.0663
B	Normal	hom	.314	1.43	.263	.0678	.427	.00390	3.42	34.4	8.56	2.21	2.22	.212	3.53	.0746
C	Normal	dir	.377	1.14	.263	.0534	.345	.00391	6.06	6.53	3.99	.947	.308	.241	2.65	.0977
D	Normal	dir	.345	1.42	.267	.0596	.381	.00405	3.82	37.9	6.65	3.01	3.47	.669	4.12	.0945
E	Normal	dir	.311	1.12	.269	.0552	.415	.00287	2.39	55.0	6.83	2.81	3.27	.424	2.96	.0865
	Mean		.343	1.25	.264	.0547	.382	.00361	5.06	76.4	7.91	2.62	3.35	.372	3.14	.0839
	$T\frac{1}{2}$			.56d		12.7d		192d		13min		6.3hr		1.9d		83d
F	Haemochrom. depleted	hom	.307	1.45	.237	.114	.464	.00410	3.07	97.1	11.5	2.03	3.23	.228	2.74	.0932
G	Haemochrom. depleted	dir					.480	.00413								
	Mean						.472	.00412								
	$T\frac{1}{2}$			.48d		6.08d		168d		10.3min		8.19hr		3.04d		7.43d
H	Haemochrom.	dir	.366	1.25	.240	.0554	.396	.00337	2.35	129	6.06	2.72	1.96	.334	2.52	.0900
	$T\frac{1}{2}$			.55d		12.5d		206d		7.7min		6.12hr		2.07d		7.7d
I	Haemochrom. relative	hom	.572	2.42	.200	.0836	.245	.00373	8.13	40.6	6.91	2.66	2.09	.517	.650	.0616
J	Haemochrom. relative	hom	.739	2.23	.145	.0882	.129	.00357	10.2	83.2	6.43	3.60	.945	.391	.728	.0764
	Mean		.655	2.33	.173	.0859	.187	.00365	9.16	61.9	6.67	3.13	1.52	.391	.689	.0690
	$T\frac{1}{2}$			.30d		8.07d		190d		16.1min		5.31hr		1.77d		10.0d
K	Haemochrom.	hom					.147	.00517							.550	.0898
L	Haemochrom.	dir	.616	3.42	.193	.0257	.183	.00322	5.45	145	5.65	11.0	2.89	1.10	.966	.0826
M	Haemochrom.	dir	.605	2.10	.216	.119	.191	.00423	6.45	33.7	3.14	1.98	1.28	.243	.338	.0633
N	Haemochrom.	dir	.643	2.49	.158	.0774	.215	.00555	6.05	29.7	2.28	1.56	.437	.201	.223	.0518
O	Haemochrom.	het	.573	2.42	.196	.106	.238	.00440	17.9	12.8	6.49	1.55	2.99	.164	.395	.0364
P	Haemochrom.	het	.473	1.46	.205	.0388	.324	.00410	7.76	126	12.6	4.81	4.29	.223	.896	.0423
	Mean		.582	2.38	.194	.0834	.216	.00444	8.88	69.4	6.03	4.18	2.38	.386	.563	.0610
	$T\frac{1}{2}$			.29d		8.3d		156d		14.4min		3.98hr		1.80d		11.4d

NOTES:

(1)   Data from Sargent et al. (1979)

(2)   Where:

$$R(t) = \Sigma_{ij} \, A_i e^{-r_j t}$$

The fitting for the whole-body retention data was performed independently of the blood data. The half-times ($T_{\frac{1}{2}}$) are calculated from $T_{\frac{1}{2}} = \ln 2/A_i$ and are given for the mean value of each r: for cases where there is only a single value for r, the $T_{\frac{1}{2}}$ is for that single value.

(3)   dir = direct injection of Cr-51

hom = injection of Cr-51 after incubation with patients own plasma

het = injection of Cr-51 after incubation with donor plasma

TABLE 21 (contd)

TABLE 22

IN VITRO REMOVAL OF CHROMIUM FROM SUBCELLULAR FRACTIONS
OF LIVER, KIDNEYS AND BLOOD CELLS OF CHROMIUM INTOXICATED
RATS BY CHELATING AGENS

	Removal of Cr, % (1)				
	Liver		Kidneys		
Chelating agent (2)	Mitochrondria	Post-mitochondrial supernatant	Mitochondria	Post-mitochondrial supernatant	Blood cells
EDDA	27.80±6.09	41.04±11.48	64.33±6.04	41.80±12.10	35.93±15.22
EDDHA	20.08±1.78	28.18± 3.09	19.35±1.31	6.25± 1.63	30.93± 2.75
HEDTA	19.68±3.99	17.70± 8.37	20.42±8.55	44.23±19.98	29.33±10.15
HDTA	65.10±2.30	68.83± 5.45	38.60±5.41	43.45± 7.74	84.43± 2.03
TTHA	77.58±2.41	75.13± 4.72	47.80±7.88	38.53± 8.39	72.98± 2.80

Notes: (1) Data from Behari and Tandon (1980). Each value represents the mean ±1 s.e. from four rats and is based on a control value taken as 0%.

(2) For full chemical names of each chelating agent see Section 6.

TABLE 23

IN VIVO REMOVAL OF CHROMIUM FROM ORGANS OF CHROMIUM - INTOXICATED RATS BY TREATMENT WITH CHELATING AGENTS (1)

Concentration ($\mu gCrg^{-1}$ fresh tissue) (2)

Treatment	Liver	Kidney	Heart	Brain
K_2CrO_4 exposed	25.68±2.07	40.61±2.82	7.56±0.72	4.18±0.51
Normal saline	17.46±2.92	28.62±3.96	5.38±0.37	3.33±0.30
EDDA	8.45±1.65(51.66) (5)	25.75±1.74(10.0)	3.74±0.52(30.5) (5)	2.37±0.45(28.8)
EDDHA	13.98±2.79(20.0)	13.87±2.48(51.5) (4)	2.41±0.60(55.2) (4)	1.09±0.28(67.2) (3)
HEDTA	9.64±1.02(44.84) (5)	6.22±1.23(78.2) (3)	4.90±0.43(8.9)	3.75±0.62
HDTA	8.38±1.88(52.0) (5)	10.66±1.17(62.7) (3)	4.31±0.61(19.9)	1.53±0.19(54.0) (3)
TTHA	11.15±0.27(36.21) (5)	25.88±8.21(9.6)	5.36±1.28(0.4)	3.28±0.71(1.5)
EGATA	13.96±0.85(20.1)	24.17±3.75(15.5)	4.69±1.26(12.8)	2.57±0.39(22.8)

Notes: (1) Data from Behari and Tandon (1980).

(2) Each value represents the mean ± 1 s.e. from 10 animals in K_2CrO_4 and normal-saline treated groups, and from 5 animals in experimental groups. Figures in parentheses are % Cr mobilized by the chelating agent, based on the mobilization by normal saline as 0%.

(3) <0.001
(4) <0.01 when compared to normal saline control as evaluated by student's t-test.
(5) <0.05

6.6   EFFECTS OF STATE OF HEALTH, ADMINISTRATION OF TOXIC
LEVELS AND THERAPEUTIC PROCEDURES

Chronic effects of chromium poisoning have already been summarily discussed (Section 6.1). Ulceration of the nasal septum or of exposed areas of skin are the most commonly reported lesions (Langard 1980), and, for Western males, chromium appears to be one of the most important causes of skin allergy (Fregert et al. 1969). Chromium may also induce pneumoconiosis in chromite miners (Sluis-Cremer and du Toit 1968), but experimental work by Swensson (1977) could not confirm these human findings. Bronchial asthma due to sensitisation to chromite-dust, chromic acid fumes or ferro-chromium dust is well documented (e.g. Joules 1932, cited in Langård 1980; Broch 1949; Williams 1969). Although irritive, such responses are unlikely to alter chromium metabolism.

In his review of data, Langård (1980) stated that, "no reports can be found in the literature indicating severe toxic effects of chromic salts in man". Consequently, consideration of the implications of administration of acutely toxic amounts of chromium is limited to the hexavalent form, although trivalent chromium is likely to be the more typical form for exposure at high levels (Mancuso and Hueper 1951).

A number of early publications showed that chromates cause nephrotoxic, hepatotoxic and cardiotoxic effects in man (e.g. Brieger 1920; Goldman and Karotkin 1935). These early findings have been confirmed subsequently in animals (e.g. Hunter and Roberts 1933; Mosinger and Fiorenti 1954; Schubert et al. 1970; Evan and Dail 1974). In fatal cases of chromate poisoning, patients may show symptoms similar to those of hepatic coma. Kaufman (1970) reported on one case of a 14 year old boy ingesting 1.5 g potassium dichromate. He died 8 days later. Autopsy revealed pale, enlarged, necrotic kidneys with leucocytic infiltrations in the interstitium. Necrosis was primarily in the tubules of the kidney, the glomeruli were near normal. The liver was congested with marked diffuse necrosis, haemorrhage and loss of architecture. In cases of acute poisoning, with associated nephrotoxicity, it is likely that the chromium clearance rates will be significantly altered, but there are not sufficient data available to quantify such a modification to the metabolic model proposed (Section 6.4.3.2). Tandon et al. (1979) tested for the effects of dose level and duration of treatment on the distribution of chromium in chromium poisoned rats. Male albino rats were given daily intraperitoneal injections of trivalent chromium at dose levels of 1, 2 or 3 mg kg^{-1} in 1 ml normal saline at pH 6.5. Results are presented in Tables 17 and 18, from which it can be seen that at the organ or sub-cellular level, the duration of treatment is of relatively little importance by comparison with the dose level. At all dose levels, the liver and kidney were the critical organs for accumulation (Table 17). As the dose increased, a greater proportion of the chromium in liver was associated with the mitochondrial fraction of the cells, and proportionately less with the nuclear fraction (Table 18).

Disorders involving the metabolic functions of glucose tolerance are known to modify the retention and clearance rates of chromium from the whole-body. Glinsmann et al. (1966) challenged diabetics and controls with glucose or chromium, and summarised their results as follows:

- normal glucose tolerance tests resulted in a rise in the plasma concentration of chromium;

- chromium supplementation in four diabetic patients resulted in elevated plasma chromium levels regardless of whether it improved glucose tolerance;
- two diabetic patients with impaired glucose tolerance failed to show elevation in plasma chromium levels after a challenge with glucose.

Doisy et al. (1971) studied glucose metabolism in normal, elderly and diabetic subjects. After oral administration of chromium-51 the plasma chromium levels were elevated in insulin-requiring diabetics relative to other subjects, as indicated in Table 19. Following oral administration urinary excretion of chromium was also higher in the insulin-requiring diabetics, as shown in Table 20. It is not known whether the fractional gastrointestinal absorption of chromium varied significantly between the groups, but similar results for urinary excretion were obtained following intravenous injection. In all cases, the blood plasma levels of chromium were somewhat depressed in elderly subjects, as indicated in Table 19, but urinary excretion levels were similar for both age groups.

Sargent et al. (1979) studied glucose metabolism in patients suffering from haemochromatosis. This iron storage disease is characterised by "hepatomegaly, bronze skin colouration, diabetes and various other symptoms, some or all of which may be present in any one patient. The symptoms result from excessive stores of iron in body tissues and in the idiopathic or primary form this has been shown to result from abnormally increased absorption of iron in the diet. The most characteristic sign of haemochromatosis is a high saturation of the plasma iron concentration" (Sargent et al. 1979).

It is known that trivalent chromium is carried in the blood bound to transferrin, as is iron, and that the binding is competitive between iron and chromium. However, transferrin has two binding sites, A and B (Harris 1977), and chromium binds only to site B; whereas iron may bind at either site, but at low levels of saturation is bound preferentially to site A (Harris 1977). Thus, when binding of iron to transferrin exceeds 50% saturation, as in haemochromatosis, one would expect the binding and transport of chromium to be affected. On this topic, Sargent et al. (1979) reported that the biological half-lives of chromium retention in blood or whole-body do not vary significantly between normal subjects and haemochromatosis patients, but that the relative amounts associated with the various components do differ, resulting in less long-term retention of chromium. Results obtained are presented in Table 21, and indicate a long-term component of whole-body retention of 156 days in haemochromatosis patients compared with 192 days in normal subjects. Fractions of 0.58, 0.20 and 0.22 were associated with short, medium and long-term retention respectively in haemochromatosis patients.

Therapeutic procedures following chromium poisoning have been discussed in detail by Langard (1980) and Behari and Tandon (1980). Langard (1980) stated that "so far no effective treatment has been found for the acute effects following chromate ingestion". Attempts to treat chromate-intoxicated patients with chelating agents, haemodialysis or peritoneal dialysis have had little therapeutic effect (Schlatter and Kissling 1973). This is presumably a consequence of hexavalent chromium being the toxic form. As discussed in Section 6.4.3.1, hexavalent chromium is rapidly taken up and bound by target organs or erythrocytes (Gray and Sterling 1950; Mertz 1969; Langard 1977) and only dialysable chromium in blood is available for excretion in the urine (Collins et al. 1961; NAS 1974). Consequently to be effective, chelation or haemodialysis would be effective only if applied soon after ingestion of chromate. Clincial data reported for haemodialysis by Reichelderfer (1968) and summarised by Langárd (1980), appear to support this view.

Ascorbic acid administered to young rats immediately following an otherwise lethal dose of potassium dichromate was effective in reducing the chromium toxicity (Samitz et al. 1962). However, a delay of 3 hours in administering the ascorbic acid virtually eliminated its effectiveness and the rats died. The apparent efficacy of ascorbic acid is due to its reducing properties. Thus, it transforms the toxic hexavalent form of chromium into the less toxic trivalent form (Samitz et al. 1962). Langárd (1980) commented that no cases of treating humans with ascorbic acid have been reported, but that there is no 'a priori' reason why such treatment should not be effective. However, "since colloidal complexes may be formed from trivalent salts present in the blood, intravenous injection of ascorbic acid is not recommended" (Langárd 1980). Several reports in the literature appear to suggest that hexavalent chromium is reduced by proteins present in milk to less absorbable compounds (e.g. Conn et al. 1932; Donaldson and Barreras 1966; Samitz et al. 1968; and reviewed in Langard 1980). Since prevention of chromium absorption will reduce toxicity, immediate consumption of milk may be of use following accidental ingestion of chromate.

Behari and Tandon (1980) also noted that chelating agents, haemodialysis or peritoneal dialysis have proved largely ineffectual in the treatment of chromate poisoning. However, they commented that "since some of the hexavalent chromium taken up in lungs is transferred to blood in the same state....and is dialysable to a certain extent from the isolated cells,.... some mobilization of chromium even after the accumulation of chromates in tissues appears possible." A few polyaminocarboxylic acids and ascorbic acid have been reported to be useful in removing trivalent chromium from organs and cells of chromium pre-treated rats (Tandon and Gaur 1977). Behari and Tandon (1980) screened the potential of six polyamino carboxylic acids for removing the metal from selected organs of chromate poisoned rats. The six acids were, ethylenediamine N,N'-diacetic acid (EDDA), ethylenediamine N,N'-di(o-hydroxyphenyl) (acetic acid (EDDHA), N-(2-hydroxyethyl)ethylenediamine triacetic acid (HEDTA), hexamethylene 1,6-diamino N,N,N'N'-tetraacetic acid (HDTA), ethyleneglycol-bis-(2-aminoethyl)tetraacetic acid (EGATA) and triethylene tetramine N,N,N'N'N''N'' -hexaacetic acid (TTHA).

In vitro tests were performed to estimate the efficiency of the various polyaminocarboxylic acids in removing chromium from the subcellular fractions of liver and kidney, and results are presented in Table 22. HDTA and TTHA were found to be highly, and almost equally, effective in dialysing the metal from the mitochondrial and post-mitochondrial supernatant fractions of both organs and from red blood cells. Data for the 'in vivo' removal of chromium from liver, kidneys, heart and brain are presented in Table 23, from which it can be seen that HDTA and EDDHA are the most consistently successful, removing more than 50% of the chromium from three of the four organs tested. HEDTA was extremely effective mobilising chromium from the kidneys, but was not so effective on the other organs. The performance of TTHA was very poor 'in vivo' compared with results obtained 'in vitro'. Behari and Tandon (1980) concluded that, "the remarkable success of HDTA and TTHA in the 'in vitro' and of HDTA in the 'in vivo' removal of chromium suggests that the chelating agents having more amino or carboxyl groups as complexing centres may be highly effective. Further, the effectiveness of EDDHA and HEDTA in the 'in vivo' study indicates that the presence of hydroxyl groups in the chelators may be of additional advantage". Th poor performance of TTHA in the 'in vivo' study, or that of EDDHA and HEDTA in the 'in vitro' study, is not well understood. Behari and Tandon (1980) suggested that the complex of chromium with TTHA (a comparatively large molecule) might dissociate in the presence of other biological ligands before excretion. Similarly, it is possible that metabolic modifications to the chelating agents, in the biological system, will alter their metal binding ability. The comparatively poor metal-mobilising ability of HEDTA and EDDHA in the 'in vitro' study may reflect the short time for which the chromium-bound subcellular fractions of blood cells were dialysed against the chelators. Alternatively, the resulting complexes may be of limited stability under such conditions. Clearly, further work is required in this area, but it is noted by Behari and Tandon (1980) that the particular effectiveness of HDTA, TTHA and EDDHA in removing chromium from organs and cells of chromate poisoned rats demonstrates the potential of these compounds in reducing chromium intoxication.

6.7   MODEL SUMMARY

     The following model for uptake and metabolism of chromium is recommended on the basis of data presented in the foregoing sections.

6.7.1   Intake of chromium

     A typical dietary intake of chromium in food is taken to be 75 µg d^{-1} (range ~30 to 200 µg d^{-1}). Diets giving daily intakes in excess of 500 µg are uncommon but have been reported. An additional intake of 0.8 to 8 µg d^{-1} probably occurs through drinking water and 1 to 2 µg d^{-1} may be inhaled by non-smoker. However, for a smoker of 20 cigarettes per day) the inhalation intake may be ~10 to 15 µg d^{-1}. Occupational exposure may result in inhalation of in excess of 200 µg of chromium in a working day, unless respiratory protection is employed.

6.7.2   Fractional gastrointestinal absorption

     An f_1 value of 0.05 is recommended for all inorganic salts of chromium. No distinction is made between intakes of trivalent or hexavalent chromium. Dietary, or biologically incorporated chromium, is absorbed more efficiently and an f_1 value of 0.25 is assigned to all dietary intakes of chromium.

6.7.3   Retention in, and translocation from, the lungs.

     Chromium is assigned to the following inhalation classes, in accordance with ICRP recommendations:

Chemical Group	Inhalation class
oxides and hydroxides	Y
halides and nitrates	W
all other compounds	D

Chromium entering the gastrointestinal tract following clearance from the lungs is assumed to be present in inorganic form, probably trivalent, and an f_1 value of 0.05 is taken to be applicable.

6.7.4   Retention in the body

Following entry of a unit quantity of chromium into the systemic circulation retention in the bone of man is adequately represented by:

$$R_{bone}t = 0.05e^{-0.693t/10000}$$

where t is in days

Retention of chromium in tissues other than bone is taken to be represented by:

$$R_{other}(t) = 0.95\ a[0.35e^{-0.693t/0.5} + 0.26e^{-0.693t/13} + 0.39e^{-0.693t/200}]$$

where t is in days and

a takes values of to 0.2, 0.02, 0.04, 0.02 and 0.72 for lung, liver, kidneys, spleen and all other tissues respectively.

No modification to the retention function is recommended for high levels of dietary chromium intake. However, the following assumptions are recommended for patients with haemochromatosis:

- retention in bone is unaffected;
- biological half-lives of retention in soft-tissues are not significantly modified, although data suggest that a long-term component of retention of 160 d may be more appropriate;
- fractions of 0.58, 0.2 and 0.22 are assigned to short, medium and long-term components of retention respectively;
- clearance of chromium from the blood is more rapid, due to a reduction in the long-term retained fraction.

6.7.5   Excretion of chromium

In view of the wide variability in reported concentrations of chromium in both urine and faeces, no model is proposed relating body burden to urinary excretion. However, it is noted that in excess of 80% of chromium absorbed to the systemic circulation is excreted in the urine. Glomerular filtration and tubular reabsorption are both of significance in the renal excretion of chromium. Nearly all chromium in urine is incorporated in low molecular weight complexes, protein-bound chromium is excreted only to a very small degree.

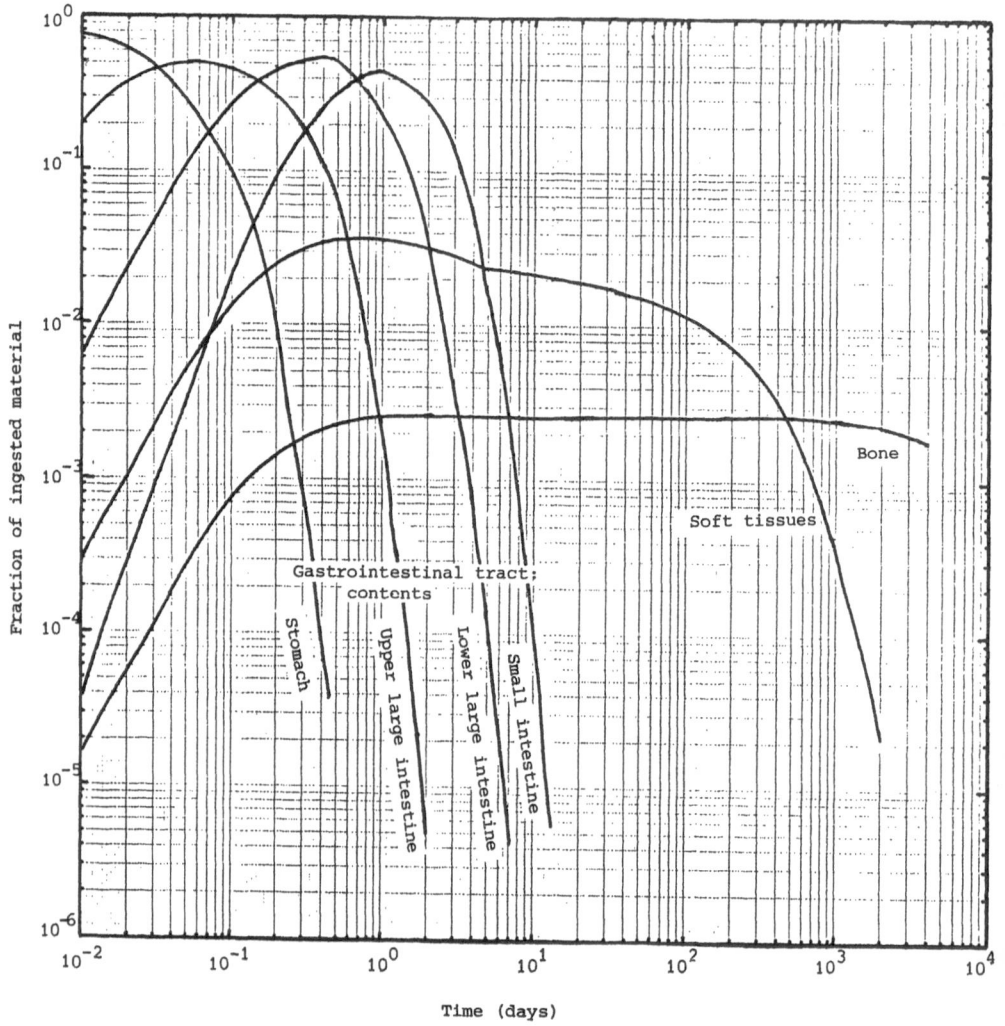

FIGURE 7.   CHROMIUM RETENTION FOLLOWING INGESTION OF A
UNIT QUANTITY OF AN INORGANIC COMPOUND

6.7.6   Skin absorption of chromium

Up to 23% of chromium in a solution of sodium chromate administered to the intact skin may be absorbed over one hour, depending on the molarity of the solution. A typical fractional absorption of 0.1 is taken to be appropriate for all forms of hexavalent chromium in contact with skin for appreciable periods. Absorption of trivalent chromium is assumed to be negligible.

6.7.7   Cross placental transfer and transfer in milk

Insufficient data are available to modify the proposed retention function in respect of physiological changes associated with pregnancy and lactation. However, it is clear that substantial depletion of maternal chromium stores may occur during both pregnancy and subsequent lactation. Plasma chromium levels in pregnant women are almost half those in healthy non-pregnant women of similar age. In cows, it has been estimated that over 40% of maternal chromium may be lost in milk, but this conclusion is very tentative and its relevance to the case of lactating women is not readily determined.

6.8   ILLUSTRATIVE CALCULATIONS

The distribution of chromium in the body following a single oral intake of an inorganic salt is shown in Fig. 7, illustrating the long-term retention in bone relative to other tissues.

6.9   REFERENCES

Aas, K.A. and Gardner, F.H., 1958. Survival of blood platelets labelled with chromium. J. Clin. Invest., 37, 1257-1268.

Abdulla, M. and Svensson, S., 1979. Chromium and nickel, Scan. J. Gastro-enterol., 14, (Suppl. 52): 176-180.

Alexander, J., Aaseth, J. and Norseth, T., 1982. Uptake of chromium by rat liver mitochondria. Toxicol., 24: 115-122.

Baetjer, A.M., 1950a. Pulmonary carcinoma in chromate workers. I. A review of the literature and report of cases. AMA Arch. Hyg. Occup. Med., 2, 487-504.

Baetjer, A.M., 1950b. Pulmonary carcinoma in chromate workers. II. Incidence on basis of hospital records. AMA Arch. Ind. Hyg. Occup. Med., 2, 505-516.

Baetjer, A.M., 1956. Relation of chromium to health. In: Udy, M.J. (Ed.). Chemistry of Chromium and Compounds. Reinhold Pub. Corp., New York; pp. 76-104.

Baetjer, A.M., Damron, C.M., Clark, J.H. and Budacz, V., 1955. Reaction of chromium compounds with body tissues and their constituents. AMA Arch. Industr. Health, 12, 258-261.

Baetjer, A.M., Damron, C. and Budacz, B.A., 1959. The distribution and retention of chromium in men and animals. AMA Arch. Industr. Health, 20, 136-150.

Baranowska-Dutkiewicz, B., 1981. Absorption of hexavalent chromium by skin in man. Arch. Toxicol., 47, 46-50.

Behari, J.R. and Tandon, S.K., 1980. Chelation in metal intoxication. VIII. removal of chromium from organs of potassium chromate administered rats. Clin. Toxicol., 16, 33-40.

Bourne, H.G. and Yee, H.T., 1950. Occupational cancer in a chromate plant - an environmental appraisal. Ind. Med. Surg., 19, 563-567.

Bourne, H.G. Jr. and Rushin, W.R., 1950. Atmospheric pollution in the vicinity of a chromate plant. Ind. Med. Surg., 19, 568-569.

Bowen, H.J.M., 1979. Environmental Chemistry of the Elements. Academic Press, London.

Breeze, V.G., 1973. J. Appl. Ecol., 10; 513-

Brieger, H., 1920. Zur Klinik der akuten Chromatvergiftung. Z. Exp. Path. Therap., 21, 393-408.

Broch, C., 1949. Bronchial asthma caused by chromium trioxide fumes. Nord. Med., 41: 996-997. [Translated in Arch. Ind. Hyg. Occup. Med., 1, 588, 1950].

Casey, C.E. and Hambidge, K.M., 1980. Trace element difficiencies in man. In: Draper, H.H. (Ed.) Advances in Nutritional Research. Vol. 3. Plenum Press, New York, pp. 23-63.

Chah, C.C., Caster, W.O., Combs, G.F., Hames, C.G., Heyden, S. and Jone, J.B., 1976. Macro- and micro-elements and the epidemiology of cardiovascular disease. In: Hemphill, D.D. (Ed.) Trace substances in Environmental Health. Volume 10, University of Missouri, Columbia, pp. 31-40.

Christian, R.A., Baker. J.R.J. and Bullock, G.R., 1977. The use of [51]Chromium for autoradiography at all levels. Acta pharmacol. et toxicol., 41, (Suppl. 1): 30-31.

Cirkt, M. and Bencko, V., 1979. Biliary excretion and distribution of 51-Cr (III) and 51-Cr (VII) in rats. J. Hyg. Epidemiol Microbiol. Immunol., 23, 241-246.

Collins, R.J., Fromm, P.O., and Collings, W.D., 1961. Chromium excretion in the dog. Am. J. Physiol., 201, 795-798.

Conn, L.W., Webster, H.L. and Johnson, A.H., 1932. Chromium toxicology. Absorption of chromium by the rat when milk containing chromium was fed. Am. J. Hyg., 15, 760-765.

Coughtrey, P.J., and Thorne, M.C., 1983. Radionuclide Distribution in Terrestrial and Aquatic Ecosystems: A Critical Review of Data. Volume 2. A.A. Balkema, Rotterdam.

Curl, H. Jr., Cutshall, N., and Osterberg, C., 1965. Uptake of chromium (III) by particles in sea-water. Nature, 205, 275-276.

Cutshall, N., Johnson, V. and Osterberg, C., 1966. Chromium-51 in sea water: chemistry. Science, 152, 202-203.

Davidson, I.W.F. and Burt, R.L., 1973. Physiologic changes in plasma chromium of normal and pregnant women: effect of a glucose load. Am. J. Obstet. Gynecol., 116, 601-608.

Davies, J.M., 1978. Lung cancer mortality of workers making chrome pigments. Lancet, 1, 384.

DeFlora, S., 1979. Metabolic deactivation of mutagens in the Salmonella - microsome test. Nature (Lond.), 271, 455-456.

DeGrooot, A.J. and Allersma, E., 1975. Field observations on the transport of heavy metals in sediments. In: Krendel, P.A. (Ed.) Heavy Metals in the aquatic Environment. Pergamon Press, New York, 85-95.

Dick, G.L., Hughes, J.T., Mitchell, J.W. and Davidson, F., 1978. Survey of trace elements and pesticide residues in the New Zealand diet. 1. Trace element content. N.Z. J. Sci., 21, 57-69.

Davis, G.K., 1956. Chromium in soils, plants and animals. In: Udy, M.J. (Ed.). Chromium, Vol.1, New York, NY, Reinhold, 105-109.

Doisy, R.J., Strecten, D.H.P., Souma, M.L., Kalafer, M.C., Rekant, S.I. and Dalakos, T.G., 1971. Metabolism of [51]chromium in human subjects normal, elderly, and diabetic subjects. In: Mertz, W., and Carnattzer (Eds.) Newer Trace Elements in Nutrition. Marcel Dekker, New York (USA), 155-168.

Donaldson, R.M. Jr. and Barreras, R.F., 1966. Intestinal absorption of trace quantities of chromium. J. Lab. Clin. Med., 68, 486-493.

Dutkiewicz, T. and Konczalik, K., 1966. The kinetics of ^{51}Cr distribution and elimination in rats. Int. Congress on Occup. Health, Vienna. Proceeding A III-34. Verlag der Wiener Medizinischen Akademie, Wien, 281-284.

Ebaugh, F.G. Jr., Emerson, C.P., Ross, J.F., Aloia, R., Halperin, P. and Richards, H., 1953. The use of radioactive chromium-51 as an erythrocyte tagging agent for the determination of red cell survival in vivo. J. Clin. Invest., 32, 1260-1276.

Edwards, C., Olsen, K.B., Heggen, G. and Glenn, J., 1961. Intracellular distribution of trace elements in liver tissue. Proc. Soc. Exptl. Biol. Med., 107, 94-97.

Evan, A.P. and Dail, W.G. (1974). The effects of sodium chromate on the proximal tubules of rat kidney. Fine structural damage and lysozymuria. Lab. Invest., 30: 704-715.

Fishbein, L., 1976. Environmental metallic carcinogens: an overview of exposure levels. J. Toxicol. Environ. Health., 2, 77-109.

Frank, R., Brown, H.E., Holdrinet, M. and Stonefield, K.I., 1977. Metal contents and insecticide residues in tobacco soils and cured tobacco leaves collected in Southern Ontario. Tobacco Sci., 21, 74-80.

Fregert, S., 1971. Contact Dermatitis Newsletter, 1, 10.

Fregert, S., Hjorth, N., Magnusson, B., Bandmann, H.J., Calnan, C.D., Cronin, E., Malten, K., Meneghini, C.L., Pirila, V., and Wilkinson, D.S., 1969. Epidemiology of contact dermatitis. Trans. St. John's Hosp. Dermatol. Soc., 55, 17-35.

Fukai, R., 1967. Valency state of chromium in seawater. Nature, 213, 901.

Gabrieli, E.R., Heckert, P., Elliot, A., and Pyzikiewicz, T., 1963. Kinetics of plasma hemoglobin catabolism in the rat. II. Cr^{51} - tagged hemoglobin. Proc. Soc. Exp. Biol. Med., 113, 206-213.

Gafafer, N.M., (Ed.), 1953. Health and Workers in Chromate Producing Industry: A study. US Public Health Service, Division of Occupational Health, Publication No. 192. Washington DC.

Gandolfo, N. and Sampaola, A., 1963. Rivievi analitici e tossicologici sul crome e suci derivati. Rend. 1st. Sup San., 26: 947-987.

Garcia, J.D. and Jennette, K.W., 1981. Electron-transport cytochrome P-450 system is involved in the microsomal metabolism of the carcinogen chromate. J. Inorg. Biochem., 14, 281-295.

Gentile, J.M., Hyde, K. and Schubert, J., 1981. Chromium genotoxicity as influenced by complexation and rate effects. Toxicol. Letters, 7, 439-448.

Glinsmann, W.H., Feldman, F.J. and Mertz, W., 1966. Plasma chromium after glucose administration. Science, 152, 1243-1245.

Glinsmann, W.H. and Mertz, W., 1966. Effect of trivalent chromium on glucose tolerance. Metab. Clin. Med., 15, 50-520.

Goldman, M. and Karotkin, R.H., 1935. Acute potassium bichromate poisoning. Amer. J. Med., Sci., 189, 400-403.

Gomes, E.R., 1972. Incidence of chromium-induced lesions among electroplating workers in Brazil. Ind. Med., 41, 21-25.

Gormican, A., 1970. Inorganic elements in foods used in hospital menus. J. Am. Diet. Assoc., 56, 397-403.

Gray, S.J. and Sterling, K., 1950. The tagging of red cells and plasma proteins with radioactive chromium. J. Chem. Invest., 29, 1604-1613.

Grogan, G.H., 1957. Experimental studies on metal carcinogenesis. Cancer (NY), 10, 625-630.

Guillemin, M.P. and Berode, M., 1978. A study of the difference in chromium exposure in workers in two types of electroplating process. Ann. Occup. Hyg., 21, 105-112.

Guthrie, B.E., 1973. Daily dietary intakes of zinc, copper, manganese, chromium and cadmium by some New Zealand women. Proc. Univ. Otago Med. Sch., 51, 47-49.

Guthrie, B.E., 1975. Chromium, manganese, copper, zinc and cadmium content of New Zealand foods. N.Z. Med. J., 82, 418-424.

Guthrie, B.E., 1982. The nutritional role of chromium. Chapter 6 of: Langard, S. (Ed.), Biological and Environmental Aspects of Chromium. Elsevier Biomedical Press, Amsterdam, pp. 117-148.

Gylseth, B., Gundersen, N. and Langård, S., 1977. Evaluation of chromium exposure based on a simplified method for urinary chromium determination. Scand. J. Work Environ. Health, 3, 28-31.

Hadjimarkos, D.M., 1967. Effect of trace elements in drinking water on dental caries. J. Pediat., 70, 967-969.

Hambidge, K.M., 1971. Chromium nutrition in the mother and growing child. In: Mertz, W. and Cornatzer, W.E. (Eds.) Newer Trace Elements in Nutrition. Marcel Dekker Inc., New York.

Hambidge, K.M and Baum, J.D., 1972. Hair chromium concentrations of human newborn and changes during infancy. Am. J. Clin. Nutr., 25, 376-379.

Harris, D.C., 1977. Different metal binding properties of the two sites of human transferrin. Biochem., 16, 560-564.

Hartford, W.H., 1979. Chromium compounds. In: Kirk, R.E. and Othmer, D.F. (Eds.). Kirk-Othmar Encyclopedia of Chemical Technology. 3rd Edit. Vol. 6: Chocolate and Cocoa to Copper. John Wiley & Sons, New York, 82-120.

Hayes, R.B., 1982. Carcinogenic effects of chromium. Chapter 10 of: Langård, S. (Ed.), Biological and Environmental Aspects of Chromium. Elsevier Biomedical Press, Amsterdam, pp. 221-247.

Hopkins, L.L. Jr., 1965. Distribution in the rat of physiological amounts of injected Cr^{51}(III) with time. Am. J. Physiol. 209, 731-735.

Hopkins, L.L. Jr., and Schwarz, K., 1964. Chromium (III) binding to serum proteins, specifically siderophilin. Biochim. Biophys. Acta. <u>90</u>, 484-491.

Hueper, W.C., 1966. Occupational and environmental cancers of the respiratory system. Recent Results Cancer Res., <u>3</u>, 1-214.

Hunter, W.C. and Roberts, J.M., 1933. Experimental study of the effects of potassium bichromate on the monkey's kidney. Amer. J. Path., <u>9</u>, 133-147.

IARC, 1979. Chemicals and Industrial Processes Associated with Cancer in Humans. IARC Monographs, Volumes 1 to 20 (Supplement 1). WHO International Agency for Research on Cancer, Lyon, Switzerland.

IARC, 1980. IARC Monographs on the Evaluation of the Carcinogenic Risk of Chemicals to Humans. Volume 23, Some Metals and Metallic Compounds. WHO International Agency for Research on Cancer, Lyon, Switzerland.

ICRP Task Group On Lung Dynamics, 1966. Deposition and retention models for internal dosimetry of the human respiratory tract. Health Phys., <u>12</u>, 173-207.

ICRP Publication 23, 1975. Report of the Task Group on the Reference Man. Pergamon Press, Oxford.

ICRP Publication 30, 1980. Limits for Intakes of Radionuclides by Workers. Part 2. Pergamon Press, Oxford.

Imbus, H.R., Cholak, J., Miller, L.H. and Sterling, T., 1963. Boron, cadmium, chromium and nickel in blood and urine: a survey of American Working men. Arch. Environ. Health, <u>6</u>, 296-295.

Ingrand, J., 1964. Contribution á l'étude des propertiés biologiques des composés marqués au radiochrom Cr-51. CEA-R-2585.

Ivankovic, S. and Preusmann, R., 1975. Absence of toxic and carcinogenic effects after administration of high doses of chromic oxide pigments in subacute and long-term feeding experiments in rats. Fd. Cosmet. Toxicol., <u>13</u>, 347-351.

Iyengar, G.V., Kollmer, W.E. and Bowen, H.J.M., 1978. The Elemental Composition of Human Tissues and Body Fluids. Verlag Chemie, Weinheim.

Jennette, K.W., 1979. Chromate metabolism in liver microsomes. Biol. Trace Elem. Res., <u>1</u>, 55-62.

Jett, R. Jr., Pierce, J.O. II and Stemmer, K.L., 1968. Toxicity of alloys of ferrochromium III. Transport of Chromium (III) by rat serum protein studied by immunoelectrophoretic analysis and autoradiography. Arch. Environ. Health, <u>17</u>, 29-34.

Joseph, K.T., Panday, V.K., Raut, S.J. and Soman, S.D., 1968. Per capita daily intake of trace elements from vegetables, fruits, and drinking water in India. Atom. Absorpt. Newslett., <u>7</u>, 25-27.

Kaufman, D.B., DiNicola, W., and McIntosh, R., 1970. Am. J. Dis. Child., 119, 374-376.

Joules, 1932. Cited in: Langárd, 1980. No bibliographic details provided.

Kelly, W.F., Ackrill, P., Day, J.P., O'Hara, M., Tye, C.T., Burton, I., Orton, C. and Harris, M., 1982. Cutaneous absorption of trivalent chromium: tissue levels and treatment by exchange transfusion. Br. J. Ind. Med., 39, 397-400.

Kirchgessner, M., 1959. Wecselbeziehungen zwischen Spurenelementen in Futtermitteln und tierischen Substanzen sowie Abhängigkeitsverhältnisse zwischen einzelnen Elementen bei der Retention. II. Mitteilung Wechselbeziehungen zwischen einzelnen Spurenelementen im Wiesengras und-Leu. Z. Tierphysiol. Tierern. Futtermittelkunde, 14, 165-175.

Kirkpatrick, D.C. and Coffin, D.E., 1974. The trace metal content of representative Canadian diets in 1970 and 1971. J. Inst. Can. Sci. Technol. Aliment., 7, 56-58.

Kirkpatrick, D.C. and Coffin, D.E., 1975a. J. Sci. Food Agric., 26, 99-

Kirkpatrick, D.C. and Coffin, D.E., 1975b. J. Sci. Food Agric., 26, 43-

Kleinfeld, M. and Rosso, A., 1965. Ulcerations of the nasal septum due to inhalation of chromic acid mist. Ind. Med. Surg., 34, 242-243.

Knopp, R.H., 1982. Altered chromium excretion in pregnancy: a physiological change? Am. J. Clin. Nutr., 35, 776-778.

Korst, D.R., 1968. Blood volume and red blood cell survival. Radioactive chromium (^{51}Cr). In: Wagner, H.J. Jr. (Ed.) Principles of Nuclear Medicine. W.B. Saunders, Philadelphia, 429-443.

Kretzschmar, J.G., Delespual, I., De Rijick, T.H. and Verduyn, G., 1977. The Belgian network for the determination of heavy metals. Atmos. Environ., 11, 263-271.

Kumpulainen, J.T., Vuovi, E., Makinen, S. and Kara, R., 1980. Dietary chromium intake of lactating Finnish mothers: effect on the Cr content of their breast milk. Br. J. Nutr., 44, 257-263.

Kumpulainen, J.T., Wolf, W.R., Veillon, C. and Mertz, W., 1979. Determination of chromium in selected United States diets. J. Agric. Food Chem., 27, 490-494.

Lane, B.P. and Mass, M.J., 1977. Carcinogenicity and co-carcinogenicity of chromium carbonyl in heterotrophic tracheal grafts. Cancer Res., 37, 476-1479.

Langárd, S., 1977. The fate of chromium after intravenous administration of Na$_2$ ^{51}CrO$_4$ and CrCl$_3$. 6H$_2$O to the rat. M.Sc. Thesis Toxicol., Univ. of Surrey. Guildford, 66p.

Langárd, S., 1979. The time-related subcellular distribution of chromium in the rat liver cell after intravenous administration of $Na_2{}^{51}CrO_4$. Biol. Trace Elem. Res., 1, 45-54.

Langárd, S., 1980. Chromium. In: Weldon, H. (Ed.). Metals in the Environment. Academic Press, New York (USA), 111-132.

Langárd, S., 1982. Absorption, transport and excretion of chromium in man and animals. Chapter 7 of: Langárd, S. (Ed.) Biological and Environmental Aspects of Chromium, Elsevier Biomedical Press, Amsterdam, pp. 149-169.

Langárd, S., Gundersen, N., Tsalev, D.L. and Gylseth, B., 1978. Whole blood chromium excretion in the rat after zinc chromate inhalation. Acta pharmacol. et toxicol., 42, 142-149.

Langárd, S. and Hensten-Pettersen, A., 1981. Chromium toxicology. In: Williams, D.F. (Ed.) Systemic Aspects of Biocompatibility, Vol. 1. CRC Press, Boca Rato, Florida, pp. 143-161.

Langárd, S. and Norseth, T., 1975. A cohort study of bronchial carcinomas in workers producing chromate pigments. Br. J. Ind. Med., 32, 62-65.

Leland, H.V., Luoma, S.N., Elder, J.F. and Wilkes, D.J., 1978. Heavy metals and trace elements. J. Water Pollut. Control Fed., 50, 1469-1514.

Léonard, A. and Lauwerys, R.R., 1980. Carcinogenicity and mutagenicity of chromium. Mutation Res., 76, 227-239.

Levander, O.A., 1975. Selenium and chromium in human nutrition. J. Am. Diet. Assoc., 66, 338-344.

Levine, R.A. Streeten, D.H.P. and Doisy, R.J., 1968. Effects of oral chromium supplementation on the glucose tolerance of elderly human subjects. Metab. Clin. Exp., 17, 114-125.

Lidén, S. and Lundberg, E., 1979. Penetration of chromium in intact human skin in vivo. J. Invest. Dermetol., 72, 42-45.

Lilien, D.L., Spivak, J.L. and Goldman, I.D., 1970. Chromate transport in human leucocytes. J. Clin. Invest., 49, 1551-1557.

Löfroth, G., 1978. The mutagenicity of hexavalent chromium is decreased by microsomal metabolism. Naturwissenschaften, 65, 207-208.

Mackenzie, R.D., Anwar, R.A., Byerrum, R.U. and Hoppert, G.A., 1959. Absorption and distribution of Cr^{51} in the albino rat. Arch. Biochem. Biophys., 79, 200-205.

Machle, W. and Gregorias, F., 1948. Cancer of the respiratory system in the United States chromate-producing industry. Publ. Health Rep. (Wash.), 63, 1114-1127.

Mancuso, T.F., and Hueper, W.C., 1951. Occupational cancer and other health hazards in a chromate plant: 1. Lung cancers in chromate workers. Ind. Med. Surg., 20, 358-363.

Masironi, R., Wolf, W. and Mertz, W., 1973. Chromium in refined and unrefined sugars - possible nutritional implications in the aetiology of cardiovascular diseases. Bull, W.H.O., 49, 322-324.

Medvedeva, V.I., 1966. Chromium content in newborn blood and maternal venous and retroplacental blood and milk. Chem. Abstr., 64: 20136. (Translated from, Dokl. Akad. Belorussk. SSR, 10, 98-100).

Mertz, W., 1969. Chromium occurrence and function in biological systems. Physiol. Rev., 49, 163-239.

Mertz, W. and Roginski, E.E., 1971. Chromium metabolism: the glucose tolerance factor. In: Mertz, W. and Cornatzer, W.E. (Eds.). Newer Trace Elements in Nutrition. Marcel Dekker, New York (USA), 123-153.

Mertz, W., Roginski, E.E., Feldman, F.J., and Thurman, D.E., 1970. Dependence of chromium transfer into the rat embryo on the chemical form. J. Nutr., 99, 363-367.

Mertz, W., Roginski, E.E. and Reba, R.G., 1965. Biological activity and fate of trace quanities of intravenous chromium (III) in the rat. Am. J. Physiol., 209, 489-494.

Mertz, W., and Schwarz, K., 1954. Effect of adrenaline and glucose on the terminal phase of dietary necrotic liver degenration. Federation Proc., 13, 469.

Mertz, W. Toepfer, E., Roginski, E.E. and Polansky, M.M., 1974. Present knowledge of the role of chromium. Fed. Proc., 33, 2275-2280.

Moeschlin, S., 1972. Klinik and Therapie der Vergiflungen 5th Edit. Georg Thieme Verlag, Stuttgart, 109-112.

Morrow, P.E., Gibb, F.R., Davies, H., and Fisher, M., 1968. Dust removal from the lung parenchyma: an investigation of clearance stimulants. Toxicol. Appl. Pharmacol., 12, 372-396.

Mosinger, M., and Fiorentini, H., 1954. On the pathology of chromates. First experimental researches. Arch. Mal. Prof. Med. Trav. Secur. Soc., 15, 187-199.

Murakami, Y., Suzuki, Y., Yamagata, T. and Yamagata, N., 1965. Chromium and manganese in Japanese diet. J. Radiat. Res., 6, 105-110.

Mutti, A., Cavatorata, A., Pedroni, C., Borghi, A., Giaroli, C. and Franchini, I., 1979a. The role of chromium accumulation in the relationship between airborne and urinary chromium in welders. Int. Arch. Occup. Environ. Health, 43, 123-133.

Mutti, A., Cavatorta, A., Borghi, L., Canal, M., Giarol, C. and Franchini, I., 1979. Distribution and urinary excretion of chromium. Studies on rats after administration of single and repeated doses of potassium dichromate. Med. Lavaro, 3, 171-179.

Nater, J.P., 1962. Possible causes of chromate eczema. Ned. Tijdschr. Geneeskd., 706, 1429-1431.

National Academy of Sciences of the United States, 1974. Chromium. NAS, Washington, 155p.

National Institute for Occupational Safety and Health, 1975. Criteria for a recommended standard. Occupational exposure to chromium (VI). NIOSH-76-129, Cincinnati, Ohio.

Norseth, T., 1981. The carcinogenicity of chromium. Environ. Health Perspect., 40, 121-130.

Norseth, T., Alexander, J., Aaseth, J. and Langard, S., 1982. Biliary excretion of chromium in the rat: a role of glutathione. Acta Pharmacol. et Toxicol., 51, 450-455.

Onkelinx, C., 1977. Compartment analysis of metabolism of chromium (III) in rats of various ages. Am. J. Physiol., 232, E478-E484.

Oshaki, Y., Abe, S., Kimura, K., Tsuneta, Y., Mikami, H. and Murao, M., 1978. Lung cancer in Japanese chromate workers. Thorax, 33, 372-374.

Pedersen, N.B., 1982. The effects of chromium on the skin. Chapter 11 of: Langárd, S. (Ed.) Biological and Environmental Aspects of Chromium. Elsevier Biomedical Press, Amsterdam, pp. 249-275.

Pedersen, N.B., Bertilson, G., Fregert, S., Lidén, K. and Rosman, H., 1969. Disappearance of chromium injected intracutaneously. Int. Arch. Allerg., 36, 82-88.

Pedersen, N.B., Fregert, S., Naversten, Y. and Rosman, H., 1970. Patch testing and absorption of chromium. Acta Dermatovener, 50, 431-434.

Pedersen, N.B. and Naversten, Y., 1973. Disappearance of chromium (III) trichloride injected intravenously. Acta Dermatovener, 53, 127-132.

Pierce, J.O. II. and Cholak, J., 1966. Lead chromium and molybdenum by atomic absorption. A.M.A. Arch. Environ. Health, 13, 208-212.

Piver, M.S., Barlow, J.J., Lele, S.B., Bakshi, S., Parthasarathy, K.L and Bender, M.A., 1982. Intraperitoneal chromic phosphate in peritoneoscopic-ally confirmed Stage I ovarian adenocarcinoma. Am. J. Obstet. Gynecol., 144, 836-840.

Pokrovskaya, L.V. and Shabynina, N.K., 1973. Carcinogenic hazard in the production of chromium ferroalloys. NTC 80-10898-06J. (Translated from Gig. Tr. Prof. Zabol., 17, 23-26).

Polak, L., Turk, J.L. and Frey, J.R., 1973. Studies on contact hypersensitivity to chromium compounds. Progr. Allergy, 17, 145-226.

Pribulada, L.A., 1963. The chromium content of hollow bones of the human fetus. Chem. Abs., 59, 3142. (Translated from Dokl. Acad. Belorussk. SSR, 7, 135-136).

Prins, H.K., 1962. The binding of ^{51}Cr by human erthrocytes. Vox Sang., 7, 370-372.

Rao, C.M. and Rao, B.S., 1980. Nutr. Metab., 24, 244-254.

Rao, B.S., Vijaysarathy, C., Rao, C.N. and Nagarajan, V., 1977. Absorption of chromium from chromium treated parboiled rice. Indian J. Med. Res., 65, 82-88.

Reichelderfer, T.E., 1968. South Med. J., 61, 96-97.

Rollinson, C.L. (1973). Chromium, molybdenum and tungsten. In: Comprehensive Inorganic Chemistry. Pergamon Press, Oxford, 623-769.

Royle, H., 1975. Toxicity of chromic acid in the chromium plating industry. Environ. Res., 10, 39-53.

Salmon, L., Atkins, D.H.F., Fischer, E.M.R. and Law, D.V., 1977. Retrospective analysis of air samples in the UK. 1957-1974. J. Radioanal. Chem. 37, 867-880.

Samitz, M.H., 1955. Some dermatologic aspects of the chromate problem. J. Industrial Health, 11, 361-367.

Samitz, M.H., Katz, S. and Shrager, J., 1967. Studies of the diffusion of chromium compounds through skin. J. Invest. Dermatol., 48, 514-520.

Samitz, M.H., Scheiner, D.M. and Katz, S.A., 1968. Ascorbic acid in the prevention of chrome dermatitis. Mechanism of inactivation of chromium. Arch. Environ. Health, 17, 44-45.

Samitz, M.H., Shrager, J. and Katz, S., 1962. Studies on the prevention of injurious effects of chromates in industry. Ind. Med. Surg., 31, 427-432.

Sanderson, C.J., 1976. The uptake and retention of chromium by cells. Transplant., 21, 526-529.

Sanderson, C.J., 1982. Applications of [51]Chromium in cell biology and medicine. Chapter 5 of: Langård, S. (Ed.) Biological and Environmental Aspects of Chromium. Elsevier Biomedical Press, Amsterdam, pp. 101-116.

Saner, G., 1981. Urinary chromium excretion during pregnancy and its relationship with intravenous glucose loading. Am. J. Clin. Nutr., 34, 1676-1679.

Sargent, T. III, Lim, J.H. and Jenson, R.L., 1979. Reduced chromium retention in patients with haemochromatosis, a possible basis of haemochromatic diabetes. Metab., 28, 70-79.

Sayato, Y., Nakamuro, K., Matsui, S. and Ando, M., 1980. Metabolic fate of chromium compounds. 1. Comparative behaviour of chromium in rat administered with Na_2[51]CrO_4 and [51]$CrCl_3$. J. Pharm. Dyn., 3, 17-23.

Schelenz, R., 1977. Dietary intake of 25 elements by man estimated by neutron activation analysis. J. Radional. Chem., 37, 539-548.

Schlatter, C. and Kissling, U., 1973. Beitr. Gericht. Med., 30, 382-388.

Schlettwein-Gsell, D. and Mommsen-Straub, S., 1971. Übersicht spuren-elemente in Lebensmitteln III. Chrom. Int. Z. Vitaminforsch., 41, 116-123.

Schroeder, H.A., 1968. The role of chromium in mammalian nutrition. Am. J. Clin. Nutr., 21, 230-244.

Schroeder, H.A., 1970. Chromium. Air Quality Monograph No. 70-15. American Petroleum Institute, Washington, 28p.

Schroeder, H.A., 1971. Losses of vitamins and trace minerals resulting from processing and preservation of foods. Am. J. Clin. Nutr., 24, 562-573.

Schroeder, H.A., Balassa, J.J. and Tipton, I.H., 1962. Abnormal trace metals in man - chromium. J. chron. Dis., 15, 941-964.

Schroeder, H.A., Balassa, J.J. and Vinton, W.H. Jr., 1964. Chromium, lead, cadmium, nickel and titanium in mice: effect on mortality, tumors and tissue levels. J. Nutr., 83, 239-250.

Schroeder, H.A., Balassa, J.J. and Vinton, W.H. Jr., 1965. Chromium, cadmium and lead in rats: effects on life span, tumors and tissue levels. J. Nutr., 86, 51-66.

Schubert, G.E., Gebhard, K. and Honlëin, F., 1970. Virchows. Arch. A., 351, 68-82.

Sklan, D., Dubrov, D., Eisner, U. and Hurwitz, S., 1975. ^{51}Cr-EDTA, ^{91}Y and ^{141}Ce as nonabsorbed reference substances in the gastrointestinal tract of the chicken. J. Nutr., 105, 1549-1552.

Sluis-Cremer, G.K. and DuToit, R.S.J., 1968. Pneumoconiosis in chromite mines in South Africa. Brit. J. Ind. Med., 25, 63-67.

Soman, S.D., Panday, V.K., Joseph, K.T. and Raut, S.J., 1969. Daily intake of some major and trace elements. Health Phys., 17, 35-40.

Stern, R.M., 1982. Chromium compounds, production and occupational exposure. Chapter 2 of: Langárd, S. (Ed.) Biological and Environmental Aspects of Chromium. Elsevier Biomedical Press, Amsterdam, pp.5-47.

Stocks, P., Comminis, B.T. and Aubrey, K.V., 1961. A study of polycyclic hydrocarbons and trace elements in smoke in Merseyside and other northern localities. Int. J. Air Water Poll., 4, 141-153.

Sunderman, F.W., Jr., 1979. Mechanisms of metal carcinogenesis. Biol. Trace Element Res., 1, 63-86.

Swensson, O., 1977. Experimentella Undersökningar över Fibrigenetiska Effekten av Kromit. Arbete och Hälse No. 2., Stockholm.

Tabor, E.C. and Warren, W.V., 1958. Distribution of certain metals in the atmosphere of some American cities. Arch. Industr. Health, 17, 145-151.

Tandon, S.K., Behari, J.R. and Kachru, D.N., 1979. Distribution of chromium in poisoned rats. Toxicol., 13, 29-34.

Tandon, S.K. and Gaur, J.B., 1977. Chelation in metal intoxication. IV. Removal of chromium from organs of experimentally poisoned animals. Clin. Toxicol., 11, 257-

Tipton, I.H. and Stewart, P.L. 1967. Long-term study of intake and excretion of stable elements. Health Physics Division Annual Progress Report for Period Ending July 31, 1967. ORNL-4168, 283-287.

Tipton, I.H. and Stewart, P.L., 1969. In: Hemphill, D.D. (Ed.) Trace Substances in Environmental Health, Vol. 3. University of Missouri, Columbia, pp. 305-330.

Tipton, I.H., Stewart., P.L. and Kickson, J., 1969. Patterns of elemental excretion in long term balance studies. Health Phys., 16, 455-462.

Tipton, I.H., Stewart, P.L. and Martin, P.G., 1966. Trace elements in diet and excreta. Health Phys., 12, 1683-1689.

Underwood, E.J., 1977. Trace Elements in Human and Animal Nutrition. 4th Edit. Academic Press, New York.

Varo, P. and Koivistoinen, P., 1980. Mineral element composition of Finnish foods XII. General discussion and nutritional evaluation. Acta Agric. Scand. Suppl., 22, 165-171.

Visek, M.J., Whitney, I.B., Kuhn, U.S.G. III and Comar, C.L., 1953. Metabolism of Cr[51] by animals as influenced by chemical state. Proc. Soc. Exp. Biol. Med., 84, 610-615.

Vittorio, P.V. and Wight, E.W., 1963. The effect of x-irradiation on the chromium-51 content of liver nucleic acids and proteins. Can. J. Biochem. Physiol., 41, 1349-1354.

Vittorio, P.V., Wight, E.W. and Sinnott, B.E., 1962. The distribution of chromium 51 in mice after intraperitoneal injection. Can. J. Biochem. Physiol., 40, 1677-1683.

Wahlberg, J.E., 1965. "Disappearance measurements", a method for studying percutaneous absorption of isotope-labelled compounds emitting gamma-rays. Acta Dermatovener, 45, 397-414.

Wahlberg, J.E., 1968a. Percutaneous absorption from chromium (^{51}Cr) solutions of different pH, 1.4-12.8. Dermatologica, 137, 17-25.

Wahlberg, J.E., 1968b. The effect of anionic, cationic, and nonionic detergents on the percutaneous absorption of sodium chromate (^{51}Cr) in the guinea pig. Acta Dermatovener, 48, 549-555.

Wahlberg, J.E. and Skog, E., 1965. Percutaneous absorption of trivalent and hexavelent chromium. Arch. Dermatol., 92, 315-318.

Walker, M.A. and Page, L., 1977. J. Am. Diet. Assoc., 70, Nutritive content of college meals. 260-266.

Walsh, E.N., 1953. Chromate hazards in industry. J. Amer. med. Ass., 153, 1305-1308.

Waterhouse, J.A.H., 1975. Cancer among chromium platers. Br. J. Cancer, 32, 262.

White, H.S., 1969. Inorganic elements in weighted diets of girls and young women. J. Am. Diet. Assoc., 55, 38-43.

Williams, C.D., 1969. Asthma related to chromium compounds: report of two cases and review of the literature on chromate diseases. N.Z. Med. J., 30, 482-490.

World Health Organization, 1973. Trace Elements in Human Nutrition. WHO Tech. Rep. Ser., 532, Geneva.

Yoshikawa, H. and Hara, N., 1980. Distribution of chromium in organs of mice injected subcutaneously daily with trivalent and hexavalent chromium. Jap. J. Ind. Health, 22, 126-127.

Zook, E.G., Green, F.E. and Morris, E.R., 1970. Nutrient composition of selected wheats and wheat products. VI. Distribution of manganese, copper, nickel, zinc, magnesium, lead, tin, cadmium, chromium, and selenium as determined by atomic absorption spectroscopy and colorimetry. Cereal Chem., 47: 720-

Zvaifler, N., 1944. Chromic poisoning resulting from inhalation of mist developed from 5% chromic acid solution; medical aspects of chromic acid poisoning. J. Industr. Toxicol., 26, 124-126.

Appendix 7
Asbestos

CONTENTS

7.1 INTRODUCTION

There is an immense literature on asbestos and it has been possible to consider only a small fraction of it herein. Emphasis has been on the use of reviews, supplemented by recent research papers. However, the primary literature on metabolism has been discussed in greater detail.

7.1.1 Physical and chemical properties of asbestos

The physical and chemical properties of asbestos have been discussed in several major reviews (Harington, 1965; 1976; Harington et al., 1975; International Agency for Research on Cancer, 1977; Langer and Wolff, 1977; Speil and Leineweber, 1969; Zielhuis, 1977). Asbestos is a generic term for a variety of hydrated silicate minerals with the common attribute of being able to be separated into relatively soft silky fibres (Speil and Leineweber, 1969). Two general types are recognised. These are the serpentines and amphiboles. The sole member of the serpentine class is chrysotile, which is by far the most common of the asbestiform minerals and, in 1969, accounted for more than 95% of asbestos fibre produced (Speil and Leineweber, 1969). There are five recognised asbestiform varieties of amphibole; crocidolite, amosite, anthophyllite, tremolite and actinolite. Although the amphiboles are common rock forming minerals, their asbestiform varieties are much less abundant than chrysotile (Speil and Leineweber, 1969).

With respect to occurrence, chrysotile and amphibole fibres are found in entirely different geological formations. Chrysotile was most probably formed as a result of two separate metamorphic changes of ultrabasic origin, involving recrystallisation of serpentine as part of the second change. In contrast, asbestiform amphibole minerals are found in metamorphised rocks of sedimentary origin (Speil and Leineweber, 1969).

7.1.1.1 Properties of chrysotile

Chrysotile has a layered structure in which a silicate sheet is attached to a brucite, $Mg(OH)_2$, layer in which two out of every three hydroxyls are replaced by the apical oxygens of the silica tetrahedra. Because of a dimensional mismatch between the silica and brucite layers, the resulting double layer structure is curved, with the brucite being on the outside of the curve (Speil and Leineweber, 1969). It is this curvature which gives fibrils of chrysotile their characteristic tubular form [see the electron micrographs presented by Speil and Leineweber (1969); Langer et al. (1978) and Kannerstein et al. (1978)]. The centre of the fibril is thought to be filled with amorphous material, but some voids may occur (Harington et al., 1975). Chrysotile fibres tend to consist of bundles of fibrils which are often curvilinear with splayed ends. Fibril dimensions range in the following manner (Langer et al., 1974):

-    diameter of central capillary (if present)   2-4.5 nm
-    average fibril diameter   30-35 nm

TABLE 1

THE CHEMICAL COMPOSITION OF CHRYSOTILE ASBESTOS[1]

Chemical	Percentage composition					
	Theoretical	Jeffrey Mine, Quebec	New Idria, California[2]	Arizona	Africa, Transvaal	Russian
SiO_2	43.4	44.1	38.4	41.07	41.83	42.09
MgO	43.5	41.6	39.9	42.35	41.39	41.68
Fe_2O_3	-	0.92	1.1	0.42	1.29	4.01
FeO	-	0.80	2.4	0.14	0.08	-
Al_2O_3	-	0.34	0.44	0.55	0.30	0.79
Cr_2O_3	-	0.019	0.31	0.03	-	-
NiO	-	0.010	0.18	Trace	-	-
Mn_2O_2	-	0.03	0.10	0.07	0.04	-
CaO	-	0.04	0.96	1.02	Trace	-
TiO_2	-	0.01	0.05	0.01	0.02	-
Na_2O	-	0.06	0.04	Trace	-	-
K_2O	-	0.04	0.04	0.03	-	-
H_2O	13.1	13.2	14.0	13.97	13.66	12.9

Notes:

(1)   From Speil and Leineweber (1969)

(2)   Coalinga chrysotile, which is morphologically different
      from other chrysotiles

More detailed information on fibril diameters for different grades of chrysotile was given by Harington et al. (1975). The normal morphology which is ascribed to chrysotile is modified substantially by processes such as ball milling (Langer et al. 1974) and this needs to be taken into account when considering its metabolism.

The chemical composition of chrysotiles varies with their place of origin and some illustrative data on this topic have been given by Speil and Leineweber (1969). These data are presented in Table 1. Physical properties of chrysotile have been summarised by Zielhuis (1977) and were discussed in detail by Speil and Leineweber (1969). The material is usually flexible, silky and tough, is usually white to pale green in colour, has a density of 2.55 g cm^{-3}, and decomposes at 450 to 700°C. It undergoes fairly rapid attack in acids, but exhibits very good resistance to alkalis.

7.1.1.2   Properties of the amphiboles

The basic crystal form of the amphibole minerals is less complicated than that of the serpentines. The basic structural unit is a double silica chain, Si_4O_{11}. These chains are paired 'back-to-back' with a layer of hydrated cations between, to satisfy the negative charges of the silica chains. The final structure is formed by the stacking of these sandwich ribbons in an ordered array (Speil and Leineweber, 1969). The various minerals in the amphibole group are characterised by the cations which occur in the structure. The principal cations are magnesium, iron, calcium and sodium. Because the bonding between the ribbons is rather weak, the crystals are easily cleaved. If the cleavage is very facile, the result is an asbestiform mineral (Speil and Leineweber, 1969). Chemical compositions for the various asbestiform amphiboles are listed in Table 2 and are discussed in an IARC Publication (International Agency for Research on Cancer, 1977). Physical properties of the various amphiboles have been summarised by Zielhuis (1977) and are listed in Table 3. Individual amphibole fibres tend to be straight and to exhibit very wide distributions in length and width. In addition to straight fibres, curved fibres are occasionally observed. Crocidolite appears to form curved fibres more often than the other amphibole asbestos types and, in all cases, the thinnest fibres predominate in the curved population (Langer et al., 1974).

7.1.1.3   Surface characteristics

The external surface of chrysotile fibres consists of magnesium hydroxide, so it is not surprising that the fibres behave in some respects as though they were composed of that substance (Speil and Leineweber, 1969). This is manifested in the electrokinetic behaviour of chrysotile, which exhibits a negative surface charge above a pH value of 11.8. Below this pH value the surface charge is positive; being relatively constant down to pH 6, increasing to a peak at ~pH 3.5 and then decreasing. The increase between pH 6 and pH 3.5 has been attributed to the removal of hydroxyl groups from the surface with the resultant exposure of the magnesium ions. At lower pH, the magnesium ions are removed and the silica surface is exposed (Speil and Leineweber, 1969).

TABLE 2

THE CHEMICAL COMPOSITION OF AMPHIBOLE ASBESTOS

Chemical	Percent composition				
	Crocidolite	Amosite	Anthophyllite	Actinolite	Tremolite
SiO_2	49-53	49-53	56-58	51-56	55-60
MgO	0-3	1-7	28-34	15-20	21-26
FeO	13-20	34-44	3-12	5-15	0-4
Fe_2O_3	17-20	-	-	0-3	0-0.5
Al_2O_3	0-0.2	-	0.5-1.5	1.5-3	0-2.5
CaO	0.3-2.7	-	-	10-12	11-13
K_2O	0-0.4	0-0.4	-	0-0.5	0-0.6
Na_2O	4.0-8.5	Trace	-	0.5-1.5	0-1.5
H_2O	2.5-4.5	2.5-4.5	1.0-6.0	1.5-2.5	0.5-2.5

Note:

From Speil and Leineweber (1969)

TABLE 3

PHYSICAL CHARACTERISTICS OF AMPHIBOLE FORMS OF ASBESTOS

Characteristics	Crocidolite	Amosite	Anthophyllite	Tremolite	Actinolite
Colour	Blue	Light grey to pale brown	White to grey pale grey	White to grey	Pale to dark green
Decomposition temperature(°C)	400–600	600–800	600–850	950–1040	620–960
Density g cm^{-3}	3.3–3.4	3.4–3.5	2.85–3.1	2.9–3.1	3.0–3.2
Resistance to acids	Good	Attacked slowly	Very good	Very good	Attacked slowly
Resistance to alkalis	Good	Good	Very good	Good	Good
Texture	Flexible to brittle and tough	Usually brittle	Usually brittle	Usually brittle	

Note:

From Zielhuis (1977)

Chemically, the surface of the amphiboles is similar to that of silica. The electrokinetic charge is negative and smaller in magnitude than the positive charge of chrysotile (Speil and Leineweber, 1969).

The adsorption of materials to the surface of asbestos fibres has been discussed in detail by Speil and Leineweber (1969). Of particular interest, in the context of toxic effects, is the observation that oils, waxes and amino acids can be associated with asbestos either naturally or by contamination (Harington, 1965). Also, occasionally, impurities such as nickel-steel fragments are added to the product during the processing of chrysotile asbestos (International Agency for Research on Cancer, 1977).

7.1.1.4   Effects of milling

Langer et al. (1978) noted that mechanical milling of chrysotile asbestos is commonly used to produce short fibres for experimental purposes. They pointed out that such manipulation also decreases fibre crystallinity, alters Si-O and Mg-O interlayer bonding, induces co-ordination of changes in the brucite layer, diminishes the ability of the fibre to reduce specific free radicals and absorb organic molecules, and decreases haemolytic potency and antagonist sorption capabilities. In view of this, they suggested that results of biological experimentation with these materials must be interpreted with caution.

7.1.1.5   Standard reference samples

As can be seen from the above discussion, different samples of asbestos from different sources can have significantly different characteristics. Because of this, the Working Group on Asbestos and Cancer recommended, in October 1964, the preparation of standard reference samples of the main types of asbestos, i.e. amosite, anthophyllite, chrysotile and crocidolite. It was intended that such samples could be used as reference material for comparison with other asbestos types in which investigators might be especially interested and could do much to establish uniformity of experimental methods and procedures. It was also thought that information on the chemical and physical nature of the reference samples would lead to a better understanding of various factors involved and their relation to the biological response (Timbrell et al., 1968).

With respect to implementation of this recommendation, the principal asbestos mining companies in South Africa, Finland, Canada and Rhodesia were approached and, with their full co-operation, 3000 lb (1360 kg) of each of the following types were sent to Johannesburg to form the basis of the standard samples:

-   South African amosite;
-   Finnish anthophyllite;
-   Canadian chrysotile; one reference sample derived from material from eight mines pooled roughly in proportion to their annual production;
-   Rhodesian chrysotile;
-   South African crocidolite.

The samples were milled using a new mill. Settings of this mill were chosen so that the different standard samples would contain high, and approximately equal, proportions of respirable dust, would be distinctly fibrous, and would contain fibres up to 150 to 200 μm long, such as are found in mine and mill atmospheres and in lungs (Timbrell et al., 1968).

Properties of the various UICC standard reference samples have been summarised by Rendall (1970) and Timbrell (1970). Particular aspects considered included homogeneity, metal contamination, oil content, chemical composition, fibre length distributions, aerodynamic characteristics, specific surface area, effects of reagents, optical properties and electron diffraction properties. The reader is referred to Rendall (1970) and Timbrell (1970) for detailed data on these aspects.

7.1.2   History and production

Asbestos was known to the ancient Chinese and Egyptians, and, in prehistoric and classical times, was used in Finland to strengthen pots. The early Greeks called it a "fabulous stone", its non-combustible character and spinning qualities being well known (Harington, 1976).

Modern use of asbestos started in the last quarter of the nineteenth century and production increased with great rapidity. In sixty years, output increased over one thousand times, compared with fifty times for oil (Harington, 1976). Quantitatively, a cumulative total of somewhat less than 5×10^9 kg had been mined by 1930 (International Agency for Research on Cancer, 1977). More recent production figures, derived from the International Agency for Research on Cancer (1977) review, are tabulated below.

Year	World production (kg)	Percentage of production	
		Canada	USSR
1960	2.210×10^9	45	29
1970	3.490×10^9	44	30
1973	4.093×10^9	41	31
1974	4.115×10^9	40	33
1975	4.560×10^9	23	48
1976	5.178×10^9	29	44

Chrysoltile accounts for approximately 90% of the world production of asbestos. This fibre is found in several parts of the world (see Harington, 1976), with the main deposits being in Canada, the USSR and Southern Africa. Most amphibole asbestos is mined in South Africa, primarily crocidolite and some amosite. Some crocidolite is also found in Western Australia and Bolivia. Finland is the major source of anthophyllite (Harington, 1976). The distribution of asbestos production and utilisation has been illustrated by Becklake (1976). Major users are the USA, USSR, Japan and the various countries comprising the EEC.

7.1.3   Utilisation

In general, the construction industry accounts for two-thirds of asbestos usage. Over 3000 applications have been identified and important ones include asbestos cement, sheets and pipes, insulation materials, taping compounds, and floor and ceiling tiles. Sprayed asbestos materials are used for decorative and acoustic purposes, as well as for the fireproofing of structural elements in buildings (International Agency for Research on Cancer, 1977).

Friction materials constitute an important class of asbestos products. These include not only clutch facings and brakes for cars, lorries, railway carriages and aeroplanes, but also braking materials used widely in industry for machinery. Asbestos-containing gaskets are also often used (International Agency for Research on Cancer, 1977).

An extraordinary variety of other uses of asbestos are known, including papier maché materials used by school children, fire-proof clothing and gloves, and fillers for plastics. The International Agency for Research on Cancer (1977) has given a breakdown of the mass of asbestos used in various applications in the USA in 1974 and this is tabulated below.

Application	Use (in units of 10^6 kg)			
	Chrysotile	Crocidolite	Amosite	Anthophyllit
Asbestos cement pipe	168	33	0.9	0.18
Asbestos cement sheet	82		3.9	
Flooring products	139			
Roofing products	66		1.5	
Packing and gaskets	26	0.09		
Insulation, thermal	6.6		1.6	
Insulation, electrical	4.2			
Friction products	72			0.18
Coatings and compounds	34			
Plastics	15	0.18		0.63
Textiles	18			
Paper	57	0.18		
Other	33	0.36	0.45	
Total	720.8	33.81	8.35	0.99

7.2   EFFECTS OF ASBESTOS

The major effects of asbestos on man can be defined as fibrotic and carcinogenic. Major fibrotic effects include asbestosis, a progressive fibrosis of the lungs akin to silicosis, asbestos corns on the skin, the development of pleural plaques or pleural thickening, and benign pleural effusion. Cancer induction by asbestos is well established with respect to lung cancer and mesotheliomas of the pleura and peritoneum. There is an indication of an excess of cancers of the gastrointestinal tract and larynx in some exposed human populations, while excess cancers at other sites have been identified tentatively in individual epidemiological studies. A brief review of the effects of asbestos has been given by Becklake (1976). Other reviews which may be consulted include those of

Cooper (1967), Kannerstein et al. (1977), Casey et al. (1981) and Zaloga (1981). Cralley and Lainhart (1973) have discussed asbestos toxicology in relation to trace metal content, while Rahman et al. (1977) have discussed the biochemical basis of asbestos toxicity and have commented that the diverse biological effects of asbestos could be interrelated and explained in terms of a unified molecular mechanism in which silicic acid has a central role.

7.2.1   Asbestosis

Diffuse interstitial fibrosis of the lung associated with asbestos exposure was recognised in the early years of the twentieth century, but the term "asbestosis" to describe this pneumoconiosis was not suggested until 1927 (Becklake, 1976). It is usual to include fibrosis of the associated visceral pleura under this term, but not that of the parietal pleura. As Becklake (1976) has commented, "there is merit in maintaining this specific usage in line with the widely accepted use of the term 'pneumoconiosis', rather than to use the term 'asbestosis' in a generic sense to describe all asbestos-related diseases of the lung and pleura, even neoplasms."

In asbestosis, macroscopic changes of the lungs range from small areas of basal fibrosis to the fully developed case of a diffuse fine fibrosis affecting both lungs. This diffuse fibrosis appears to affect sub-pleural areas first, often quite extensively, before advancing into other lobes with the extension of the disease process. Lower lobes tend to be affected first, then middle lobes and eventually upper lobes. Small honeycomb cysts may be seen, in the lower lobes particularly, and honeycombing also tends to be concentrated sub-pleurally. The pleural surface is almost invariably involved in the fibrosis, but the hilar lymph nodes are not usually enlarged, or otherwise affected (Becklake, 1976). At a microscopic level, the early reaction in the interstitial tissue resembles that of other forms of interstitial pneumonia, with mixed leukocyte infiltration of the alveolar walls, moderate numbers of phagocytes in the alveoli, and varying degrees of organisation with fibrosis. In some cases, the early changes are concentrated at the level of the respiratory bronchiole, where reticulin fibres, macrophages and dust particles collect, leading subsequently to what has been termed the basic lesion of asbestosis, namely a peribronchiolar fibrosis. From here, the process extends outward to involve the surrounding alveoli, leading to diffuse alveolar wall thickening, with peribronchiolar and perivascular fibrosis (Becklake, 1976). Kannerstein et al. (1977) considered that the unit lesion is located in the alveoli arising from the respiratory bronchiole. In their view, it consists of an effusion of macrophages that engulf asbestos fibres. Reticulin is deposited with disintegration of macrophages and ultimate collagenisation. There is spreading of the fibrosis, with eventual linkage of the individual lesions and the formation of a fibrotic network.

It is noted that the fibrotic reaction of asbestosis almost certainly derives from the longer asbestos fibres. Gross (1974) has stated, "it has been the finding of research laboratories in Germany, England, South Africa and the United States that short-fibred asbestos dust, i.e. less than 5 μm in length, is incapable of causing fibrosis or cancer". This seems to be generally true, but some conflicting data on

the matter do exist (Holt et al., 1965). Distinctions in fibre size are
also thought to explain observations that different types of asbestos
give rise to different exposure-response relationships for fibrosis in
animals (Reeves et al., 1974, Davis et al., 1978) and man (Weill et al.,
1977), though effects of fibre structure and macrophage response may also
be involved (Hiett, 1978a).

For more information on the origin and pathogenesis of asbestosis,
the reader is referred to the reviews cited above and also to the
extensive original literature. Experimental asbestosis has been discussed
by many authors including Vorwald et al. (1951), Holt et al. (1965),
Davis (1965), Gross et al. (1967), Reeves et al. (1974), Davis et al.
(1978), Hiett (1978; 1978a). Epidemiological studies include those of
Enterline and Kendrick (1967), Rossiter et al. (1972), McDonald et al.
(1974), Elmes and Simpson (1977), Weill et al. (1977), and Liddell et al.
(1982). Changes in immunological status, subsequent to the induction of
pleural thickening and asbestosis, have been discussed by Kagan et al.
(1977).

7.2.2   Benign pleural disease

The pleural changes associated with asbestos were first noted in
1931. Several pleural reactions to asbestos exposure have subsequently
been described. Pleural thickening, particularly a discrete localised
thickening known as pleural plaque, is often the only radiogenic evidence
of exposure (Casey et al., 1981). Studies in occupationally exposed
populations have indicated that the prevalence of pleural plaques
increases with increasing exposure and that such plaques do not appear
before at least twenty years after the first exposure to asbestos. All
forms of asbestos appear to be capable of producing plaques, although
anthophyllite may be associated with the highest rates (Casey et al.,
1981). Pleural plaques occur as discrete, raised, grey-white lesions on
the inner surface of the rib cage and on the diaphragm (Casey et al.,
1981). Their distribution is irregular; they tend to be more marked over
the lower ribs, may follow or cross rib lines and may be concentrated in
the posterior, lateral, or anterior surfaces, but not the cartilaginous
portions. The diaphragm is usually involved, frequently in the area of
the central tendon. Plaques do not occur in the costophrenic angles or
over the apices. Also, mediastinal plaques have not been observed, but
the pleural surface of the pericardium is not infrequently involved,
particularly in the advanced case (Becklake, 1976).

Plaque formation appears, generally, to occur in areas free of adhe-
sions. Their thickness varies greatly and calcification, which is common,
appears unrelated to plaque thickness. Microscopically, plaques consist
of a 'basket weave' of cell-poor, collagenous, connective tissue, often
with calcium granules along the course of the collagen fibres (Becklake,
1976; Kannerstein et al., 1977). Elastic staining results suggest that
plaques are extra-pleural, developing between the pleura and its covering
layer of mesothelial cells (Becklake, 1976).

Coated asbestos fibres do not appear to have been found in
association with pleural plaques, but uncoated fibres have been observed
and electron microscopy has revealed that most plaques contain many small
fibres. Concentrations of these fibres are higher in the calcified zones
(Becklake, 1976).

For more detailed discussion on the pathology and epidemiology of pleural plaques, the reader is referred to reviews by Gross et al. (1970), Becklake (1976), Kannerstein et al. (1977) and Casey et al. (1981). In addition, it is noted that recent studies have implicated genetic factors (Charpin et al., 1981) and smoking habits (Weiss et al., 1981) as important aetiological factors.

With respect to the mechanism of induction of pleural plaques and pleural thickening, the situation is not clear. The comment by Gross et al. (1970) that "it almost seems as though the pleural involvement is metastatic" has been rendered invalid by the observation of sub-microscopic fibres in plaques. Becklake (1976) discussed two major hypotheses concerning the formation of plaques. These were:

- traumatisation of the parietal pleura during breathing by the penetration of sharp asbestos spicules; and
- intracellular transport via pulmonary lymphatics and retrograde spread via the chest wall lymphatics due to the massaging action of the respiratory muscles.

She also cited a descriptive model of asbestos movement and pleural involvement, but the mechanisms driving this movement were not identified. Overall, she concluded that it is most realistic to accept the conclusion that the pathogenesis of pleural plaques, that occur in association with asbestos exposure, is unknown. This conclusion has also been reached, more recently, by Casey et al. (1981).

Other benign pleural diseases which have been identified include pleural effusion and pulmonary pseudo-tumours. Exudative pleural reactions may occur in association with all the asbestos-related lung diseases, but may also be the primary, or most prominent, manifestation. Examination by thoracotomy shows variable pleural thickening, increased vascularity and varying degrees of interstitial pneumonitis (Sluis-Cremer and Webster, 1982; Becklake, 1976). On the basis of this associated pathology, benign pleural effusion is probably best considered as a limited manifestation of the fibrotic reactions of the lung and pleura to asbestos. Similar remarks can be made concerning clinical reports on pseudo-tumours (Hillerdal and Hemmingsson, 1980), described as localised fibrotic lesions of the visceral pleura with involvement of the underlying lung parenchyma.

7.2.3   Other non-carcinogenic effects

A variety of other non-carcinogenic effects of asbestos have been reported. These include early obstruction of the small airways of the lung (Di Menza et al., 1976), changes in lung function associated with fibrotic reactions (Kleinfeld et al., 1973; Weill et al., 1975; Weill et al., 1977; Lumley, 1977), changes in cAMP and alkaline phosphatase levels in bronchoalveolar lavage fluids of sheep exposed to asbestos for six months (Lemaine et al., 1981), inflammatory responses in rabbit skin (Hamilton et al., 1981) and biochemical changes associated with the presence of asbestos in the gut of the rat (Amacher et al., 1975; Jacobs et al., 1977; Jacobs and Richards, 1980). These are of limited significance and are not discussed further.

7.2.4   Lung cancer

The relationship between asbestos exposure and lung cancer incidence has been established unequivocally on the basis of a number of epidemiological studies of occupationally exposed groups of workers and a wide variety of animal experiments. These data have been discussed in a variety of reviews of asbestos toxicology (Wagner et al., 1971; Harington et al., 1975; Harington, 1976; Becklake, 1976; Selikoff, 1977; Kannerstein et al., 1977, International Agency for Research on Cancer, 1977; Zielhuis, 1977; Wagner et al., 1980; Casey et al., 1981).

With respect to epidemiological studies, Doll (1955) performed the first retrospective cohort study on a population of British asbestos textile workers. Subsequent studies included that of Selikoff et al. (1972), which demonstrated that exposure to amosite asbestos was associated with an increased risk of lung cancer; those of McDonald et al. (1974) and Dement et al. (1982), which demonstrated a relation between cumulative exposure and lung cancer mortality; those of Enterline and Henderson (1973) and Weill et al. (1977), which distinguished between risks in different occupations with exposures to different types of asbestos; as well as those of Knox et al. (1968), Elmes and Simpson (1977), Peto et al. (1977) and Newhouse et al. (1982).

Two important areas which have been investigated epidemiologically are the relation between ingestion of asbestos in drinking water and cancer mortality, and the interactions between smoking and asbestos in the induction of lung cancer.

With respect to asbestos in drinking water, Wigle (1977) reported that the mortality experience of twenty two municipalities in Quebec, grouped by evidence of asbestos fibres in water, did not reveal any evidence of excess cancer mortality that could be attributed to exposure to asbestos in drinking water.

Evidence for an interaction between asbestos and smoking in the induction of lung cancer has been discussed by Selikoff and his co-workers (Selikoff et al., 1968; Selikoff, 1974; Selikoff and Hammond, 1979) and by Berry et al. (1972). The data available were analysed by Saracci (1977) in terms of the following three models:

-     the excess incidence of lung cancer due to asbestos and due to smoking adds together when both agents are present (additive model);
-     the addition of each one of the two agents produces an effect which is proportional to the effect of the other (multiplicative model);
-     asbestos can only increase lung cancer incidence in the presence of smoking (amplifier model).

The additive model was found to be the least plausible of the three examined. Of the two other models, the amplifier model was contradicted by one sub-set of data, while the multiplicative model was not refuted, at the probability level p=0.05, by any one of the sets of data examined. Saracci (1977) also noted that there is some general and experimental support for the multiplicative model and, therefore, concluded that "at the present time, and in the absence of new evidence to the contrary, the multiplicative model stands as the more plausible interpretation of the asbestos-smoking interaction on human lung cancer production". Support for the hypothesis of an interactive effect between smoking and asbestos in the induction of lung cancer comes from the observations of Whitwell et al. (1974). These authors reported that in male, asbestos exposed, smokers suffering from lung cancer, adenocarcinomas were the commonest tumour type, whereas, in general, among smokers, squamous cell carcinomas dominate: On the basis of this observation, and from the knowledge that squamous, or oat cell, carcimonas are produced proximally, and adenocarcinomas distally, in the lungs, Whitwell et al. (1974) suggested that asbestos lying in the distal parts of the lung may exert a co-carcinogenic, perhaps multiplicative, effect with tobacco smoke. These data should be treated with caution, since the availability of special techniques to classify poorly differentiated tumours can affect the proportion of a specific cell type recorded and because there is evidence that adenocarcinoma is becoming the most common cell type of lung cancer (Casey et al., 1981).

Other data on man derive from case studies. In this area, attention is drawn to the observation of Dohner et al. (1975) that multiple primary tumours may occur in asbestos exposed individuals, and the correlations in asbestosis and lung cancer incidence in two pairs of monozygotic twins reported by Charpin et al. (1981). Taken together, these observations suggest significant individual variations in the risk from asbestos exposure and the possibility that these variations may have, at least in part, a genetic basis.

As Harington (1976) has stated, comparatively few tests for the carcinogenity of asbestos in the lungs of experimental animals have been made. However, the available data are of interest. They demonstrate the following points:

- pulmonary tumours can be produced in rats by chrysotile, amosite, anthophyllite, and crocidolite (Reeves et al., 1974; Reeves, 1976; Wagner, 1976);
- it is probably the fibrous nature of asbestos rather than its surface characteristics which gives rise to its carcinogenic potential (Pott et al., 1976; Kuschner and Wright, 1976), though in some circumstances trace metals, introduced by milling, may be implicated (Gross et al., 1967);
- benzo(a)pyrene and asbestos act as co-carcinogens with respect to lung cancer and pre-cancerous lesion induction in rats (Shabad et al., 1974; Harington et al., 1975), this may be because asbestos delays clearance of benzo(a)pyrene from the lower respiratory tract and/or because it augments carcinogenesis in that site (Smith et al., 1968);
- chrysotile asbestos has been variously reported as similar in effectiveness to the amphiboles (Wagner, 1976), or much more effective (Davis et al., 1978); these differences may be attributable to differences in fibre length distribution (Davis et al., 1978);
- intermittent, or uniform, exposure of rats to amosite or chrysotile gave similar incidences of pulmonary neoplasms (Davis et al., 1980).

7.2.5 Mesothelioma

Undoubtedly, the most characteristic carcinogenic response to asbestos exposure is the induction of mesotheliomata of various types. This subject has been discussed in numerous reviews (e.g. Cooper, 1967; Harington, 1967; Wagner et al., 1971; Harington et al., 1975; Harington, 1976; Becklake, 1976; Selikoff, 1977; Kannerstein et al., 1977;

International Agency for Research on Cancer, 1977; Zielhuis, 1977; Kannerstein et al., 1978; Wagner et al., 1980; Davis, 1981; Casey et al., 1981).

Diffuse malignant mesothelioma is an uncommon and uniformly fatal neoplasm of the serosal lining of the pleural cavity, peritoneum and, rarely, other sites. Prior to 1950, it was extremely rare, but there is evidence that the incidence is increasing (Casey et al., 1981). The tumours are thought to arise from a pluripotent mesothelial cell, or a primitive mesenchymal cell associated with the mesothelial tissue. The pluripotent nature of the cell of origin creates a variety of histologic patterns in the resulting neoplastic tissue which has confounded recognition of this tumour as a distinct entity (Casey et al., 1981).

On gross examination, diffuse malignant mesothelioma appears ivory white to grey-yellow in colour. The tumour characteristically spreads along serosal surfaces and invades local tissues, such as the chest wall and mediastinum, encasing underlying tissue in a bulky mass which may grow very rapidly. The tumour spreads predominantly by local extension, but distant metastases also occur, especially to hilar and abdominal lymph nodes. Both visceral and parietal pleura are involved. Areas of necrosis occur, forming cystic spaces filled with gelatinous fluid. Pleural effusion and ascites are common features (Kannerstein et al., 1978; Casey et al., 1981). A detailed pathological and histological study of 54 mesothelioma cases was given by De Lajartre et al. (1976).

Numerous epidemiological studies and case reports have demonstrated the existence of a relationship between asbestos exposure and mesothelioma incidence, e.g. Wagner et al. (1960), Selikoff et al. (1965), Knox et al. (1968), Godwin and Jagatic (1970), McEwen et al. (1971), Selikoff et al. (1972), McDonald et al. (1974), Peto et al. (1977), Elmes and Simpson (1977), Sebastien et al. (1977), Cochrane and Webster (1978), Selikoff and Seidman (1981), Argouarch et al. (1981), McDonald et al. (1982), Newhouse et al. (1982). It is noted that in one recent study (Dement et al., 1982) of chrysotile asbestos textile workers, only one death out of 191 was attributed to mesothelioma. The authors of this study noted that it was possible that mesothelioma was underdiagnosed in this cohort and that certain deaths mentioning 'cancer of the abdomen' were suspect. However, they also commented that others have also found lower mortalities due to mesothelioma among cohorts exposed only to chrysotile.

Overall, human experience has been well summarised by Casey et al. (1981) as follows.

"The relative risk of developing diffuse malignant mesothelioma varies with occupation, probably as a result of differing intensities of exposure and also because of the specific types of asbestos fibres being used. Crocidolite seems to be the most potent type followed by amosite and then chrysotile. Anthophyllite very rarely produces diffuse malignant mesothelioma, if at all. Despite the frequent occurrence of benign pleural lesions in Finland, where only anthophyllite was mined, diffuse malignant mesothelioma remains very rare. This observation is evidence against the notion that pleural plaques are a direct precursor of diffuse malignant mesothelioma.

There does not appear to be any interaction between
cigarette smoking and asbestos exposure in producing
diffuse malignant mesothelioma. Pleural and peritoneal
mesotheliomas are clearly associated with asbestos
exposure. Mesotheliomas arising in other sites such
as pericardium and tunica vaginalis are extremely rare
and have not been linked conclusively to asbestos."

In addition to the available human data, it is noted that
mesotheliomas have been induced in various mammalian species by several
different routes of exposure. These experiments demonstrate the following
points:

- there are distinctions between fibre types and animal models in
  terms of the incidence of mesotheliomata, e.g. Reeves et al. (1971)
  and Bolton et al. (1982);
- rat mesotheliomas also exhibit considerable variations in cell type;
  early tumours tend to be mainly connective or epithelial, but later
  tumours consist of a mixture of cell types (Davis, 1979);
- in the rat, peritoneal mesotheliomas are made up primarily of
  'connective' type tissue, whereas, in the pleura, 'epithelial' cells
  predominate (Davis, 1976);
- mesotheliomas can be induced by materials other than asbestos and by
  asbestos from which oils have been removed; this suggests strongly
  that it is the shape of the fibre which is important in mesothelioma
  induction (Smith et al., 1972; Stanton and Wrench, 1972; Wagner
  et al., 1973; Pott et al., 1976; 1976a; Wagner, 1976; Stanton
  et al., 1977);
- interactions of asbestos with benzo(a)pyrene and Moloney murine
  sarcoma virus can enhance its neoplastic potential with respect to
  mesothelioma induction (Shabad et al., 1974; Kanazawa et al., 1979)
  and absorption of benzo(a)pyrene onto asbestos fibres could be of
  significance (Lakowicz and Bevan, 1980).

7.2.6   Other malignant neoplasms

Evidence for association of asbestos with a variety of other
malignant neoplasms has been summarised by Casey et al. (1981). Several
studies have revealed an association between asbestos exposure and
laryngeal carcinoma. However, the number of cases is small and it has
been difficult to exclude the effect of numerous other factors, including
smoking, which can influence this tumour. In this respect, it is noted
that Hinds et al. (1979), in a retrospective study of 47 cases of
laryngeal cancers in males of three counties of Washington State, were
unable to find any relationship with asbestos exposure, but did establish
clear dose-response relationships for smoking and alcohol consumption.
Several studies of the mortality of asbestos workers have concluded
that death rates from cancers of the gastrointestinal tract are excessive
(Miller, 1978; Casey et al., 1981). In some of these studies, the excess
was small and in two other studies no excess was found (Casey et al.,
1981). From their review of the data, Casey et al. (1981) concluded as
follows.

"Data regarding the prevalence of gastrointestinal cancer must be regarded with some caution. On the one hand, falsely negative results may be obtained if the study is performed early in the period of latency and cancers resulting from past exposures have not had sufficient time to develop. On the other hand, it is frequently argued that peritoneal mesothelioma may be underdiag- nosed because of inaccurate classification as metastatic gastrointestinal carcinoma .... Nevertheless, it appears likely that occupational exposure to asbestos increases the risk of developing cancers of the gastrointestinal tract. This risk is increased to a lesser degree than is the risk of bronchogenic carcinoma. Smoking does not seem to have a signi- ficant impact upon gastrointestinal carcinogenesis, except perhaps in the oesophagus, but the interaction requires further study".

These comments are in agreement with those of Miller (1978) who stated that "exposure to asbestos is associated with the subsequent development of gastrointestinal malignancies". He also stated that "all anatomical sites of the gastrointestinal tract appear to be affected" and that "there is no evidence that any other factor either contributes or sub- tracts from the causal relationship between asbestos exposure and cancer of the gastrointestinal tract".

With respect to non-occupational exposure, Casey et al. (1981) concluded that there is no conclusive evidence of a relationship between such exposure and cancer of the gastrointestinal tract.

With respect to other cancers, excess mortality associated with cancer of the kidney has been demonstrated. Associations with ovarian and breast cancer are generally discounted, but reports on asbestos-related neoplasms of B-cell lineage, such as lymphocytic leukaemia, multiple myeloma and Waldenström's macroglobulinaemia are more difficult to discount (Casey et al., 1981).

7.3   EXPOSURE TO ASBESTOS

As discussed by the International Agency for Research on Cancer (1977), the occurrence of asbestos in the general or occupational environment has been reported in various units of measurement. In work places, air units include millions of particles per cubic foot (mppcf), or, more recently, number of fibres of length >5 μm per ml and millions of fibres per m^3. In ambient air samples, values are generally recorded on a gravimetric basis, e.g. ng m^{-3}. Attempts to formulate a conversion factor between ambient and occupational levels have generally been unsuccessful because of large variability. This is to be expected, since ambient levels are generally determined by transmission electron microscopy, whereas phase contrast optical microscopy is used to measure occupational exposures. Measurements of asbestos in fluids have been expressed as fibres per ml, fibres per litre, or ng per g of sample. These comments on the different, and not necessarily compatible, methods of asbestos assay should be taken into account when considering the data given below.

From the point of view of individuals at risk from asbestos exposure, four general groups can be distinguished. These are:

- those exposed occupationally either as a result of their work or the work of others in their vicinity;
- individuals exposed in the neighbourhood of asbestos producing or utilising facilities;
- individuals exposed because of their residence in the same accommodation as asbestos workers, e.g. close family relatives;
- individuals exposed to asbestos present in the general environment.

7.3.1 Occupational exposure

Becklake (1976) identified a wide variety of occupations that may involve exposure to asbestos. These include mining, milling and transport of the material; spray insulation in construction and ship-building, manufacture of textiles, cement products and paper products; production of friction materials; installation of insulation for boilers, pipes and ship bulkheads; building construction, repair and demolition; ship construction, repair and refitting; car manufacture and repair.

The International Agency for Research on Cancer (1977) quoted the following levels for asbestos in air, as measured by electron microscopy:

near asbestos spraying	10-1000 ng m^{-3}
during a milling operation	10-5000 ng m^{-3}
in other occupational exposures	1000-100000 ng m^{-3}

Fibre concentrations in various asbestos using industries in the US, prior to 1971, were given as:

Industry	Range of means (fibres >5µm ml^{-1})	Range of individual samples (fibres >5 µm ml^{-1})
Textile	0.1-29.9	0.0-143.9
Insulation	0.1-74.4	0.0-208.4
Paper packing and asphalt production	0.2-13.6	0.0-18.9
Cement, shingles millboard and gasket	0.1-4.4	0.0-16.6
Friction	0.1-14.4	0.1-32.4
Cement pipe	0.2-6.3	0.0-13.4

Studies on drywall taping (Verma and Middleton, 1980) gave similar air concentrations of 0.3 to 26.5 fibres (>5µm) ml^{-1}, with mean values of 4.3 to 8.0 and median values of 2.7 to 5.9. Hammad et al. (1979) evaluated exposure in asbestos-cement manufacturing operations and recorded the following results.

Dust zone	Concentration (mppcf)		Concentration (fibres >5μm ml^{-1})	
	Mean ±.s.d.	Range	Mean ± s.d.	Range
Forming	0.50±0.34	0.15-1.3	0.23±0.068	0.14-0.46
Mixing	0.91±0.92	0.17-4.0	1.2±1.9	0.31-9.2
Shingle finishing	0.40±0.18	0.22-0.94	0.38±0.11	0.18-0.55
Corrugated finishing	1.3±1.5	0.23-4.0	3.5±5.5	0.28-20
Panel plant	0.64±0.62	0.10-2.0	0.46±0.21	0.24-0.86
All samples	0.79±0.94	0.10-4.0	1.3±3.0	0.14-20

Nicholson (1977) reviewed the history of US national standards for asbestos exposure. In 1969, the standard was set at 2 mppcf or 12 fibres (>5 μm) ml^{-1}, but, by 1976, had been reduced to 2 fibres ml^{-1} as a mandating time-weighted average.

7.3.2   Neighbourhood and domestic exposure

As Nicholson (1977) noted, the US ambient air standard for asbestos simply states that there can be no visible emissions from any facility producing or utilising asbestos minerals. He also commented on levels of asbestos in the vicinity of facilities using asbestos and in the homes of asbestos workers. Recorded levels were as follows.

Location	Number of samples	Range of asbetos concentration (ng m^{-3})
1/8 to 1/4 mile from asbestos spraying activities	11	10-400
1/4 to 1 mile from asbestos mines and mills	3	10-10000
Air around a taconite processing plant	6	20-5000
Homes of asbestos workers	4	100-5000

7.3.3   Environmental exposure

Levels of asbestos in ambient air have been discussed by the International Agency for Research on Cancer (1977). They commented that such levels do not normally exceed 100 ng m^{-3} and are usually less than 10 ng m^{-3}. Typical levels for urban air were summarised as 0.1 to 100 ng m^{-3} in the USA and 0.1 to 10 ng m^{-3} in Paris. Potential environmental exposures were identified as being due to the presence of asbestiform fibres in various geological formations, in asbestos mine tailings used on roads, in the vicinity of waste dumps and in stucco used for building cladding.

Average concentrations of asbestos in drinking waters have been quoted as ranging from 0.3 to 1.5 µg l^{-1}. Levels of $2x10^6$ to $1.73x10^8$ fibres l^{-1} have been reported in Canadian tap water, the highest levels being found in unfiltered tap water near a mining area. Levels of up to 12.46 µg l^{-1} of chrysotile, as determined by electron microscopy, were found in the Jumata and Connecticut rivers, while a study of the Great Lakes and St. Lawrence River bywaters showed average concentrations of about $1.7x10^6$ fibres l^{-1}. Locations with higher counts were found along the north shore of Lake Superior between Silver Bay and Duluth; along the St. Clair River, downstream from Montreal ;and in the asbestos mining district in the province of Quebec (International Agency for Research on Cancer, 1977). Levels of asbestos in drinking waters and their implications are considered in more detail in Section 7.6.

The asbestos contents of foods have not been well investigated, but asbestos filters, and talc, which contains asbestos as an impurity, may be used in the manufacture of some processed foods. Asbestos filters may also be used in the production of wines and spirits. The following levels have been recorded (International Agency for Research on Cancer, 1977).

Beverage	Comment	Concentration (fibres l^{-1})
Spirits	Fibrils thought to be chrysotile	$(1.3-2.4)x10^7$
Beer	British, Canadian, US	$(1.6-6)x10^6$
Sherry, port, vermouth, soft drinks		$(1.7-12.2)x10^6$

More detailed data on levels in drinking water and beverages have been given by Zielhuis (1977).

Other routes of potential exposure include the presence of asbestos in some pharmaceutical and dental products (International Agency for Research on Cancer, 1977).

7.4   INTERACTIONS IN VITRO AND IN VARIOUS TISSUE PREPARATIONS

One of the key factors in asbestos carcinogenesis has been identified as the interaction of fibres with cells and cell components. This topic has often been investigated using cell or tissue culture systems. Because many of the data gained in these studies are of relevance to the general question of asbestos distribution and retention in the body, it is appropriate to review this information as a preliminary to discussion of results from in vivo experiments. The data available can generally be classified into four broad areas. These are:

- studies on haemolysis;
- interactions with macrophages;
- interactions with fibroblasts and other cell types;
- interactions in tracheal grafts.

Individual areas are discussed below.

7.4.1   Studies on haemolysis

Although haemolysis of erythrocytes plays no part in the pathogenesis of dust diseases, the technique provides a simple and rapid way of studying the effects of dusts and fibres on biological membranes. The general topic of haemolysis by dusts and fibres was discussed by Harington (1976) and this section is based on his review, supplemented by some more recent reports.

In the case of silica, at least two types of haemolytic effect operate. These are:

- direct haemolysis caused by contact of the erythrocyte with silica as a powder or, in certain circumstances, as a solution;
- indirect haemolysis in which colloidal silicic acid and certain soluble silicate polymers sensitise the erythrocyte to lysis by complement.

These two types of effect are also found in haemolysis by various forms of asbestos. Chrysotile has a marked direct haemolytic action, but various other forms of asbestos, notably crocidolite and amosite, are relatively inactive. Differences in activity of the various forms of asbestos are not directly related to their surface area, but are almost completely determined by their Mg:Si ratio. This explains both the high activity of chrysotile and the, otherwise anomalously, high activities of magnesium rich actinolites.

Experiments on the prevention of haemolysis using a wide range of chelating agents, some with specific affinity for Mg^{2+}, in conjunction with the observed correlation between Mg:Si ratio and haemolytic activity, have left little room for doubt that the magnesium groups on the surface of the fibres are mainly responsible for the interaction with erythrocyte membranes and, presumably, with other membranes also (Harington, 1976). More recent data on the haemolytic activity of magnesium-depleted chrysotile asbestos support this hypothesis (Morgan et al., 1977) in that the haemolytic activity declined until about half the magnesium had been removed, after which there was little further change. Morgan et al. (1977) attributed the residual haemolytic activity in the leached chrysotile to the silica skeleton which remained. Reduction in the haemolytic activity of acid-leached chrysotile was confirmed by Jaurand et al. (1979), but these authors also found that acid-leaching enhanced the haemolytic effect of amphibole asbestos. These results were in agreement with those from studies by Light and Wei (1977; 1977a), who found that the strength of the haemolytic effect was correlated with surface charge and commented that while there is an apparent correlation between the magnesium concentration in fibres and haemolytic activity, strict adherence to this correlation is questionable. They noted that Desai et al. (1975) had found that 20 and 80% magnesium-depleted chrysotiles were still potently haemolytic and that magnesium is not required for haemolysis by silica and glass fibres. For these reasons, they concluded that, although magnesium may be involved in determining the ion-adsorption characteristics of fibres, particularly chrysotiles, it is the adsorption or desorption of hydrogen ions which probably gives the fibres the surface potential that seems to be the critical factor in haemolysis by asbestos.

Light and Wei (1977) also noted that, compared with chrysotiles, amphiboles had a much less effective lysing mechanism and suggested that this could explain why amphiboles are less acutely cytotoxic than chrysotiles. They also commented that, in respect of carcinogenicity, the activity of chrysotiles is reduced relative to the amphiboles and suggested that this might be due to the leaching of chrysotile in vivo, with the consequent reduction in surface charge and lytic effectiveness.

7.4.2   Interactions with macrophages

The interaction of asbestos with alveolar macrophages almost certainly plays a part in the pathogenesis of asbestosis and it may be involved in other chronic effects of asbestos, as well as in the clearance of fibres from the lung. Many of the relevant data on asbestos interactions with macrophages are included in the reviews by Harington (1976) and Allison (1976). More recent papers of interest include those by Beck (1976), Jaurand et al. (1977), Morgan et al. (1977), Jaurand et al. (1979), McLemore et al. (1979; 1980), Johnson and Davies (1981), Kagan and Miller (1981) and Kaw et al. (1982).

With respect to phagocytosis, Allison (1976) commented that, independent of the type of asbestos, short fibres (<5 μm) were readily and completely taken up by phagocytosis, whereas long fibres (>30 μm) were never completely ingested. The cells were closely attached to, or enveloped, the ends of the latter type of fibre, but part of these fibres remained outside the cells. The reflection of the plasma membrane over the fibres was demonstrable. With long fibres, two or more cells could be seen attached to a single fibre, sometimes with apparent continuity of cytoplasm, and the presence in the culture of multinucleate cells containing long fibres suggested to Allison (1976) that the process could lead to cell fusion. Allison (1976) also commented that long-term contact with the plasma membrane might be implicated in the biological effects of asbestos. Effects of asbestos on macrophages were recorded as including cell death and release of lysosomal enzymes (Allison, 1976; Harington, 1976). Harington (1976) distinguished two types of cytotoxicity. The first was an early lytic reaction occurring within minutes of adding asbestos to macrophages or other cells. This reaction was reported to be inhibited by the presence in the medium of decomplemented serum and may have been accelerated by complement-sufficient serum. Harington (1976) considered that early cytotoxicity of this type is due to the interaction of asbestos fibres with plasma membranes.

The second type of asbestos induced cytotoxicity reactions occur many hours after incubation of macrophages with asbestos, are associated with selective releases of lysosomal hydrolases into the medium (e.g. Davies et al., 1974) and have been attributed to interactions of phagocytosed asbestos particles with the membranes surrounding secondary lysosomes (Harington, 1976).

Harington (1976) also commented that, of all types of asbestos fibres, greatest early and late cytotoxicity is shown by chrysotile. He discussed morphological and biochemical effects of various types of asbestos and concluded that there are distinct similarities between the cytotoxic behaviour of chrysotile and silica, both being phagocytosed like inert particles and eventually localised inside discrete phagosomes. However, beyond this stage, mechanisms of interaction differ.

More recent work is relevant to the comments of Harington (1976). Beck (1976) demonstrated delayed/incomplete phagocytosis of long fibres and showed that incomplete incorporation of the fibre causes a local discontinuity in the cell membrane, resulting in continuous liberation of intra-cellular enzymes, which is compensated for by increasing glycolytic metabolism. Beck (1976) also showed that fibrous dusts, such as asbestos and glass fibres, induce the formation of polykaryotic giant cells by way of fusion. He also suggested that in the process of asbestos induced cell fusioning, integrated virus genomes are activated and infectious virus are released. On the basis of his results, Beck (1976) suggested that there seems to be a causal relationship between the fibrogenic and carcinogenic effects of inorganic dusts and their length and diameter, regardless of their chemical composition. In his view, the fibrogenic and carcinogenic effect is likely to be limited by a minimal length and a maximal diameter (see also Brunch, 1974).

Jaurand et al. (1979) studied asbestos fibre interactions with alveolar macrophages in vitro. They commented that unleached amphiboles and commercial attapulgites were both cytotoxic, but chrysotile was not. However, acid treated chrysotile was found to be cytotoxic.

McLemore at al. (1979; 1980) examined the phagocytosis of asbestos fibres and asbestos bodies by human alveolar macrophages. In the case of fibres, it was demonstrated that both complete and incomplete phagocytosis occurred by similar processes of fibre engulfment. The presence of proteinaceous material at the point of entry of the fibre into the cell was also noted. In the case of asbestos bodies, it was demonstrated that complete phagocytosis could occur and that phagocytosed asbestos bodies were only very slightly cytotoxic, as assayed by Trypan Blue exclusion (see Section 7.7.3 for a detailed discussion of the formation of asbestos bodies).

Johnson and Davies (1981) studied the effects of crocidolite and chrysotile asbestos on lavaged mouse peritoneal macrophages by both scanning (SEM) and transmission (TEM) electron microscopy. They reported partial engulfment of long fibres, with occurrences of several macrophages on a single fibre. TEM observations demonstrated fibres in, and protruding from, membrane-bound vacuoles; free in cytoplasm; and penetrating the nucleus. In the TEM studies, a space between the cell membrane and the fibre was evident.

In another experiment on mouse peritoneal macrophages, Kaw et al. (1982) reported on cytotoxicity, release of lactate dehydrogenase and uptake of tritiated amino acids according to weight, surface area, or fibre length. In all reactions tested, chrysotile was more active than the amphiboles, particularly on a weight basis. Long-fibred asbestos proved more cytotoxic than short fibres when used on the basis of equal mass. In contrast, in acid leaching studies, while the haemolytic activity of chrysotile decreased with increasing magnesium loss, the selective release of acid hydrolases from macrophages in culture increased (Morgan et al., 1977). The authors found this result surprising, but concluded that it may be explained by the mechanisms involved in the interaction of asbestos with specific groups on the plasma membrane. It is noted that both chrysotile fibres from human lung and those incubated in vitro with alveolar macrophages have shown an increase in the Si:Mg ratio relative to standard fibres (Jaurand et al., 1977). This may be taken as evidence of magnesium leaching by the macrophage.

In terms of interactions with other materials, Jaurand et al. (1978) reported that UICC chrysotile asbestos and SO_2 sorbed UICC chrysotile

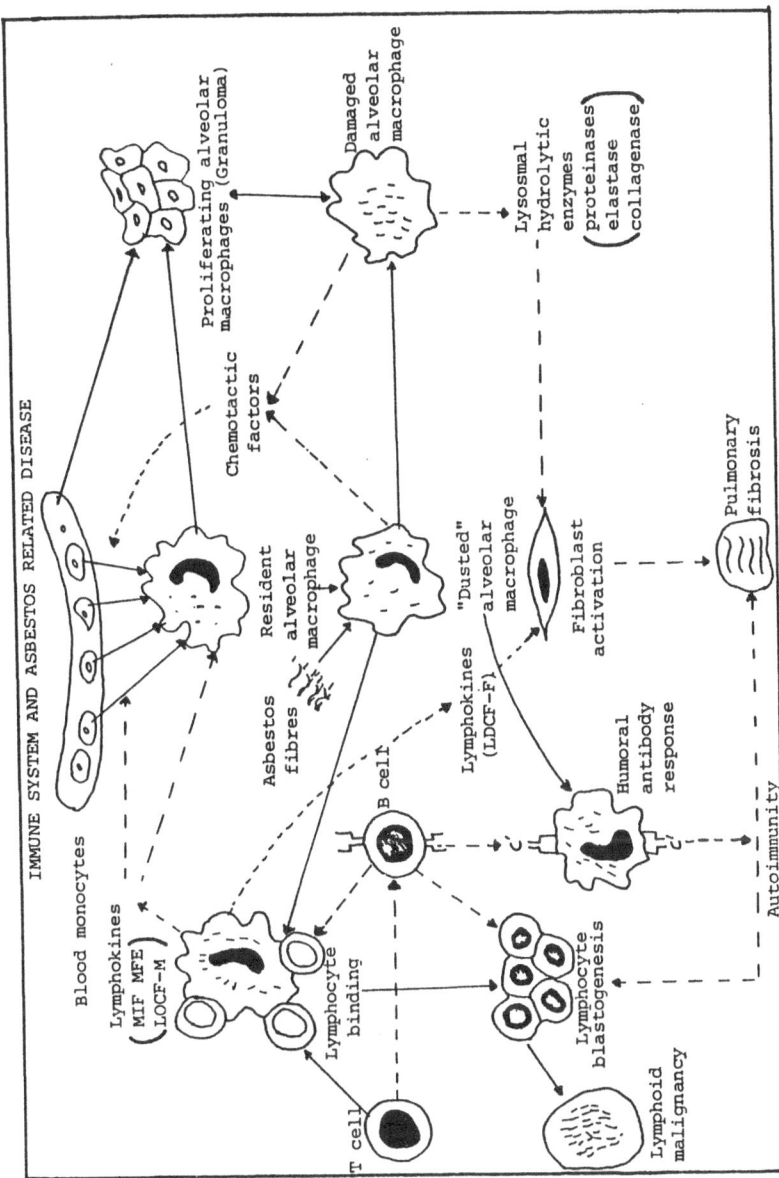

FIGURE 1. THE POSSIBLE CONTRIBUTION OF IMMUNOLOGIC PROCESSES TO THE PATHOGENSIS OF
ASBESTOS -RELATED DISEASE. LDCF-F AND LDCF-M = LYMPHOCYTE-DERIVED
CHEMOTACTIC FACTORS FOR FIBROBLASTS AND MACROPHAGES, RESPECTIVELY.
MFF = MACROPHAGE FUSION FACTOR, MIF = MIGRATION INHIBITION FACTOR.
FROM KAGON AND MILLER (1981).

asbestos could not be distinguished, in terms of cytotoxicity to alveolar macrophages, either in vivo or in vitro, though some changes in enzyme levels were recorded in the in vivo studies.

Finally, in respect of macrophage interactions, it is noted that Kagan and Miller (1981) have shown that alveolar macrophages obtained from asbestos-exposed rats can initiate a vigorous in vitro splenic lymphocytic proliferative response. They commented that the induction of cellular immunity in the lung might initiate a complex series of reactions involving the interplay of lymphokines, lysosomal hydrolytic enzymes and complement activation, with pulmonary fibrosis reflecting the end-stage of these events (Fig. 1 and see also Miller, 1979).

7.4.3   Interactions with fibroblasts and other cell types

Effects of asbestos on a variety of cell lines have been investigated. The effects studied include cytotoxicity, cellular ageing and the induction of chromosome aberrations. A comprehensive review of these aspects is not given here, but reference is made to a variety of recent studies of interest.

With respect to cytogenetic effects, Lavappa et al. (1975) reported that single oral doses of 100 or 500 mg kg⁻¹ of chrysotile failed to induce chromosome aberrations in bone marrow cells of Rhesus monkeys. Similarly, oral or intraperitoneal administration, over a range of 0.4 to 400 mg kg⁻¹, failed to induce micronuclei formation in the bone marrow of mice. In contrast, chrysotile was found to induce a significant and dose-related increase in chromosome aberrations and a dose-related inhibition of mitotic index in cultured Syrian hamster embryo cells. Farulla et al. (1978) reported that, while the endocellular incorporation of asbestos fibres seemed to be capable of inducing chromosome aberrations in Chinese hamster cell cultures, this effect was not observed in human cultured lymphocytes. Livingston et al. (1980) reported that chrysotile was more effective in preventing growth of Chinese hamster ovary cells than either amosite or crocidolite. They also found that crocidolite was more effective than amosite in inducing sister chromatid exchanges in these cells and that, where sister chromatid exchanges did occur, they were restricted to long and medium length chromosomes.

Finally, on this topic, Babu et al. (1980) reported that chrysotile asbestos exposure of Chinese hamster ovary cells gave rise to high vacuolisation of cytoplasm, as well as flattening of cells with increased size and chromosomal aberrations. Both cytological and cytogenetic effects were dependent on dose and period of exposure.

With respect to cytotoxic and other reactions, Beck (1976) has shown that phagocytosis of asbestos and release of lysosomal enzymes occurs in mouse fibroblasts as well as macrophages. This gives a basis for the cytogenetic effects discussed above and the cytotoxic effects reported by various authors (e.g. Chamberlain and Brown, 1978; Brown et al. 1978; 1979; Neugut et al., 1978; Reiss et al., 1980). Of particular interest are the following points made by the various authors.

-    Fibrous dusts which are cytotoxic in in vitro systems (V79-4 cells) are those which produce mesotheliomata in experimental animals; non-fibrous dusts are not toxic in these systems (Brown et al., 1979).

-   The biological activity of three types of amphibole asbestos, in respect of plating efficiency of V79-4 cells, correlated best with the number of fibres above a threshold length of 6.5 μm (Brown et al., 1978).
-   Using embryonic-human-intestine derived and adult-rat-liver derived epithelial cells, and assaying for cytotoxicity by inhibition of colony formation in cell culture, the order of cytotoxicity was chrysotile > amosite > crocidolite. Leaching in HCl greatly decreased the cytotoxicity of chrysotile and slightly increased the toxicity of amosite and crocidolite (Reiss et al., 1980).

With respect to cellular ageing, Richards et al. (1977) reported that chrysotile asbestos induces rapid cellular ageing in lung fibroblast cultures. These authors also gave a speculative account of the mechanisms of action on lung fibroblasts in vitro. This included:

-   coating of crysotile asbestos by a range of biological substances prior to any contact with the cells (see also Hasselbacher, 1979; Valerio et al., 1980);
-   phagocytosis of the 'non-foreign' coated asbestos;
-   enzyme release and effects on collagen synthesis;
-   binding of RNA to chrysotile, leading to cytosol depletion of RNA, nuclear stimulation, increased RNA synthesis and hence protein or proteoglycan synthesis.

Evidence for these various phenomena, and in particular the sequence of RNA interactions, is very limited.

Finally, two other papers on cellular interactions are noted. Maroudas et al. (1973), on the basis of experiments on fibroblasts in culture and from a consideration of mesothelioma induction by short and long fibres, postulated that solid foreign bodies induce two basic types of hyperplastic reaction, according to size. The effects of fibres above 40 μm depends on the provision of anchorage, which predominantly stimulates the mesenchyme, while particles of <20 μm stimulate only phagocytosis in monocytes. Long fibres would, by this mechanism, stimulate persistent hyperplasia in fibroblasts or reticuloendothelial cells and thus might be a necessary, but perhaps not sufficient, component in the induction of cancers.

In respect of interactions with other materials, Hahon et al. (1977) have shown that both chrysotile and amphibole asbestos have a depressive action on interferon induction by influenza virus in cell cultures, but that this effect is significantly diminished, or abolished completely, when the cells are pre-treated with poly(4-vinylpyridine-N-oxide). The mechanism of this effect is not clear.

7.4.4.   Interactions in tracheal grafts

In addition to the cell culture studies reviewed above, there have been a limited number of studies on various model systems other than the intact animal. Thus, Mossman et al. (1977) reported on the retention of crocidolite asbestos fibres in an organ culture of hamster trachea. Much of the asbestos was cleared by mucocilliary action. At 3h post-exposure, some short (<10 μm) fibres were lodged on the surfaces of non-ciliated and mucin secreting cells. Asbestos fibres were seen in the cytoplasm of epithelial cells and protruding through the plasma membrane. At a later stage, there was sloughing of the superficial necrotic epithelium and phagocytosis of the crocidolite by a hyperplastic basal layer. Crocidolite fibres were also found interposed between cells in this layer. The authors commented that particles appeared to be transported to the basement membrane both within and between cells. Observation of this transport is likely to be relevant in the context of a mechanism for the induction of bronchogenic carcinoma. Further results on this system have recently been reported by Mossman and Craighead (1981; 1982) who have suggested that the enhanced co-carcinogenic response of 3-methyl cholanthrene absorbed onto asbestos fibres may be due to the cytotoxicity of the asbestos and the resultant stimulation of the proliferative response.

Other papers on tracheal graft systems have been primarily concerned with tumourigenic response (Topping and Nettesheim, 1980; Topping et al., 1980) and are not discussed further.

7.5   DETECTION OF ASBESTOS IN TISSUES

Because of the extensive use of asbestos and asbestos products and because of its wide distribution in the environment, it is not surprising that significant levels have been recorded in various tissues and fluids, but most particularly in the lung. In the lung, and in other tissues, the presence of asbestos is demonstrated by detection of the presence of uncoated asbestos fibres and/or by the presence of asbestos bodies, i.e. asbestos fibres coated with proteinaceous material. The genesis of asbestos bodies is discussed elsewhere (Section 7.7.3), but their presence in human tissues is reviewed below.

Asbestos bodies have been described as elongated yellow-brown structures 20-150 μm long and 3-5 μm wide and are formed as a result of the coating of asbestos fibres by an iron-protein complex (Goldstein and Rendall, 1970). However, such bodies can be formed around fibres other than asbestos and, for this reason, many authors have preferred to term these structures 'ferruginous bodies' (Goldstein and Rendall, 1970; Becklake, 1976). The situation is complicated by the observation that chrysotile asbestos can be chemically altered in vivo (Langer et al., 1970), rendering identification of the core fibre of an asbestos body more difficult. In the case of workers exposed to asbestos, this is of limited significance, but it is of more concern in respect of observations of asbestos bodies in the non-occupationally exposed. Thus, Langer et al. (1977) commented as follows.

> "In recent years a number of investigations ... have demon-
> strated the presence of what appear to be 'asbestos bodies'
> in the lungs (both in tissue sections and in expressed tissue
> fluid) of a large proportion of urban dwellers who had no
> recorded occupational exposure to asbestos.... The question
> whether the cores of 'asbestos bodies' observed in these
> non-occupationally exposed individuals are necessarily
> asbestos has been revived. Although 'asbestos bodies'
> occurring in the general population appear morphologically
> identical to asbestos bodies observed in asbestos workers,
> this does not guarantee that they necessarily have the same
> core. For epidemiological studies it would be useful to have

unequivocal identification of the fibrous core. This has not been easily accomplished because of technical factors."

To investigate this problem, Langer et al. (1971) investigated asbestos body and asbestos fibre levels in 28 consecutive autopsies of long-term residents of New York city, both by optical and electron microscopy. They reported that electron microscopy showed chrysotile asbestos to be present in all examined, but did not address themselves to the problem of whether the ferruginous bodies, which were also seen, were nucleated on asbestos fibres (see also Selikoff et al., 1972a). Following these investigations, the question of the core fibre in ferruginous bodies has been answered by the application of electron microprobe analysis.

Thus, Langer et al. (1972) reported that analyses of asbestos body cores from lung tissues of individuals in the general population indicated that they could be composed of a number of materials including chemically degraded chrysotile, extruded silicate fibre and amphibole asbestos. Because of sampling biases inherent in the micromanipulation techniques used, the authors cautioned that the meaning and significance of their results was limited. More recently, Churg et al. (1977) reported analyses on lung samples from 23 autopsy cases or surgical patients. None of the individuals involved had been engaged in a primary asbestos-handling operation. The authors found that all morphologically typical ferruginous bodies were nucleated on asbestos and almost always on amphibole fibres. Although the nature of cores in bodies with protein coats too thick for diffraction was not generally determinable, such cores always occurred in association with bodies nucleated on amphibole fibres. Furthermore, in some instances, electron beam heating removed sufficient of the coating to demonstrate the amphibole fibre within.

In a second study, Churg et al. (1979) analysed a variety of 'atypical' bodies, in contrast to those analysed previously which had exhibited optically transparent straight cores. A total of 83 bodies was selected by light microscopy, encompassing the entire morphological spectrum seen. These bodies were analysed by transmission electron microscopy, electron diffraction and electron microprobe analysis. Of these bodies, 43 contained asbestos cores; included in this group were bodies with unusual branched and curved transparent cores. Microprobe analysis demonstrated that some of the cores were amosite or crocidolite, whereas others were anthophyllite. Of the remaining 40 bodies, 20 were probably carbon, 13 had characteristics consistent with sheet silicates and a few were apparently formed on diatomaceous earth. The authors concluded that, in human lungs, most ferruginous bodies containing asbestos can be separated, by light microscopic morphology, from bodies which do not contain asbestos. However, they also emphasised that their conclusions applied only to structures visible by light microscopy and that such ferruginous bodies represent only a fraction of the fibrous inorganic particulate material in the lungs. For this reason, they commented that future work needed to be directed to analysis of uncoated fibres visible by light microscopy and to the numerous fibres visible only by electron microscopy. This point is emphasised by the observation of Pooley (1972) that, because of their shape, chrysotile fibres are much less likely to act as cores for asbestos bodies than are amphibole asbestos fibres.

Examination of uncoated fibres in the lungs has, in fact, been undertaken in several studies (e.g. Langer et al., 1972a; Fondimare et al., 1976; Rowlands et al., 1982; Wagner et al., 1982; McDonald et al., 1982). The relatively low levels of chrysotile asbestos found in these studies indicate that its deposition, and/or retention, in the lungs is limited in comparison with the amphiboles (e.g. Wagner et al., 1982). In this context, it is of interest to note that Sebastien et al. (1977a) recorded that, in cases where observations were made a long time after the onset of exposure, amphibole fibres were more commonly found than chrysotile in the lung parenchyma, but chrysotile, in the form of ultimate fibrils, was more often found in pleural plaques.

Sebastien et al. (1977a) also quantified the proportion of coated fibres relative to total fibres in a light microscope study. This value was typically ~48% in highly exposed individuals, ~66% in less exposed individuals and 100% in unexposed individuals. For comparison, Ashcroft and Heppleston (1973) gave a proportion of 26.1% in asbestotic individuals. While there is a clear trend in these results, it should be treated with caution, in view of the vast number of fibres which are not visible by optical microscopy. Thus, for example, Fondimare and Desbordes (1974) recorded the following results for patients suffering from severe asbestosis.

Case no.	Number of asbestos bodies in 4 g of lung tissue (optical microscopy)	Number of uncoated fibres in 4 g of lung tissue (electron microscopy)	Ratio
30.606	11×10^4	12×10^6	109
A.481	69×10^4	30×10^6	43
A.691	1.5×10^4	3.0×10^6	200
A.1384	47×10^4	13.5×10^6	29
A.382	11×10^4	16×10^6	145
A.1154	22×10^4	31×10^6	141
Mean ± s.d.	-	-	111±60

Finally, it is noted that, in a recent paper, Auerbach et al. (1980) have demonstrated that when people have such a degree of exposure to asbestos dust that a great many asbestos bodies are formed in the lungs, then asbestos bodies are very likely to be present in one, or several, other organs as well. These authors noted that there are two different possibilities concerning the presence of asbestos bodies in other organs:

-   they may have been formed in the lungs and then migrated to another organ; or
-   asbestos fibres may have migrated to another organ and been coated there, thus forming an asbestos body.

Auerbach et al. (1980) stated that they were inclined to favour the second of these hypotheses, but gave no reason for this statement.

7.6   UPTAKE FROM THE GASTROINTESTINAL TRACT

Because of the presence of asbestos fibres in human drinking waters and beverages, (Section 7.3.3) and the association of occupational exposure to asbestos with an enhanced incidence of cancers of the gastrointestinal tract (Section 7.2.6), there has been considerable attention to the passage of asbestos through, and uptake from, the gastrointestinal tract. In discussing this topic, it is necessary to bear in mind that the discussion centres throughout on the uptake of a very small fraction of asbestos from the gut contents and that a persorbative mechanism for the uptake of a small fraction of a variety of large particles from the gut has been demonstrated in an extensive series of experiments by Volkheimer (1974; 1977).

The earliest account of asbestos absorption from the gastrointestinal tract appears to be that of Westlake et al. (1965) who reported on studies in which rats were fed for 3 months on a diet containing 6% asbestos. These authors reported that occasional asbestos particles were found near the luminal surface of the cells, and, by scanning many sections, were detected in intercellular and interstitial locations. The particles usually measured from 0.5 to 1.0 μm in length and had a typical chrysotile structure of two concentric tubes. In most instances, entrance of the particles seemed to be through the goblet cells and some appeared to be penetrating the membrane at the base of the cell. Similar fibres were found in the cytoplasm of the cell, with no apparent isolating membrane. Asbestos was also found in the lamina propria in both interstitial substance and smooth muscle cells. Sections of the regional lymph nodes and spleen were examined, with the thought that the particles might be carried by the lymphatics, but no fibres were found in these areas. At this time, no alterations could be found that were inconsistent with normal mucosa. The possibility that the asbestos fibres had been introduced during processing and sectioning were discussed and discounted. Subsequent to this, Cunningham and Pontefract (1973), and Pontefract and Cunningham (1973) injected 9.4×10^9 or 9.4×10^{10} fibres directly into the stomachs of rats and reported that ~0.1% of the dose was present in blood 2 d later and ~0.003% was present 4 d later. They also noted that the omentum around the small intestine contained most of the retained activity. It is almost impossible to interpret the results of this experiment, since the possibility of leakage of fibres back along the track of the injection needle cannot be discounted.

In response to these reports of asbestos penetrating the gut wall, Gross et al. (1974) reported on several experiments in which rats were exposed to various types of asbestos in their diets. These authors summarised their results as follows.

- Twenty one months of intimate contact of rat G.I. mucosa with very high concentrations of chrysotile asbestos failed to produce cancer, or any other kind of lesion. In earlier work, different modes of exposure resulted in cancer production within 16 to 17 months.
- Twenty one months of high-dosage chrysotile feeding of rats resulted in no evidence of penetration of G.I. mucosa by the mineral fibres and no incontrovertible proof of transmigration, as judged from electron microscopic studies.
- Administration of a single dose of 400 mg of either amosite or taconite tailings by gavage provided no evidence of transmigration of fibres.
- The voluntary intake by rats, over six days, of 2 to 10 g of amosite or taconite tailings mixed in oleomargarine provided no evidence of transmigration of mineral fibres.

- Short-term and long-term feeding of chrysotile and crocidolite by a second laboratory resulted in no tumour production in the G.I. tract or mesothelium during the lifetime of the animals. Light microscopic studies provided no evidence that penetration of tissues by ingested asbestos fibres occurred.
- A partially completed light and electron microscopic study in a third laboratory provided data that supported the results and conclusions of the other two laboratories with regard to the failure of ingested asbestos fibres to penetrate tissues.

In addition, Gross et al. (1974) pointed to the lack of mesenteric lymph node involvement in particulate uptake in miners as evidence of the formidible barrier that the gastrointestinal tract poses to particle uptake. This argument was also given by Davis et al. (1974) who pointed out that morphological considerations, at the electron microscopic level, indicate that the gut wall is a substantial barrier to particle uptake. These authors also reported on experiments in which rats were fed asbestos mixed with butter and killed after three months feeding. In respect of these studies, Davis et al. (1974) stated that their early experimental results suggested that asbestos fibres ingested along with normal quantities of food do not cause damage to the gut linings in rats nor penetrate into the gut epithelial cells. These results were confirmed in a later paper (Bolton and Davis, 1976) where it was also calculated that, following consumption of asbestos in margarine at a rate of 250-300 mg per week for a year, the maximum penetration of the rat intestine, in terms of fibre number, would be less than 100 for amosite, 550 for crocidolite and 1500 for chrysotile (90% confidence level). These figures suggest fractional uptakes $<10^{-9}$, very much less than the figure of 2×10^{-5} (±50%) suggested by Volkheimer (1977) for persorption. In the view of Bolton and Davis (1976), persorption of large particles could only occur following breakdown in the intestinal mucosal barrier.

In contrast to the results summarised above, Webster (1974) reported that, in baboons fed with crocidolite, small numbers of asbestos needles of length 0.5 to 1.0 µm could be found in the ashed tissue of the gut wall. It was suggested that these needles came from iron containing macrophages in the mucosa of the gut wall and that these macrophages could migrate to serosal tissues. However, no evidence was presented concerning passage of asbestos fibres across the gut wall. Similarly, Westlake (1974) found asbestos fibres in the colonic wall of rats fed a chrysotile containing diet. He reported that these particles were found in the mucus of goblet cells, within the cytoplasm of the epithelial cells and down in the smooth muscle layers. No membrane appeared to surround the fibres in cells, i.e. the fibres were not situated in lysosomes or phagosomes.

Sebastien et al. (1977; 1980) reported that, in studies in which rats were exposed to UICC asbestos samples by gavage or feeding, significant quantities of both long and short fibres could be recovered in fluids obtained by catheterisation of the thoracic lymph duct. Fractional transfers are listed below (Sebastien et al., 1980).

Exposure	No. positive: No. total	Fractional recovery
Chrysotile-gavage	5:5	$6.9 \times 10^{-7} - 3 \times 10^{-5}$
Crocidolite-gavage	3:5	$5.7 \times 10^{-8} - 5.6 \times 10^{-7}$
Crysotile-diet (short fibred)	13:15	$2.1 \times 10^{-7} - 2.1 \times 10^{-6}$ (*)
Crysotile-diet (long fibred)	4:8	$1.9 \times 10^{-5} - 2.1 \times 10^{-4}$ (*)
Control	0:2	-

Note: * Maximum daily recovery rate

Storeygard and Brown (1977) reported on the injection of 20 ml of a physiologic saline solution containing ~1.9×10^{11} amosite asbestos fibres into a closed jejunal cannula system. One hour later, segments of jejunal muscosa were taken for examination by scanning electron microscopy. Fibres were seen penetrating the epithelial surface in three of the five rats exposed to the amosite suspension. Fibres were also present in the lamina propria. However, the volume of fluid used in these experiments renders them difficult to interpret.

Cunningham et al. (1977) fed rats on a diet containing 1% chrysotile asbestos and 5% corn oil (to reduce the chance of inhaling free asbestos fibres) or 5% molasses. Asbestos levels in tissue were given as follows.

Tissues	Concentration (millions of fibres g^{-1})	
	Control	Asbestos treated
Blood	0.00	0.57±0.43
Omentum	1.08±0.58	9.66±3.18
Lung	0.29±0.08	1.02±0.20
Kidney	0.17±0.03	0.36±0.03
Liver	0.13±0.06	0.62±0.30
Brain	0.22±0.11	1.25±0.34

These data indicate that a small fraction of asbestos fibres can penetrate the walls of the gastrointestinal tract, in agreement with previous work presented by this group (Cunningham and Pontefract, 1973; Pontefract and Cunningham, 1973).

Two recent papers on this subject have given data for the gastrointestinal absorption of asbestos in baboons. Thus, Patel-Mandlik et al. (1979) reported on an experiment in which neonatal baboons were bottle-fed chrysotile asbestos suspended in a milk formula. These authors reported that tissues from control animals showed no fibres, but that a significant number of fibres were present in the kidney cortex of the test animal. The applicability of these data to adult animals or humans should be considered with care, bearing in mind changes in gut physiology over the period of weaning. This point is emphasised by the failure of this group of workers to detect any uptake of asbestos from the gastrointestinal tract of an adult baboon gavaged with both chrysotile and crocidolite asbestos (Hallenbeck et al., 1981).

With respect to experience in man, Cook and Olson (1979) reported that sediment in human urine examined by transmission electron microscopy contained amphibole fibres which originated from the ingestion of drinking water contaminated with these mineral fibres. They also found that the ingestion of filtered water resulted in the eventual disappearance of amphibole fibres from the urine. In quantitative terms, ingestion of water contaminated with amphibole fibres was observed to result in $\sim 10^{-3}$ of these fibres being excreted in the urine. In subjects transferred to filtered water, asbestos concentrations in urine dropped substantially, but significant levels were still present 2 months later.

In view of the available data, it must be concluded that the question of asbestos transfer across the gut mucosa is an unresolved issue. Persorption studies indicate that $\sim 10^{-5}$ of ingested particles might be absorbed, but these could also be excreted rapidly rather than retained in the body. In baboons, absorption may be significant in the neonate, but low in the adult. However, this conclusion is based on a total of four animals and should not be given undue weight. In man, a single study on urinary excretion suggests a fractional uptake of $\sim 10^{-3}$ with excretion on a timescale of days to months. This rapid loss by excretion reduces the weight of the argument concerning the build-up of particulate matter in the mesenteric lymph nodes. Data on rats are difficult to interpret, but, overall, there is evidence that some penetration of the gut wall may occur, either as a result of macrophage involvement, or due to mechanical penetration of fibres into mucosal cells. In view of the uncertainties in the data, further, more extensive, experimental work is required, preferably on animals with a gut physiology closely analagous to that of man, concentrating on processes of uptake, distribution and retention of different sized fibres in the body following intake. In the absence of such data, no recommendations can be made concerning a model for the distribution and retention of ingested asbestos.

7.7   EXPOSURE BY INHALATION

Exposure by inhalation is the major route by which asbestos enters the body and virtually all the toxic effects of asbestos fibres have been attributed to exposure via this route (see Section 7.2). For this reason, it merits detailed attention. For convenience, four broad areas of study can be defined. These are:

-      deposition in the lung;
-      interactions with lung tissues at the cellular level;
-      formation of asbestos bodies;
-      retention in the lung and translocation to other tissues.

These topics are discussed in detail below.

7.7.1   Deposition in the lung

Asbestos fibres are not compact entities, being elongated particles, or, in the case of chrysotile, bundles of fibrils, often with splayed ends. For this reason, their passage through the airways of the lung and their deposition in lung tissue needs to be given special consideration. This can be achieved by a consideration of two types of information, i.e.:

- model calculations;
- deposition data for asbestos in various animal models and man.

7.7.1.1 Model calculations

Various considerations determining the deposition of fibrous material in the lungs have been discussed by Timbrell (1970; 1976). The mechanisms operating and the relevant particle parameters were defined as follows (Timbrell, 1970).

Mechanism	Particle parameter
Gravitational settlement	free falling speed
Inertial impaction	free falling speed
Interception	size
Diffusion	size

Timbrell (1970) noted that diffusion is efficient only for particles smaller than 0.5 μm diameter and is of little importance for the long fibres that can penetrate deeply into the lung. For fibres, in contrast to compact particles, interception can be very important. A long fibre, if it is slender, may avoid deposition in the upper respiratory tract from gravitational settlement and inertial impaction, and penetrate deeply into the pulmonary air spaces. In these regions, the length of the fibre may be comparable with the diameters of the airways and interception becomes a major mechanism (Timbrell, 1970). While these comments are directly applicable to glass fibres and amphibole asbestos, they are less valid for chrysotile, the fibres of which generally resemble a stretched coil (Timbrell, 1970). For this reason, Timbrell (1970) suggested that for the purpose of categorisation each chrysotile fibre could be categorised by a cylinder with its axis parallel to the preferred orientation of the fibre and a diameter just sufficient to entirely enclose the fibre in the cylinder. On this basis, the fibre is categorised by the length of the cylinder and its aspect ratio. Although Timbrell (1970) reported some experimental studies analysed using this concept, mathematical models of deposition involving these fibre parameters do not appear to have been developed.

With respect to modelling of asbestos deposition in the lungs, it is also relevant to note that Timbrell (1976), in studies using an aerosol spectrometer, reported that, in comparison with glass fibres, even clean asbestos fibres showed a reduced tendency to align with the airflow. Timbrell (1976) noted that the implication of this was that industrial asbestos would tend to be randomly orientated. Calculations on the deposition of randomly oriented rectilinear fibres in airway models pointed to the respiratory bronchioles, especially the bifurcations in them, as preferred deposition sites for long fibres (Timbrell, 1976). These comments indicate that the deposition models given by Harris (1976) for fibrous glass, and Harris and Fraser (1976) for fibres in general, may have limited application to asbestos, since they deal only with straight rigid rods (Harris and Fraser, 1976). Nevertheless, results from the model are useful in giving a comparison with experimental studies and are, for this reason, listed in Table 4. Finally, in respect of models,

TABLE 4

FRACTION OF UNIT DENSITY RODS DEPOSITED IN EACH
RESPIRATORY COMPARTMENT - TIDAL VOLUME 1450 CC

Rod length μ	Rod diam. μ	Equiv. diam. μ	Fraction deposited			
			Naso-pharynx	Tracheo-bronchial	Pulmonary spaces	Fraction exhaled
0.5	0.03	0.068	0.008	0.024	0.365	0.603
1.0	0.03	0.074	0.016	0.022	0.329	0.632
3.0	0.03	0.083	0.049	0.030	0.288	0.633
3.0	0.10	0.245	0.049	0.029	0.289	0.633
3.0	0.20	0.448	0.048	0.029	0.309	0.613
10	0.03	0.092	0.151	0.069	0.264	0.517
10	0.10	0.277	0.150	0.069	0.272	0.510
10	0.20	0.519	0.147	0.068	0.300	0.485
10	0.40	0.959	0.329	0.067	0.307	0.296
25	0.03	0.098	0.325	0.057	0.275	0.344
25	0.10	0.300	0.327	0.021	0.299	0.353
25	0.20	0.566	0.323	0.030	0.309	0.338
25	0.40	1.06	0.492	0.048	0.274	0.186
25	1.0	2.40	0.709	0.099	0.152	0.040
25	2.0	4.36	0.850	0.107	0.039	0.004
50	0.03	0.102	0.545	0.021	0.227	0.207
50	0.10	0.315	0.549	0.025	0.214	0.211
50	0.20	0.599	0.543	0.034	0.219	0.204
50	0.40	1.13	0.660	0.047	0.190	0.104
50	1.0	2.59	0.795	0.082	0.104	0.018
50	2.0	4.79	0.904	0.075	0.019	0.001
50	4.0	8.73	1.000	-	-	-
100	0.03	0.106	0.793	0.023	0.116	0.069
100	0.10	0.330	0.793	0.025	0.114	0.069
100	0.20	0.631	0.782	0.031	0.124	0.063
100	0.40	1.20	0.830	0.035	0.105	0.029
100	1.0	2.77	0.891	0.051	0.053	0.004
100	2.0	5.19	0.955	0.038	0.007	<0.001
100	4.0	9.59	1.000	-	-	-
200	0.03	0.111	0.949	0.012	0.035	0.005
200	0.10	0.345	0.948	0.013	0.035	0.004
200	0.20	0.661	0.945	0.014	0.037	0.004
200	0.40	1.26	0.956	0.014	0.028	0.002
200	1.0	2.94	0.971	0.016	0.013	<0.001
200	2.0	5.5	0.990	0.009	0.001	<0.001
200	4.0	10.4	1.000	-	-	-

Note:

From Harris (1976)

Lippman et al. (1976) compared predicted and calculated depositions of fibres at airway bifurcations and in daughter tubes. Theoretical calculations were based on consideration of impaction and sedimentation, while deposition was measured in a hollow cast of a human lung. Results of this study are shown in Fig. 2. On the basis of these results, Lippman et al. (1976) concluded that the calculated and measured depositions were in reasonable agreement at a respiration rate of 15 l min^{-1}, but that at 30 l min^{-1} and 60 l min^{-1} the theoretical relations underestimated deposition in the larger bronchi. The authors tentatively attributed this to a change from laminar to turbulent flow at the higher respiration rates.

7.7.1.2 Experimental data

There have been several studies in which the deposition of inhaled asbestos was measured in the lungs of rats. Thus, Wagner and Skidmore (1965) exposed rats to clouds of asbestos and glass dusts for 7.5 h per day, 5 days per week over a period of six weeks. On the day after exposure, the rats were killed and the lung contents assayed in terms of total silica content. Results were also obtained from a gravitational thermal precipitator sampling at 0.1 l min^{-1} (which was stated to approximate to the minute volume of the rats). Results from this study are summarised below.

	Chrysotile	Dust type Crocidolite	Amosite	Glass
Gravitational thermal precipitator (mg)	36.4	38.9	41.8	43.4
Lung (mg) - background	0.72	2.79	3.59	6.69
Lung:precipitator ratio	0.020	0.072	0.086	0.154

These data indicate the relatively low deposition/retention of asbestos relative to glass and chrysotile relative to amphibole asbestos.
Timbrell et al. (1970) exposed rats to the UICC amosite, crocidolite, anthophyllite and Canadian chrysotile asbestos samples. They demonstrated that fibres in terminal air sacs were generally shorter than fibres in air ducts which in turn were shorter than fibres in the dust cloud to which the animals were exposed. Comparison with results from animals allowed to survive for some time after exposure indicated that, with time, the fibre in the air ducts became coarser, suggesting a fibre transport mechanism that is sensitive to fibre length. This conclusion is rendered more attractive by data from a further experiment in which rats were exposed to 180 mg m^{-3} of glass fibres for eight hours per day over ten days. Fibres were categorised as straight, curved and aggregated. Deposition of the various fibre types was very similar, decreasing rapidly with increasing particle length to ~20 μm and then decreasing considerably less steeply out to 90 μm. The authors suggested that a possible explanation for this change of slope is that clearance processes are less efficient for fibres longer than 20 μm. This is in line with the suggestion of Morgan et al. (1978) that long fibres are more liable than short to penetrate the alveolar wall, since they tend to bridge the alveolar ducts and alveoli.

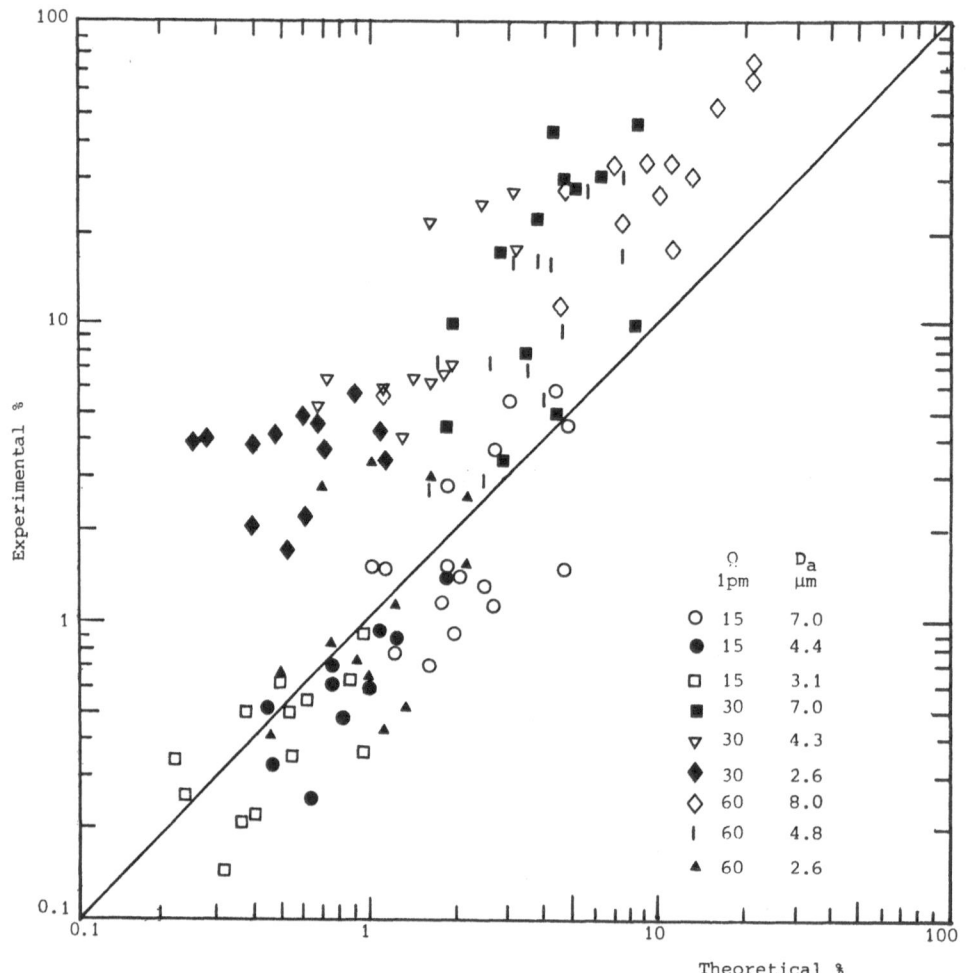

FIGURE 2.   PREDICTED AND EXPERIMENTALLY MEASURED DEPOSITION
            ON A SPECIFIC AIRWAY BIFURCATION AND ALONG ITS
            DAUGHTER TUBES, FOR A SPECIFIC PARTICLE SIZE
            AND INSPIRATORY FLOW.

            NOTE: FROM LIPPMANN ET AL. (1976); Ω = RESPIRATION RAT
                    D_a= AERODYNAMICAL
                         DIAMETER

Wagner et al. (1974) exposed rats to the various UICC reference samples of asbestos and reported the following data on exposure and lung retention.

Length of exposure	Mean exposure (mg h m^{-3})	Dust retained in lungs (mg)		
		Amosite	Anthophyllite	Crocidolite
5 weeks	1880	1.0	1.3	1.1
8 weeks	2450	0.9	1.6	1.6
10 weeks	3290	2.0	2.8	2.1
3 months	5050	3.7	3.5	3.0
6 months	8470	4.7	4.4	4.5
12 months	17100	8.3	9.6	9.3
24 months	33400	16.8	13.8	14.9

Length of exposure	mean exposure (mg h m^{-1})	Dust retained in lungs (mg)	
		Canadian chrysotile	Rhodesian chrysotile
5 weeks	1880	0.1	0.1
8 weeks	2450	0.1	0.3
10 weeks	3290	0.5	0.5
3 months	5050	0.6	0.7
6 months	8470	0.4	0.4
12 months	17100	0.8	1.4
24 months	33400	0.3	0.6

Using a minute volume for rats of 0.1 l (see above) these results can be re-expressed as fraction of inhaled material retained in the lungs. This is done below.

Length of exposure	Fraction retained				
	Amosite	Anthophyllite	Crocidolite	Canadian chrysotile	Rhodesian chrysotile
5 weeks	0.089	0.115	0.098	0.009	0.009
8 weeks	0.061	0.109	0.109	0.007	0.020
10 weeks	0.101	0.142	0.106	0.025	0.025
3 months	0.122	0.116	0.099	0.020	0.023
6 months	0.092	0.087	0.089	0.008	0.008
12 months	0.081	0.094	0.091	0.008	0.014
24 months	0.084	0.069	0.074	0.001	0.003

These results are very consistent and indicate little clearance from the lung, except possibly over the 24 month exposure period. Clearance on a 24 month timescale is also indicated by comparison of lung contents in animals exposed for six months and assayed immediately or 18 months later (Wagner et al., 1974). These results are listed below.

Asbestos type	Lung content (mg)		
	Immediate	After 18 months	Ratio
Amosite	4.7	1.3	0.28
Anthophyllite	4.4	2.6	0.59
Crocidolite	4.5	1.2	0.27
Canadian chrysotile	0.4	0.0	0.00
Rhodesian chrysotile	0.4	0.1	0.25

Excluding the 24 month exposure data from consideration, mean fractional retentions are estimated to be 0.091, 0.111, 0.099, 0.013 and 0.017 for amosite, anthophyllite, crocidolite, Canadian chrysotile and Rhodesian chrysotile respectively.

Evans et al. (1973) exposed rats to neutron activated crocidolite asbestos and reported the following results for animals killed immediately after exposure.

Organ	Deposition (μg)			
	Experiment 1 (elutriated)		Experiment 2 (unelutriated)	
	Rat 1	Rat 3	Rat 5	Rat 7
Skinned head	4.6	2.1	1.7	1.1
Larynx	0.6	0.1	<0.1	0.8
Oesophagus	1.0	0.1	0.2	0.2
Stomach	12.2	9.9	6.4	6.3
Small+Large intestine	6.3	7.2	6.4	14.7
Upper respiratory tract	24.7	19.4	14.7	23.1
Lower respiratory tract	22.0	16.4	20.9	23.1

The exposures to asbestos in air in the two experiments were 544 and 725 μg min l^{-1} respectively (Evans et al., 1973). Using these values, together with a minute volume of 0.1 l, the fractional deposition in the upper+lower respiratory tract can be calculated. These values are 0.86, 0.66, 0.49 and 0.64 respectively. It is noted that the median fibre length for this asbestos, as measured by electron micrographic techniques, was between 1 and 2 μm. In a later paper, Morgan et al. (1977a) demonstrated linear relationships between amount of fibre deposited in the respiratory tract and amount inspired during 30 minute exposures to various UICC asbestos samples and synthetic fluoramphibole. Fractional depositions have been estimated from these results as follows.

Fibre type	Fractional deposition	
	Total respiratory tract	Lower respiratory tract
Crocidolite	0.50	0.17
Anthophyllite	0.65	0.19
Fluoramphibole	0.65	0.20
Chrysotile A	0.30	0.12
Chrysotile B	0.45	0.15
Amosite	0.50	0.15

Morgan et al. (1978) also reported separately on the retention of anthophyllite in the lungs of rats, following exposure on three consecutive days, and gave data from which an initial fractional deposition of 0.11 can be estimated. This deposition was mainly in the alveolar region, but with a small amount in the conducting airways.

Middleton et al. (1979) exposed rats to UICC chrysotile 'A', amosite and crocidolite, at concentrations close to 1, 5 and 10 mg m^{-3} of respirable fibre, for a total of 210 h over a 6 week period. They gave the following aggregate exposures and asbestos recoveries at 5 d after exposure.

Type of asbestos	Exposure level (mg m^{-3})	Inhalation intake (µg)	Asbestos recovery (µg per rat)	Fractional retention
Chrysotile	7.8	9828	245	0.025
	3.8	4788	112	0.023
	1.2	1512	70	0.046
	10.1*	15908	724	0.046
Amosite	9.4	11844	1448	0.122
	4.6	5796	693	0.120
	1.4	1764	79	0.045
Crocidolite	11.8	14868	1052	0.071
	5.9	7434	1012	0.136
	1.4	1764	146	0.083
	12.9*	20318	1695	0.083

Note: * nocturnal exposure

Mean values of deposition for the three types of asbestos are calculated to be 0.035, 0.096 and 0.093 for chrysotile, amosite and crocidolite respectively.

Davis et al. (1980) studied the effects of intermittent, relative to uniform, asbestos exposure on the lungs of rats. Animals were exposed for 7 h per day, either 1 day per week (intermittent exposure) or 5 days per week (uniform exposure), for a period of 12 months. Using a minute volume of 0.1 l, the following results can be calculated for retention two days after the end of the exposure period.

Asbestos type	Exposure type	Total mass inhaled (µg)	Mean lung content (µg)	Fractional retention
Chrysotile	uniform	21840	526	0.024
	intermittent	19656	501	0.025
Amosite	uniform	109200	9169	0.084
	intermittent	107453	11226	0.104

Hammad et al. (1982) exposed rats to man-made mineral fibres. The animals were exposed for 6 h per day for six consecutive days and killed 5 d after the last exposure. Mean concentrations in the exposure chamber were 300 ± 82 fibres cm^{-3} (±1 s.d.), implying a total inhalation intake ~6.5×10^7 fibres. The mean number of fibres per rat lung recorded was from 1.8×10^5 to 2.5×10^5, i.e. 0.0028 to 0.0038 of those inhaled. It is noted that the count median diameter of the fibres used in this study was 13 µm and that only ~1% were less than 2 µm long. These fibres were, therefore, relatively long and this may have explained their poor penetration into the lung.

Finally, with respect to rats, Brody and Hill (1981) reported that, following nose-only inhalation of chrysotile by rats, the vast majority of particles inhaled beyond the terminal bronchioles impacted initially upon bifurcations of alveolar ducts. The farther the alveolar duct bifurcation was from its bronchiole, the less asbestos was observed. Duct bifurcations in the lungs of animals recovering in room air for five hours clearly exhibited less asbestos. Transmission electron microscopy demonstrated that numerous small asbestos fibrils were taken into the cytoplasm of underlying type I epithelial cells. Twenty-four hours after the one-hour exposure, asbestos was found in epithelial cells, basement membranes, interstitial cells and connective tissue, as well as in endothelial cells, capillary lumina and numerous alveolar macrophages. Four to eight days after exposure, fibres were rarely observed on alveolar duct surfaces.

Data on the deposition of asbestos in mammals other than the rat are much less extensive. Wehner et al. (1975) reported that, in Syrian golden hamsters, exposure to an asbestos aerosol of concentration 35 µg l^{-1} for 3.5 h per day for four to eight weeks resulted in a lung deposit of 100 to 500 µg. This is indicative of a retention of a few percent of the inhaled asbestos, but, in the absence of minute volumes for these animals, this statement cannot be quantified further.

Griffis et al. (1983) reported on the deposition of UICC standard crocidolite and similar size glass fibres in beagle dogs, as a result of a 60 minute nose-only inhalation exposure. Results were as listed below.

	Total inhaled (mg)	Total deposited		Total retained at 4 d	
		mg	fraction	mg	fraction
Asbestos:					
Dog A	10.3	6.9	0.67	1.3	0.13
Dog B	8.1	4.4	0.54	1.5	0.18
Dog C	7.3	4.3	0.59	1.2	0.12
Dog D	9.5	6.8	0.72	1.8	0.19
Mean ± s.d.			0.63±0.08		0.17±0.03
Glass					
Dog E	9.2	4.1	0.45	0.5	0.05
Dog F	9.3	6.0	0.64	0.5	0.06
Dog G	4.7	2.4	0.51	0.7	0.15
Dog H	4.9	2.6	0.54	0.8	0.17
Mean ± s.d.			0.54±0.08		0.11±0.06

Depositions per unit weight in all lung lobes were recorded as being very similar.

For man, Timbrell (1982) reported on electron microscope measurements of distributions of the diameters and lengths of fibres recovered from lung specimens related to the Paakkila anthophyllite mine. These distributions were compared with samples of airborne dust taken at the mine. Conclusions from this study were:

- clearance of long fibres decreased inversely with length up to ~5 to 17 µm, i.e. comparable with the diameter of an alveolar macrophage;
- no direct relation between clearance and fibre diameter had to be invoked to explain the differential removal of thinner fibres; and
- asbestosis can impair clearance.

7.7.1.3   Discussion

With respect to deposition of asbestos fibres a clear distinction must be made between that material which is deposited initially in the lungs and that which is retained there for extended periods. The available evidence suggests that ~50 to 60% of inhaled asbestos is initially deposited in the lung. This value is compatible with the fractional deposition of compact particulate material in the sub-micron to micron size range. All the evidence indicates that the degree of deposition is inversely related to fibre length, but the limited data do not allow this statement to be quantified further.

Following deposition, a considerable fraction of the deposited asbestos is cleared rapidly, primarily via the gastrointestinal tract. Thus, from the point of view of accumulation, it is that material which is retained in the lung for more than a few days that is of particular interest. With respect to this material, there is almost complete uniformity in the available results and it is possible to conclude that, expressed on a mass basis, ~0.1 of inhaled amphibole asbestos is well retained in the lung, whereas the corresponding figure for chrysotile is in the range 0.01 to 0.04 with a best estimate of 0.025. From the data of

Timbrell et al. (1970), it can be seen that this material will be strongly depleted in long fibres. For calculations on the fibre length distribution of material retained in the lungs it is recommended that the fibre length/ diameter distribution in air be weighted by deposition factors interpolated from those for pulmonary spaces given by Harris (1976; see also Table 4).

7.7.2   Interaction with macrophages and other cells

Removal of asbestos from the lung is considered later in this appendix (Sections 7.7.4, 7.7.5 and 7.7.6). Here it suffices to note that the phagocytic action of macrophages and other cells, discussed above (Sections 7.4.2 and 7.4.3) may be a major component in this migration. Phagocytic action by alveolar macrophages and movement out of the lung via ciliary action and mucus flow in the bronchii is too well known to require further comment (International Commission on Radiological Protection, 1966). However, other processes occur. Thus, Davis (1981) noted that many dust containing macrophages are cleared from the lung tissue, but others become incorporated into the lung parenchyma. These cells may die and liberate their contained fibres, but these will be rephagocytosed by new populations of macrophages and cells containing fibre can be found in the alveolar septa years after the end of dust inhalation. Cells other than macrophages, e.g. alveolar epithelial type I cells, can also be involved in this process (Section 7.7.1). Furthermore, some transport to the pleura may be macrophage mediated via lymphatics (Davis, 1981). This may lead to preferrential transport of short fibres of asbestos to the pleura, since Wright and Kuschner (1977) observed that when guinea pigs were injected intratracheally with crocidolite asbestos, a synthetic fluoramphibole and glass fibre, short, but not long, fibres, were translocated to the hilar lymph nodes. A particular interesting observation in this regard is that of Holt (1980) who reported that, apparently, alveolar macrophages containing dust reach the cilia of the larger bronchioles not by following the airways, but by a route through alveolar and bronchiolar walls. The implications of this movement through tissue, rather than via interstitial spaces, should be investigated further, in contexts other than transport to the ciliated epithelium of the bronchii.

7.7.3.   The formation of asbestos bodies

The occurrence and identification of asbestos bodies is discussed elsewhere in this review (Section 7.5). The formation of these bodies has been discussed by several authors. Davis (1965) reported that, in human lung material, asbestos bodies were found in three sites only; in alveolar macrophages, in fibroblasts, or embedded among collagen fibres in areas of fibrosis. He also noted that, in guinea pig lung, asbestos bodies were found in extracellular locations, or with one end inside a cell, but under the electron microscope such bodies were usually seen to be covered by very thin layers of macrophage cytoplasm. He concluded that asbestos body production is an intracellular process involving the deposition of ferritin containing material around the fibre. With amosite asbestos there was a suggestion that fine fibrils of this material could be incorporated in the coat.

Botham and Holt (1968) studied the formation of asbestos bodies in guinea pigs. They identified haemorrhage of capillaries close to dust laden macrophages as the primary process involved. They noted that iron from the haemoglobin of leaking erythrocytes is very soon found in the macrophages, but the details of the transfer process were not elucidated and it was uncertain whether it was the haemoglobin, or a decomposition product, that was being digested by the macrophages.

Iron from the haemoglobin was found to diffuse throughout the cytoplasm of the macrophage, before concentrating into particular areas. About three days after exposure there was evidence that asbestos fibres in the stained cell were absorbing iron. After ~16 d, two types of fibre coating were found. On some fibres the coating was mottled and on others even. After ~1 month, the coating showed signs of organisation and beaded asbestos bodies first occurred. After ~6 months, many fully-developed asbestos bodies were observed. Botham and Holt (1968) commented that beading of the asbestos body appeared to require the deposition of cytoplasmic contents over the ferroprotein coating and that some structures appeared to show a macrophage shrinking onto the developing asbestos body, the cell membrane disintegrating at some stage. Break-up of the beaded asbestos body can, in the guinea pig, begin as early as ~13 weeks after exposure, though it is not common at this stage.

In a second, comparative, study on guinea pigs and rats, Botham and Holt (1972) reported that, within a month after inhalation of anthophyllite some fibres develop into asbestos bodies in the lungs of guinea pigs, but that asbestos bodies are rarely found in the lungs of similarly exposed rats, even when these animals are observed to 19 months after exposure. In both species, diapedesis of erythrocytes through pulmonary capillary walls was observed as a source of ferruginous material. It was noted that in the guinea pig, but seldom in the rat, some macrophages fused in the alveolar region to form giant cells. It was suggested that these cells inhibit macrophage-mediated clearance of asbestos fibres and ferruginous material and consequently leave more material available for asbestos body formation.

Morphgenesis of the asbestos body in hamsters was discussed in detail by Suzuki and Churg (1969; 1969a). The following successive steps were identified:

-    phagocytosis of asbestos by alveolar macrophages, and other phagocytic cells, and incorporation into phagolysosomes;
-    accumulation of iron micelles around the fibres, possibly by fusion of asbestos-containing phagosomes with haemosiderin granules;
-    compaction of the micelles and clearing of the peripheral zone to form a mature asbestos body.

Suzuki and Churg (1969a) noted that formation of asbestos bodies seems to be a continuous process, with old bodies growing in thickness and uncoated fibres being converted into bodies months or years after instillation of asbestos. In contrast to the studies of Davis (1965), these authors found that the intracellular organelles of phagocytic cells, especially alveolar macrophages, were well developed and suggested that they played a role in the formation of the asbestos body.

A detailed analysis of asbestos bodies formed in human lung tissues was given by Pooley (1972a) who concluded that:

-    a pre-requisite for formation of such a body in most cases is a straight rigid fibre;

- two predominant asbestos body shapes prevail, these being sheath and segmented forms;
- it is likely that some of the more rectangular segmented varieties are derived from sheath types due to splitting and breaking away of sections of sheath as the body ages; this may be due to a slow hardening and shrinkage of the body because of protein denaturation;
- the process of fragmentation cannot explain the great majority of segmented asbestos bodies which have obviously grown by the formation of individual segments only;
- the texture of asbestos bodies suggests that material is incorporated in the form of aggregates or floccules of different sizes.

With respect to asbestos body composition, Pooley (1972a) commented that the material forming the body is definitely biological in origin. Its diffraction patterns were found to match those obtained from ferritin extracts. However, the protein content of asbestos bodies is likely to be variable and, on this basis, Pooley (1972a) thought it appropriate to classify them as haemosiderin formations. Phosphorus and calcium were also found in the bodies and Pooley (1972a) suggested that it is probable that the calcium content accounts for their structural stability and has an important role in body formation, by acting as an aggregating agent for ferritin or haemosiderin granules.

More recently, Das et al. (1977) studied the formation of asbestos bodies in guinea pigs and concluded that ferric iron, associated with protein in ferritin or haemosiderin, is deposited on intracellular asbestos fibres, probably as a monolayer by physical adsorption, and that the thick coating of fibres is formed by attachment of Perl's positive globules to this thin layer. These authors considered that major steps in the generation of asbestos body material are diapedesis of erythrocytes, phagocytosis of insoluble compounds formed from the haemoglobin of these erythrocytes, intracellular conversion of those compounds to soluble forms in secondary lysosomes and fusion of these lysosomes to form the Perl's positive granules.

It is noted that there is general agreement that it is longer asbestos fibres which are preferrentially coated to form asbestos bodies (Das et al., 1977; Holmes and Morgan, 1980; Morgan, 1980). This is illustrated by the data of Morgan (1980) listed below.

Subject	Type of fibre	Probability of fibre of stated length being coated*					
		2-4.9	5-9.9	10-19.9	20-39.9	40-79.9	>80
Rat	Anthophyllite	0	0	0.1	0.6	7	~100
Human	Crocidolite	0	0.3	3.1	5.8	8.1	+
Human	Crocidolite	0	2.2	8.1	8.8	15.4	38
Human	Crocidolite	0	2.8	16.7	33.7	41.4	56
Guinea pig	Anthophyllite	0.3	3.1	27.4	63.8	+	+

Notes: * Fibre lengths in μm, probabilities as percentages
          + Insufficient fibres to determine probability

Arul and Holt (1980) considered clearance of asbestos bodies from the lungs of mesothelioma patients and concluded that two routes were involved. Transparent structures could break up to give small fragments that were phagocytosed and dissolved by macrophages. Alternatively, ferroprotein could be converted into haemosiderin, the structure then fragmenting into granules smaller than 0.5 µm. Initially, the haemosiderin may have been phagocytosed and heavy deposits were found near some blood vessels. However, later, phagocytosis was less important because of a lack of macrophages.

7.7.4   Retention in the lung and translocation to other tissues

The short-term retention in the lungs following inhalation is discussed in the context of deposition in the lung (Section 7.7.1.2). This section contains a discussion of long-term retention in the lung and translocation to other tissues, including the pleura.

Some studies on long-term lung retention are discussed in the context of estimating initial deposition (Section 7.7.1.2). Thus, the results of Wagner et al. (1974) indicate relatively little clearance, except in rats exposed for 24 months, or exposed for 6 months and assayed after a further 18 months. It is noted that exposure levels in these studies were sufficient to induce asbestosis and that the degree of asbestosis increased with increasing exposure. This may explain why lung retention of amphibole asbestos in the 24 month exposed group is higher than would be expected by comparison with the data for the 6 month exposed group. Results for chrysotile clearance in the two groups are comparable, possibly reflecting an enhanced importance of in vivo dissolution relative to macrophage clearance in the case of chrysotile asbestos. From the 6 month exposure studies, the following half-lives for lung retention can be calculated.

Asbestos type	Half-life (d)
Amosite	300
Anthophyllite	720
Crocidolite	290
Rhodesian chrysotile	270

These half-lives are for mass retention and are subject to considerable, unquantifiable, uncertainty. Half-lives at higher levels of exposure would, almost undoubtedly, be longer, at least for amphibole asbestos types.

Wagner and Skidmore (1965) gave the following data for retention of asbestos and glass fibre in rat lungs following inhalation exposure.

| Time after exposure(d) | Sex | Mass of dust in lungs (mg): mean ± s.e.* | | | |
		Chrysotile	Crocidolite	Amosite	Glass
1	Male	0.98±0.05	2.98±0.39	4.10±0.28	8.04±0.52
	Female	0.68±0.12	2.90±0.61	3.26±0:32	5.60±0.56
29	Male	0.33±0.07	3.34±0.09	3.32±0.37	5.60±0.20
	Female	0.37±0.15	2.80±0.41	2.78±0.15	4.30±0.18
58	Male	0.18±0.02	1.76±0.21	2.88±0.62	6.60±1.27
	Female	0.15±0.03	1.76±0.18	2.18±0.16	3.50±0.49

Note: * 4 animals in each group

These data indicate that chrysotile was lost from the lungs with a half-life of 25 d, whereas half-lives for the other forms of asbestos and fibrous glass were ~80 to 200 d. Initial levels of asbestos in the lungs of these animals were comparable with those obtained by Wagner et al. (1974), but the animals were exposed for 6 weeks rather than 6 months.

Davis et al. (1980) reported on the retention of asbestos in rats exposed to 'uniform' or 'intermittent' exposure regimes (see Section 7.7.1.2). The animals were exposed over a period of 1 year and the following results were recorded.

Asbestos type	Exposure type	Time after exposure(d)	Mean lung content (µg)	Percentage clearance between 7 and 182 d
Chrysotile	uniform	7	526	66
		182	180	
	intermittent	7	501	47
		182	270	
Amosite	uniform	7	9169	24
		182	7020	
	intermittent	7	11226	35
		182	7331	

Corresponding half-lives of retention, on a mass basis, are as follows.

Asbestos type	Exposure type	Half-life (d)
Chrysotile	uniform	112
	intermittent	191
Amosite	uniform	442
	intermittent	282

Morgan and his co-workers have undertaken an extensive series of experiments on the clearance of asbestos from the rat lung following inhalation and intrapleural injection (Holmes and Morgan, 1967; Morgan and Holmes, 1970; Morgan et al., 1971; Evans et al., 1973; Morgan et al., 1977a; Morgan et al., 1978; Morgan, 1980; Holmes and Morgan, 1980). Using neutron activated asbestos, Morgan and Holmes (1970) concluded that radiometric methods are not suitable for detecting the translocation of relatively small amounts of asbestos following subcutaneous injection, but that they may be used with advantage after dusting or intratracheal administration. They demonstrated that the faecal clearance of Fe-59, following intratracheal injection of radioactive crocidolite is well described by a three-component function:

$$E_f(t) = 27\ e^{-0.693t/1} + 0.4\ e^{-0.693t/14} + 0.1\ e^{-0.693t/240}$$

where $E_f(t)$ is the percentage of injected Fe-59 excreted each day; and t is in days.

Morgan and Holmes (1970) noted that the half-life of the first component (1 d) represents transfer delay through the gut and should not be related to lung clearance. They also demonstrated that whole-body retention, as estimated by integrating the faecal excretion curve, was in good agreement with directly measure values to 100 d after injection. In this context, it is noted that the measured faecal excretion curve integrated over all time would represent only 81.7% of the injected activity.

In a second experiment, Evans et al. (1973) exposed rats to either elutriated or unelutriated crocidolite asbestos. In this case, a two component function was found to fit the faecal excretion results to 30 d after exposure. Representing this function in the form:

$$E_f(t) = A_1 e^{-\lambda_1 t} + A_2 e^{-\lambda_2 t}$$

values of A_1, λ_1, A_2 and λ_2 for individual rats were as listed below.

Rat number	A_1 (µg)	λ_1 (d^{-1})	A_2 (µg)	λ_2 (d^{-1})
2	60	1.68	0.21	0.022
4	60	1.67	0.23	0.025
6	62	1.41	0.25	0.019
8	64	1.75	0.32	0.035

The authors also reported on the distribution of fibres in the lungs at 30 d after exposure. In the conducting airways, the largest number of fibres were located at bifurcations of the smaller bronchioles just downstream from the carina. This can be accounted for by interception effects. Fibres on the bronchiolar epithelium were frequently associated with macrophages. Fibres in the lung parenchyma tended to occur at the ends of alveolar ducts and at the entrances to alveolar sacs, though some were seen within alveoli. In general, it was clear that fibres deposited in the bronchioles were longer and thicker than those found in the alveolar region.

In a further experiment, Morgan et al. (1977) used serial killing to estimate long-term half-lives for UICC standard reference samples and synthetic mineral fibres in rat lungs. Results from these studies were summarised as follows.

Fibre type	Clearance half-life (d)	Duration of experiment (d)
Chrysotile A	62	101
Chrysotile B	46	101
Amosite	56	171
Crocidolite	76	138
Anthophyllite	55	129
Fluoramphibole	58	101

The authors noted that these results were based on radioactivity measurements. For this reason, half-lives for chrysotile, which is readily leached in vivo, may have been underestimated. Morgan et al. (1977) also reported on the whole body retention of a synthetic fluoramphibole by in vivo counting. The retention curve found was:

$$R(t) = 0.865\ e^{-0.693t/0.38} + 0.053\ e^{-0.693t/8} + 0.082\ e^{-0.693t/118}$$

where t is in days.

For comparison, differentating this function and assuming that faecal excretion predominates, it is possible to calculate a faecal excretion function. Thus;

$$E_f(t) = 158.7\ e^{-0.693t/0.38} + 0.46\ e^{-0.693t/8} + 0.048\ e^{-0.693t/118}$$

where $E_f(t)$ has units of percent per day; and t is in days.

Throughout the above discussion, retention in the lung, or excretion in the faeces, has been expressed on a mass basis. However, as has been noted, fibre clearance is related to size (primarily length). For this reason, retention expressed on a mass basis is not related directly to retention expressed on a fibre number basis. For anthophyllite, this has been studied by Morgan et al. (1978) and Holmes and Morgan (1980). Morgan et al. (1978) concluded that fibres of <5 μm length were removed more rapidly than longer fibres, probably as a result of processes mediated by alveolar macrophages (Morgan, 1980), and noted that fibres longer than ∿100 μm could not be recovered from the lung by lavage procedures. The count median length of anthophyllite fibres in the lungs of rats at various times after exposure was given by Holmes and Morgan (1980) as follows:

Time after exposure (d)	Count median length (μm)
100	4.7
247	6.0
332	6.5
730	11.0

These results are similar to those recorded for human lungs by Timbrell (1982) following unspecified regimes of exposure in a mine environment. In the study of Morgan et al. (1978), the half-life of anthophyllite in the lungs was estimated to be 76 d. The mean content of anthophyllite per lavaged macrophage also fell rapidly dropping from 9 to 2 pg over the first 90 d after exposure, corresponding to a half-life of 41.5 d. In the absence of further information on the cell kinetics of the macrophage population, the implications of this result cannot be assessed.

With respect to their intrapleural injection studies on rats, Morgan et al. (1971) reported that clearly visible asbestos granuloma formed on the right thoracic surface of the diaphragm and that ultramicroscopic fibrils were observed in the underlying liver tissue, in Kupffer cells of the right and median lobe areas. These were associated with the oesophagal and vascular openings and a zone equivalent to the 'bare area' in the human liver.

Other studies on asbestos retention in rat lung have been reported by Middleton et al. (1977; 1979). Middleton et al. (1977) gave the following data for retention following a six week period of exposure (see also Section 7.7.1.2).

Asbestos type	Exposure level (mg m^{-3})	Asbestos content (µg per rat)				
		5 d	32 d	66 d	102 d	128 d
Amosite	1.4	78	72	45	47	38
	4.6	646	309	160	138	119
	9.4	1498	605	410	332	371
Crocidolite	5.9	1012	645	442	337	268
	11.8	1338	1267	1114	884	583
Chrysotile	3.8	109	52	42	36	-
	7.8	245	93	113	63	55

In some cases, a rapid fall in lung content between 5 and 32 d after exposure was observed. This may have represented clearance corresponding to the intermediate phase recognised by Morgan and Holmes (1970) and Morgan et al. (1977). Retention half-lives for long-term retention have been calculated using the remainder of the data and are listed below.

Asbestos type	Exposure level (mg m^{-3})	Half-life (d)*		
		32-66 d	32-102 d	32-128 d
Amosite	1.4	50	114	104
	4.6	36	60	70
	9.4	61	81	136
Crocidolite	5.9	62	75	76
	11.8	183	135	86
Chrysotile	3.8	110	132	-
	7.8	∞	125	127

Note: * Half-life estimated for clearance over a specified interval.

Middleton et al. (1979) gave similar data for retention in rats following a six week period of exposure. These data are listed below (see also Section 7.7.1.2).

Type of asbestos	Exposure level (mg m^{-3})	Asbestos content (µg per rat)				
		5 d	40 d	70 d	97 d	125 d
Chrysotile	7.8	245	98	113	72	54
	3.8	112	58	43	35	51
	1.2	70	27	27	23	20
	10.1*	724	458	279	243	253
		5 d	32 d	66 d	102 d	128 d
Amosite	9.4	1448	605	410	332	385
	4.6	693	309	160	138	124
	1.4	79	69	46	45	43
		5 d	35 d	67 d	96 d	126 d
Crocidolite	11.8	1052	1267	1114	742	546
	5.9	1012	772	396	352	276
	1.4	146	105	95	43	40
	12.9*	1695	1195	1028	762	661

Note: * nocturnal exposure

Again, the reduction in body content between 5 and 32 to 40 d is relatively large. Half-lives computed from the rest of the data are listed below.

Type of asbestos	Exposure level (mg m^{-3})	Half-life (d)*		
		40-70 d	40-97 d	40-125 d
Chrysotile	7.8	∞	128	99
	3.8	69	78	458
	1.2	∞	246	196
	10.1	42	62	99
		32-66 d	32-102 d	32-128 d
Amosite	9.4	61	81	147
	4.6	36	60	73
	1.4	58	114	141
		35-67 d	35-96 d	35-126 d
Crocidolite	11.8	172	79	75
	5.9	33	54	61
	1.4	222	47	65
	12.9	147	94	107

These data do not indicate that chrysotile asbestos is cleared from the lung any faster than the amphiboles and the long term half-life of retention in all cases is typically ~100 d.

With respect to translocation from the lung to other tissues, data are very limited and the mechanisms of transport are almost totally obscure. Thus, for example, in case reports, asbestos has been found in hilar and mediastinal lymph nodes, lymphatics, the spleen, abdominal tumours and small intestinal wall (Godwin and Jagatic, 1970) and, in workers, asbestos fibres have been observed in liver, pancreas, kidney, adrenal gland and spleen (Langer, 1974). However, the current lack of quantitative knowledge is reflected in the statement by Davis (1981) that "some of the asbestos deposited in the lung tissue reaches the pleura probably by both lymphatic transport within macrophages and by the direct penetration of free fibres." Davis (1981) went on to comment that "experimental studies have so far been unable to elucidate the exact processes involved." In this context, some results of studies using other routes of exposure are of interest. Thus, Roe et al. (1967) reported that, following subcutaneous injection of asbestos into mice, fibres were disseminated widely from the sites of injection, but in a highly selective fashion. In the chest, the main sites of accumulation were the visceral and parietal pleura, and pericardium, with involvement of the adjacent parts of the lungs. In the abdomen, asbestos was seen on the serosal surfaces of the stomach, intestine, liver and spleen, in the mesentery and also in retroperitoneal structures, particularly around the pancreas and kidneys. It was also noted that, in contrast to other tissues, serosal tissues reacted vigorously to the presence of asbestos fibres, exhibiting a wide range of histological changes. Cunningham and Pontefract (1974) using intravenous injection of chrysotile asbestos into pregnant rats, reported that asbestos could cross the placenta and enter the foetus. The data available are not sufficient to quantify this process, but the variations in results suggest that this may have been a pathological effect in some cases. Finally, it is noted that Monchaux et al. (1982) have demonstrated the transport of intrapleurally injected asbestos and glass fibres to the lung parenchyma. However, as the authors state, "the route which the fibres follow to reach the mediastinal lymph nodes and the lung are still unknown and cannot be ascertained by this study."

7.7.5   A model for asbestos retention following inhalation

On the basis of the data reviewed in this section, the following recommendations are made concerning asbestos retention in the body following inhalation.

- Of inhaled asbestos, 50% can be assumed to be deposited in the lung, including both upper and lower components of the respiratory tract.
- Of inhaled amphibole asbestos, 10% can be assumed to be retained in the lung with a half-life of 200 d and the rest rapidly excreted.
- Of inhaled chrysotile asbestos, 2.5% can be assumed to be retained in the lung with a half-life of 200 d and the rest rapidly excreted.
- For the purpose of monitoring, all asbestos leaving the lungs may be assumed to be lost from the body via faecal excretion though a small amount is undoubtedly translocated to other tissues.

- For assessment of intakes of asbestos by inhalation the following retention functions are recommended.

Chrysotiles:

$$R(t) = 0.925e^{-0.693t/1} + 0.05e^{-0.693t/10} + 0.025e^{-0.693t/200}$$

Amphiboles:

$$R(t)\ 0.85e^{-0.693t/1} + 0.05e^{-0.693t/10} + 0.1e^{-0.693t/200}$$

The corresponding faecal excretion functions are as follows.

Chrysotiles:

$$E_f(t) = 64e^{-0.693t/1} + 0.35e^{-0.693t/10} + 0.0087e^{-0.693t/200}$$

Amphiboles:

$$E_f(t) = 59e^{-0.693t/1} + 0.35e^{-0.693t/10} + 0.035e^{-0.693t/200}$$

where $E_f(t)$ is the percentage excretion per day; and t is in days.

It is noted that there is undoubtedly a small fraction of asbestos which is retained in the lung with a biological half-life of much more than 200 d.   This asbestos is probably long-fibred and it is emphasised that neither the period of its retention, nor the processes of its transfer from the lung, can currently be quantified.

8.   REFERENCES

Allison, A.C., 1976. Effects of silica, asbestos and other pollutants on macrophages. In: Aharonson, E.F., Ben-David, A. and Klingberg, M.A. (Eds.). Air Pollution and the Lung, John Wiley and Sons, New York, US, pp.114-134.

Amacher, D.E., Alarif, A. and Epstein, S.S., 1975. The dose-dependent effects of ingested chrysotile on DNA synthesis in the gastrointestinal tract, liver and pancreas of the rat. Environ. Res., 10, 208-216.

Argouarch, L.P., Borel, B., Justum, A.M., Davy, A., Verwaerde, J.C. and Valla, A., 1981. Mésothéliome primitif du péritoine et exposition à l'amiante. Médecine et Chirurgie Digestives, 10, 583-586.

Apul, K.J. and Holt, P.F., 1980. Clearance of asbestos bodies from the lung: a personal view. Br. J. Ind. Med., 37, 273-277.

Ashcroft, T. and Heppleston, A.G., 1973. The optical and electron micros-copic determination of pulmonary asbestos fibre concentration and its relation to the human pathological reaction. J. Clin. Path., 26, 224-234.

Auerbach, O., Conston, A.S., Garfinkel, L., Parks, V.R., Kaslow, H.D. and Hammond, E.C., 1980. Presence of asbestos bodies in organs other than the lung. Chest, 77, 133-137.

Babu, K.A., Lakkad, B.C., Nigam, S.K., Bhatt, D.K., Karnik, A.B., Thakore, K.N., Kashyap, S.K. and Chatterjee, S.K., 1980. In vitro cytological and cytogenic effects of an Indian variety of Chrysotile asbestos. Environ. Res., 21, 416-422.

Beck, E.G., 1976. Interaction between fibrous dust and cells in vitro. Ann. Anat. Pathol. (Paris), 21, 227-236.

Becklake, M.R., 1976. Asbestos related diseases of the lung and other organs: their epidemiology and implications for clinical practice. Am. Rev. Resp. Dis., 114, 187-227.

Berry, G. Newhouse, M.L. and Turok, M., 1972. Combined effect of asbestos exposure and smoking on mortality from lung cancer in factory workers. Lancet, 2, 476-479, 2 September.

Bolton, R.E., Davis, J.M.G., Donaldson, K. and Wright, A., 1982. Variations in the carcinogenicity of mineral fibres. Ann. occup. Hyg., 26, 569-582.

Botham, S.K. and Holt, P.F., 1968. The mechanism of formation of asbestos bodies. J. Path. Bact., 96, 443-453.

Botham, S.K. and Holt, P.F., 1972. Asbestos body formation in the lungs of rats and guinea pigs after inhalation of anthophyllite. J. Pathol., 107, 245-252.

Brody, A.R. and Hill, L.H., 1981. Deposition pattern and clearance pathways of inhaled chrysotile asbestos. Chest, 80, Suppl., 64S-67S.

Brown, R.C., Chamberlain, M., Griffiths, D.M. and Timbrell, V., 1978. The effect of fibre size on the in vitro biological activity of three types of amphibole asbestos. Int. J. Cancer, 22, 721-727.

Brown, R.C., Chamberlain, M. and Skidmore, J.W., 1979. In vitro effects of man-made mineral fibres. Ann. occup. Hyg., 22, 175-179.

Bruch, J., 1974. Response of cell cultures to asbestos fibers. Environ. Health Perspect., 9, 253-254.

Casey, K.R., Rom, W.N. and Moatamed, F., 1981. Asbestos-related diseases. Clinics in Chest Medicine, 2, 179-202.

Charpin, D., Vervloet, D., Poirier, R., Charpin, J. and Laval, P. 1981. Manifestations thoraciques de l'amiante et génétique: a propos de deux paires de jumeaux univitellins. Rev. fr. Mal. Resp., 9, 55-59.

Churg, A and Warnock, M.L., 1977. Analysis of the cores of ferruginous (asbestos) bodies from the general population. I. Patients with and without lung cancer. Lab. Invest., 37, 280-286.

Churg, A., Warnock, M.L. and Green, N., 1979. Analysis of the cores of ferruginous (asbestos) bodies from the general population: II. True asbestos bodies and pseudoasbestos bodies. Lab. Invest., 40, 31-38.

Cochrane, J.C. and Webster, I., 1978. Mesothelioma in relation to asbestos fibre exposure. S. Afr. Med. J., 54, 279-281.

Cook, P.M. and Olson, G.F., 1979. Ingested mineral fibers: elimination in human urine. Science, 204, 195-198.

Cooper, W.C., 1967. Asbestos as a hazard to health. Arch. Environ. Health, 15, 285-290.

Cralley, L.J. and Lainhart, W.S., 1973. Are trace metals associated with asbestos fibers responsible for the biologic effects attributed to asbestos? J. Occup. Med., 15, 262-266.

Cunningham, H.M. and Pontefract, R.D., 1973. Asbestos fibers in beverages, drinking water and tissues: their passage through the intestinal wall and movement through the body. J. Assoc. Off. Anal. Chem., 56, 976-981.

Cunningham, H.M. and Pontefract, R.D., 1974. Placental transfer of asbestos. Nature (Lond.), 249, 177-178.

Cunningham, H.M., Moodie, C.A., Lawrence, G.A. and Pontefract, R.D., 1977. Chronic effects of ingested asbestos in rats. Arch, Environm. Contam. Toxicol., 6, 507-513.

Das, R.M., Holt, P.F. and Horne, M.C., 1977. The formation of asbestos bodies. Medna Lav., 68, 431-436.

Davies, P., Allison, A.C., Ackerman, J., Butterfield, A. and Williams, S., 1974. Asbestos induces selective release of lysosomal enzymes from mononuclear phagocytes. Nature (Lond.), 251, 423-425.

Davis, J.M.G., 1965. Electron microscope studies of asbestosis in man and animals. Ann. N.Y. Acad. Sci., 132, 98-111.

Davis, J.M.G., 1976. Structural variations between pleural and peritoneal mesotheliomas produced in rats by the injection of crocidolite asbestos. Ann. Anat. Pathol. (Paris), 21, 199-210.

Davis, J.M.G., 1979. The histopathology and ultrastructure of pleural mesotheliomas produced in the rat by injections of crocidolite asbestos. Br. J. exp. Path., 60, 642-652.

Davis, J.M.G., 1981. The biological effects of mineral fibres. Ann. occup. Hyg., 24, 227-234.

Davis, J.M.G., Bolton, R.E. and Garrett, J., 1974. Penetration of cells by asbestos fibers. Environ. Health Perspect., 9, 255-260.

Davis, J.M.G., Beckett, S.T., Bolton, R.E., Collings, P. and Middleton, A.P., 1978. Mass and number of fibres in the pathogenesis of asbestos-related lung disease in rats. Br. J. Cancer, 37, 673-688.

Davis, J.M.G., Beckett, S.T., Bolton, R.E. and Donaldson, K., 1980. The effects of intermittent high asbestos exposure (peak dose levels) on the lungs of rats. Br. J. exp. Path., 61, 272-280.

DeLajartre, A.Y., Mussini-Montpellier, J. and Lenne, Y. 1976. Étude anatomo-pathologique de 54 cas de mésothéliomes pleuraux diffus observés dans les régions portuaires de Nantes, Saint-Nazaire et Lorient. Ann. Anat. Pathol. (Paris), 21, 247-260.

Dement, J.M., Harris, R.L. Jr., Symons, M.J. and Shy, C., 1982. Estimates of dose-response for respiratory cancer among chrysotile asbestos textile workers. Ann. Occup. Hyg., 26, 869-887.

Desai, R., Hext, P. and Richards, R., 1975. The prevention of asbestos-induced hemolysis. Life Sci., 16, 1931-1938.

Di Menza, L., Ruff, F., Bignon, J., Bonnaud, G. and Brouet, G., 1976. Obstruction des voies aériennes peripheriques au cours de l'exposition professionnelle à l'amiante. Ann. Anat. Pathol. (Paris), 21, 261-268.

Dohner, V.A., Beegle, R.G. and Miller, W.T., 1975. Asbestos exposure and multiple primary tumors. Am. Rev. Resp. Dis., 112, 181-199.

Doll, R., 1955. Mortality from lung cancer in asbestos workers. Br. J. Ind. Med., 12, 81-86.

Elmes, P.C. and Simpson, M.J.C., 1977. Insulation workers in Belfast. A further study of mortality due to asbestos exposure (1940-1975). Br. J. Ind. Med., 34, 174-180.

Enterline, P.E. and Henderson, V., 1973. Types of asbestos and respiratory cancer in the asbestos industry. Arch. Environ. Health, 27, 312-317.

Enterline, P.E. and Kendrick, M.A., 1967. Asbestos-dust exposures at various levels and mortality. Arch. Environ. Health, 15, 181-186.

Evans, J.C., Evans, R.J., Holmes, A., Hounam, R.F., Jones, D.M., Morgan, A. and Walsh, M., 1973. Studies on the deposition of inhaled fibrous material in the respiratory tract of the rat and its subsequent clearance using radioactive tracer techniques. I. UICC crocidolite asbestos. Environ. Res., 6, 180-201.

Farulla, A., Naro, G., Alimena, G., Delfini, A.M., Ogis, M., Pugliese, D. and Zingarelli, S., 1978. Studio dell'effetto in vitro di fibre di asbesto su colture a breve termine di linfociti umani. Ann. Ist. Super. Sanità, 14, 655-658.

Fondimare, A. and Desbordes, J., 1974. Asbestos bodies and fibers in lung tissues. Environ. Health Perspect., 9, 147-148.

Fondimare, A., Sebastien, P., Monchaux, G., Bignon, J., Desbordes, J. and Bonnaud, G., 1976. Variations topographiques des concentrations pulmonaires et pleurales en fibres d'amiante chez des sujets diversement exposés. Ann. Anat. Pathol. (Paris), 21, 277-284.

Godwin, M.C. and Jagatic, J., 1970. Asbestos and mesothelioma. Environ. Res., 3, 391-416.

Goldstein, B. and Rendall, R.E.G., 1970. Ferruginous bodies. In: Shapiro H. (Ed.) Pneumoconiosis. Oxford University Press, London, pp. 92-98.

Griffis, L.C., Pickrell, J.A., Carpenter, R.L., Wolff, R.K., McAllen, S.J. and Yerkes, K.L., 1983. Deposition of crocidolite asbestos and glass microfibers inhaled by the beagle dog. Am. Ind. Hyg. Assoc. J., 44, 216-222.

Gross, P., 1974. Is short fibered asbestos dust a biological hazard? Arch. Environ. Health, 29, 115-117.

Gross, P., 1977. The biologic response to inhaled mineral fibers: facts and fancies. Rev. Environ. Health, II, 167-175.

Gross, P., de Treville, R.T., Tolker, E.B., Kaschak, M. and Babyak, M.A., 1967. Experimental asbestosis. The development of lung cancer in rats with pulmonary deposits of chrysotile dust. Arch. Environ. Health, 15, 343-355.

Gross, P., de Treville, R.T.P., Cralley, L.J. and Pundsack, F.L., 1970. Problems in the pathology of asbestosis. In: Shapiro, H. (Ed.) Pneumoconiosis Oxford University Press, London, pp.126-132.

Gross, P., Harley, R.A., Swinburne, L.M., Davis, J.M.G. and Greene, W.B., 1974. Ingested mineral fibers. Do they penetrate tissue or cause cancer? Arch. Environ. Health, 29, 341-347.

Hahon, N., Booth, J.A. and Eckert, H.L., 1977. Antagonistic activity of poly(4-vinylpyridine-N-oxide) to the inhibition of viral interferon induction by asbestos fibres. Br. J. Ind. Med., 34, 119-125.

Hallenbeck, W.H., Markey, D.R. and Dolan, D.G., 1981. Analyses of tissue, blood, and urine samples from a baboon gavaged with chrysotile and crocidolite asbestos. Environ. Res., 25, 349-360.

Hamilton, J.A., Vadas, P. and Hay, J.B., 1981. Measurement of blood flow and vascular permeability changes in response to 12-0-tetradecanoyl-phorbol-13-acetate and to asbestos fibers. J. Toxicol. Environ. Health, 8, 205-214.

Hammad, Y.Y., Diem, J. and Weill, H., 1979. Evaluation of dust exposure in asbestos cement manufacturing operations. Am. Ind. Hyg. Assoc. J., 40, 490-495.

Hammad, Y., Diem, J., Craighead, J. and Weill, H., 1982. Deposition of inhaled man-made mineral fibres in the lungs of rats. Ann. occup. Hyg., 26, 179-187.

Harington, J.S., 1965. Chemical studies of asbestos. Ann. N.Y. Acad. Sci., 132, 31-47.

Harington, J.S., 1967. Mesothelioma. In: Raven, R.W. and Roe, F.J.C. (Eds.) Prevention of Cancer, Butterworth, London, pp.207-211.

Harington, J.S., 1976. The biological effects of mineral fibres, especially asbestos, as seen from in vitro and in vivo studies. Ann. Anat. Pathol. (Paris), 21, 155-198.

Harington, J.S., Allison, A.C. and Badami, D.V., 1975. Mineral fibers: chemical, physicochemical and biological properties. Adv. Pharmacol. Chemother., 12, 291-401.

Harris, R.L. Jr., 1976. Aerodynamic considerations; what is a respiratory fiber of fibrous glass. In: Proc. Symp. Occup. Exposure to Fibrous Glass, HEW-PHS, pp.51-56.

Harris, R.L. and Fraser, D.A., 1976. A model for deposition of fibers in the human respiratory system. Am. Ind. Hyg. Assoc. J., 37, 73-89.

Hasselbacher, P., 1979. Binding of immunoglobulin and activation of complement by asbestos fibers. J. Allergy Clin. Immunol., 64, 294-298.

Hiett, D.M. 1978. Experimental asbestosis: an investigation of functional and pathological disturbances. I. Methods, control animals and exposure conditions. Br. J. Ind. Med., 35, 129-134.

Hiett, D.M., 1978a. Experimental asbestosis: an investigation of functional and pathological disturbances. II. Results for chrysotile and amosite exposures. Br. J. Ind. Med., 35, 135-145.

Hillerdal, G. and Hemmingsson, A., 1980. Pulmonary pseudotumours and asbestos. Acta Radiol. Diagnosis, 21, 615-620.

Hinds, H.W., Thomas, D.B. and O'Reilly, H.P., 1979. Asbestos, dental x-rays, tobacco, and alcohol in the epidemiology of laryngeal cancer. Cancer, 44, 1114-1120.

Holmes, A. and Morgan, A. 1967. Leaching of constituents of chrysotile asbestos in vivo. Nature (Lond.), 215, 441-442.

Holmes, A. and Morgan, A., 1980. Clearance of anthophyllite fibers from the rat lung and the formation of asbestos bodies. Environ. Res., 22, 13-21.

Holt, P.F., 1980. Dust elimination from pulmonary alveoli. Environ. Res., 23, 224-227.

Holt, P.F., Mills, J. and Young, D.K., 1965. Experimental asbestosis with four types of fibers: importance of small particles. Ann. N.Y. Acad. Sci., 132, 87-97.

International Agency for Research on Cancer, 1977. Monograph Series on the Evaluation of Carcinogenic Risk of Chemicals to Man, 14, Asbestos. IARC, Lyon.

International Commission on Radiological Protection 1966. Deposition and retention models for internal dosimetry of the human respiratory tract. Health Phys., 12, 173-207.

Jacobs, R. and Richards, R.J., 1980. Distribution of 6-6(n)-³[H] sucrose and its radiolabeled degradation products from isolated, perfused rat small intestine loops following prolonged ingestion of chrysotile asbestos. Environ. Res., 21, 423-431.

Jacobs, R., Dodgson, K.S. and Richards, R.J., 1977. A preliminary study of biochemical changes in the rat small intestine following long-term ingestion of chrysotile asbestos. Br. J. Exp. Path., 58, 541-548.

Jaurand, M.C., Bignon, J., Sebastien, P. and Goni, J., 1977. Leaching of chrysotile asbestos in human lungs. Correlation with in vitro studies using rabbit alveolar macrophages. Environ. Res., 14, 245-254.

Jaurand, M.C., Bignon, J., Gaudichet, A., Magne, L. and Oblin, A., 1978. Biological effects of chrysotile after SO_2 sorption. II. Effects on alveolar macrophages and red blood cells. Environ. Res., 17, 216-227.

Jaurand, M.C., Bignon, J., Magne, L., Renier, A. and Lafuma, J., 1979. Interaction des fibres avec les globules rouges et les macrophages alveo- laires in vitro. Rev. fr. Mal. Resp., 7, 717-722.

Johnson, N.F. and Davies, R., 1981. An ultrastructural study of the effects of asbestos fibres on cultured peritoneal macrophages. J. exp. Path., 62, 559-570.

Kagan, E. and Miller, K., 1981. Asbestos inhalation and the induction of splenic lymphocytic proliferation in the rat. Chest, 80, July Supplement, 11S-12S.

Kagan, E., Webster, I., Cochrane, J.C. and Miller, K., 1977. The immunology of asbestosis. In:Walton, W.H. (Ed.) Inhaled Particles IV. Pergamon Press, Oxford, pp.429-433.

Kanazawa, K., Yamamoto, T. and Yuasa, Y., 1979. Enhancement by asbestos of oncogenesis by Moloney murine sarcoma virus in CBA mice. Int. J. Cancer, 23, 866-874.

Kannerstein, M., Churg, J., McCaughey, W.T.E. and Selikoff, I.J., 1977. Pathogenic effects of asbestos. Arch. Pathol. Lab. Med., 101, 623-628.

Kannerstein, M., Churg, J. and Elliott-McCaughey, W.T., 1978. Asbestos and mesothelioma: a review. Pathol. Ann., 1, 81-129.

Kaw, J.L., Tilkes, F. and Beck, E.G., 1982. Reaction of cells cultured in vitro to different asbestos dusts of equal surface area but different fibre length. Br. J. exp. Path., 63, 109-115.

Kleinfeld, M., Messite, J. and Langer, A.M., 1973. A study of workers exposed to asbestiform minerals in commercial talc manufacture. Environ. Res., 6, 132-143.

Knox, J.F., Holmes, S., Doll, R. and Hill, I.D., 1968. Mortality from lung cancers and other causes among workers in an asbestos textile factory. Br. J. Ind. Med., 25, 293-303.

Kuschner, M. and Wright, G., 1976. The effects of intratracheal instillation of glass fiber of various sizes in guinea pigs. In: Proc. Symp. Occup. Exposure to Fibrous Glass, HEW-PHS, pp.151-167.

Lakowicz, J.R. and Bevan, D.R., 1980. Benzo[α]pyrene uptake into rat liver microsomes: effects of adsorption of benzo[α]pyrene to asbestos and non-fibrous mineral particulates. Chem.-Biol. Interactions, 29, 129-138.

Langer, A.M., 1974. Inorganic particles in human tissues and their association with neoplastic disease. Environ. Health Perspect., 9, 229-233.

Langer, A.M. and Wolff, M.S., 1977. Asbestos carcinogenesis. Chapter 3 (pp.29-55) of G.N. Schrauzer (Ed.) Inorganic and Nutritional Aspects of Cancer. Plenum Press, New York.

Langer, A.M., Rubin, I. and Selikoff, I.J., 1970. Electron microprobe analysis of asbestos bodies. In: Shapiro, H. (Ed.), Pneumoconiosis. Oxford University Press, London, pp.57-69.

Langer, A.M., Selikoff, I.J. and Sastre, A., 1971. Chrysotile asbestos in the lungs of persons in New York City. Arch. Environ. Health, 22, 348-360.

Langer, A.M., Rubin, I.B. and Selikoff, I. J., 1972. Chemical characterisation of asbestos body cores by electron microprobe analysis. J. Histochem. Cytochem., 20, 723-734.

Langer, A.M., Rubin, I.B., Selikoff, I.J. and Pooley, F.D., 1972a. Chemical characterisation of uncoated asbestos fibers from the lungs of asbestos workers by electron microprobe analysis. J. Histochem. Cytochem., 20, 735-740.

Langer, A.M., Mackler, A.D. and Pooley, F.D., 1974. Electron microscopical investigation of asbestos fibers. Environ. Health Perspect., 9, 63-80.

Langer, A.M., Wolff, M.S., Rohl, A.N. and Selikoff, I.J., 1978. Variation of properties of chrysotile asbestos subjected to milling. J. Toxicol. Environ. Health, 4, 173-188.

Lavappa, K.A., Fu, M.M. and Epstein, S.S., 1975. Cytogenetic studies on chrysotile asbestos. Environ. Res., 10, 165-173.

Lemaire, I., Nadeau, D. and Bégin, R., 1981. Significant increases of cyclic AMP and alkaline phosphatase in bronchoalveolar lavage fluids of sheep exposed to asbestos. Res. Comm. Chem. Pathol. Pharmacol., 33, 567-570.

Liddell, F.D.K., Gibbs, G.W. and McDonald, J.C., 1982. Radiological changes and fibre exposure in chrysotile workers aged 60-69 years at Thetford Mines. Ann. occup. Hyg., 26, 889-898.

Light, W.G. and Wei, E.T., 1977. Surface charge and haemolytic activity of asbestos. Environ. Res., 13, 135-145.

Light, W.G. and Wei, E.T., 1977a. Surface charge and asbestos toxicity. Nature (Lond.), 265, 537-539.

Lippman, M., Bohning, D.E. and Schlesinger, R.B., 1976. Deposition of fibrous glass in the human respiratory tract. In: Proc. Symp. Occup. Exposure to Fibrous Glass, HEW-PHS, pp.57-61.

Livingston, G.K., Rom, W.N. and Morris, M.V., 1980. Asbestos-induced sister chromatid exchanges in cultured chinese hamster ovarian fibroblast cells. J. Environ. Pathol. Toxicol., 4, 373-382.

Lumley, K.P.S., 1977. Physiological changes in asbestos pleural disease. In: Walton, W.H. (Ed.) Inhaled Particles IV. Pergamon Press, Oxford, pp. 781-788.

McDonald, J.C., Becklake, M.R., Gibbs, G.W., McDonald, A.D. and Rossiter, C.E., 1974. The health of chrysotile asbestos mine and mill workers. Arch. Environ. Health, 28, 61-68.

McDonald, A.D., McDonald, J.C. and Pooley, F.D., 1982. Mineral fibre content of lung in mesothelial tumours in North America. Ann. Occup. Hyg., 26, 417-422.

McEwen, J., Finlayson, A., Mair, A. and Gibson, A.A.M., 1971. Asbestos and mesothelioma in Scotland: an epidemiological study. Int. Arch. Arbeitsmed., 28, 301-311.

McLemore, T., Corson, M., Mace, M., Arnott, M., Jenkins, T., Snodgrass, D., Martin, R., Wray, N. and Brinkley, B.R., 1979. Phagocytosis of asbestos fibers by human pulmonary alveolar macrophages. Cancer Lett., 6, 183-192.

McLemore, T.L., Mace, M.L. Jr., Roggli, V., Marshall, M.V., Lawrence, E.C., Wilson, R.K., Martin, R.R., Brinkley, B.R. and Greenberg, S.D., 1980. Asbestos body phagocytosis by human free alveolar macrophages. Cancer Lett., 9, 85-93.

Maroudas, N.G., O'Neil, C.H. and Stanton, N.F., 1973. Fibroblast anchorage in carcinogenesis by fibres. Lancet 1, 807-809, 14 April.

Middleton, A.P., Beckett, S.T. and Davis, J.M.G., 1977. A study of the short-term retention and clearance of inhaled asbestos by rats using UICC standard reference samples. In: Walton, W.H. (Ed.). Inhaled Particles IV. Pergamon Press, Oxford, pp.247-258.

Middleton, A.P., Beckett, S.T. and Davis, J.M.G., 1979. Further observations on the short-term retention and clearance of asbestos by rats, using UICC reference samples. Ann. occup. Hyg., 22, 141-152.

Miller, A.B., 1978. Asbestos fibre dust and gastrointestinal malignancies. Review of literature with regard to a cause/effect relationship. J. chron. Dis., 31, 23-33.

Miller, K., 1979. Alterations in the surface-related phenomena of alveolar macrophages following inhalation of crocidolite asbestos and quartz dusts: an overview. Environ. Res., 20, 162-182.

Monchaux, G., Bignon, J., Hirsch, A. and Sebastien, P., 1982. Translocation of mineral fibres through the repiratory system after injection into the pleural cavity of rats. Ann. occup. Hyg., 26, 309-318.

Morgan, A., 1980. Effect of length on the clearance of fibres from the lung and on body formation. IARC Sci. Publ., 30, 329-335.

Morgan, A. and Holmes, A., 1970. Neutron activation techniques in investigations of the composition and biological effects of asbestos. In: Shapiro, H. (Ed.). Pneumoconiosis, Oxford University Press, London, pp.52-56.

Morgan, A., Holmes, A. and Gold, C., 1971. Studies of the solubility of constituents of chrysotile asbestos in vivo using radioactive tracer techniques. Environ. Res., 4, 558-570.

Morgan, A., Davies, P., Wagner, J.C., Berry, G. and Holmes, A., 1977. The biological effects of magnesium-leached chrysotile asbestos. Brit. J. Exp. Pathol., 58, 465-473.

Morgan, A., Evans, J.C. and Holmes, A., 1977a. Deposition and clearance of inhaled fibrous minerals in the rat. Studies using radioactive tracer techniques. In: Walton, W.H. (Ed.). Inhaled Particles IV. Pergamon Press, Oxford, pp.259-274.

Morgan, A., Talbot, R.J. and Holmes, A., 1978. Significance of fibre length in the clearance of asbestos fibres from the lung. Br. J. Ind. Med., 35, 146-153.

Mossman, B.T. and Craighead, J.E., 1981. Mechanisms of asbestos carcinogenesis. Environ. Res., 25, 269-280.

Mossman, B.T. and Craighead, J.E., 1981. Comparative cocarcinogenic effects of crocidolite asbestos, hematite, kaolin and carbon in implanted tracheal organ cultures. Ann. occup. Hyg., 26, 553-567.

Mossman, B.T., Kessler, J.B., Ley, B.W. and Craighead, J.E., 1977. Interaction of crocidolite asbestos with hamster respiratory mucosa in organ culture. Lab. Invest., 36, 131-139.

Neugut, A.I., Eisenberg, D., Silverstein, M., Pulkrabek, P. and Weinstein, I.B., 1978. Effects of asbestos on epithelioid cell lines. Environ. Res., 17, 256-265.

Newhouse, M.L., Berry, G. and Skidmore, J.W., 1982. A mortality study of workers manufacturing friction materials with chrysotile asbestos. Ann. occup. Hyg., 26, 899-909.

Nicholson, W.J., 1977. Occupational and environmental standards for asbestos and their relation to human disease. In: Hiatt, H.H., Watson, J.D. and Winsten, J.A. (Eds.), Origins of Human Cancer, Cold Spring Harbor Laboratories, Cold Spring Harbor, NY, US, pp.1785-1796.

Patel-Mandlik, K.J., Hallenbeck, W.H. and Millette, J.R., 1979. Asbestos fibers: 1. A modified preparation of tissue samples for analysis by electron microscopy. 2. Presence of fibers in tissues of baboon fed chrysotile asbestos. J. Environ. Pathol. Toxicol., 2, 1385-1395.

Peto, J., Doll, R., Howard, S.V., Kinlen, L.J. and Lewinsohn, H.C., 1977. A mortality study among workers in an English asbestos factory. Br. J. Ind. Med., 34, 169-173.

Pontefract, R.D. and Cunningham, H.M., 1973. Penetration of asbestos through the digestive tract of rats. Nature (Lond.), 243, 352-353.

Pooley, F.D., 1972. Electron microscope characteristics of inhaled chrysotile asbestos fibre. Br. J. Ind. Med., 29, 146-153.

Pooley, F.D., 1972a. Asbestos bodies, their formation, composition and character. Environ. Res., 5, 363-379.

Pott, F., Dolgner, R., Friedrichs, K.-H. and Huth, F., 1976. L'effect oncogène des poussières fibreuses. L'expérimentation animale et ses relations avec la carcinogénèse humaine. Ann. Anat. Pathol. (Paris), 21, 237-246.

Pott, F., Friedrichs, K.H. and Huth, F., 1976a. Ergbnisoe aus Tierversuchen zur kanzerogenen Wirkung faserförmiger Staübe und ihre Deutung in Hinblick auf die Tumorentstehung bein Menschen. Zentralbl. Bakteriol. Hyg. Abt., 162, 467-505.

Rahman, Q., Viswanathan, P.N. and Zaidi, S.H., 1977. Some new perspectives on the biological effects of asbestos. Environ. Res., 14, 487-498.

Reeves, A.L., 1976. The carcinogenic effect of inhaled asbestos fibers. Ann. Clin. Lab. Sci., 6, 459-466.

Reeves, A.L., Puro, H.E., Smith, R.G. and Vorwald, A.J., 1971. Experimental asbestos carcinogenesis. Environ. Res., 4, 496-511.

Reeves, A.L., Puro, H.E. and Smith, R.G., 1974. Inhalation carcinogenesis from various forms of asbestos. Environ. Res., 8, 178-202.

Reiss, B., Solomon, S., Weisburger, J.H. and Williams, G.M., 1980. Comparative toxicities of different forms of asbestos in a cell culture assay. Environ. Res., 22, 109-129.

Rendall, R.E.G., 1970. The data sheets on the chemical and physical properties of the UICC standard reference samples. In: Shapiro, H.A. (Ed.). Pneumoconiosis, Oxford University Press, London, pp. 23-27.

Richards, R.J., Hext, P.M., Desai, R., Tetley, T., Hunt, J., Presley, R. and Dodgson, K.S., 1977. Chrysotile asbestos: biological reaction potential. In: Walton, W.H. (Ed.). Inhaled Particles IV. Pergamon Press Oxford, pp. 477-493.

Roe, F.J.C., Carter, R.L., Walters, M.A. and Harington, J.S., 1967. The pathological effects of asbestos fibres in mice: migration of fibres to submesothelial tissues and induction of mesotheliomata. Int. J. Cancer, 2, 628-638.

Rossiter, C.E., .Bristol, L.J., Cartier, P.H., Gilson, J.G., Grainger, T.R., Sluis-Cremer, G.K. and McDonald, J.C., 1972. Radiographic changes in chrysotile asbestos mine and mill workers of Quebec. Arch. Environ. Health, 24, 388-400.

Rowlands, N., Gibbs, G.W. and McDonald, A.D., 1982. Asbestos fibres in the lungs of chrysotile miners and millers - a preliminary report. Ann. occup. Hyg., 26, 411-415.

Saracci, R., 1977. Asbestos and lung cancer: an analysis of the epidemiological evidence on the asbestos-smoking interaction. Int. J. Cancer, 20, 323-331.

Sebastien, P., Janson, X., Riba, G., Masse, R., Bonnaud, G. and Bignon, J., 1977. Translocation of asbestos fibers through respiratory tract and gastrointestinal tract according to fiber type and size. In: Occupational Exposures to Fibrous and Particulate Dusts and their Extension into the Environment. Conference of the Society for Occupational and Environmental Health, Washington, D.C., pp.65-85.

Sebastien, P., Fondimare, A., Bignon, J., Monchaux, G., Desbordes, J. and Bonnaud, G., 1977a. Topographic distribution of asbestos fibres in human lung in relation to occupational and non-occupational exposure. In: Walton, W.H. (Ed.). Inhaled Particles IV. Pergamon Press, Oxford, pp. 435-446.

Sebastien, P., Masse, R. and Bignon, J., 1980. Recovery of ingested asbestos fibers from the gastrointestinal lymph of rats. Environ. Res., 22, 201-216.

Selikoff, I.J., 1974. Epidemiology of gastrointestinal cancer. Environ. Health Perspect., 9, 299-305.

Selikoff, I.J., 1977. Cancer risk of asbestos exposure. In: Hiatt, H.H., Watson, J.D. and Winsten, J.A. (Eds.). Origins of Human Cancer, Cold Spring Harbor Laboratories., Cold Spring Harbor, NY, US, pp.1765-1784.

Selikoff, I.J. and Hammond, E.C., 1979. Asbestos and smoking. J. Am. Med. Assoc., 242, 458-459.

Selikoff, I.J. and Seidman, H., 1981. Cancer of the pancreas among asbestos insulation workers. Cancer (Philadelphia), 47, 1469-1473.

Selikoff, I.J., Churg, J. and Hammond, E.C., 1965. Relation between exposure to asbestos and mesothelioma. New Engl. J. Med., 272, 560-565.

Selikoff, I.J., Hammond, E.C. and Churg, J., 1968. Asbestos exposure, smoking and neoplasia. J Amer. Med. Assoc., 204, 106-112.

Selikoff, I.J., Hammond E.C. and Churg, J., 1972. Carcinogenicity, of amosite asbestos. Arch. Environ. Health, 25, 183-186.

Selikoff, I.J., Nicholson, W.F. and Langer, A.M., 1972a. Asbestos air pollution. Arch. Environ. Health, 25, 1-13.

Shabad, L.M., Pylev, L.M., Krivosheeva, L.V., Kulagina, T.F. and Nemenko, B.A., 1974. Experimental studies on asbestos carcinogenicity. J. Natl. Cancer Inst., 52, 1175-1187.

Sluis-Cremer, G.K. and Webster, I., 1972. Acute pleurisy in asbestos exposed persons. Environ. Res., 5, 380-392.

Smith, W.E., Miller, L. and Churg, J., 1968. Respiratory tract tumors in hamsters after intratracheal benzo(a)pyrene with and without asbestos. Proc. Amer. Assoc. Cancer Res., 9, p.65.

Smith, W.E., Hubert, D.D. and Badollet, M.S., 1972. Biologic differences in response to long and short asbestos fibers. Am. Ind. Hyg. Assoc. J., 33, p.67.

Speil, S. and Leineweber, J.P., 1969. Asbestos minerals in modern technology. Environ. Res., 2, 166-208.

Stanton, M.F. and Wrench, C., 1972. Mechanisms of mesothelioma induction with asbestos and fibrous glass. J. Natl. Cancer Inst., 48, 797-821.

Stanton, M.F., Layard, M., Tegeris, A., Miller, E., May, M. and Kent, E., 1977. Carcinogenicity of fibrous glass: pleural response in the rat in relation to fiber dimension. J. Natl. Cancer Inst., 58, 587-597.

Storeygard, A.R. and Brown, A.L. Jr., 1977. Penetration of the small intestinal mucosa by asbestos fibers. Mayo Clin. Proc., 52, 809-812.

Suzuki, Y. and Churg, J., 1969. Structure and development of the asbestos body. Am. J. Pathol., 55, 79-108.

Suzuki, Y. and Churg, J., 1969a. Formation of the asbestos body. A comparative study with three types of asbestos. Environ. Res., 3, 107-118.

Timbrell, V., 1970. Characteristics of the International Union against Cancer standard reference samples of asbestos. In: Shapiro, H.A. (Ed.). Pneumoconiosis. Oxford University Press, London, pp.28-36.

Timbrell, V., 1970a. The inhalation of fibers. In: Shapiro, H.A. (Ed.) Pneumoconiosis. Oxford University Press, London, pp.3-9.

Timbrell, V., 1976. Aerodynamic considerations and other aspects of glass fiber. In: Proc. Symp. Occup. Exposure to Fibrous Glass, HEW-PHS, pp. 34-50.

Timbrell, V., 1982. Deposition and retention of fibres in the human lung. Ann. occup. Hyg., 26, 347-369.

Timbrell, V., Gibson, J.C. and Webster, I., 1968. UICC standard reference samples of asbestos. Int. J. Cancer, 3, 406-408.

Timbrell, V., Pooley F. and Wagner, J.C., 1970. Characteristics of respirable asbestos fibers. In: Shapiro, H.A. (Ed.) Pneumoconiosis. Oxford University Press, London, pp.120-125.

Topping, D.C. and Nettesheim, P., 1980. Two-stage carcinogenesis studies with asbestos in Fischer 344 rats. J. Natl. Cancer Inst., 65, 627-630.

Topping, D.C. Nettesheim, P. and Martin, D.H., 1980. Toxic and tumorigenic effects of asbestos on tracheal mucosa. J. Environ. Pathol. Toxicol., 3, 261-275.

Valerio, F., Veggi, M. and Santi, L., 1980. Absorption isotherms of albumin and ferritin on Rhodesian Chrysotile. Effects of magnesium depletion. Environ. Res., 21, 186-189.

Verma, D.K. and Middleton, C.G., 1980. Occupational exposure to asbestos in the drywall taping process. Am. Ind. Hyg. Assoc. J., 41, 264-269.

Volkheimer, G., 1974. Passage of particles through the wall of the gastrointestinal tract. Environ. Health Perspect., 9, 215-225.

Volkheimer, G., 1977. Persorption of particles: physiology and pharmacology. Advan. Pharmacol. Chemother., 14, 163-187.

Vorwald, A.J., Durkan, T.M. and Pratt, D.E., 1951. Experimental studies of asbestosis. AMA Arch. Ind. Hyg. Occup. Med., 3, 1-43.

Wagner, J.C., 1976. Tumours in experimental animals following exposure to asbestos dust. Ann. Anat. Pathol. (Paris), 21, 211-214.

Wagner, J.C. and Skidmore, J.W., 1965. Asbestos dust deposition and retention in rats. Ann. N.Y. Acad. Sci., 132, 77-86.

Wagner, J.C., Sleggs, C.A. and Marchand, P., 1960. Diffuse pleural mesothelioma and asbestos exposure in the North-West Cape Province. Brit. J. Ind. Med., 17, 260-271.

Wagner, J.C., Gilson, J.C., Berry, G. and Timbrell, V., 1971. Epidemiology of asbestos cancers. Br. Med. Bull., 27, 71-76.

Wagner, J.C., Berry, G. and Timbrell, V., 1973. Mesothelioma in rats after innoculation with asbestos and other materials. Br. J. Cancer, 28, 173-185.

Wagner, J.C., Berry, G., Skidmore, J.W. and Timbrell, V., 1974. The effects of the inhalation of asbestos in rats. Br. J. Cancer, 29, 252-269.

Wagner, J.C., Berry, G. and Pooley, F.D., 1980. Carcinogenesis and mineral fibres. Br. Med. Bull., 36, 53-56.

Wagner, J.C., Pooley, F.D., Berry, G., Seal, R.M.E., Munday, D.E., Morgan, J. and Clark, N.J., 1982. A pathological and mineralogical study of asbestos-related deaths in the United Kingdom in 1977. Ann. occup. Hyg., 26, 423-431.

Webster, I., 1974. The ingestion of asbestos fibers. Environ. Health Perspect., 9, 199-202.

Wehner, A.P., Busch, R.H., Olson, R.J. and Craig, D.K., 1975. Chronic inhalation of asbestos and cigarette smoke by hamsters. Environ. Res., 10, 368-383.

Weill, H., Ziskind, M.M., Waggenspack, C. and Rossiter, C.E., 1975. Lung function consequences of dust exposure in asbestos cement manufacturing plants. Arch. Environ. Health, 30, 88-97.

Weill, H., Rossiter, C.E., Waggenspack, C., Jones, R.N. and Ziskind, M.M., 1977. Differences in lung effects resulting from chrysotile and crocidolite exposure. In: Walton, W.H. (Ed.) Inhaled Particles IV. Pergamon Press, Oxford, pp.789-798.

Weiss, W., Levin, R. and Goodman, L., 1981. Pleural plaques and cigarette smoking in asbestos workers. J. occup. Med., 23, 427-430.

Westlake, G.E., 1974. Asbestos fibers in the colonic wall. Environ. Health Perspect., 9, p.227.

Westlake, G.E., Spjut, H.J. and Smith, M.N., 1965. Penetration of colonic mucosa by asbestos particles, an electron microscopic study in rats fed asbestos dust. Lab. Invest., 14, 2029-2033.

Whitwell, F., Newhouse, M.L. and Bennett, D.R., 1974. A study of the histological cell types of lung cancer in workers suffering from asbestosis in the United Kingdom. Br. J. Ind. Med., 31, 298-303.

Wigle, D.T., 1977. Cancer mortality in relation to asbestos in municipal water supplies. Arch. Environ. Health, 32, 185-190.

Wright, G.W. and Kuschner, M., 1977. The influence of varying lengths of glass and asbestos fibres on tissue reponse in guinea pigs. In: Walton, W.H. (Ed.) Inhaled Particles IV. Pergamon Press, Oxford, pp.455-474.

Zaloga, G., 1981. Asbestos related diseases: a review. Military Medicine, 146, 413-419.

Zielhuis, R.L. (Ed.), 1977. Public Health Risks of Exposure to Asbestos. Pergamon Press, Oxford.

Appendix 8
Benzene

CONTENTS

8.1   INTRODUCTION

Benzene was discovered by Michael Faraday in 1825, but it was not until the 1920's that the unusual chemical behaviour and stability of this compound began to be understood (Solomons, 1980). Benzene consists of a ring of six carbon atoms with a single hydrogen atom attached to each (Fig. 1). Spectroscopic measurements show the molecules of benzene are planar and all the carbon-carbon bonds are of equal length, i.e. individual bonds between carbon atoms cannot be categorised as single or double (Solomons, 1980). The stability of the benzene ring is such that the primary reactions of benzene almost exclusively involve substitution reactions such as bromination, nitration and alkylation (Solomons, 1980).

Physically, benzene is a clear, colourless, highly flammable liquid with a melting point of 5.5°C and a boiling point of 80.1°C. The vapour pressure is 74.6 mm Hg at 20°C and inhalation of benzene vapour is the primary route of human exposure (International Agency for Research on Cancer, 1974; 1982). Benzene is only slightly soluble in water, but is miscible with acetone, alcohol, carbon disulphide, carbon tetrachloride, chloroform, ether, glacial acetic acid and oils (International Agency for Research on Cancer, 1974). In animal experiments, exposure is generally to the vapour or by injection of benzene in vegetable oil.

Various petroleum refining techniques are used in the production of benzene, which takes place in most industrialised nations. Benzene is used as a chemical intermediate in the production of a large number of compounds including ethylbenzene, phenol, cyclohexane, maleic anhydride, detergent alkylate, aniline, dichlorobenzenes and DDT. Several of these materials are used in the manufacture of plastics and resins (International Agency for Research on Cancer, 1974; 1982).

There have been a substantial number of major reviews of benzene toxicity and metabolism produced during the last decade (Braun, 1974; Brief et al., 1980; Cohen et al., 1978; International Agency for Research on Cancer, 1974; 1982; Laskin and Goldstein, 1977; NIOSH, 1974; Snyder and Kocsis, 1975; Rusch et al., 1977; Snyder et al., 1977; Snyder et al., 1981) and these have been used extensively herein.

8.2   LEVELS OF EXPOSURE TO BENZENE

8.2.1   Air

Concentrations of benzene in air are generally given as ppb, ppm, $mg\,l^{-1}$ or $mg\,m^{-3}$. The relevant conversion factor is that 1 ppm is equal to $0.0035\,mg\,l^{-1}$.

With respect to occupational exposure to benzene in air, the International Agency for Research on Cancer (1982) has summarised available data as follows.

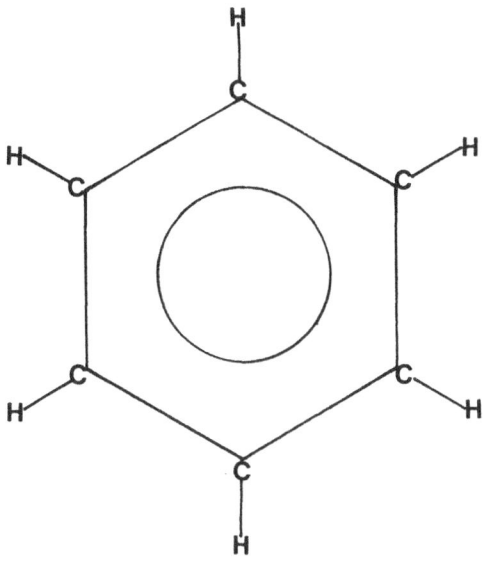

FIGURE 1.   THE STRUCTURE OF BENZENE

Industry	Concentration Range (ppm)	Year
Rubber coating	65-260	1935-1937
Rubber factory	100 (500 peak)	1942
Rubber coating	25-125	1961
	20-25 (140 peak)	1960-1963
Printing	10-1060	1939
Artificial leather, rubber goods or shoe manufacture	100-500	1936-1939
Leatherette factory	47-310	1953-1957
(+ improved control)	25-47	1953-1957
Shoe factory	318-470	1956
	31-156	1960-1963
	41-44	1964
	150-650	1966-1978
Chemical plant producing hexabromocyclododecane and dialkylaminoethyl chloride hydrochlorides	0.1-0.4	1979
Petroleum refinery (quality control laboratory)	0.6-32	1978
Waste water treatment plant at petroleum refinery	<0.02-7.22	1978
Coal liquefaction plant	0.02	1980
Australian Air Force Workshop	10-35 (1400 peak)	1947
Paint Manufacture	trace - 78.5	1963
Painting of metal products	0.17-3.1	1978
US tyre production (personal breathing sample)		1973-1977
Cement mixing	0.2-4.8	
Extrusion	<0.1-5.1	
Tyre building	0.1-2.4	
Curing preparation	<0.1-5.9	
Inspection and repair	<0.1-1.9	
Maintenance	0.2-0.5	

These values should be seen in the context of the various national occupational exposure limits for benzene. These have been tabulated by the International Agency for Research on Cancer (1982) and are summarised below, converted to a common basis of ppm.

Country	Year	Concentration (ppm)	Interpretation*	Status+
Australia	1978	10	TWA	G
Belgium	1978	10	TWA	R
Czechoslovakia	1976	14	TWA	R
		23	Ceiling (10 min.)	R
Finland	1972	10	TWA	R
Hungary	1974	6	TWA	R
Italy	1978	10	TWA	G
Japan	1978	25	Ceiling	G
Netherlands	1978	10	TWA	G
Poland	1976	9	Ceiling	R
Romania	1975	14	Maximum	R
Sweden	1978	5	TWA	G
		10	Maximum (15 min.)	G
Switzerland	1978	2	TWA	R
USA **	1980	10	TWA	R
(Occuptional		25	Ceiling	R
Safety and Health		50	Peak	R
Administration)				
USSR	1980	1.4	Ceiling	R
Yugoslavia	1971	15	Ceiling	R

Notes:
* TWA = Time weighted average
+ G = guideline, R = regulation
** Other guidelines include a recommendation of a ceiling of 1 ppm

(National Institute for Occupational Safety and Health, 1980)

These data indicate that, in most industries, average exposure levels are unlikely to exceed 5 ppm (0.0175 mg l^{-1}) for extended periods. For a man breathing 20 l of air per minute over an 8 h working day (International Commission on Radiological Protection, 1975), this corresponds to a daily intake rate of 168 mg. Averaged over a working year, including week-ends and holidays, this drops to ~100 mg d^{-1}. However, higher intakes could occur in individuals involved in strenuous occupations.

With respect to benzene in ambient air, the International Agency for Research on Cancer (1982) quoted normal levels of 10^{-4} to 1.7×10^{-2} ppm in rural air and 2×10^{-2} ppm in urban air. Values for Los Angeles range from 0.005 to 0.182 ppm, for London from 0.087 to 0.179 ppm and for other cities from 0.001 to 0.098 ppm (International Agency for Research on Cancer, 1982). From these data, and assuming an inhalation rate of 23 m^3 d^{-1} (International Commission on Radiological Protection, 1975), it is calculated that a typical urban dweller inhales 1.6 mg of benzene per day. Inhalation rates in rural areas are likely to be substantially lower than this, but inhalation rates in some urban areas could be as high as 15 mg d^{-1}.

It is noted that the levels discussed above do not apply to specific areas around industries producing or utilising benzene. However, levels in these areas are generally comparable with those in general urban environments (International Agency for Research on Cancer, 1982) and do not usually require special consideration, though there may be isolated instances of levels in ambient air similar to those typical of occupational exposure (International Agency for Research on Cancer, 1982).

Finally, with respect to inhalation exposure, it is noted that benzene has been found in cigarette smoke at levels of 47 to 64 ppm (International Agency for Research on Cancer, 1982). Evaluation of the significance of this concentration is difficult, but it could correspond to an intake ~10 mg d^{-1} and be the major source of inhalation exposure in the non-occupationally exposed.

8.2.2   Water

Levels of benzene in various water samples have been summarised by the International Agency for Research on Cancer (1982). Rainwater in the UK is quoted as exhibiting a concentration of 87.2 µg l^{-1}, with lake, stream and river waters exhibiting concentrations of between 6.5 and 18.6 µg l^{-1}. Concentrations of benzene in US and Czechoslovakian drinking waters were quoted as 0.1 to 0.3 µg l^{-1}, though a value of 1 µg l^{-1} was used for calculational purposes. On the basis of a water concentration of 1 µg l^{-1} and a daily fluid intake of 1.65 l (International Commission on Radiological Protection, 1975), a daily benzene intake of 1.65 µg is calculated. This is three orders of magnitude lower than typical intakes of urban dwellers by inhalation (Section 8.2.1).

8.2.3   Beverages and diet

Benzene has been reported in several foods and beverages. Values have been summarised by the International Agency for Research on Cancer (1982) as follows:

Food	Concentration (µg kg^{-1})
Eggs	500-1900
Jamaican rum	120
Irradiated beef	19, <100
Heat treated or canned beef	2

Taking daily food consumption to be 1.38 kg f.w. (International Commission on Radiological Protection, 1975; Table 121, UK data) an average dietary content of benzene of 100 µg kg^{-1} would correspond to a daily intake of 140 µg. This is consistent with the US National Research Council (1980) estimate that the dietary intake of benzene may be as high as 250 µg d^{-1}.

8.2.4   Summary

On the basis of the data reviewed in this section, the following daily intakes of benzene are estimated.

Medium	Intake ($\mu g\ d^{-1}$)	Comment
Air	$\leq 10^5$	Occupational exposure
	1600	Typical urban dweller
	1.5×10^4	Urban dwellers in some specific locations
	$\sim 10^4$	Cigarette smoking
Water	0.17-17	Based on drinking water concentrations of 0.1 to 10 $\mu g\ l^{-1}$
Beverages and diet	<250	

This table indicates that inhalation of benzene will almost invariably be the main route of intake.

8.3   TOXIC EFFECTS

Benzene toxicity has been classified as two distinct phenomena, acute and chronic. The symptoms of acute toxicity have generally been related to the central nervous system. Manifestations include euphoria, dizziness, weakness, headache, muscle tremors, ataxia, convulsions, salivation, nystagmus, cardiac arrhythmias and phenomena of very intense asphyxiation due to paralysis of the medullary respiratory centre (Cohen et al., 1978; International Agency for Research on Cancer, 1982; Vale and Meredith, 1983). Single exposures to concentrations of 20000 ppm have been reported to be fatal to man within 5 to 10 minutes (International Agency for Research on Cancer, 1982). Chronic benzene toxicity, on the other hand, is predominantly a disorder of the haemopoietic system, although chronic central nervous system, cardiovascular and gastrointestinal effects have been suggested. The most frequently reported findings, on history and physical examination, include loss of weight, weakness, fatigue, epitaxis, dryness of mucosa, flatulence and/or pyrosis, nausea and/or vomiting, colic, palpitations, dyspnea, headache, dizziness, insomnia, lethargy, irritability and rash (Cohen et al., 1978). As Vale and Meredith (1983) have commented, anaemia (including aplastic anaemia), leukopenia, thrombocytopenia, pancytopenia, chromosome abnormalities and cerebral atrophy have all been reported. Some effects on blood have been recorded at relatively low levels of exposure. Thus, in workers exposed to about 25 ppm benzene over several years, increases in mean corpuscular volume and minimal decreases in mean haemoglobin and haematocrit levels were seen. Values of these quantities returned to normal after cessation of exposure. Having reviewed these data, the International Agency for Research on Cancer (1982) commented that "it has not been possible to establish with certainty the degree of exposure below which no adverse haematological effects of benzene in humans would occur". Effects of benzene on immune competence, taken together with the well-known ability of benzene to depress leucocytes, may explain why benzene-intoxicated individuals readily succumb to infection and why the terminal event in severe benzene toxicity is often an acute, overwhelming, infection (International Agency for Research on Cancer, 1982).

A detailed discussion of chronic benzene toxicity in humans has been given by Snyder and Kocsis (1975). These authors presented a reconstruction of the progress of the disease, based on a synthesis of observations made on people at various stages of toxicity, supplemented with inferences from animal studies. In its initial stages, benzene toxicity is manifested as a parodoxical alteration of the blood picture. Polycythaemia and anaemia, leucocytosis and leucopenia, thrombocytosis and thrombocytopenia have all been reported in the same studies. However, with continuing exposure, the trend is toward decreasing levels of circulating erythrocytes, leucocytes and thrombocytes. As the disease intensifies, circulating blood cell levels decrease further as pancytopenia develops. With respect to circulating lymphocytes, depression is mainly of B-cells with immunoglobulin surface-receptor-negative cells, presumably T-lymphocytes, little affected (Irons and Moore, 1980).

In man, decreases in erythrocyte levels are a frequent indicator of early chronic benzene poisoning. This anaemia is described as macrocytic and hyperchromic and may be associated with the appearance of foetal haemoglobin (Snyder and Kocsis, 1975).

Although there is some evidence of an increase in haemolysis in benzene toxicity, the anaemia is most commonly thought to be the result of decreased erythrocyte production. The long mean lifetime of circulating erythrocytes (~120 d) implies that early detection of their production is not possible by cell counting techniques, though animal studies have demonstrated that depression of Fe-59 uptake into the haemoglobin of maturing erythrocytes can be used as an early indicator of reduced production (Snyder and Kocsis, 1975).

In contrast to the situation with erythrocytes, the shorter lifespan of the leucocytes in the bloodstream implies that detecting decreased white cell production should be simpler than detecting changes in erythrocytes and leucopenia has been described as the earliest and most frequent sign of benzene toxicity (Snyder and Kocsis, 1975).

Apart from the chronic effects described above, the main long-term sequelae of benzene exposure have been identified as cancers of the haemopoietic system and there is now no reasonable doubt that benzene causes leukaemia in man (Goldstein and Snyder, 1982). In agreement with this, the International Agency for Research on Cancer (1982) concluded as follows.

-    There is limited evidence that benzene is carcinogenic in experimen-
     tal animals.
-    It is established that human exposure to commercial benzene, or
     benzene-containing mixtures, can cause damage to the haematopoietic
     system, including pancytopenia. The relationship between benzene
     exposure and the development of acute myelogenous leukaemia has been
     established in epidemiological studies.
-    Reports linking exposure to benzene with other malignancies were
     inadequate for evaluation.

It was also noted that, although most of the leukaemias associated with benzene exposure in case reports and epidemiological studies were of the myelogenous type, some monocytic, erythroblastic and lymphocytic leukaemias, as well as some lymphomas, have been identified.

Similarly, Kocsis and Snyder (1975) commented that chronic exposure to high concentrations of benzene may lead to one of several types of leukaemia, the most prevalent of which is acute, or subacute, myeloblastic leukaemia. Chronic granulocytic, lymphatic, aleukaemic and erythroleukaemic leukaemia, as well as Hodgkin's disease, have also been reported to result from chronic benzene toxicity, but there are fewer of these and, in some cases, they are inadequately documented. Snyder and Kocsis (1975) also commented on the difficulty of diagnosing leukaemia without the study of bone marrow aspirates. In such circumstances, pancytopenia could be erroneously equated with aplastic anaemia rather than aleukaemic leukaemia. From the available data, there is a strong possibility that leukaemia induction by benzene is related to the effects of this material as a bone marrow depressant and it has been suggested that the association between benzene and leukaemia may be of a promotional nature, with benzene potentiating the carcinogenic action of other chemicals, or facilitating the induction of viral leukaemias (Snyder et al., 1977).

Original reports on leukaemia induction by benzene in man include those of Vigliani and co-workers (Vigliani, 1976; Vigliani and Forni, 1976) from the provinces of Milan and Pavia, those of Aksoy and co-workers (Aksoy et al., 1976; Aksoy and Erdem, 1978; Aksoy, 1980) from Turkey, those of Infante et al. (1979) from Ohio and those of Greene et al. (1979) on employees at the US Government Printing Office. It is also of note that Goldstein et al. (1982) have recently reported that benzene may induce myelogenous leukaemia in CD-1 mice and Sprague-Dawley rats, and have suggested that CD-1 mice are a suitable strain for developing an experimental model of benzene leukaemogenesis. Benzene induction of Zymbal gland carcinomas in rats following ingestion and inhalation has also been reported (Maltoni et al., 1982), but the significance of these results, in terms of effects on man, is not clear.

The importance of benzene as a bone marrow depressant and leukaemogenic agent has resulted in a large number of studies of its effects on the cell cycle and, in particular, of its effects on cells at different levels of differentiation. Also, the early identification of benzene as an agent capable of inducing alterations in the erythroblast analogous to those found in erythraemias, led to its use as an investigative tool in studies of erythroblastic mitosis (Rondanelli et al., 1970).

A detailed discussion of the effects of benzene at the cellular level is beyond the scope of this review, but it is noted that a variety of cell types have been implicated. Steinberg (1949) undertook marrow regeneration experiments in rabbits and commented that at least one part of the mechanism by which benzene induces aplasia of bone marrow is probably inhibition of cell division and maturation past the level of the primitive reticular cell. More recently, use of Fe-59 labelling has indicated that benzene inhibits the multiplication of pronormoblasts and normoblasts, but does not interfere with the incorporation of iron into haem (Lee et al., 1973; 1974; Snyder and Kocsis, 1975; Snyder et al., 1977a). Similar conclusions have been drawn from a study of [H-3]thymidine uptake in the marrow of rabbits (Moeschlin and Speck, 1967). Finally, a variety of studies (Uyeki et al., 1977; Gill et al., 1980; Green et al., 1981; 1981a; Tunek et al., 1981; Harigaya et al., 1981) have demonstrated that benzene is cytotoxic to bone marrow and spleen stem cells, as assayed by their capacity to form colonies either in vitro or in vivo, and Irons et al. (1979) have suggested that such cells are blocked in G_2 or M phase by benzene.

At the subcellular level, chromosomal and chromatid aberrations have been observed amongst benzene exposed workers (International Agency for Research on Cancer, 1982) and in experimental animals (e.g. Tice et al., 1980; 1982).

With respect to other effects, Mehlman et al. (1980) reviewed experimental studies on teratogenesis associated with exposure to benzene by oral, parenteral or inhalation routes. They concluded that administration of benzene to pregnant experimental animals did not produce marked developmental effects in the foetus at concentrations which did not cause concomitant maternal toxicity and that, at maternally non-toxic levels, benzene does not constitute a teratogenic hazard. This is particularly interesting, since Dowty et al. (1976) reported that benzene is present in cord blood at concentrations equal to, or higher than, those in maternal blood.

8.4   METABOLISM

The metabolism of benzene and its derivatives has been studied extensively. Individual studies are discussed in detail below, but it is convenient to first give a brief summary of the major features so that the results of various studies can be seen in context. Thus, major features of benzene metabolism are as follows.

- Benzene absorption through the intact skin is limited.
- The vapour is well absorbed from the lungs, but a large fraction of that absorbed is eventually re-excreted, unmodified, in the exhaled air.
- A small amount of benzene is metabolised to CO_2 which is excreted in the exhaled air.
- Most of the benzene which is metabolised is transformed to phenol. This transformation almost undoubtedly takes place through the formation of the unstable intermediate benzene epoxide. In the liver, and possibly other tissues, the tranformation is mediated by the mixed function oxidase system and involves cytochrome P-450.
- High levels of benzene exposure depress the transformation of benzene to phenol, probably because enhanced phenol levels act to suppress mixed function oxidase mediated metabolism.
- Phenol is further metabolised to water soluble compounds such as catechol and hydroquinone. This metabolism can involve glutathione.
- Phenol is the main metabolite of benzene to be excreted in the urine, but small amounts of other water-soluble metabolites are also excreted.
- Compounds such as phenobarbital and DDT which affect the mixed function oxidase system can have an effect on the degree of benzene metabolism. This effect is larger in in vitro systems than it is in vivo and is enhanced in acute exposures relative to chronic exposures. This is because of the depressant effect of benzene on its own metabolism.
- Metabolites of phenol can bind covalently to macromolecules, including proteins and nucleic acids.

These various aspects of benzene metabolism are discussed in detail and quantified, as appropriate, in the remainder of this section.

8.4.1   Absorption through the skin

As Cohen et al. (1978) noted, exposure to benzene can be by direct contact, although benzene absorption through the skin is not very great. Cohen et al. (1978) also pointed out that, when direct contact is achieved, the significant toxicity is usually due to inhalation rather than skin absorption.

In terms of quantifying skin absorption, the International Agency for Research on Cancer (1982) cited data of Hanke et al. (1961) as showing that, when benzene was placed on the skin in a closed cup, it was absorbed at a rate of 0.4 mg cm^{-2} h^{-1}; this was stated to be a rate equal to 2% of that for ethylbenzene absorption and 2 to 3% of that for toluene absorption.

Other data relevant to the skin absorption of benzene include a study by Conca and Maltagliati (1955), who reported that three men were subjected to the immersion of their hands and forearms in commercial benzene for 25 to 35 minutes. Assays of urinary sulphates and expired air failed to reveal any evidence of benzene uptake via the percutaneous route. In experiments on rabbits, Wolf et al. (1956) reported that benzene caused slight to moderate irritation of the skin, but was not absorbed in acutely toxic amounts.

8.4.2   Absorption from the lung, loss in exhaled air and retention following inhalation

The retention of benzene following inhalation exposure was reviewed by Docter and Zielhuis (1967) who concluded that "the retention of benzene .... may be regarded as constant, and to be about 1 mg min.$^{-1}$ when the subject is exposed to 80 mg m^{-3} with a ventilation of 25 l min.$^{-1}$ ". This conclusion corresponds to a fractional retention of 0.5 of inhaled benzene vapour. Similarly, Hunter (1966) commented that on exposure to the vapour of benzene, a human subject absorbs benzene and a steady state is reached in which the concentration of vapour in the exhaled air is some 50% of that in the inhaled air. Commenting on the studies of Srbova et al. (1950), Hunter (1966) noted that, while the mean retention was 54%, the amount of benzene in exhaled air varied from 45 to 80% of that in the inhaled air. In his own studies, Hunter (1966) recorded an absorption of 47% in a healthy adult male with a ventilation rate of 16.2 l min.$^{-1}$.

There have been a considerable number of additional human studies on the loss of benzene in expired air since the early work discussed above. Thus, Hunter (1968) reported that a steady rate of absorption of benzene occurs quickly after the start of an exposure, the time to attain this state and the proportion of intake absorbed being a reflection of the individual and his energy expenditure. At the end of several exposures to concentrations of benzene vapour in the order of 300 mg m^{-3}, the expired air contained concentrations of 180 to 220 mg m^{-3}. Hunter (1968) also presented data on the time course of benzene concentration in expired air up to 24 h after the cessation of exposure. These data can be fitted by a two component loss curve.

$$C_a(t) = 30e^{-18t} + 1.0e^{-1.8t}$$

where $C_a(t)$ is the concentration in exhaled air in mg m^{-3}; and

t is in days.

Unfortunately, in the absence of data on concentrations of benzene in air, or exposure period, this function cannot be related to the rate, or total amount, of intake.

Sherwood and Carter (1970) reported on concentrations of benzene in exhaled air subsequent to sedentary exposure to 25 ppm benzene for 4.5 h. The results shown indicate two phases of clearance with intercept ratios and rate coefficients similar to those recorded by Hunter (1968). However, the limited data presented preclude any more exact quantification. In a more recent paper, Sherwood (1976) described a three compartment model with biological half-lives of 2.5, 28 and 90 h.

Nomiyama and Nomiyama (1974; 1974a) reported on the respiratory retention, uptake and excretion of several organic solvents, including benzene, in men and women volunteer students. Nomiyama and Nomiyama (1974) defined retention, R, by:

$$R = (C_i - C_e)/C_i$$

where C_i was the organic solvent concentration in inspired air; and
C_e was the organic solvent concentration in expired air during exposure.

Excretion, E, was defined by:

$$E = C_e(0)/C_i$$

where $C_e(0)$ was the organic solvent concentration in expired air immediately after cessation of exposure.

Uptake, U, was then defined by

$$U = R + E.$$

For benzene, values of R decreased from ~0.5 after 1 h of exposure to ~0.3 after 3 h of exposure. Values of R, U and E in percent after 3 h exposure are listed below.

Group	R	U	E
Men	29.5±5.8	45.8±3.9	16.3±2.0
Women	30.9±7.7	48.0±4.0	17.2±2.0
All	30.2±6.7	46.9±3.7	16.8±1.8

Results were very similar for the closely related compound toluene.

In a subsequent paper, Nomiyama and Nomiyama (1974a) reported on the elimination of benzene from the body in the first 17 h following cessation of exposure. Three components of loss in expired air were identified. These were reported to exhibit half-lives of 0.19, 0.94 and 43.9 h in men, and 0.23, 0.64 and 16.2 h in women. However, examination of the data presented indicates that differences in respiratory excretion between men and women could not have been statistically significant and that the biological half-life of the long-term component was determined completely by a single data point which was subject to considerable uncertainty. Overall, the data are well fitted by an excretory function of the form:

$$C_a(t) = 5e^{-3.5t} + 4e^{-0.9t} + e^{-0.03t}$$

where $C_a(t)$ is the concentration of benzene in expired air
(ppm) for a person exposed to ~60 ppm for 3 h; and
t is in hours.

The presence of long-term components in this function indicates that equilibrium between intake and respiratory loss would not be reached in a 3 h exposure. For this reason, and in view of uncertainties concerning the relative magnitude and half-lives of the long-term components of benzene excretion, these data are difficult to interpret further.

More recently, Sato and Nakajima (1979) have reported on the concentration curves for benzene and toluene in blood and end-tidal air for humans inhaling the materials separately, or as a mixture, for a period of 2 h. The benzene and toluene concentrations used in these studies were 25 ppm and 100 ppm respectively. No significant interaction between the substances was found at this level of exposure. Also, the blood and end-tidal air concentration curves showed very similar time dependences. Sato and Nakajima did not give retention functions based on their data, but they can be fitted by a curve of the form:

$$C_a(t) = 0.1e^{-10t} + 0.08\ e^{-1.5t} + 0.022e^{-0.2t}$$

where $C_a(t)$ is the concentration in breath (μm); and
t is the time in hours.

However, in this fit, the exponent of the rapidly excreted component is extremely uncertain.

Finally, with respect to human experience, Berlin et al. (1980) reported on studies in which they exposed subjects to known concentrations of benzene in air for single and repeated daily periods. Breath concentrations, measured during repeated exposures, approached saturation after 3 d, as illustrated by the data listed below.

Morning breath concentration (ppb)

Day	Subject 1	Subject 2	Subject 3	Subject 4
1	4	-	10.7, 12.5	9.5, 14
2	8	8	9	13, 35
3	14, 17	11, 21	21	17, 34
4	12, 21	21, 27	13, 23	26, 29
5	16.5, 21	17, 17	9, 22	24, 30

Mean daily benzene exposures (ppm h) were 26.4, 26.2, 42.2 and 38.4 for subjects 1 to 4 respectively. Because the samples were taken 16 h after cessation of exposure and because of the slow build up in breath concentration, these data indicate a component of loss by exhalation with a half-life ~1 d. The existence of such a component was confirmed by a study of the decay of benzene in breath after the 5 d exposure period. The concentration of benzene in breath over the next 5 days was well fitted by:

$$C_a(t) = 0.2835e^{-0.263t} + 0.033e^{-0.0285t}$$

where $C_a(t)$ is the concentration in exhaled air (ppm); and t is in hours.

Berlin et al. (1980) also examined occupationally exposed workers and commented that the decay in breath concentration after prolonged occupational exposure appeared to be slower, but that the difference was not significant.

A number of animal studies are also relevant to the dynamics of benzene loss in exhaled air. Thus, Andrews et al. (1977) found that simultaneous subcutaneous injection of benzene and toluene reduced urinary excretion of benzene metabolites relative to benzene alone, but increased loss of benzene in the exhaled air. However, the levels used, 880 mg kg^{-1} of benzene and 1720 mg kg^{-1} of toluene, are of little relevance to human exposure. For comparison, a man exposed to 10 ppm of benzene for 8 h will typically inhale ~340 mg or ~5 mg kg^{-1}.

In rabbits exposed to [C-14]benzene via stomach tube (Parke and Williams 1953a) between 34.0 and 48.4% of the C-14 was eliminated as unchanged benzene in the expired air, whereas between 0 and 1.75% of the C-14 was eliminated as respiratory CO_2. Similarly, in rats given various pre-treatments to stimulate or inhibit microsomal enzymes and injected subcutaneously with [C-14]benzene, only 1.6 to 6.6% of the C-14 was exhaled as CO_2, whereas 43.3 to 60.1% was exhaled as benzene.

In more detailed studies in rats, Rickert et al. (1979) reported on the build-up of benzene in various tissues during a 6 h exposure to an air concentration of 500 ppm benzene. Rickert et al. (1979) also studied the loss of benzene from these tissues over the first 9 h subsequent to exposure (see also Rickert et al., 1981). The following results were obtained.

Sample	Steady state concentration ($\mu g\ g^{-1}$ or $\mu g\ ml^{-1}$)	Half-times (h) Approach to steady state	Elimination
Blood	11.5±0.7	1.4	0.7
Bone marrow	37.0±2.2	very short	0.5
Fat	164.4±15.0	2.0	1.6
Liver	9.9±0.7	1.9	0.4
Lung	15.1±0.9	1.5	0.4
Kidney	25.3±1.3	1.3	0.6
Spleen	4.9±0.5	0.9	0.8
Brain	6.5±0.6	2.6	0.6

Elimination in expired air was studied to 36 h post-exposure and was biphasic, the two components exhibiting half-lives of 0.7 and 13.1 h, with the long-term component contributing ~4% of the benzene lost in expired air.

Finally, in dogs, Schrenk et al. (1941) reported that, during a single inhalation exposure of 4 to 7 h, benzene concentrations

FIGURE 2.   PATHWAYS OF BENZENE METABOLISM (1)

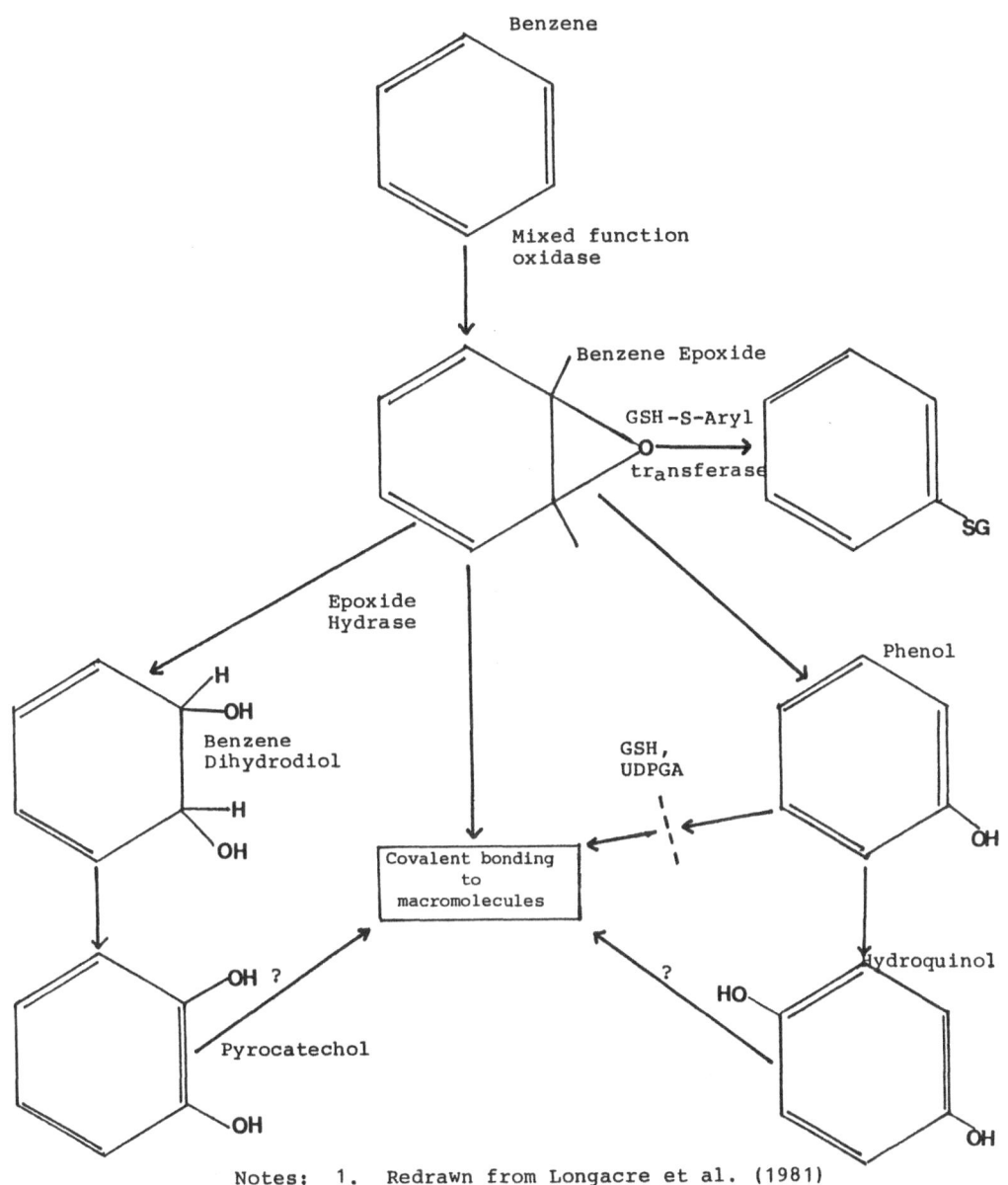

Notes: 1.   Redrawn from Longacre et al. (1981)
         GSH = Glutathione
       UDPGA = Uridine - 5 - diphosphoglucuronic acid.

equilibrated very rapidly between arterial blood and inspired air. However, in longer-term exposures, benzene levels in blood appeared to increase for several days, indicating a less rapid component of equilibration with a half-time ~1 d. Such a component was also identified in studies of the decrease in blood concentrations following cessation of exposure.

Schrenk et al. (1941) also gave data on the distribution of benzene in tissues following various exposure regimes. Concentrations in most organs, tissues and fluids were similar to those in blood. Exceptions to this were urine, surface fat, peritoneal fat and bone marrow, which exhibited concentrations an order of magnitude higher.

8.4.3   Pathways of benzene metabolism

The various possible pathways of benzene metabolism have recently been discussed by Longacre et al. (1981) and are shown in Fig. 2. Benzene is oxidised to the epoxide by the mixed function oxidase system. The epoxide is further metabolised to phenol, binds glutathione or binds hydroxyl groups to form pyrocatechol. Phenol is further metabolised to hydroquinone. Phenol and other benzene derivates may be present conjugated with sulphates. It is noted that, even excluding sulphate conjugation, Fig. 2 is not exhaustive. Thus, Tunek et al. (1981) commented that p-benzoquinone and/or p-benzosemiquinone are the metabolites of benzene causing covalent binding to macromolecules in incubations with rat liver microsomes. They also noted that the dihydrodiol could give rise to catechol, o-benzosemiquinone or a dihydrodiol epoxide. A detailed illustration of many potential pathways of benzene metabolism was given by Rasch et al. (1977).

8.4.3.1   Excretion of benzene metabolites in urine

The primary step in benzene metabolism is identified as the formation of the epoxide (e.g. Sato et al., 1963). In this respect, benzene is very similar to other arenes (see Jerina and Daly, 1974). However, the instability of the expoxide means that the metabolites detected in urine are various derivatives of the epoxide, and, in particular, conjugated phenols. This excretion can be assayed directly, but historically was at first measured in terms of the ratio of free to bound sulphates (e.g. Callow and Hele, 1926; Yant et al., 1936; Hough et al., 1944; Li et al., 1945; Hammond and Hermann, 1960). Excretion of phenol in benzene-intoxicated experimental animals and man has been variously reported. Brewer and Weiskotten (1916) studied the excretion of free and total phenol in the urine of rabbits given three successive daily injections of a benzene/olive oil mixture. Results from this study (Fig. 3) demonstrate the rapid excretion of phenol in urine (half-life ≤1 d) and the limited sensitivity of the free to total phenol ratio to benzene exposure.

Porteous and Williams (1949) studied the excretion of phenol, conjugated glucuronic acid, ethereal sulphate and neutral sulphur in rabbits administered oral doses of 500 mg kg^{-1}, or 1000 mg kg^{-1}, of benzene. Excretion of all metabolites was essentially complete by two days after exposure. From their data, the following estimates of total urinary excretion have been derived.

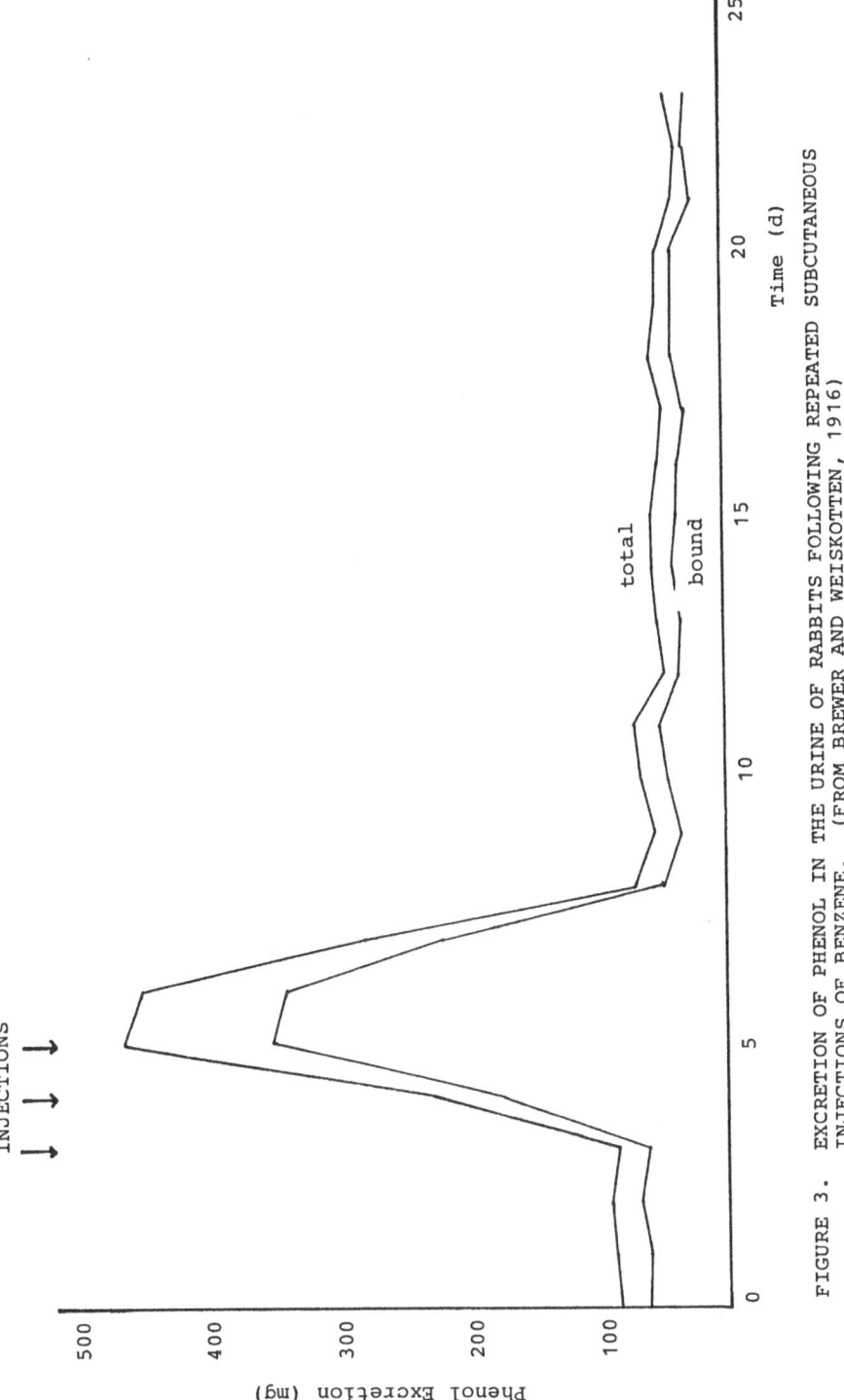

FIGURE 3. EXCRETION OF PHENOL IN THE URINE OF RABBITS FOLLOWING REPEATED SUBCUTANEOUS INJECTIONS OF BENZENE. (FROM BREWER AND WEISKOTTEN, 1916)

Substance	Percent of dose excreted (mean ± s.e.)	Number of observations
Free phenol	<1.6	6
Total phenol	9.2±1.7	6
Glucuronic acid	11.3±2.0	11
Ethereal sulphate	9.6±1.2	8
Neutral sulphur	0	8

Porteous and Williams (1949a) commented that their previous work (Porteous and Williams, 1949) had shown that about 9.5% of orally administered benzene is excreted by rabbits as ethereal sulphates. They proceeded to demonstrate that phenol, catechol, quinol and hydroxyquinol occurred in this sulphate fraction. Recovery of these substances was as listed below.

Substance	Percent of dose in urine	
	Day 1+2	Day 3+4
Phenol	2.5	0.025
Quinol	0.28	0.15
Catechol	0.3	0.11
Hydroxyquinol	trace	0.10

On the basis of their data, Porteous and Williams (1949a) suggested that the first metabolite of benzene is phenol, which is then oxidised to catechol and quinol and that one or both of these dihydric phenols may then give rise to hydroxyquinol.

Parke and Williams (1953) studied the recovery of C-14 labelled substances in the urine of rabbits given oral doses of [$^{14}C_1$]benzene. The following results were recorded.

			Percentage of dose excreted in 48 h		
Dose of benzene (mg kg^{-1})	Total phenol	Phenyl glucuronide	Phenyl sulphuric acid	Catechol	Quinol
150	21.6	8.1	13.8	-	-
500	17.6	6.3	11.1	-	-
350	18.2	-	-	4.4	7.5

Labelled substances present in urine after oral administration of [^{14}C]phenol were also determined. Virtually all the phenol was excreted in the urine mainly as phenylglucuronide (~45%), phenylsulphuric acid (~45%) and quinol (~10%). Small quantities (≤1%) of catechol and hydroxyquinol were also excreted. These authors also demonstrated that orally administered phenol does not give rise to any of the isomers of muconic acid or phenyl-mercapturic acid.

Parke and Williams (1953a) also studied the excretion and tissue distribution of radioactivity in rabbits following the administration of [$^{14}C_1$]benzene. Excretion of total radioactivity in urine was very rapid, corresponding to a biological half-life ~0.5 d. The distribution of label between different compounds in urine, expressed as percentage of administered activity, was summarised as follows.

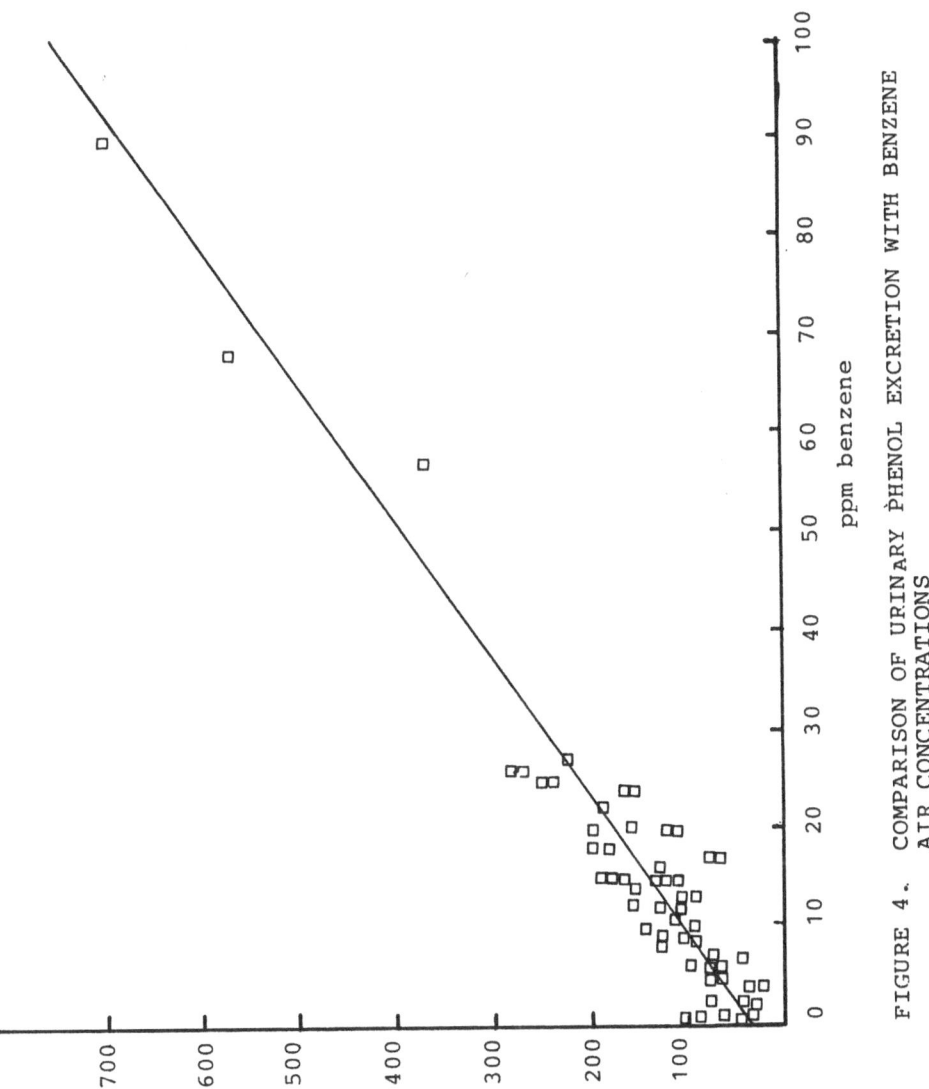

FIGURE 4. COMPARISON OF URINARY PHENOL EXCRETION WITH BENZENE AIR CONCENTRATIONS

	Duration of experiment (d)				
Form	2	2	2	3	5
Phenol	16.7	23.7	30.8	22.8	22.9
Catechol	1.2	2.1	2.6	2.8	2.9
Quinol	6.2	4.8	4.9	3.5	3.6
Hydroxyquinol	0.35	<0.1	0.4	0.3	0.32
Resorcinol	≦0.3	≦0.2	≦0.2	-	-
Pyrogallol	0	-	-	0	0
Phenylmercapturic acid	0.7	-	0.4	0.4	0.4
Diphenyl	0	-	-	-	-
p-diphenylglucuronide	0	-	-	-	-
Sum of aromatic compounds plus trans-trans-muconic acid	27.25	31.6	40.4	30.9	31.2
Total radioactivity of urine	35.0	34.8 (41.7)	39.7	28.5	28.7 (28.8)

Note: totals in parentheses are for 7 d urine collections.

With respect to C-14 not excreted in urine, ~45% of the administered activity was lost as [^{14}C]benzene in the expired air and ~1 to 2% was lost as [^{14}C]O$_2$. The total quantity of activity remaining in soft tissues was ~5 to 16% at 2 d post-exposure, but only ~1.3% at 7 d post-exposure. The label did not appear to be concentrated to any significant degree in any particular organs or tissues.

Walkley et al. (1961) studied the excretion of phenol in the urine of occupationally, or experimentally, exposed workers. With respect to occupational exposure, a linear relationship was obtained between urinary phenol levels and benzene levels in air (Fig. 4). In this study, the urine samples were obtained near the end of the work period. Because of the rapid metabolism of benzene and excretion of phenol, this relationship would not be expected to hold subsequent to the exposure period, or in the case of exposure to temporally varying concentrations of benzene.

Walkley et al. (1961) also gave data on the phenol excretion of two subjects exposed to 200 ppm of benzene for 30 minutes (Fig. 5). These data suggest a half-time for benzene metabolism to phenol of about 2 or 3 h and a half-life for phenol excretion of about 5 to 8 h.

Van Haaften and Sie (1965) gave a critical review of the studies of Teisinger and Fiserova-Bergerova (1958) and Walkley et al. (1961) concerning relationships between phenol in urine and benzene exposure. They noted that the various colourimetric methods used suffer from interference by other phenolic compounds present in urine. While this affects the 'normal' level of 'phenol' measured in urine, it does not affect the proportionality between excess phenol and benzene exposure.

Urinary excretion of phenol in relation to benzene exposure was further investigated by Rainsford and Lloyd Davies (1965) who proposed a new screening test and gave the following data for phenol levels in urine before and after 8 h shifts in various factories.

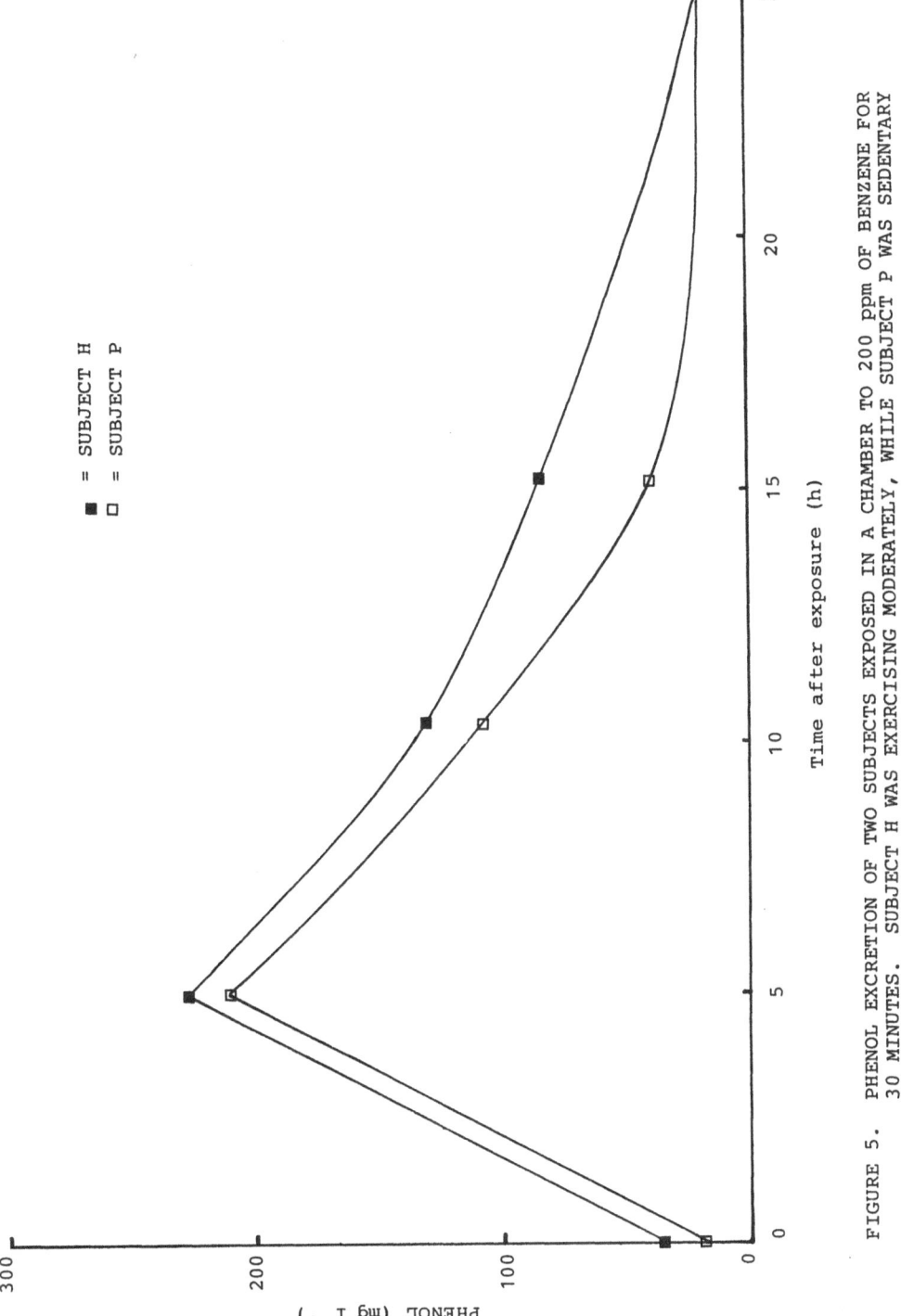

FIGURE 5.   PHENOL EXCRETION OF TWO SUBJECTS EXPOSED IN A CHAMBER TO 200 ppm OF BENZENE FOR 30 MINUTES.   SUBJECT H WAS EXERCISING MODERATELY, WHILE SUBJECT P WAS SEDENTARY

| Factory | Number of workers studied | Benzene concen- tration (ppm) | Phenol excretion (mg l^{-1}) | | | |
| | | | Before exposure | | After exposure | |
			Range	Mean	Range	Mean
1	30	<10	17-40	28	19-74	31
2	2	<10	12-29	16	19-44	31
3	5	<10	20-44	31	28-48	37
4	6	<10	21-37	27.5	19-55	37.5
5	8	7.5-50	25-46	37	52-124	74
6	10	7-15	24-144	52	14-176	87
7	8	12-15	37-98	55	60-195	100
8	7	40-60	41-91	60	61-310	126
9	6	10-70	21-56	37	50-254	129
10	5	10-70	59-117	79	107-210	140
11	5	20-80	52-111	68	87-224	140
12	14	25-150	19-69	39	113-278	177
13	3	>500	-	-	82-188	132

These data indicate generally elevated levels of phenol in the urine of the exposed populations, as well as end-of-shift elevation in these levels.

Docter and Zielhuis (1967) also discussed various studies on the relationship between benzene exposure and phenol excretion in groups of workers. When corrections for ventilation and conversions from phenol excretion in 24 h to phenol concentration in a spot sample at the end of the working shift were taken into account, various linear regressions between benzene exposure and phenol excretion showed good agreement. For spot samples at the end of the shift these were:

$$y = 0.49x - 4.28 \qquad (1)$$

$$y = 0.44x - 3.3 \qquad (2)$$

$$y = 0.44x - 13.3 \qquad (3)$$

where y (mg m^{-3}) was the concentration of benzene in air; and
x (mg l^{-1}) was the concentration of phenol in urine.

Docter and Zielhius (1967) commented that the regressions give an indication of the relationship between exposure to benzene and the average phenol concentration in the urine of groups of workers, but that individual values may have too great a variation to be used as a reliable measure for individual exposure.

Phenol levels in urine have also been used in assessing the benzene exposure of non-occupationally exposed populations (Eikmann et al., 1981).

Cornish and Ryan (1965) studied the excretion of various metabolites of benzene in fed and fasted rats, and also in animals in which β-diethylaminoethyldiphenylpropylacetate hydrochloride (β-DDH) was used to inhibit the hydroxylating enzyme system in the liver. They reported that, in the non-fasted rat, the major metabolites were conjugated phenols, other than glucuronides, whereas, in the fasted rat, the major excretory pathway was glucuronide conjugation. In rats treated with β-DDH, all excretory pathways requiring hydroxylation were depressed. In

TABLE 1

EFFECTS OF VARIOUS PRE-TREATMENTS ON THE EXCRETION OF
C-14 AFTER THE SUBCUTANEOUS ADMINISTRATION OF [C-14] BENZENE

Percentage of dose

Pre-treatment	Urine 24h	Urine 24-48h	Urine total	Carcass and faeces	Total in urine, faeces and carcass	Expired air CO_2	Expired air benzene	Overall total
None	15.8±3.8	6.7±0.8	22.4±4.6	2.2±1.1	24.6±3.5	1.6±1.4	54.4±13.6	80.6±17.7
Phenobarbital	22.2±1.9	6.6±4.9	28.9±6.6	2.5±0.7	31.4±7.3	6.6±8.4	43.3±17.6	80.4±12.5
Piperonyl butoxide	13.5±5.1	12.8±2.9	26.1±7.9	2.3±0.6	28.3±8.5	2.2±1.8	60.1±14.7	90.6±15.8
Cobalt chloride	14.0±2.3	12.1±8.3	26.2±9.9	4.4±3.4	30.6±13.2	1.8±2.7	52.2±13.4	84.6±12.2
Benzene	23.1±2.7	5.4±2.2	28.5±4.3	2.1±0.8	30.6±5.0	4.2±3.4	45.4±6.6	80.2±5.9

Note:

From Timbrell and Mitchell (1977); mean ± s.d. (3 animals in each group)

TABLE 2

EFFECTS OF VARIOUS PRE-TREATMENTS ON THE CONJUGATED URINARY
METABOLITES OF [C-14]BENZENE EXCRETED IN URINE OF RATS

Pre-Treatment	Metabolites as percent of dose in 24h urine				
	Quinol and catechol glucuronide	Phenyl glucuronide	Phenyl mercapturate	Phenyl sulphate	Total
None	0.35±0.21	0.45±0.18	0.73±0.31	7.52±3.11	9.45±3.92
Phenobarbital	1.60±0.24	1.35±0.15	1.23±0.12	11.60±1.41	15.78±1.88
Piperonyl butoxide	0.50±0.44	2.20±1.31	0.67±0.46	7.98±1.97	11.58±4.18
Cobalt chloride	1.00±0.35	2.33±0.89	0.77±0.29	7.90±1.06	12.19±1.76
Benzene	3.44±1.50	3.66±0.34	1.32±0.09	7.78±1.90	16.57±0.18

Note:

From Timbrell and Mitchell (1977): mean ± s.d. (3 animals in each group)

all cases, excretion peaked during the day after exposure and was essentially complete by the second day post-exposure.

Sherwood and Carter (1970) reported on the excretion of phenol in human urine after a 4.5 h exposure to 25 ppm benzene in air. The data presented are consistent with a half-life for phenol excretion of about 8 h.

Hunter and Blair (1972), took note of the high solubility of benzene in fat and studied phenol excretion in relation to the body fat content of human subjects. Results of these studies are summarised below.

Subject No.	Body fat (% wt.)	Post-exposure time of obser- vation (h)	Dose of benzene (mg)	Phenol excretion (% dose)
1	8.3	24.7	33.0	50.6
		49.8	118.0	59.4
		30.8	184.0	75.7
2	13.0	31.9	116.0	73.3
3	16.0	48.0	117.0	77.6
4	18.2	30.5	75.0	85.9
		38.2	167.0	82.4
5	19.7	28.9	99.0	72.0
		29.5	217.0	78.5
		23.0	58.0	84.6
		43.5	52.0	87.1

No clear trend with percentage body fat is exhibited by these data.

Timbrell and Mitchell (1977) studied the effects of microsomal enzyme inducers and inhibitors on the metabolism of C-14 labelled benzene in the rat. They reported that pre-treatment of animals with the inhibitors piperonyl butoxide and cobaltous chloride tended to reduce the urinary excretion of metabolites in 24 h, but increased the overall urinary excretion. Furthermore, piperonyl butoxide tended to increase expired benzene. Pre-treatment with the inducer phenobarbital, or with benzene itself, tended to increase urinary excretion of metabolites, but decreased expired benzene. Detailed examination of the results of this experiment (listed in Tables 1 and 2), reveals that the various effects identified are of marginal significance.

Snyder et al. (1977a) investigated benzene metabolism in mice. Following the subcutaneous administration of [H-3]benzene at several dose levels between 440 and 8800 mg kg^{-1}, labelled benzene metabolites were collected in the urine over a 24 h period. A double-reciprocal plot of dose of benzene against total metabolites of benzene in urine (Fig. 6) indicates that the mouse is capable of metabolising about 2 mmoles of benzene per day.

Snyder et al. (1977a) also performed a chromatographic separation of the urinary metabolites. These analyses were performed on two pooled 24 h urine samples, each sample being collected from three mice. Results were as listed below.

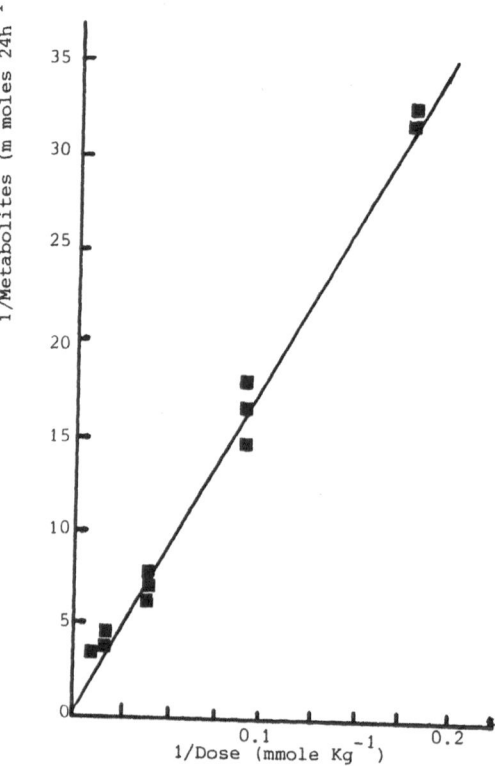

NOTE: From Snyder et al. (1977a); each value
         obtained from the analysis of pooled urine
         from six or more animals (r = 0.95)

FIGURE 6   URINARY EXCRETION OF [³H]BENZENE METABOLITES
            IN MICE AS A FUNCTION OF DOSE

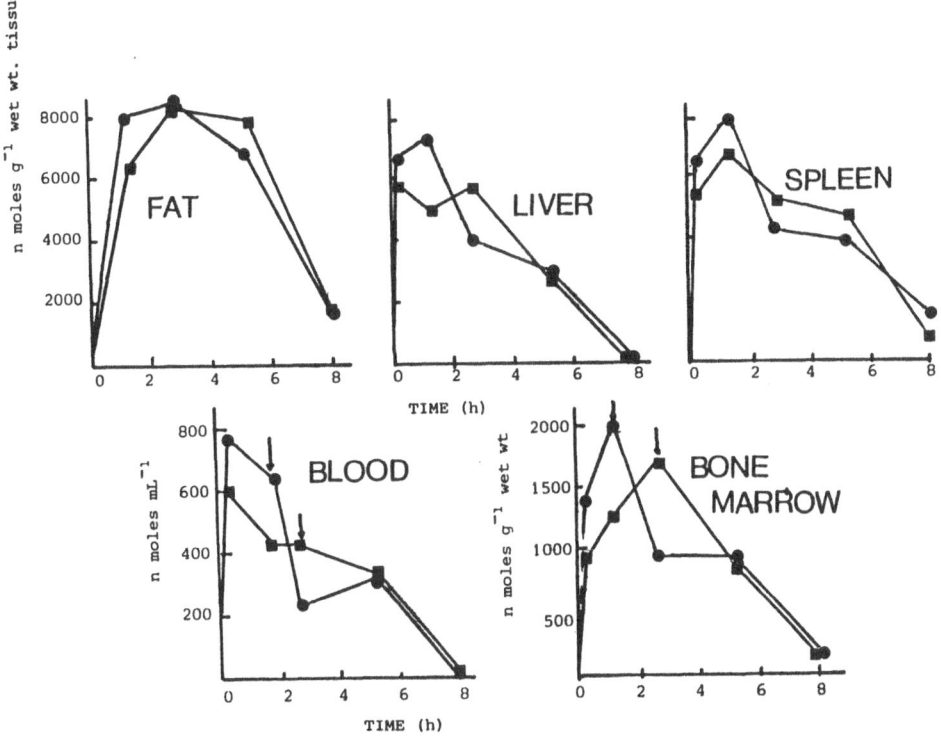

NOTES: From Snyder et al. (1977a)
         [^{3}H] Benzene (880 mg kg^{-1}) (●) or [^{3}H] benzene
         (800 mg kg^{-1}) plus toluene (1720 mg kg^{-1}) (■) was
         given subcutaneously in olive oil solutions. Tissues
         were removed and weighed, toluene - extractable
         radioactivity was determined, and the amount of [^{3}H]
         benzene present was assayed. Each point represents
         a mean value obtained from six mice.

FIGURE 7.   CONCENTATIONS OF [^{3}H] BENZENE IN MOUSE TISSUES

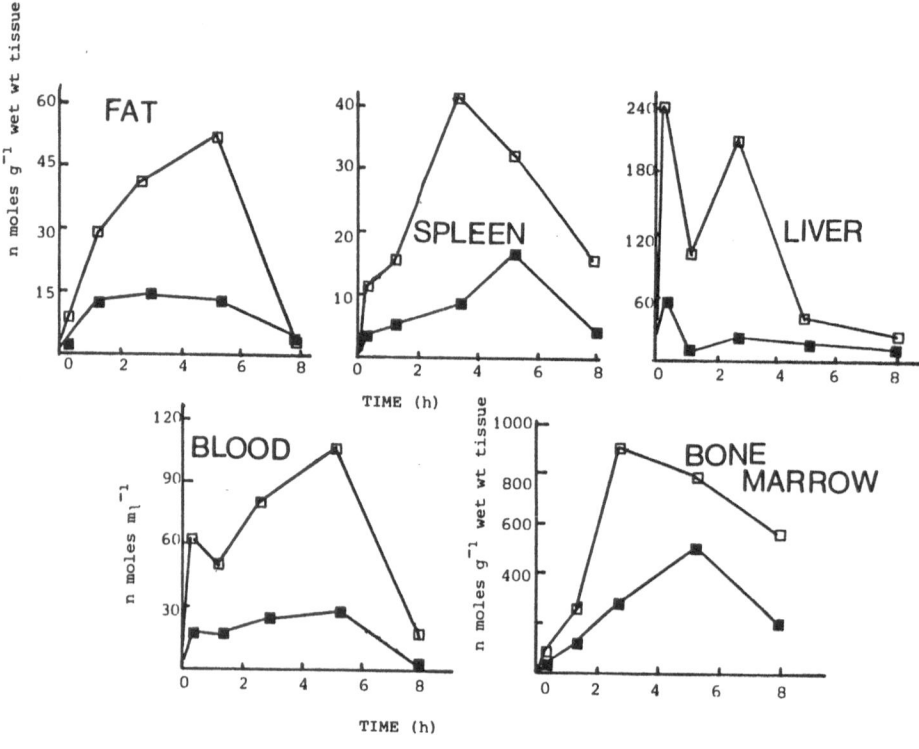

NOTES: From Snyder et al. (1977a)
         Following subcutaneous administration of [³H] benzene (880 mg kg⁻¹)
         (■) or [³H] benzene (880 mg kg⁻¹) plus talvene (1760 mg kg⁻¹) (□) to
         mice, the water-soluble radioactivity present in various tissues
         was determined and n mel [³H] benzene metabolites present was cal-
         culated using the specific activity of the injected [³H] benzene.
         Each point represents a mean value obtained from six mice.

FIGURE 8.   CONCENTRATIONS OF METABOLITES OF [³H] BENZENE IN MOUSE
              TISSUES.

Dose (mg kg^{-1})	Percent sample composition		
	Free phenol	Glucuronides	Sulphates
440	33.3	26.8	39.8
880	7.0	52.7	40.4
2200	0.75	68.4	30.9
4400	6.1	58.4	35.7
8800	5.1	67.8	27.1

The authors reported that no free phenol metabolite, other than phenol, was detected. Further analysis of the glucuronide and sulphate fractions showed that conjugated phenol was the major metabolite and that a small quantity of catechol was also present.

Extending their studies to investigations of the effects of benzene metabolism on benzene toxicity, Snyder et al. (1977a) investigated the effects of toluene as a modifier of benzene metabolism. Administration of toluene with [H-3]benzene was found to enhance the cumulative pulmonary excretion of unchanged [H-3]benzene (see Section 8.4.2) and depressed substantially the urinary excretion of benzene metabolites, as shown below.

Teatment	Precent of [H-3]benzene recovered in urine in 24 h (mean ± s.d. for six animals)
880 mg kg^{-1} [H-3]benzene	20.1 ± 4.5
880 mg kg^{-1} [H-3]benzene + 1720 mg kg^{-1} toluene	7.9 ± 2.7

This effect was demonstrably due to competitive inhibition of the metabolism of benzene and not to an effect of toluene on the distribution of benzene in the body. This was shown by a study of the effect of toluene on benzene metabolism in a mouse liver microsomal preparation (see Section 8.4.3.2) and by showing that, while the distribution of benzene in mouse tissues following subcutaneous injection was unaffected by simultaneous administration of toluene, levels of benzene metabolites in mouse tissues were substantially depressed at all times after exposure (see Figs. 7 and 8). Similar results on the effects of toluene on urinary phenol excretion after intraperitoneal injection of benzene into rats were reported by Van Rees (1972).

In the report on their studies, Snyder et al. (1977a) noted that the concentration of benzene metabolites in bone marrow far exceeded the level in blood. Indeed they were comparable with, or in excess of, those recorded for liver, as illustrated below.

TABLE 3

[H-3]BENZENE AND ITS WATER SOLUBLE AND COVALENTLY BOUND
METABOLITES IN ORGANS OF C57BL/6 AND DBA/2 MICE GIVEN
MULTIPLE DOSES OF [H-3] BENZENE(1)

Organ or tissue	[H-3]benzene(2)		Water soluble metabolites(2)		Covalently bound(3)	
	C57BL/6	DBA/2	C57BL/6	DBA/2	C57BL/6	DBA/2
Bone marrow	-	-	2480±668	4529±270	33±12	52±9
Liver	5±2	7±2	843±197	1258±237	534±87	577±117
Kidney	8±1	6±1	807±135	1134±165	539±70	650±45
Blood	4±3	4±2	1051±127	1389±46	77±9	244±42
Spleen	16±5	27±6	416±44	639±130	105±18	146±28
Lung	9±2	10±4	722±160	1070±210	215±70	150±13
Muscle	8±1	7±2	588±36	771±76	38±3	35±7

Notes:

(1) From Longacre et al. (1981): [H-3]benzene administered subcutaneously at 880 mg kg^{-1}, two doses per day, for 3 days; mice killed 16 h after last dose.

(2) nmol benzene equivalents per g wet weight tissue or per ml of blood: mean ± s.d. (3 to 4 values except for liver where 10 to 12 values were obtained)

(3) nmol benzene equivalents per g dry tissue residue: mean ± s.d. (3 to 4 values)

Tissue	Time after injection (h)	Concentration (ng g^{-1} w.w.)		
		Free phenols	Conjugated phenol	Conjugated catechol
Femoral bone marrow	0.25	21	140	-
	1.0	34	245	-
	3.0	24	760	34
	5.0	105	1170	38
Liver	0.25	21	120	3.3
	1.0	54	598	3.4
	3.0	17	512	31
	5.0	32	973	59

In more recent experiments (Longacre et al., 1981), Snyder and his co-workers studied differences in the metabolism of benzene between DBA/2 and C57BL/6 mice, since DBA/2 mice are more susceptible to benzene intoxication than are C57BL/6 mice. They reported that, following subcutaneous administration of benzene, no differences in the total amounts of urinary metabolites were noted, but that differences in specific metabolites were found. Thus, DBA/2 mice excreted more phenylglucuronide, but less ethereal sulphate conjugates than C57BL/6 mice. Also, DBA/2 mice excreted more phenol, but less hydroquinone than C57BL/6 mice. Total excretion of benzene metabolites was ~20% of the injected activity in the first day after injection, rising to ~24% in the first three days after injection.

Longacre et al. (1981) also studied the distribution of benzene metabolites in various organs and tissues of mice following single and repeated subcutaneous injections of benzene. Results from the single injection studies are illustrated in Fig. 10, while results from the multiple injection studies are summarised in Table 3. The single injection studies did not reveal much inter-strain difference between the levels of water soluble metabolites in any tissue except kidney. However, the repeated injection studies revealed that the more resistant C57BL/6 mice contained less water soluble benzene metabolites in bone marrow, liver, kidney, blood, spleen and lung than did the DBA/2 mice. Similarly, the C57BL/6 mice also contained less covalently bound metabolites in bone marrow, blood, spleen and muscle than did the DBA/2 mice.

Sato and Nakajima (1979) conducted a detailed study on the retention of benzene in blood and the excretion of phenol in urine after benzene was administered to rats, by intraperitoneal injection, singly, or in combination with an equimolar amount of toluene. Results from these studies are shown in Figs. 11 and 12. With respect to loss from blood, Sato and Nakajima (1979) stated that as long as the dose of benzene remained in the range 0.31 to 1.25 mmol kg^{-1}, there was no significant difference in the disappearance rate of benzene from blood, whether given alone or in combination with an equimolar amount of toluene. When the dose of benzene was increased to 5.0 mmol kg^{-1}, the rate of clearance of benzene alone was somewhat reduced and the clearance of benzene adminstered with toluene was markedly delayed. With respect to urinary excretion of phenol, there was no difference between the benzene alone and benzene plus toluene groups at the 0.31 mmol kg^{-1} level, whereas, at 1.25 mmol kg^{-1}, toluene depressed induced phenol excretion to some extent

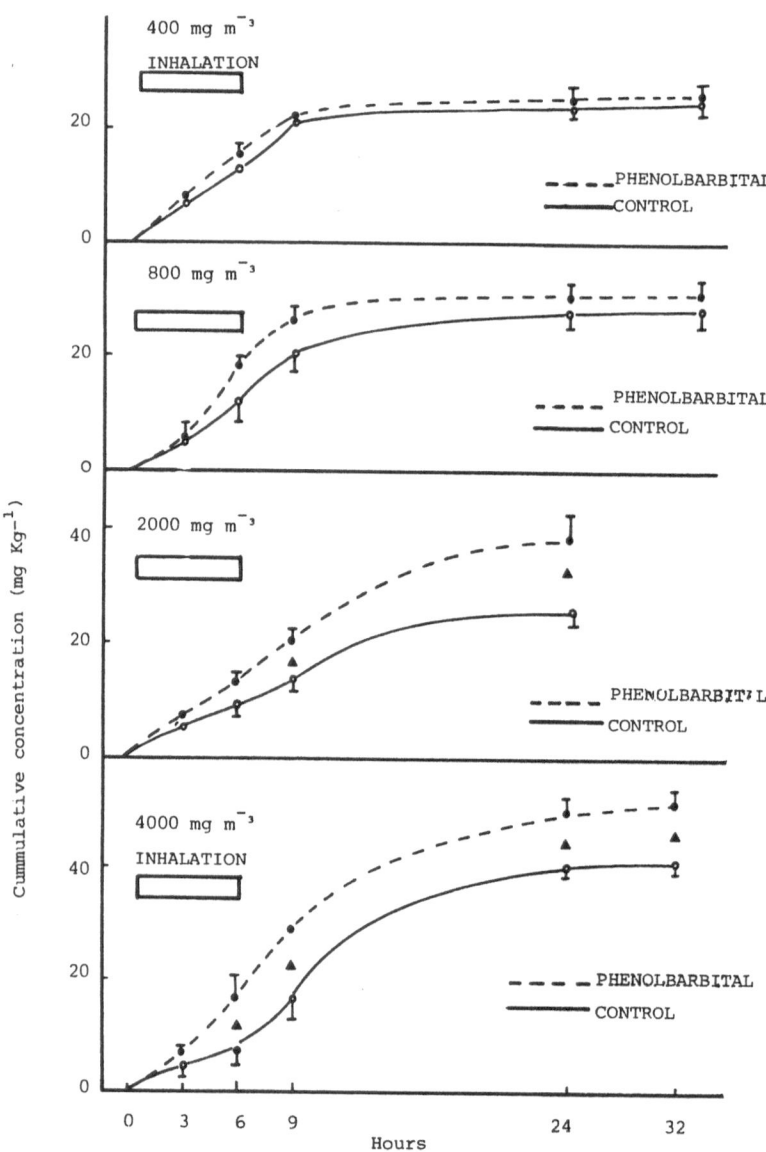

NOTE: From Gut and Frantik (1980)

FIGURE 9.   EFFECT OF BENZENE INHALATION AND PHENOBARBITAL
PRETREATMENT ON THE ELIMINATION OF PHENOL IN
URINE'OF MALE RATS

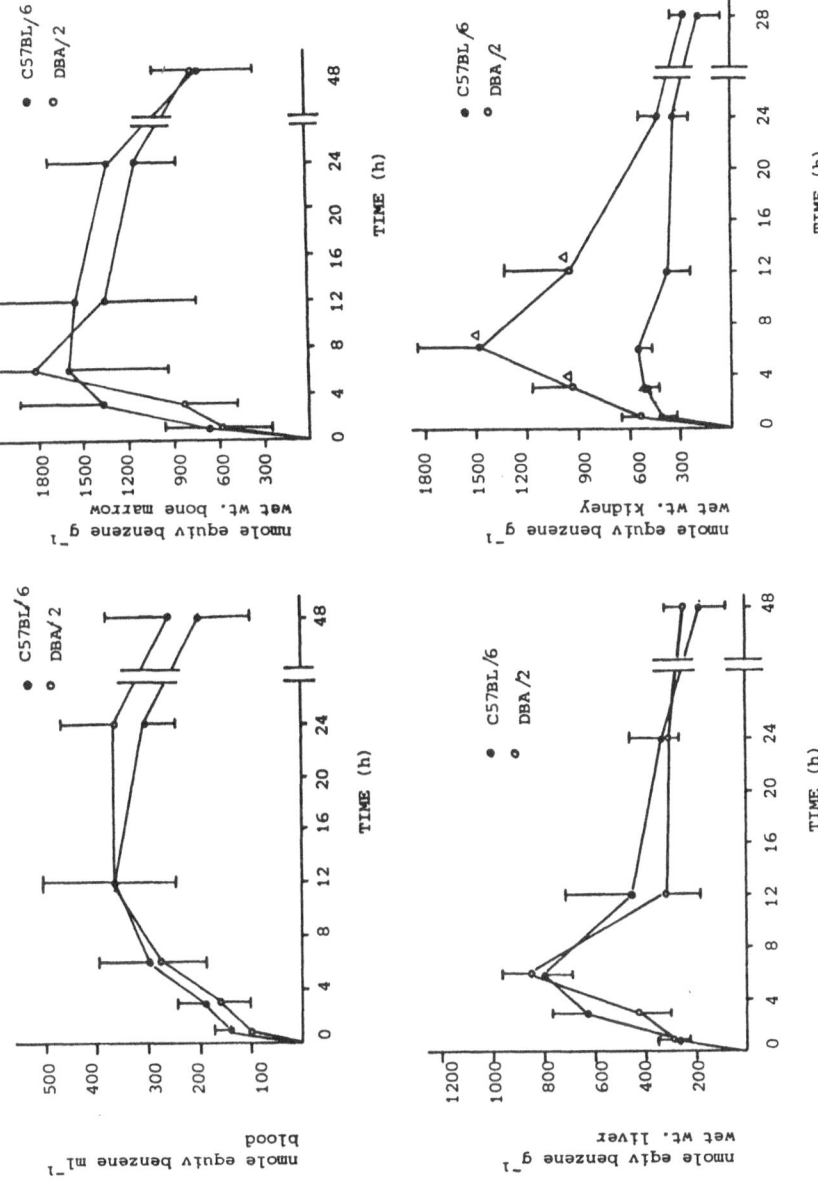

NOTE: From Longacre et al. (1981). Mice received a single injection of 880 mg kg^{-1} [^{3}H] benzene and concentrations of water-soluble metabolites were determined at various time intervals. Each data point represents the mean ± SD of four to six samples. Δ significantly different from C57BL/6 mice (p<0.05)

FIGURE 10.   RECOVERY OF WATER SOLUBLE METABOLITES FROM VARIOUS ORGANS OF [^{3}H] BENZENE TREATED C57BL/6 AND DBA/2 MICE.

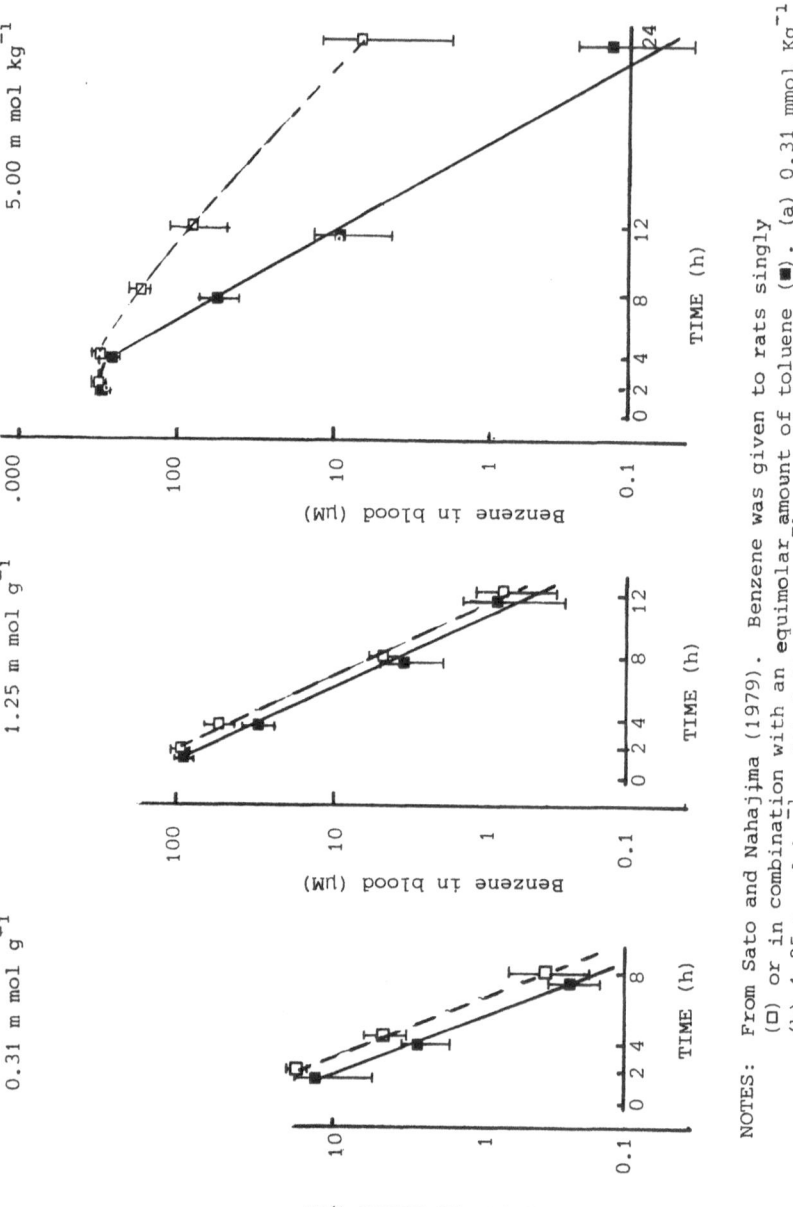

NOTES: From Sato and Nahajima (1979). Benzene was given to rats singly
        (□) or in combination with an equimolar amount of toluene (■). (a) 0.31 mmol Kg^{-1}
        (b) 1.25 m mol kg^{-1} : (C) 5.00 m mol kg^{-1}. Vertical lines depict Sd (n=4)

FIGURE 11. TIME COURSES OF BENZENE CONCENTRATION IN BLOOD

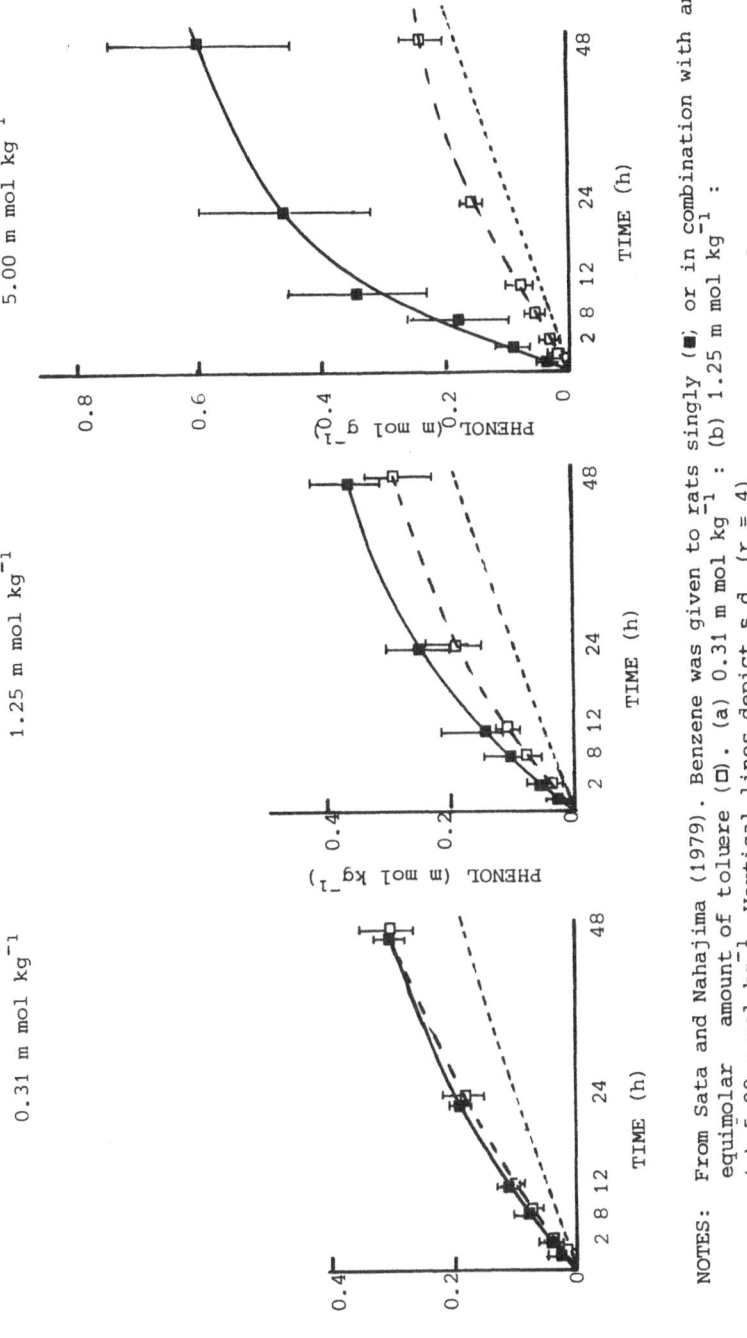

NOTES: From Sata and Nahajima (1979). Benzene was given to rats singly (■), or in combination with an equimolar amount of toluere (□). (a) 0.31 m mol kg⁻¹ : (b) 1.25 m mol kg⁻¹ : (c) 5.00 m mol kg⁻¹. Vertical lines depict s.d. (r = 4) The naturally occurring background amount of plenol is shown by a dotted line.

FIGURE 12.   CUMULATIVE AMOUNT OF PHENOL EXCRETED IN URINE

and at 5.0 mmol kg^{-1}, this effect was very marked, particularly in the first 12 to 24 h after exposure.

Gut and Frantik (1980) studied the excretion of phenol in the urine of rats inhaling benzene concentrations of 400 to 4000 mg m^{-3} (114 to 1140 ppm) for 6 h. Rates of phenol excretion were similar at all levels of administration, demonstrating that benzene metabolism was already capacity limited at the lowest exposure levels used. Pre-treatment with phenobarbital was used to enhance mixed function oxidase metabolism. This pre-treatment enhanced phenol excretion in the urine at benzene exposure levels of 800 mg m^{-3} and above (see Fig. 9). However, pre-treatment with phenobarbital only increased excretion in the first six hours of a 12 h exposure. Gut and Frantik (1980) concluded that phenobarbital pre-treatment may significantly increase the metabolism of inhaled benzene, but only at high concentrations of benzene. They also commented that the effect is diminished, or reversed, by a high induction caused by benzene and, possibly, by a metabolite of benzene.

Denton et al. (1981) studied the excretion of phenol in urine of rats exposed to various levels of lead in drinking water for 23 weeks prior to exposure to 400 mg kg^{-1} of benzene injected intraperitoneally. The following results were recorded.

Pb treatment (µg ml^{-1} in drinking water	Pre-injection	Time after injection of benzene (d)			
		0-1	1-2	2-3	3-4
		Free phenol (µg/d)			
0.00	5.3±3.2	13.2	2.2	1.5	0.6
0.05	5.1±5.2	23.2±21.1	2.9±0.8	1.1±0.2	1.5±0.9
0.58	2.1±1.5	15.3±9.7	2.1±0.7	0.8±0.0	4.0±0.5
17.00	6.2±5.3	7.4±0.8	0.6±0.3	1.5±1.2	0.9±0.3
352.00	2.7±2.6	56.9±21.0	2.3±2.0	1.0±0.1	2.4±2.8
		Conjugated phenol (mg d^{-1})			
0.00	0.5±0.1	23.2	14.4	0.41	0.43
0.05	0.5±0.3	33.3±16.1	1.2±0.6	0.4±0.4	0.2±0.1
0.58	0.3±0.2	28.7±4.9	18.2±10.8	0.4±0.2	0.6±0.2
17.00	0.3±0.1	39.9±4.1	17.8±5.0	0.3±0.0	0.3±0.1
352.00	0.3±0.2	23.6±2.4	11.1±12.2	0.2±0.0	0.2±0.2

Values are means ± one standard error (9 animals at each data point) and Denton et al. (1981) reported that statistical analysis of the data showed that prior lead treatment had no effect on the amount of phenol excreted after the benzene injection.

Because phenol excreted in the urine can be an useful monitor of benzene exposure and metabolism, it is relevant also to consider the excretion of phenol and its metabolites following exposure to phenol. While this is not discussed in detail herein, it is noted that Ohtsuji and Ikeda (1972) demonstrated a linear relationship between phenol levels in air and conjugated phenols in urine for workers in Bakelite factories. Estimates of phenol intake and urinary excretion indicated that virtually all phenol entering the lungs was excreted in conjugated form via the urine. Levels of free phenol in urine were very low at all levels of exposure.

Similarly, Capel et al. (1972) reported that, in three men, 90% of an oral dose of [C-14]phenol was excreted in the urine within 24 h, mainly as phenyl sulphate and phenyl glucuronide. Considerable inter-species differences were observed in these studies, both with respect to the fractional excretion within 24 h and in terms of the proportion of different metabolites excreted. Examination of the data presented by Capel et al. (1972) suggests that the metabolism of phenol in the rat bears a closer resemblance to that in man, than does the metabolism of phenol in either the mouse or the rabbit.

8.4.3.2   Other studies of benzene metabolism in vivo

Many of the in vivo studies of benzene metabolism relevant to construction of a model are discussed elsewhere, either in the content of retention of inhaled benzene (Section 8.4.2), or in the context of urinary excretion of metabolites (Section 8.4.3.1). This section includes discussion of other relevant in vivo experiments.

Of particular note, are the various early studies of Garton and Williams (1948; 1949a; 1949b), who, by investigating the metabolism of catechol, quinol, resorcinol and phenol, elucidated many of the pathways of benzene metabolism illustrated in Fig. 2. More recent studies of interest include that of Longacre et al. (1981a) who demonstrated a gradual accumulation of benzene and benzene metabolites in various tissues of mice given repeated subcutaneous injections of [H-3]benzene (Figs. 13 and 14). It is noted that the data for water soluble metabolites in various tissues are not readily interpretable, since chromatographic studies of liver tissue demonstrated that the H-3 was present as tritiated water and as a non-phenolic metabolite of benzene. It is emphasised that tritiated water is very mobile in the body and that its presence in any organ or tissue does not constitute evidence for its production in that organ or tissue. Longacre et al. (1981a) also reported the following data for [H-3] benzene metabolites irreversibly bound in liver and bone marrow (nmol per g d.w.).

Site	Day of treatment			
	1	3	6	9/10
Liver	185, 185	522, 596	716, 685	808, 854
Bone marrow	7.4, 6.5	34, 28	145, 247	61

Concentrations of benzene metabolites in the blood and bone marrow of rats following inhalation exposure were studied by Longacre et al. (1979) and results of these studies are illustrated in Fig. 15. These data indicate the rapid production of phenol and other benzene metabolites.

The question of whether benzene can be metabolised by bone marrow, or whether metabolites are transported to that tissue from other parts of the body, was addressed by Irons et al. (1980) who introduced [C-14] benzene directly into the bone marrow space of rats through a hole drilled in the distal head of the femur. Irons et al. (1980) concluded that the results of the study clearly established the capability of bone marrow to metabolise benzene, independent of metabolism of the compound by the liver. While the experimental protocol used makes it impossible to

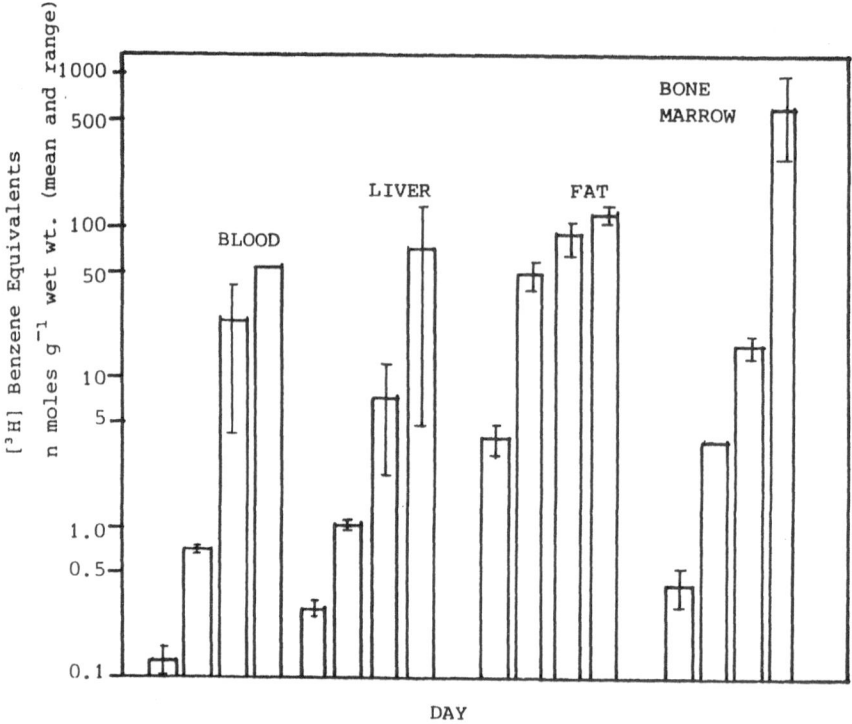

NOTE: From Longacre et al. (198 1b)Benzene was the only
        component found in these fractions.

FIGURE 13.   RESIDUAL TOLUENE - SOLUBLE RADIOACTIVITY IN
                BLOOD, LIVER TESTICULAR FAT AND BONE MARROW
                FROM MICE TREATED WITH [^{3}H] BENZENE (440 mg kg^{-1}
                TWICE A DAY) FOR 1-10d.

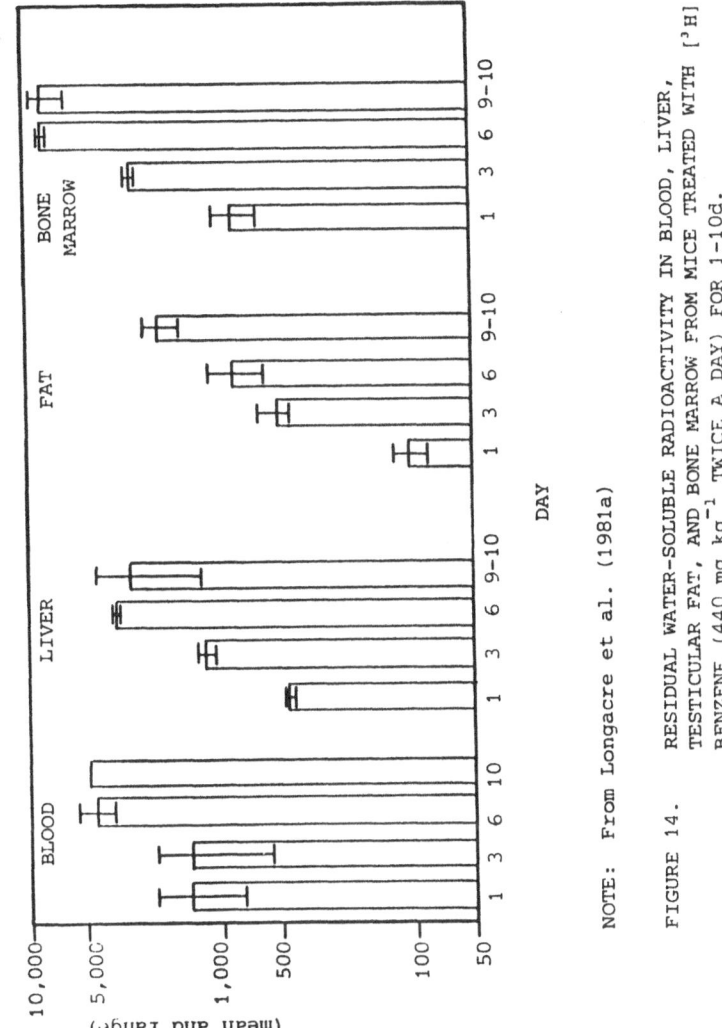

NOTE: From Longacre et al. (1981a)

FIGURE 14.   RESIDUAL WATER-SOLUBLE RADIOACTIVITY IN BLOOD, LIVER, TESTICULAR FAT, AND BONE MARROW FROM MICE TREATED WITH [³H] BENZENE (440 mg kg^{-1} TWICE A DAY) FOR 1-10d.

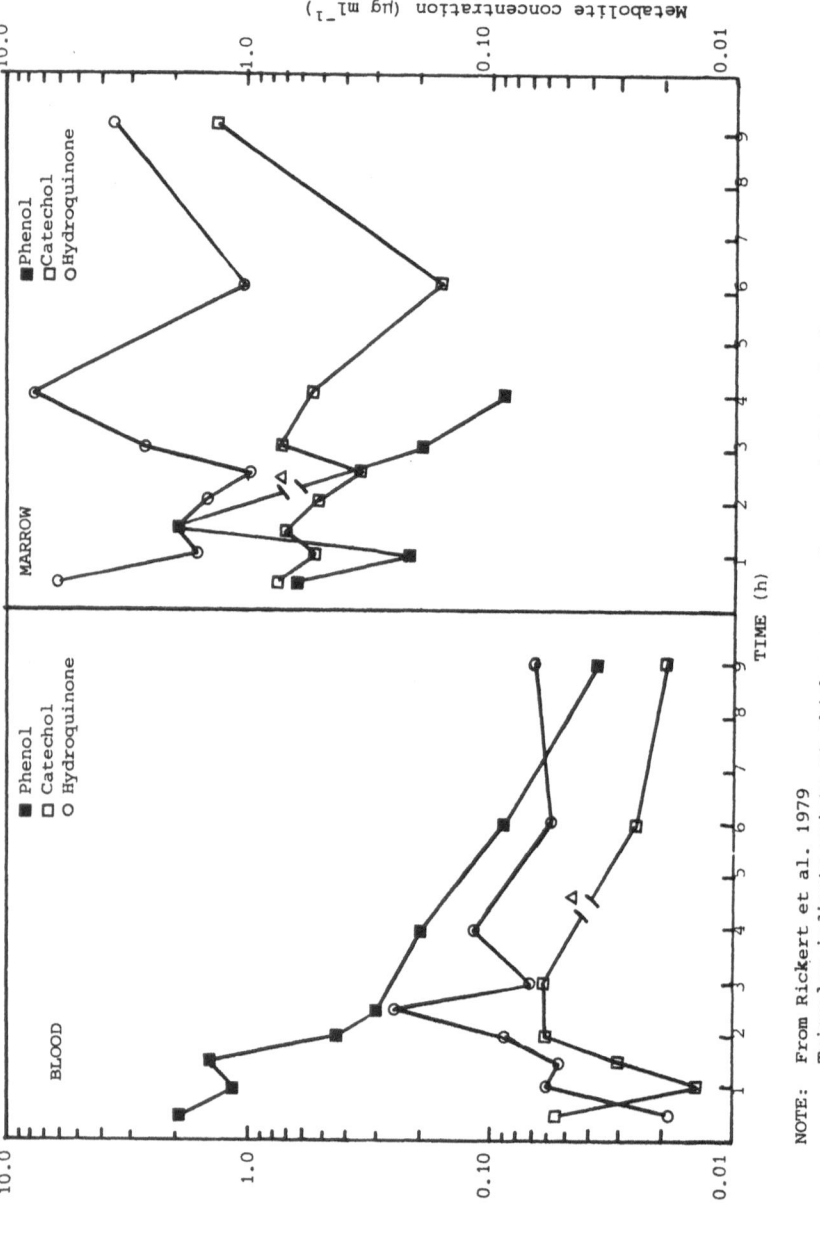

NOTE: From Rickert et al. 1979
         Triangles indicate points at which a compound was not detected due to
         technical difficulties. SE were all less than 50%. Each point is the mean for three
         animals.

FIGURE 15.   CONCENTRATION OF METABOLITES FOLLOWING A 6-HOUR INHALATION EXPOSURE TO BENZENE

interpret this result in quantitative terms, account must be taken of the comment by Irons et al. (1980) that the metabolite concentration ratio between bone marrow and blood approached 400 in this study, as compared with 7 in an inhalation experiment. This suggests that a high proportion of the metabolites formed in bone marrow are retained in that tissue.

However, more recently, Irons and co-workers (Greenlee et al., 1981a) have reported data from whole-body autoradiographic studies of rats, which indicate that the uptake and concentration of hydroquinone and catechol in bone marrow and thymus can occur independent of the metabolism of benzene in these tissues. Thus, the site of production of toxic metabolites of benzene remains an open question, particularly since Sammett et al. (1979) have demonstrated that partial hepatectomy reduces both the metabolism and toxicity of benzene.

With respect to the excretion of benzene and its derivatives in bile, Abou-el-Makarem et al. (1967) reported that, when [C-14]benzene was injected intraperitoneally into biliary cannulated female rats, only 0.8% of the administered dose was excreted in the bile within 24 h. Phenyl glucuronide comprised 16% of the metabolites found in bile, but three other, unidentified, compounds were also found.

Other in vivo studies of relevance all relate to the modification of benzene metabolism or toxicity by various agents. Thus, Nomiyama (1962) reported that 3-amino-1,2,4-triazole, which reduces the oxidation rate of benzene in liver as well as liver catalase activity, also reduces the myelotoxic effects of benzene. Similarly, Abramova and Gadaskina (1965) reported that some sulphur-containing compounds (cystine, cystamine and methionine) reduced the oxidation of benzene in rat liver homogenate, weakened the myelotoxic action of benzene in sub-acute poisoning of rabbits, and reduced excretion of benzene-derived bound sulphur and glucuronides in rabbit urine. Inversely, Kocsis et al. (1968) demonstrated that liver preparations from dimethyl sulphoxide treated rats showed an increased capacity to metabolise benzene and that animals treated with dimethyl sulphoxide plus benzene exhibited enhanced excretion of taurine relative to rats treated with benzene alone. The authors argued that because increased levels of taurine are found in urine after whole-body x-irradiation, toxic doses of colchicine, or toxic doses of carbon tetrachloride (presumably as a result of cell death and lysis), this compound can be used as an indicator of early toxicity. However, the non-specificity of the response, and its tenuous relationship to the mechanisms of benzene toxicity, make this difficult to justify for comparative, quantitative, studies.

Ikeda and Ohtsuji (1971) reported that aromatic hydroxylase activity in rats and guinea pigs was stimulated by treatment with phenobarbital, but that conjugation reactions of phenolic sulphation and glucuronidation were not stimulated markedly. In further experiments it was found that rats pre-treated with phenobarbital exhibited a different time course of phenol excretion following benzene exposure as compared with control animals. During the first two hours after benzene exposure, the phenobarbital-treated rats excreted more than twice as much phenol as the control rats. Conversely, urinary phenol from the phenobarbital treated group dropped to two-thirds that of the controls during the period 4 to 6 h after benzene exposure. Pre-treatment with phenobarbital was also found to offer effective protection against the leukopenic effects of inhalation of benzene vapour by rats.

Ikeda et al. (1972) went on to study interactions between the metabolism of benzene and toluene, and the effects of phenobarbital upon this interaction. They reported that toluene suppressed the excretion of conjugated phenol in benzene treated animals, but that pre-treatment with phenobarbital reduced this suppressive effect. In contrast, Drew and Fouts (1974) found that, whereas phenobarbital and 3-methylcholanthrene both induce benzene metabolism in liver, pre-treatment with these compounds had no effect upon the acute toxicity of benzene in rats following inhalation or intraperitoneal administration. Further studies of the effects of phenobarbital and 3-methylcholanthrene on benzene metabolism in rats were reported by Gill et al. (1979), who also studied the effects of SKF-525A, a compound which inhibits the oxidation of type I microsomal substrates by the liver and may have effects on conjugating enzyme systems. Gill et al. (1979) reported the following results.

- Phenobarbital protected animals from leucopenia and increased both total and unconjugated phenol in urine.
- 3-methylcholanthrene did not prevent leukopenia, but increased conversion of benzene to phenol and enhanced the amount of unconjugated phenol excreted.
- SKF-525A had no effect on leukopenia, reduced the conversion of benzene to phenol and did not change the excretion of unconjugated phenol.

In view of these results, Gill et al. (1979) concluded that the marrow effect of benzene is due to a metabolic product other than phenol and that the rate of production of this toxic principle is not strictly dependent on the rate of phenol production.

In another, recent, study, Greenlee and Irons (1981) reported that pre-treatment of rats with 2,4,5,2´,4´,5´,-hexachlorobiphenyl (HCB) or 3,4,3´,4´-tetrachlorobiphenyl (TCB) protected against benzene toxicity for as long as 7 days, but not after 10 days of repeated dosing. On the basis of studies on changes in enzyme levels and metabolism to phenol in treated animals, Greenlee and Irons (1981) concluded that the protection against benzene toxicity obtained by pre-treatment with HCB and TCB is a complex process involving a variety of metabolic processes, but that decreasing the production of primary metabolites, and/or increasing hepatic conjugating activity, are important factors.

Finally, it is of interest to note that Gut et al. (1981) studied phenol excretion in the urine of benzene exposed rats. Phenobarbital was found to enhance excretion in the first 12 h after exposure, but not thereafter. Gut et al. (1981) also found that the elimination of radioactive metabolites of [C-14]benzene in the urine of rats, orally administered 3 mmole kg^{-1} of benzene, was decreased by intraperitoneal administration of 1.2 mmole kg^{-1} of phenol, but was unaffected by intraperitoneal administration of pyrocatechol, resorcinol or hydroquinol at levels of 0.6 mmole kg^{-1}. In rats administered smaller amounts of benzene (1 mmole kg^{-1}) and phenol (0.1, 0.2 or 0.4 mmole kg^{-1}), no inhibition of excretion was observed. On the basis of these and other, in vitro, studies, Gut et al. (1981) concluded as follows.

- The rate of benzene metabolism to phenol in vivo appears to be influenced by factors in addition to the activity of (hepatic) microsomal monooxygenases.

- The manifestation of microsomal enzyme induction in vivo apparently requires that the benzene concentration exceeds a certain level.
- Benzene oxidation in vivo appears to be inhibited by the phenol produced as a result of this oxidisation.

8.4.3.3   Benzene metabolism in vitro

Benzene metabolism has been studied extensively in vitro, in particular, in liver homogenate and liver microsomal fractions from a variety of mammalian species. While these studies are of interest in elucidating the biochemical pathways of benzene metabolism, they are of limited relevance for the construction of a model of benzene metabolism in vivo. For a discussion of these aspects of benzene metabolism the reader is referred to papers by Hirokawa and Nomiyama (1962), Snyder et al. (1967), Gonasun et al. (1973), Harper et al. (1973), Drew et al. (1974) and Tunek et al. (1978), as well as the recent reviews by Snyder et al. (1981) and the International Agency for Research on Cancer (1982). In the context of transformation to phenol, interest has centred on metabolism by the cytochrome P-450 dependent mixed-function oxidase system which is responsible for the metabolism of many xenobiotics and can be stimulated by such agents. This enzyme system is present in liver, but also to a lesser extent, in a variety of organs (Snyder et al., 1981). It is noted that more than one enzyme of this system may be responsible for the metabolism of benzene, but that the detailed mechanisms have not yet been elucidated.

As discussed by Snyder et al. (1981), although current evidence strongly suggests that a metabolite of benzene mediates its haemopoietic toxicity, the identity and origin of the toxic metabolite or metabolites is still uncertain. Thus, while several studies have been conducted on the binding of benzene metabolites to various macromolecules including proteins and nucleic acids (see Greenlee et al., 1981; Snyder et al., 1978; Tunek et al., 1981; Lutz and Schlatter, 1977) the implications of the results of these studies with respect to benzene toxicity are not clear, though interactions of tubulin with quinones may be implicated in cell cycle effects (Irons and Pfeifer, 1982).

8.5   METABOLIC MODEL

In this section, a metabolic model for benzene is developed based on the data reviewed in Section 8.4. This model relates only to inhalation exposure to benzene, since other routes are of little significance in comparison. Furthermore, the model relates specifically to monitoring for benzene exposure, since the distribution of benzene and its metabolites in man, or any other species, have not been characterised adequately and the particular metabolites responsible for the toxic effects of benzene have not been identified clearly. The model used is shown in Fig. 16.

About 50% of inhaled benzene is retained in the body following inhalation, though some of this is rapidly re-excreted in the exhaled air, such that, in a 3 h exposure, concentrations of benzene in exhaled air are 70% of concentrations in inhaled air. Further, following cessation of exposure three components of loss are identified with rate constants ~ 5 h^{-1}, 1 h^{-1} and 0.02 h^{-1}. Benzene retained in the body will

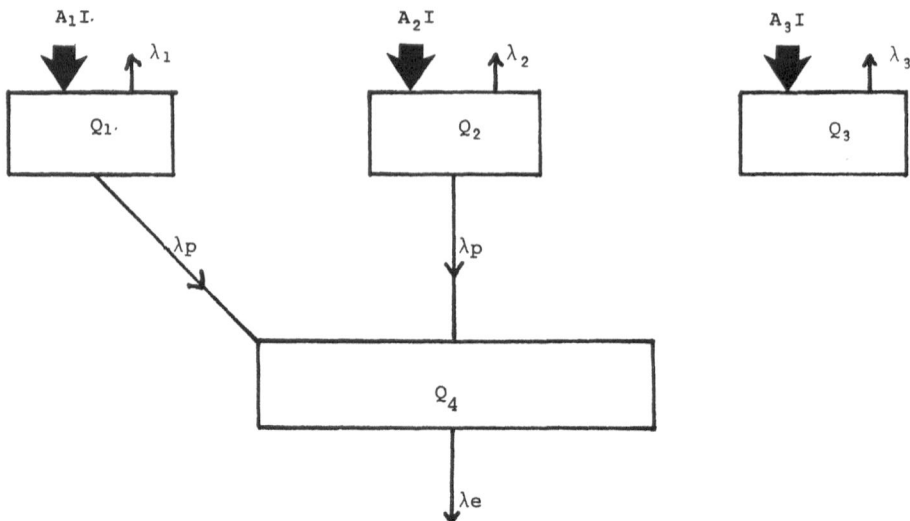

NOTES: A_1 to A_3 are the fractions of inhaled benzene deposited in the various retention compartments;

I is the rate of inhalation of benzene;

λ, to λ_3 are the rates of loss to exhalation;

λp is the rate of conversion to phenol and other metabolites of benzene;

$\lambda.e$ is the rate of excretion of benzene metabolites;

Q_1 to Q_3 are the amounts of benzene retained in the body;

Q_4 is the amount of benzene metabolites retained in the body.

FIGURE 16.   A SIMPLE MODEL FOR SIMULATING THE RETENTION OF INHALED BENZENE AND THE EXCRETION OF BENZENE METABOLITES IN URINE.

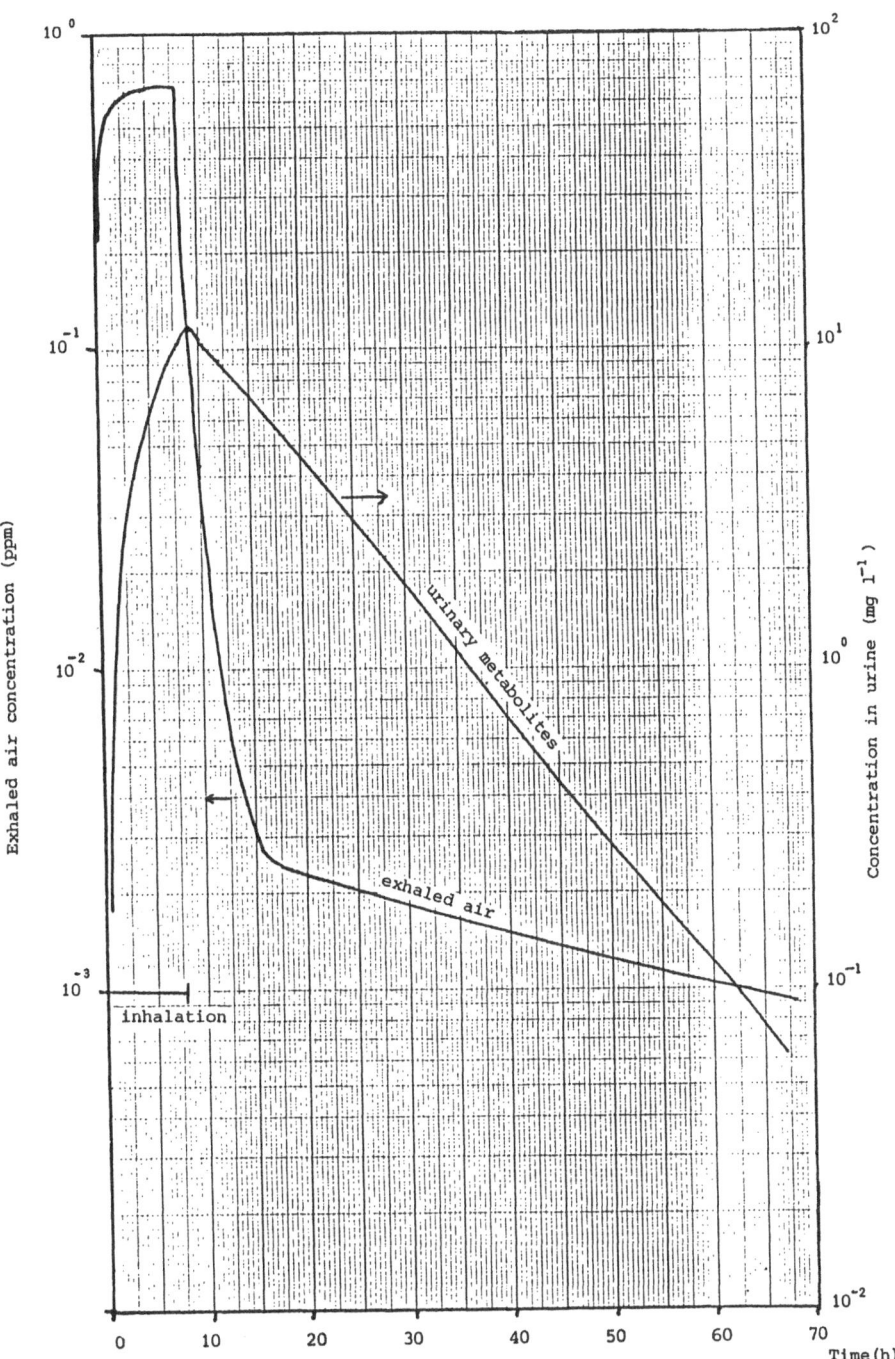

FIGURE 17.   LOSS OF BENZENE IN EXHALED AIR AND BENZENE METABOLITES IN
              URINE DURING AND AFTER AN EIGHT HOUR INHALATION EXPOSURE.

be available for excretion into the exhaled air or conversion into phenol and other derivatives for excretion in the urine. It is not clear whether the transformation to phenol operates on benzene associated with all components of retention, but as a first approach to modelling it is assumed that transformation to phenol occurs only in the two most rapidly turning-over compartments. Phenol and other metabolites produced from benzene are assumed to be excreted entirely in the urine. The reason for exclusion of the component with slow turnover is that it is probably associated with fat and is, therefore, not available for cellular oxidation. Values of the model parameters have been calculated from the data available and are listed below. The definition and application of these parameters is given in Fig. 16.

$$\lambda_1 = 4.72 \text{ h}^{-1} \qquad A_1 = 0.3$$
$$\lambda_2 = 0.5 \text{ h}^{-1} \qquad A_2 = 0.6$$
$$\lambda_3 = 0.02 \text{ h}^{-1} \qquad A_3 = 0.02$$
$$\lambda_p = 0.5 \text{ h}^{-1}$$
$$\lambda_e = 0.09 \text{ h}^{-1}$$

At high levels of exposure, phenolic inhibition of cytochrome P-450 will cause reduction in λ_p, but the data available are not sufficient to quantify this. If this effect were to be modelled, the use of a Michaelis-Menten type of saturable expression would probably be appropriate (see Appendix 9, Section 9.4.2.3).

8.6   ILLUSTRATIVE CALCULATIONS

The proposed model was used to study the concentration of benzene in exhaled air and the concentration of phenolic metabolites in urine during and after an 8 h exposure to 1 ppm benzene in air at an inhalation rate of 20 l min^{-1}. The results of this simulation are shown in Fig. 17.   For these calculations the rate of excretion of urine was assumed to be 1.4 l d^{-1}.

8.7   REFERENCES

Abou-el-Makarem, M.M., Millburn, P., Smith, R.L. and Williams, R.T., 1967. Biliary excretion of foreign compounds: benzene and its derivatives in the rat. Biochem. J., 105, 1269-1274.

Abramova, Z.I. and Gadaskina, I.D., 1966. Inhibition of oxidation of benzene by certain anti-oxidants. Fed. Prof. Trans. Suppl., 25, T91-T92.

Aksoy, M., 1980. Different types of malignancies due to occupational exposure to benzene: a review of recent observations in Turkey. Environ. Res., 23, 181-190.

Aksoy, M. and Erdem, S., 1978. Followup study on the mortality and the development of leukemia in 44 pancytopenic patients with chronic exposure to benzene. Blood, 52, 285-292.

Aksoy, M., Erdem, S. and Dincol, G., 1976. Types of leukemia in chronic benzene poisoning. A study in thirty-four patients. Acta Haemat., 55, 65-72.

Andrews, L.S., Lee, E.W., Witmer, C.M., Kocsis, J.J. and Snyder, R., 1977. Effects of toluene on the metabolism, disposition and haemopoietic toxicity of [3H]benzene. Biochem. Pharmacol., 26, 293-300.

Andrews, L.S., Sasame, H.A. and Gillette, J.R., 1979. 3H-benzene metabolism in rabbit bone marrow. Life Sci., 25, 567-572.

Berlin, M., Gage, J.C., Gullberg, B., Holm, S., Knudsen, P. and Tunek, A., 1980. Breath concentration as an index of the health risk from benzene. Scand. J. Work environ. Health, 6, 104-111.

Braun, D. (Ed.), 1974. Symposium on Toxicology of Benzene and Alkylbenzenes. Industrial Health Foundation, Pittsburgh, USA.

Brewer, R.H. and Weiskotten, H.G., 1916. The action of benzol: III. The urinary phenols with special reference to the diphasic leukopenia. J. Med. Research, 35, 71-78.

Brief, R.S., Lynch, J., Bernath, T. and Scala, R.A., 1980. Benzene in the work-place. Amer. Ind. Hyg. Assoc. J., 41, 616-623.

Callow, E.H. and Hele, T.S., 1926. Studies in the sulphur metabolism of the dog III. The effect of benzene and of some derivatives of benzene on sulphur metabolism. Biochem. J., 20, 598-605.

Capel, I.D., French, M.R., Millburn, P., Smith, R.L. and Williams, R.T., 1972. The fate of [14C]phenol in various species. Xenobiotica, 2, 25-34.

Cohen, H.S., Freedman, M.L. and Goldstein, B.D., 1978. The problem of benzene in our environment:clinical and molecular considerations. Am. J. Med. Sci., 275, 125-136.

Conca, G.L. and Maltagliati, A., 1955. Study on the absorption of benzene through the skin. Med. Lav., 46, 194-198.

Cornish, H.H. and Ryan, R.C., 1965. Metabolism of benzene in nonfasted, fasted and aryl-hydroxylase inhibited rats. Toxicol. Appl. Pharmacol., 7, 767-771.

Denton, J.E., Potter, G.D. and Santolucito, J.A., 1981. Effects of lead on benzene metabolism. J. Toxicol. Environ. Health, 7, 893-900.

Docter, H.J. and Zielhuis, R.L., 1967. Phenol excretion as a measure of benzene exposure. Ann. Occup. Hyg., 10, 317-326.

Dowty, B.J., Laseter, J.L. and Storer, J., 1976. The transplacental migration and accumulation in blood of volatile organic constituents. Pediat. Res., 10, 696-701.

Drew, R.T. and Fouts, J.R., 1974. The lack of effects of pretreatment with phenobarbital and chlorpromazine on the acute toxicity of benzene in rats. Toxicol. Appl. Pharmacol., 27, 183-193.

Drew, R.T., Fouts, J.R. and Harper, C., 1974. The influence of certain drugs on the metabolism and toxicity of benzene. In: Braun, D. (Ed.) Symposium on Toxicology of Benzene and Alkylbenzenes. Industrial Health foundation, pp.17-31.

Eikmann, K., Stinner, D. and Prajsnar, D., 1981. Haematological data relating to phenol excretion in urine with chronical benzene exposure. I. Epidemiological studies of adults. Zentralbl. Bakteriol. Microbiol. Hyg. [B], 174, 57-76.

Garton, G.A. and Williams, R.T., 1948. Studies in detoxication 17. The fate of catechol in the rabbit and the characterisation of catechol monoglucuronide. Biochem. J., 43, 206-211.

Garton, G.A. and Williams, R.T., 1949a. Studies in detoxication 21. The fates of quinol and resorcinol in the rabbit in relation to the metabolism of benzene. Biochem. J., 44, 234-238.

Garton, G.A. and Williams, R.T., 1949b. Studies in detoxication 26. The fates of phenol, phenylsulfuric acids and phenylglucuronide in the rabbit in relation to the metabolism of benzene. Biochem. J., 45, 158-163.

Gill, D.P., Kempen, R.R., Nash, J.B. and Ellis, S., 1979. Modifications of benzene myelotoxicity and metabolism of phenobarbital, SKF-525A and 3-methylcholanthrene. Life Sci., 25, 1633-1640.

Gill, D.P. Jenkins, V.K., Kempen, R.R. and Ellis, S., 1980. The importance of pluripotential stem cells in benzene toxicity. Toxicology, 16, 163-171.

Goldstein, B.D. and Snyder, C.A., 1982. Benzene leukemogenesis. In: Tice, R.R., Costa, D.L. and Schaich, K.M. (Eds.) Genotoxic Effects of Airborne Agents. Plenum Press, New York, pp.277-289.

Goldstein, B.D., Snyder, C.A., Laskin, S., Bromberg, I., Albert, R.E. and Nelson N., 1982. Myelogenous leukemia in rodents inhaling benzene. Toxicol. Lett., 13, 169-173.

Gonasun, L.M., Witmer, C., Kocsis, J.J. and Snyder, R., 1973. Benzene metabolism in mouse liver microsomes. Toxicol. Appl. Pharmacol., 26, 398-406.

Green, J.D., Snyder, C.A., LoBue, J., Goldstein, B.D. and Albert, R.E., 1981. Acute and chronic dose/response effect in benzene inhalation on the peripheral blood, bone marrow, and spleen cells of CD-1 mice. Toxicol. Appl. Pharmacol., 59, 204-214.

Green, J.D. Snyder, C.A., LoBue, J., Goldstein, B.D. and Albert, R.E., 1981a. Acute and chronic dose/response effects of inhaled benzene on multipotential hematopoetic stem (CFU-S) and granulocyte/macrophage progenitor (GM-CFU-C) cells in CD-1 mice. Toxicol. Appl. Pharmacol., 58, 492-503.

Greene, M.H., Hoover, R.N., Eck, R.L. and Fraumeni, J.F. Jr., 1979. Cancer mortality among printing plant workers. Environ. Res., 20, 66-73.

Greenlee, W.F. and Irons, R.D., 1981. Modulation of benzene-induced lymphocytopenia in the rat by 2,4,5,2´,4´,5´-hexachlorobiphenyl and 3,4,3´,4´-tetrachlorobiphenyl. Chem.-Biol. Interact., 33, 345-360.

Greenlee, W.F., Sun, J.D. and Bus, J.S., 1981. A proposed mechanism of benzene toxicity: formation of reactive intermediates from polyphenol metabolites. Toxicol. Appl. Pharmacol., 59, 187-195.

Greenlee, W.F., Gross, E.A. and Irons, R.D., 1981a. Relationship between benzene toxicity and the disposition of ^{14}C-labelled benzene metabolites in the rat. Chem.-Biol. Interact., 33, 285-299.

Gut, I. and Frantik, E., 1980. Kinetics of benzene metabolism in rats in inhalation exposure. Arch. Toxicol. (Suppl. 4), 315-317.

Gut, I., Hátle, K. and Zizkova, L., 1981. Effect of phenobarbital pretreatment on benzene biotransformation in the rat II. 9000 g supernatant and isolated perfused liver versus living rat. Arch. Toxicol., 47, 13-24.

Hammond, J.W. and Hermann, E.R., 1960. Industrial hygiene features of a petro-chemical benzene plant design and operation. Am. Ind. Hyg. Assoc. J., 21, 173-177.

Hanke, J., Dutkiewicz, T. and Piotrowski, J., 1961. The absorption of benzene through the skin in men. Med. Pracy., 12, 413-426.

Harigaya, K., Miller, M.E., Cronkite, E.P. and Drew. R.T., 1981. The detection of in vivo haematotoxicity of benzene by in vitro liquid bone marrow cultures. Toxicol. Appl. Pharmacol., 60, 346-353.

Harper, C., Drew, R.T. and Fouts, J.R., 1973. Species differences in benzene hydroxylation to phenol by pulmonary and hepatic microsomes. Drug. Metabol. Disp., 3, 381-388.

Hirokawa, T. and Nomiyama, K., 1962. Studies on poisoning by benzene and its homologues (5). Oxidation rate of benzene in rat liver homogenates. Med. J. Shinshu Univ., 7, 29-39.

Hough, V.H., Gunn, F.D. and Freeman, S., 1944. Studies on the toxicity of commercial benzene and of a mixture of benzene, toluene and xylene. J. Ind. Hyg., 26, 296-306.

Hunter, C.G., 1966. Aromatic solvents. Am. J. occup. Hyg., 9, 191-198.

Hunter, C.G., 1968. Solvents with reference to studies on the pharmaco-dynamics of benzene. Proc. R. Soc. Med., 61, 913-915.

Hunter, C.G. and Blair, D., 1972. Benzene: pharmacokinetic studies in man. Ann. Occup. Hyg., 15, 193-199.

Ikeda, M. and Ohtsuji, H., 1971. Phenobarbital-induced protection against toxicity of toluene and benzene in the rat. Toxicol. Appl. Pharmacol., 20, 30-43.

Ikeda, M., Ohtsuji, H. and Imamura, T., 1972. In vivo suppression of benzene and styrene oxidation by co-administered toluene in rats and effects of phenobarbital. Xenobiotica, 2, 101-106.

Infante, P.F., Rinsky, R.A., Wagoner, J.K. and Young, R.J., 1979. Leukemia in benzene workers. J. Environ. Pathol. Toxicol., 2, 251-257.

International Agency for Research on Cancer, 1974. Benzene. IARC Monographs on the Evaluation of the Carcinogenic Risks of Chemicals to Humans, 7, 203-221.

International Agency for Research on Cancer, 1982. Benzene. IARC Monographs on Evaluation of the Carcinogenic Risks of Chemicals to Humans, 29, 93-148.

International Commission on Radiological Protection, 1975. ICRP Publication 23. Report of the Task Group on Reference Man. Pergamon Press, Oxford.

Irons, R.D. and Moore, B.J., 1980. Effect of short term benzene administration on circulating lymphocyte subpopulations in the rabbit: evidence of a selective B-lymphocyte sensitivity. Res. Commun. Chem. Pathol. Pharmacol., 27, 147-155.

Irons, R.D. and Pfeifer, R.W., 1982. Benzene metabolites: evidence for an epigenetic mechanism of toxicity. In: Tice, R.R., Costa, D.L. and Schaich, K.M. (Eds.) Genotoxic Effects of Airborne Agents, Plenum Press, New York, pp. 241-256.

Irons, R.D. Heck, H. d'A., Moore, B.J. and Muirhead, K.A., 1979. Effects of short-term benzene administration on bone marrow cell cycle kinetics in the rat. Toxicol. Appl. Pharmacol., 51, 399-409.

Irons, R.D., Dent, J.G., Baker, T.S. and Rickert, D.E., 1980. Benzene is metabolised and covalently bound in bone marrow in situ. Chem.-Biol. Interact., 30, 241-245.

Irving, W.S. Jr. and Grumbles, T.G., 1979. Benzene exposures during gasoline loading at bulk marketing terminals. Am. Ind. Hyg. Assoc. J., 40, 468-473.

Jerina, D.M. and Daly, J.W., 1974. Arene oxides: a new aspect of drug metabolism. Science, 185, 573-582.

Kocsis, J.J., Harkaway, S., Santoyo, M.C. and Snyder, R., 1968. Dimethyl sulfoxide: interactions with aromatic hydrocarbons. Science, 160, 427-428.

Laskin, S. and Goldstein, B.D. (Eds.), 1977. Benzene toxicity, a critical evaluation. J. Toxicol. Environ. Health (Suppl. 2).

Lee, E.W., Kocsis, J. and Snyder, R., 1973. Dose dependent inhibition of ^{59}Fe incorporation into erythrocytes after a single dose of benzene. Res. Commun. Chem. Pathol. Pharmacol., 5, 547-549.

Lee, E.W., Kocsis, J.J. and Snyder, R., 1974. Acute effect of benzene on ^{59}Fe incorporation into circulating erythrocytes. Toxicol. Appl. Pharmacol., 27, 431-436.

Li, T.-W., Freeman, S., Hough, V.H. and Gunn, F.D., 1945. The increased susceptibility of protein-deficient dogs to benzene poisoning. Am. J. Physiol., 145, 166-176.

Longacre, S.L., Kocsis, J.J. and Snyder, R., 1981. Influence of strain differences in mice on the metabolism and toxicity of benzene. Toxicol. Appl. Pharmacol., 60, 398-409.

Longacre, S.L., Kocsis, J.J., Witmer, C.M., Lee, E.W., Sammett, D. and Snyder, R., 1981a. Toxicological and biochemical effects of repeated administration of benzene in mice. J. Toxicol. Environ. Health, 7, 223-237.

Lutz, W.K. and Schlatter, Ch., 1977. Mechanism of the carcinogenic action of benzene: irreversible binding to rat liver DNA. Chem.-Biol. Interact., 18, 241-245.

Maltoni, C., Cotti, G., Valgimigli, L. and Mandrioli, A., 1982. Zymbal gland carcinomas in rats following exposure to benzene by inhalation. Am. J. Ind. Med., 3, 11-16.

Mehlman, M.A., Schreiner, C.A., Mackerer, C.R., 1980. Current status of benzene teratology: a brief review. J. Environ. Pathol. Toxicol., 4, 123-131.

Moeschlin, S. and Speck, B., 1967. Experimental studies on the mechanism of action of benzene on the bone marrow (radioautographic studies using ^{3}H-thymidine). Acta haemat., 38, 104-111.

NIOSH, 1974. Criteria for a Recommended Standard - Occupational Exposure to Benzene. United States Department of Health, Education and Welfare, Public Health Service, Center for Disease Control, National Institute for Occupational Safety and Health. HEW Publication (NIOSH), 74-137.

Nomiyama, K., 1962. Studies on the poisoning by benzene and its homologues (6). Oxidation rate of benzene and benzene poisoning. Med. J. Shinshu Univ., 7, 41-48.

Nomiyama, K. and Nomiyama, H., 1974. Respiratory retention, uptake and excretion of organic solvents in man. Benzene, toluene, n-hexane, trichloroethylene, acetone, ethyl acetate and ethyl alcohol. Int. Arch. Arbeitsmed., 32, 75-83.

Nomiyama, K. and Nomiyama, H., 1974a. Respiratory elimination of organic solvents in man. Benzene, toluene, n-hexane, trichloroethylene, acetone, ethyl acetate and ethyl alcohol. Int. Arch. Arbeitsmed., 32, 85-91, 1974.

Ohtsuji, H. and Ikeda, M., 1972. Quantitative relationship between atmospheric phenol vapour and phenol in the urine of workers in Bakelite factories. Brit. J. Ind. Med., 29, 70-73.

Parke, D.V. and Williams, R.T., 1953. Studies in detoxication 54. The metabolism of benzene. (a) The formation of phenylglucuronide and phenylsulphuric acid from [^{14}C]benzene. (b) The metabolism of [^{14}C]phenol. Biochem. J., 55, 337-340.

Parke, D.V. and Williams, R.T., 1953a. Studies in detoxication 49. The metabolism of benzene containing [^{14}C$_1$] benzene. Biochem. J., 54, 231-238.

Porteous, J.W. and Williams, R.T., 1949. Studies in detoxication. 19. The metabolism of benzene I. (a) The determination of phenol in urine with 2:6 - dichloroquinonechloroimide. (b) The excretion of phenol, glucuronic acid and ethereal sulphate by rabbits receiving benzene and phenol. (c) Observations on the determination of catechol, quinol and muconic acid in urine. Biochem. J., 44, 46-55.

Porteous, J.W. and Williams, R.T., 1949a. Studies in detoxication, 20. The metabolism of benzene II. The isolation of phenol, catechol, quinol and hydroxyquinol from the ethereal sulphate fraction of the urine of rabbits receiving benzene orally. Biochem. J., 44, 56-61.

Rainsford, S.G. and Lloyd Davies, T.A., 1965. Urinary excretion of phenol by men exposed to vapour of benzene: a screening test. Brit. J. Ind. Med., 22, 21-26.

Rickert, D.E., Baker, T.S., Bus J.S., Barrow, C.S. and Irons, R.D., 1979. Benzene disposition in the rat after exposure by inhalation. Toxicol. Appl. Pharmacol., 49, 417-423.

Rickert, D.E., Baker, T.S. and Chism, J.P., 1981. Analytical approaches to the study of the disposition of myelotoxic agents. Environ. Health Perspect., 39, 5-10.

Rondanelli, E.G., Gorini, P., Gerna, G. and Magluilo, E., 1970. Pathology of erythroblastic mitosis in occupational benzene erythropathy and erythraemia. In vivo and in vitro studies. Bibliotheca Haematologica No. 35. S. Karger, Basel, Switzerland.

Rusch, G.M., Leong, B.K.J. and Laskin, S., 1977. Benzene metabolism. J. Toxicol. Environ. Health (Suppl. 2), pp. 23-35.

Sammett, D., Lee, E.W., Kocsis, J.J. and Snyder, R., 1979. Partial hepatectomy reduces both metabolism and toxicity of benzene. J. Toxicol. Environ. Health, 5, 785-792.

Sato, A. and Nakajima, T., 1979. Dose-dependent metabolic interaction between benzene and toluene in vivo and in vitro. Toxicol. Appl. Pharmacol., 48, 249-256.

Sato. T., Fukuyama, T., Suzuki, T. and Yoshikawa, H., 1963. 1,2 - dihydro-1,2-dihydroxybenzene and several other substances in the metabolism of benzene. J. Biochem. (Japan), 53, 23-27.

Schrenk, H.H., Yant, W.P., Pearce, S.J., Patty, F.A. and Sayers, R.R., 1941. Absorption, distribution and elimination of benzene by body tissues and fluids of dogs exposed to benzene vapor. J. Indust. Hyg. Toxicol., 23, 20-34.

Sherwood, R.J., 1976. Criteria for Occupational Exposure to Benzene. International Workshop on Toxicology of Benzene, Paris.

Sherwood, R.J. and Carter, F.W.G., 1970. The measurement of occupational exposure to benzene vapour. Ann. Occup. Hyg., 13, 125-146.

Solomons, T.W.G., 1980. Organic Chemistry, 2nd edit., John Wiley and Sons, New York.

Snyder, R. and Kocsis, J.J., 1975. Current concepts of chronic benzene toxicity. CR.C Critical Reviews in Toxicology, 3, 265-288.

Snyder, R., Uzuki, F., Gonasun, L., Bromfeld, E. and Wells, A., 1967. The metabolism of benzene in vitro. Toxicol. Appl. Pharmacol., 11, 346-360.

Snyder, R., Lee, E.W., Kocsis, J.J. and Witmer, C.M., 1977. Bone marrow depressant and leukemogenic actions of benzene. Life Sci., 21, 1709-1722.

Snyder, R., Andrews, L.S., Lee, E.W., Witmer, C.M., Reilly, M. and Kocsis, J.J., 1977a. Benzene metabolism and toxicity. In: Jollow, D.J., Kocsis, J.J. et al., (Eds.) Biological Reactive Intermediates, Plenum Press, New York, USA, pp.286-301.

Snyder, R., Lee, E.W. and Kocsis, J.J., 1978. Binding of labeled benzene metabolites to mouse liver and bone marrow. Res. Comm. Chem. Pathol. Pharmacol., 20, 191-194.

Snyder, R., Longacre, S.L., Witmer, C.M., Kocsis, J.J., Andrews, L.S. and Lee, E.W., 1981. Biochemical toxicology of benzene. In: Hodgson, E., Bend, J.R. and Philpot, R.M. (Eds.) Reviews in Biochemical Toxicology, Vol.3. Elsevier/North-Holland, New York, pp.123-153.

Snyder, R., Sammett, D., Witmer, C. and Kocsis, J.J., 1982. An overview of the problem of benzene toxicity and some recent data on the relationship of benzene metabolism to benzene toxicity. In: Tice, R.R., Costa, D.L. and Schaich, K.M. (Eds.) Genotoxic Effects of Airborne Agents, Plenum Press, New York, pp.225-240.

Srbova, J., Teisinger, J. and Skramovsky, S., 1950. Absorption and elimination of inhaled benzene in man. Arch. ind. Hyg., 2, 1-8.

Steinberg, B., 1949. Bone marrow regeneration in experimental benzene intoxication. Blood, 4, 550-556.

Teisinger, J. and Fiserova-Bergerova, V., 1958. Valeur comparée de la détermination des sulfates et du phénol contenus dans l'urine pour l'évaluation de la concentration du benzène dans l'air. Arch. Malad. Prof., 16, 221-232.

Tice, R.R., Costa, D.L. and Drew, R.T., 1980. Cytogenetic effects of inhaled benzene in murine bone marrow: induction of sister chromatid exchanges, chromosomal aberrations, and cellular proliferation inhibition in DBA/2 mice. Proc. Natl. Acad. Sci. USA, 77, 2148-2152.

Tice, R.R., Vogt, T.F. and Costa, D.L., 1982. Cytogenetic effects of inhaled benzene in murine bone marrow. In: Tice, R.R. Costa, D.L. and Schaich, K.M.(Eds.) Genotoxic Effects of Airborne Agents, Plenum Press, New York, pp.257-275.

Timbrell, J.A. and Mitchell, J.R., 1977. Toxicity-related changes in benzene metabolism in vivo. Xenobiotica, 7, 415-423.

Tunek, A., Platt, K.L., Bentley, P. and Oesch, F., 1978. Microsomal metabolism of benzene to species irreversibly binding to microsomal protein and effects of modifications of this metabolism. Mol. Pharmacol., 14, 920-929.

Tunek, A., Olofsson, T. and Berlin, M., 1981. Toxic effects of benzene and benzene metabolites on granulopoietic stem cells and bone marrow cellularity in mice. Toxicol. Appl. Pharmacol., 59, 149-156.

Uyeki, E.M., El-Ashkar, A., Shoeman, D.W. and Bisel, T.V., 1977. Acute toxicity of benzene inhalation to hemopoietic precursor cells. Toxicol. Appl. Pharmacol., 40, 49-57.

US National Research Council, 1980. Drinking Water and Health, Vol.3, National Academy Press, Washington, D.C., pp.80-86 and 261-262.

Vale, J.A. and Meredith, T.J., 1983. Poisoning from hydrocarbons, solvents and other inhalational agents. In: Weatherall, D.J. Ledingham, J.G.G. and Warrell, D.A. (Eds.). Oxford Textbook of Medicine, Oxford University Press, Oxford, pp.6.27-6.33.

Van Haaften, A.B. and Sie, S.T., 1965. The measurement of phenol in urine by gas chromatography as a check on benzene exposure. Am. Ind. Hyg. Assoc. J., 26, 52-58.

Van Rees, H., 1972. Mutual influence on the metabolism of some industrial solvents in rats. In: DeC. Baker, S.B. and Neuhaus, G.A. (Eds.) Proceedings of the European Society for the Study of Drug Toxicity XIII. Toxicological Problems of Drug Toxicity. Exerpta Medica Foundation, Amsterdam, 69-74.

Vigliani, E.C., 1976. Leukemia associated with benzene exposure. Ann. N.Y. Acad. Sci., 271, 143-151.

Vigliani, E.C. and Forni, A., 1976. Benzene and leukemia. Environ. Res., 11, 122-127.

Walkley, J.E., Pagnotto, L.D. and Elkins, H.B., 1961. The measurement of phenol in urine as an index of benzene exposure. Am. Ind. Hyg. Assoc. J., 22, 362-367.

Wolf, M.A., Rowe, V.K., McCollister, D.D., Hollingsworth, R.L. and Oyen, F., 1956. Toxicological studies of certain alkylated benzenes and benzene. Experiments on laboratory animals. AMA Arch. Indust. Health, 14, 387-398.

Yant, W.P., Schrenk, H.H., Sayers, R.R., Horvath, A.A. and Reinhart, W.H., 1936. Urine sulfate determinations as a measure of benzene exposure. J. Ind. Hyg. Toxicol. 18, 69-88.

Appendix 9
Vinyl Chloride

CONTENTS

VINYL CHLORIDE

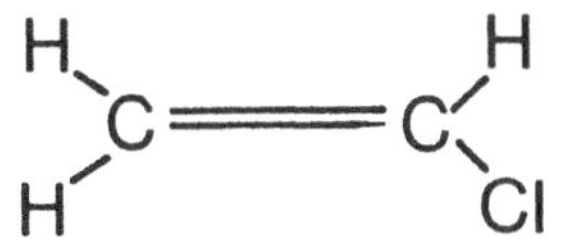

VINYL BROMIDE

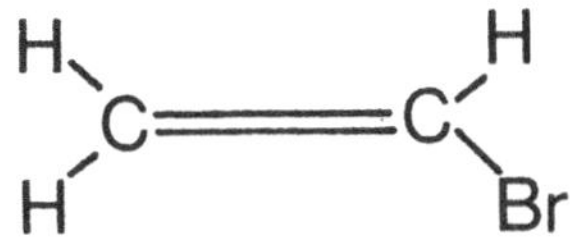

VINYLIDENE CHLORIDE

FIGURE 1. THE STRUCTURE OF VINYL CHLORIDE AND
           RELATED COMPOUNDS

9.1   INTRODUCTION

Vinyl chloride monomer (chloroethene or VCM) has the formula C_2H_3Cl and a molecular weight of 62.5. Its structure is shown in Fig. 1, together with the structures of the closely related compounds vinyl bromide and vinylidene chloride. VCM is a colourless gas at room temperature with a density a factor of 2.2 higher than that of air. The solid form melts at -153.8°C and the liquid boils at -13.37°C (International Agency for Research on Cancer, 1979).

VCM is produced in very large quantities in virtually all highly industrialised countries. The bulk of this is for use in the production of homopolymer and copolymer resins. The other major use of VCM, in some countries, is the production of methyl chloroform.

9.2   LEVELS OF EXPOSURE TO VINYL CHLORIDE MONOMER

9.2.1   Air

Concentrations of VCM in air are generally given as ppb, ppm, mg l^{-1} or mg m^{-3}. the relevant conversion factor is that 1 ppm is equal to 0.0028 mg l^{-1}.

With respect to occupational exposure, the International Agency for Research on Cancer (1979) has summarised air concentrations of VCM at various locations in industrial plant. These values are tabulated below.

Location	Air concentration (ppm)
In a polymerization reactor prior to ventilation	3000
In a polymerization reactor during scraping	50-100
Close to the hands during scraping	600-1000
Near polymerization reactors in one factory: 1950-1959	4000
Working places in polyvinyl chloride producing factories	40-312 (peak 33500)
	43-214
	>75
Russian synthetic leather plant	<44
Three UK cable factories	<0.15-0.35

Time-weighted average exposures to VCM were reported as 50-250 ppm for coagulator operators. However, general exposure levels in vinyl chloride plants have, more recently, been reported as 0.07-27 ppm, <0.01-5.89 ppm, 0.01-84.77 ppm and 0.02-21.8 ppm.

These levels should be seen in the context of the various limits which are set on exposure to VCM in different countries. These values were summarised by the International Agency for Research on Cancer (1979) and are tabulated below.

Country	Concentration (ppm)	Interpretation
USA	1	TWA
	5	Ceiling (15 min.)
Canada	10	TWA
	25	Ceiling (15 min.)
Finland	5	TWA
	10	Ceiling (10 min.)
Italy	50	TWA
	25	TWA (expected)
Japan	10	TWA (expected)
Netherlands	10	TWA
Norway	1	TWA
	5	Ceiling (15 min.)
Sweden	1	TWA
	5	Ceiling (15 min.)
USSR	12	-
France	5	TWA+
	15	Ceiling+
	1	TWA**
	5	Ceiling**
Denmark	1	TWA
Belgium	5	TWA
	15	Ceiling
Federal Republic of Germany	5	TWA
	15	Ceiling+
	2	TWA**
	15	Ceiling**
United Kingdom	10	TWA
	30	Ceiling
Switzerland	10	TWA

Note: * TWA = time-weighted average: + = existing: ** = proposed

In view of these data, it seems that some workers may have been exposed to VCM levels of about 100 ppm, but that current standards should restrict exposure of the most highly exposed personnel to ~5 ppm. Taking a breathing rate of 20 l min. (International Commission on Radiological Protection, 1975), these levels imply intakes of 2700 and 130 mg respectively over an 8 h working shift. Averaged over a year, these values imply average intake rates of 1700 and 80 mg d^{-1}.

With respect to non-occupational exposure, it has been estimated that, prior to 1975, the average VCM concentration around US polyvinyl chloride plants was 44 µg m^{-3}. In the Houston, Texas, area, where ~40% of the US production capacity is located, concentrations of 8-3200 µg m^{-3} have been measured. In the ambient air near two vinyl chloride plants in the Long Beach, California, area, concentrations were 260 to 8800 µg m^{-3}. In the air of Delaware City maximum levels were 3900 µg m^{-3} and mean levels were 2000 µg m^{-3} (International Agency for Research on Cancer, 1979).

On the basis of these figures, it seems that relatively large numbers of members of the public may have been exposed to VCM at levels ~1000 µg m^{-3}. Taking the volume of air inhaled per day to be 23 m^3

(International Commission on Radiological Protection, 1975), this concentration corresponds to a daily inhalation intake of 23 mg.

VCM has been detected in cigarettes at levels ~10 ng per cigarette (International Agency for Research on Cancer, 1979). Thus, daily intakes by this route are unlikely to exceed 0.2 mg, even in heavy smokers. VCM has been detected in some new automobile interiors, but the two studies available on this topic exhibit very different results (International Agency for Research on Cancer, 1979). However, in either case, intakes would almost certainly not exceed 10 mg d^{-1}.

9.2.2   Water

The highest concentration of VCM detected in finished drinking water in the US was 10 µg l^{-1} (International Agency for Research on Cancer, 1979). Taking the daily fluid consumption of fluids less milk to be 1.65 l (International Commission on Radiological Protection, 1975), the maximum daily intake of VCM by this route is estimated to be 17 µg.

9.2.3   Food

VCM has been found in a variety of alcoholic drinks at levels of up to 2.1 mg kg^{-1} and in vinegars at up to 9.4 mg kg^{-1}. It has also been found in edible oils at 0.05 to 14.8 mg kg^{-1}, and in butter and margarine at 0.05 mg kg^{-1}, when these items have been packaged and stored in polyvinyl containers (International Agency for Research on Cancer, 1979). For comparison, if the entire diet were contaminated at 1 mg kg^{-1}, this would only correspond to a VCM intake rate of 1.4 mg d^{-1}. This is consistent with the comment of Van Esch and Van Logten (1975) that daily intakes of VCM in food are likely to be less than 100 µg.

9.2.4   Summary

On the basis of data reviewed in this section, the following daily intakes of VCM are estimated.

Medium	Intake (µg d^{-1})	Comments
Air	≦1.7x10^6	Occupational exposure (pre-1975)
	≦8x10^4	Occupational exposure (post-1975)
	~2x10^4	Most highly exposed members of the public living near polyvinyl chloride production plants
	<200	Intake via smoking
Water	<17	Based on highest recorded water concentrations
Food	<<1400	

From these figures, it is clear that inhalation is likely to be the predominant route of exposure to VCM, both for the occupationally and the non-occupationally exposed.

9.3   EFFECTS

9.3.1   Non-neoplastic effects

The non-neoplastic effects due to chronic exposure of man to VCM have been summarised by Bartsch and Montesano (1975), Haley (1975) and Bahlman et al. (1979). Characteristic effects include liver damage and, more particularly, a sclerotic syndrome called acro-osteolysis.

The liver damage presents as enlargement and tenderness of the liver in association with jaundice. At the tissue level, it consists of parenchymal damage, fibrosis of the liver capsule, periportal fibrosis associated with hepatomegaly, splenomegaly and oesophageal varices, and impaired liver function (Bartsch and Montesano, 1975).

VCM induced fibrosis of the liver and its relation to angiosarcoma induction has been discussed by Tomas et al. (1975) who commented that there was no evidence that all cases of fibrosis proceeded to angiosarcoma, but that such a transition may occur in some cases, since focal proliferation of sinusoidal lining cells and hepatocytes is seen at the fibrotic stage.

Acro-osteolysis is generally located in the distal phalanges and seems only to have occurred in workers employed in the cleaning of autoclaves in which VCM polymerisation had taken place. Symptoms of VCM exposure in such workers included upper abdominal complaints, tiredness, dizziness, increased perspiration and numbness, tingling, and sensation of cold in fingers and toes. Pathological findings included thrombocytopenia, hepatic dysfunction, enlargement of the spleen and reticulocytosis. External changes included morphological effects on the fingers and scleroderma-like changes of the skin of the knuckles and forearm. Acro-osteolysis was particularly noted as a band at the base of the finger nail, which usually exhibited complete regression after removal from VCM exposure, Vascular changes were seen in close association with the bone changes (Potter, 1976).

With respect to subjective symptoms of VCM exposure, Lester et al. (1963) reported that, at levels of 1.2 to 2.0% VCM in air, experimental subjects, unaware of their degree of exposure, reported intoxication with dizziness, lightheadedness, nausea, dulling of auditory and visual cues, and headache. These symptoms disappeared rapidly on cessation of VCM exposure.

Other studies of the non-carcinogenic effects of VCM on man have been concerned with identification of high risk individuals and techniques for early diagnosis of pathological changes to the liver (Anderson et al., 1978; Gluzcz, 1981).

In mice, Suzuki (1980) demonstrated a variety of proliferative, hypertrophic, hypersecretory and inflammatory effects in lung after a 5 or 6 month exposure to 2500 or 6000 ppm of VCM. Also in mice, Tatrai and Ungvary (1981) demonstrated that exposures to 1500 ppm of VCM for less than 24 h can cause circulatory changes, vasomotor paralysis, and alterations in liver and lungs. Changes of this type were not observed in rats and rabbits subject to identical exposure regimes.

There have also been a substantial number of studies on the non-neoplastic effects of VCM in various strains of rats. These are summarised in Table 1. Of particular significance, in respect of VCM metabolism, are the effects of cytochrome P-450 stimulators and inhibitors in enhancing or depressing VCM toxicity.

TABLE 1

NON-NEOPLASTIC CHANGES IN RATS DUE TO EXPOSURE TO
VINYL CHLORIDE MONOMER

Reference	Effects observed
Lester et al. (1963)	Deep anaesthesia and death during 2 h exposures to 15% VCM in air. Changes in liver and spleen weight, and in red and white cell counts during chronic exposure to 2% or 5% VCM in air.
Viola et al. (1971)	Slight anaethesia, degeneration of cerebellum, severe chronic hepatitis, interstitial pneumonia and moderate swelling of kidney parenchyma during exposures to 30000 ppm VCM for 4 h d^{-1}, 5 d per week for 12 months.
Jaeger et al. (1974)	In animals pre-treated with phenobarbital and exposed to 5.0% VCM for a single 6 h period an increase of serum alanine-α-ketoglutarate transaminase (AKT) activity was found, whereas this increase did not occur in non-pretreated rats. This indicates the significance of the mixed function oxidase system in acute liver injury by VCM.
Reynolds et al. (1975; 1975a) Jaeger et al. (1977)	Serum AKT activities enhanced by pretreatment with phenobarbital and Aroclor 1254, to a lesser extent by hexachlorobenzene and not at all by 3-methylcholanthrene, spironolactone or pregnenolone-16-α-carbonitrile. SKF 525A, which inhibits the mixed function oxidase system, decreased the effects of VCM on serum AKT.
Reynolds et al. (1976a)	Phenobarbital and Aroclor 1254 enhanced VCM induced increases in liver weight and reduced glutathione content.
Watanabe et al. (1976)	Exposure to 150 to 2000 ppm of VCM for 1 to 7 h caused progressive depression of hepatic non-protein sulphydryl content. At 50 ppm depression was inconsistent and at 10 ppm did not occur. Results indicate that VCM metabolites interact with glutathione and/or cysteine.

TABLE 1 (Cont.)

Feron et al. (1979; 1979a) Feron and Kroes (1979)	Exposure to 5000 ppm of VCM for 7 h d^{-1}, 5 d per week for 52 weeks caused slight growth retardation, high mortality, slight haematological changes and various morphological changes in the liver and other organs and tissues.
Conolly and Jaeger (1979)	Trichloropropene oxide, which depletes hepatic glutathione, significantly increased VCM toxicity in fasted, but not in fed, rats. This effect was not attributable to hepatic glutathione depression. Diethylmaleate depleted hepatic glutathione, but did not modify VCM toxicity. Cysteine gáve partial protection against VCM toxicity.
Laib et al. (1979)	Newborn animals exposed for 8 h d^{-1} 5 d per week to 2000 ppm VCM exhibited focal hepatocellular deficiencies in nucleoside-5-triphosphatase. It was suggested that this could be an early sign of malignancy.
Du et al. (1979)	Changes in glucose-6-phosphatase, glucose-6-phosphatase dehydrogenase and cysteine levels in animals exposed to 15000 ppm for VCM after 70-100 h exposure. After 137 h of exposure, some dilation of rough endoplasmic reticulum was seen.
Norpoth et al. (1980)	Exposure to 500 ppm of VCM in air leads to stimulation of cell proliferation in regenerating rat liver.
Wisniewska-Knypl (1980)	After 1 and 3 month exposure to 500 and 20000 ppm VCM, cytochrome P-450 levels in liver were depressed, but recovered after 10 months exposure, in association with a slight increase in aniline p-hydroxylase activity. Liver enlargement and ultrastructural alterations were also seen after the third month of exposure.

9.3.2   Carcinogenesis and mutagenesis

The carcinogenic and mutagenic actions of VCM on man have been discussed in several reviews (Bartsch and Montesano, 1975; Haley, 1975; Potter, 1976; 1976a; Berk et al., 1976; Griciute, 1978; International Agency for Research on Cancer, 1979; 1982). On the basis of the data then available, the International Agency for Research on Cancer (1979) concluded as follows.

> " Vinyl chloride is a human carcinogen. Its target organs are the liver, brain, lung and haemolymphatic system. Similar carcinogenic effects were first demonstrated in rats and were later confirmed in mice and hamsters. Although evidence of a carcinogenic effect of vinyl chloride in humans has come from groups occupationally exposed to high doses of vinyl chloride, there is no evidence that there is an exposure level below which no increased risk of cancer would occur in humans.
>
> Epidemiological reports regarding clastogenic effects among vinyl chloride-exposed workers and a single study of increased foetal mortality among the wives of workers who had been exposed to vinyl chloride suggest that vinyl chloride could be mutagenic to humans. Additional support for this suggestion derives from experimental evidence of its mutagenicity.
>
> Studies which indicate increased rates of birth defects among the children of parents residing in communities where vinyl chloride production and polymerisation plants are located indicate the necessity for further investigation of the teratogenicity of vinyl chloride and its polymers in both animals and humans."

More recently, the International Agency for Research on Cancer (1982) stated that "vinyl chloride causes angiosarcoma of the liver; it has also been associated with tumours of the brain and lung and the haematopoietic and lymphatic systems in humans". They went on to note that "reports of increased incidence of tumours of the digestive system, urinary tract and breast (in women) are inadequate to evaluate the carcinogenicity of vinyl chloride for these sites".

It is noted that the evidence for VCM carcinogenicity in humans all dates from 1974 or later (Creech and Johnson, 1974; Monson et al., 1974; Tabershaw and Gaffey, 1974; Nicholson et al., 1975; Ott et al., 1975; Waxweiler et al., 1976; Fox and Collier, 1977; Buffler et al., 1979), following the association of angiosarcomas of the liver with VCM exposure (Creech and Johnson, 1974). Excess angiosarcoma incidence is relatively easy to detect, since this is an extremely rare tumour type. In contrast, other tumours which may be associated with vinyl chloride exposure require substantial epidemiological studies for their identification. For this reason, it is possible that the total carcinogenic risk from VCM exposure significantly exceeds the angiosarcoma risk and that not all

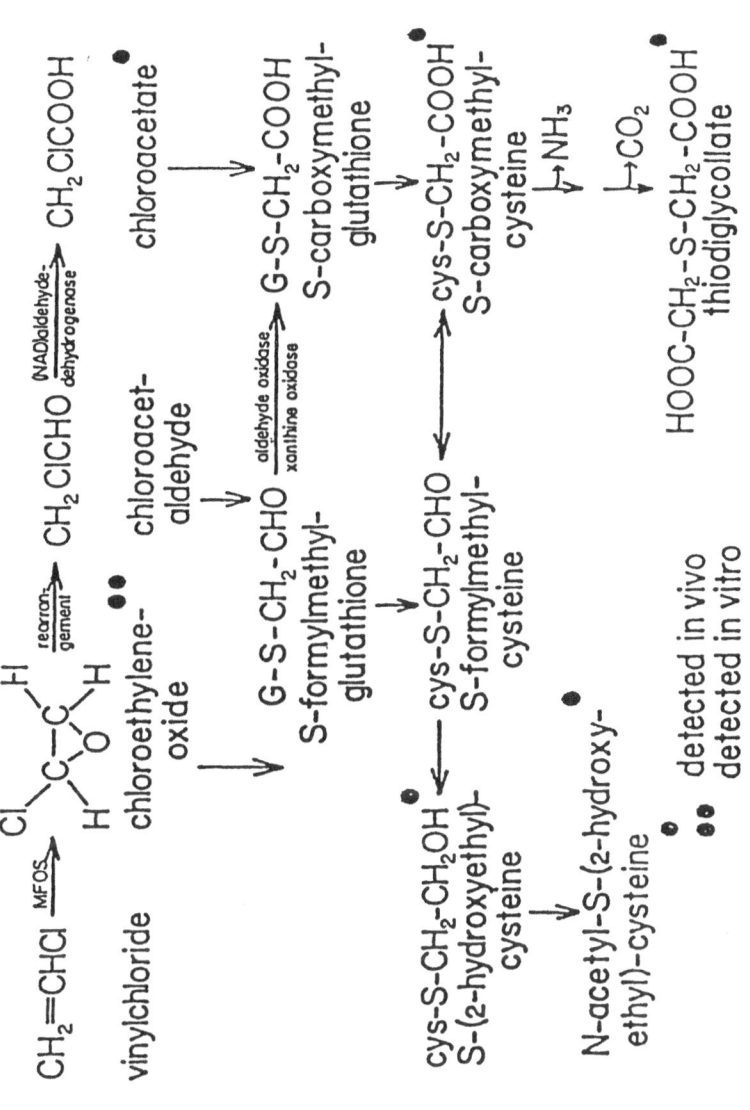

NOTE: From Plugge and Safe (1977)

FIGURE 2. MAJOR PATHWAY OF VINYL CHLORIDE METABOLISM

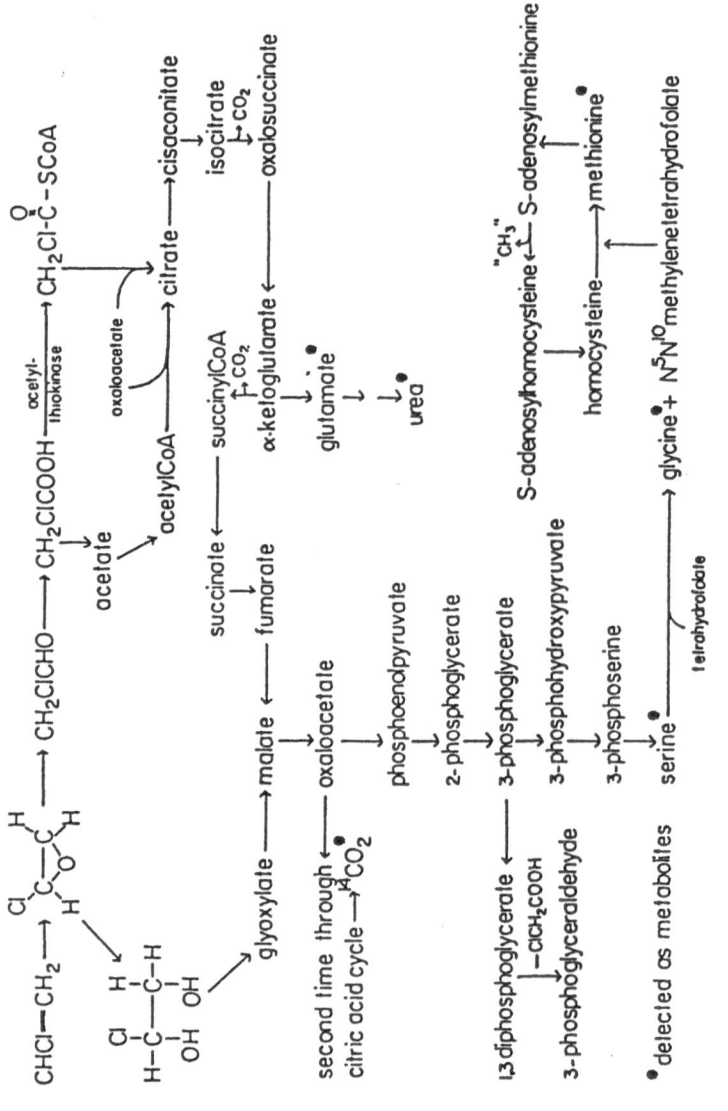

NOTE: From Plugge and Safe (1977)

FIGURE 3.   POSSIBLE MINOR PATHWAY OF VINYL CHLORIDE METABOLISM

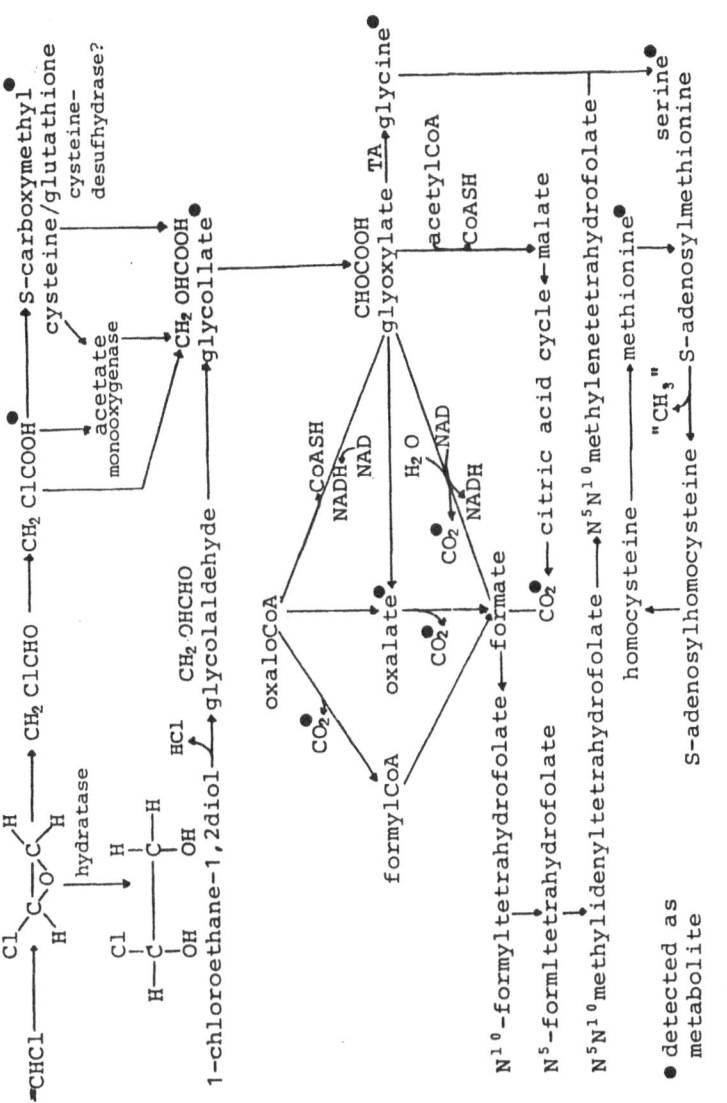

FIGURE 4. POSSIBLE MINOR PATHWAY OF VINYL CHLORIDE METABOLISM.

Note: From Plugge and Safe (1977)

potential tumourogenic sites have, as yet, been identified. In view of
the rapid increase in the vinyl chloride industry subsequent to World War
II, and the long latent period of many tumours, the status of populations
exposed to VCM needs to be kept under continuous review.

In the context of risks of other cancers, it is of interest to note
that these have been a significant feature of various animal studies.
Thus, Viola et al. (1971) obtained tumours of skin, lungs and bone in
rats exposed for 12 months to VCM vapours, Lee et al. (1978) induced
bronchioalveolar adenomas, mammary gland tumours and adenocarcinomas plus
haemangiosarcomas in mice chronically exposed to 50, 250 or 1000 ppm of
VCM, and Feron and Kroes (1979) found tumours in the brain, lungs, ceruminous glands and nasal cavity of rats exposed to 5000 ppm of VCM for
7 h d^{-1}, 5 d per week, over 52 weeks.

With respect to mutagenicity, VCM is mutagenic in various in vitro
test systems in the presence of liver extracts, particularly from
phenobarbital treated animals (Bartsch and Montesano, 1975; Hopkins,
1979a). VCM can also induce chromosome aberrations in animals and man
(Bartsch and Montesano, 1975; Fleig and Theiss, 1978; Basler and
Röhrborn, 1980). Of particular interest is the observation of excess
foetal loss in women whose husbands had been exposed to VCM (Infante
et al., 1976). This suggests the possibility that VCM is mutagenic to
germ cells at levels which have been encountered during occupational
exposure.

9.4   METABOLISM

9.4.1   Metabolic pathways

The various metabolic pathways of VCM metabolism have been described
by Plugge and Safe (1977), Bolt (1978) and Hopkins (1979). They have also
been discussed, in the context of other halogenated unsaturated hydrocarbons, by Fishbein (1979) and, in the context of chlorinated aliphatic
hydrocarbons, by Bonse and Henschler (1976). The major pathway (Fig. 2)
appears to involve formation of the epoxide, chloroethylene oxide, by the
mixed function oxidase system which is present in the liver and some
other tissues. The epoxide can spontaneously re-arrange to chloroacetaldehyde which can be oxidised to chloroacetate. All these compounds can
bind directly, or by enzyme-mediated reactions, to glutathione. Hydroxylation reactions then give various cysteine compounds and hence thiodigly-
collate, a significant urinary metabolite.

According to Plugge and Safe (1977), the metabolism of VCM in the
mixed function oxidase system is predominantly through the cytochrome
P-450 system. Some evidence for this has already been presented
(Section 9.3.1 and Table 1) and the topic is discussed more fully below.

Other pathways proposed by Plugge and Safe (1977) are shown in
Figs. 3 and 4. These pathways were proposed to explain the production of
$[\text{C-14}]\text{O}_2$ from C-14 labelled VCM.

It is noted that other pathways of VCM metabolism have also been
proposed. Thus, Fig. 5, taken from Green and Hathway (1975), shows a
scheme in which the metabolite S-(2-chlorethyl)cysteine and N-acetyl-
S(2-chloroethyl) cysteine are formed through direct interaction of
glutathione-derived cysteine with the original substance. Other pathways
shown in Fig. 5 would involve initial formation of the epoxide, as

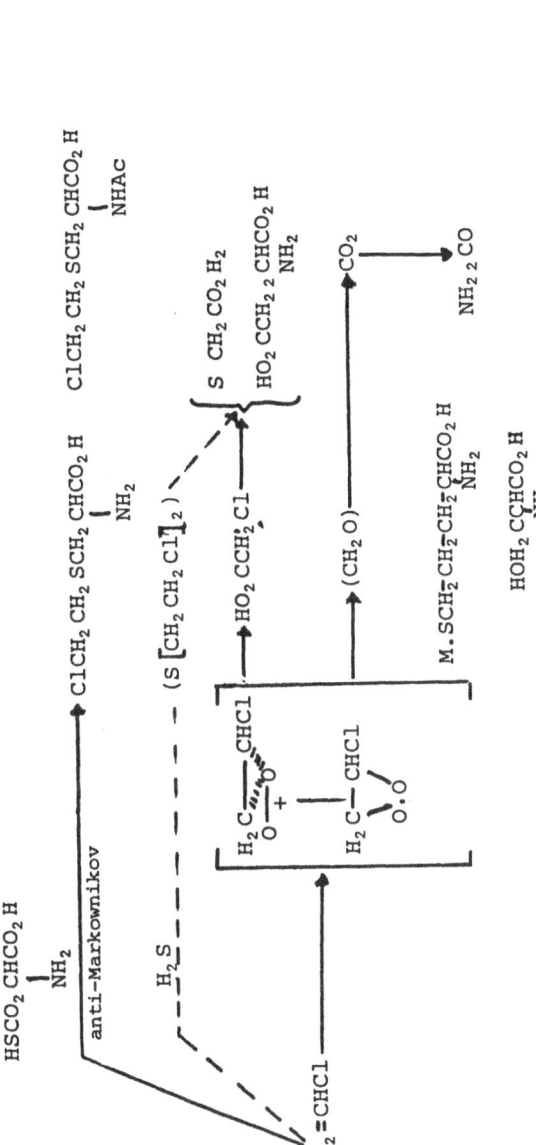

Note: From Green and Hathway (1975) and later identified as probably erroneous (see Section 9.4.1)

FIGURE 5. SCHEME FOR THE METABOLISM OF VINYL CHLORIDE IN RATS WHICH DOES NOT NECESSARILY INVOLVE EPOXIDE FORMATION.

discussed above. With repect to this figure, it is noted that Watanabe et al. (1976a) were critical of the proposed scheme, suggesting that the chlorethyl compounds were procedural artefacts. This was accepted by Green and Hathway (1977), but, nevertheless, this pathway has since been reproduced (see Fishbein, 1979).

It will be noted that the pathways set out above do not include covalent binding to proteins and nucleic acids. This is discussed in Section 9.4.3.

9.4.2   Metabolism in vivo

9.4.2.1   Absorption through the skin

Very few data are available concerning the absorption of VCM through the intact skin. In the only relevant paper, Hefner et al. (1975) reported that, when two monkeys were exposed (whole body, excluding the head) to atmospheres containing 7000 and 8000 ppm of VCM for 2.0 and 2.5 h respectively, the amounts of VCM absorbed were 0.023 and 0.031% of that available. This corresponded to 0.79 and 0.12 mg for the two exposures. For comparison, a Reference Man breathing 20 litres of air per minute (International Commission on Radiological Protection, 1975) would have inhaled 4.7×10^4 and 6.7×10^3 mg under the two exposure regimes. This indicates that, as a route of exposure, absorption through the intact skin is likely to be insignificant in comparison with inhalation. This conclusion was also reached by Hefner et al. (1975).

9.4.2.2   Retention following oral administration

The distribution and retention of VCM and its metabolites in the body following oral administration have been studied by several groups. Thus, Green and Hathway (1975) reported that the main eliminative route for C-14 labelled VCM after oral, intravenous or intraperitoneal administration to rats is pulmonary, both as unchanged VCM and as VCM related CO_2. For intragastric administration, the following results were given.

Size of dose ($mg\ kg^{-1}$)	Time (h)	Exhaled air VCM	CO_2	Urine	Faeces
0.25	0-24	3.7±1.2	12.6±1.1	71.5±5.0	2.8±2.5
	24-48	-	0.9	3.3	1.6
	48-72	-	-	0.3	0.2
	Total	3.7±1.2	13.5±1.3	75.1±4.2	4.6±3.0
450	0-24	91.9±2.5	0.6	4.5±2.3	0.4
	24-48	-	0.1	0.8	0.3
	48-72	-	-	0.1	-
	Total	91.9±2.5	0.7	5.4±2.2	0.7

Note: mean ± s.d. (4 animals)

The substantial differences in VCM metabolism at the two different dosage levels reflect the existence of a saturable pathway for VCM metabolism. Thus, at high doses, much of the VCM cannot be metabolised and is lost, unmodified, in the exhaled air. From the figures presented above, the oral saturation dose in rats is estimated to be ~30 mg kg^{-1}.

Green and Hathway (1975) also used autoradiography of whole-body sagittal sections to determine the distribution of radioactivity from 15 min. to 4 h after intragastric dosing. These studies showed liver and kidney medulla as primary sites of accumulation, but gave no quantitative information.

Urinary metabolites recorded in this study are discussed elsewhere (Section 9.4.1).

Watanabe et al. (1976a) reported on the excretion of C-14 by rats given single oral doses of 0.05, 1 and 100 mg kg^{-1} of [C-14]VCM. The percentage of activity excreted in the first 72 h post-exposure by the various routes is given below, together with the activity found in the carcass.

| | Dose (mg kg^{-1}) | | |
	0.05	1.0	100
Expired as VCM	1.43±0.13	2.13±0.22	66.64±0.67
Expired as CO_2	8.96±0.59	13.26±0.47	2.52±0.13
Urine	68.34±0.54	59.30±2.75	10.84±0.95
Faeces	2.39±0.52	2.20±0.39	0.47±0.06
Carcass and tissues	10.13±1.93	11.10±0.47	1.83±0.14
Cage wash	0	0.84±0.45	0
Total recovery	91.25±2.47	88.83±1.98	82.30±0.43

Note: mean ± s.e. (5 animals)

These data are consistent with an oral saturation dose of 16 mg kg^{-1}.

Watanabe et al. (1976a) also gave data on the loss of vinyl chloride in expired air and urine as a function of time (Figs. 6 and 7). The data for loss of vinyl chloride in expired air exhibit a very clear distinction between a biphasic curve for the 100 mg kg^{-1} dose and monophasic curves for the 0.05 and 1 mg kg^{-1} doses. This difference is explicable as a change from zero-order to first-order kinetics of metabolism as the VCM level in the body decreases below the saturation point. This hypothesis is substantiated by the observation that the second phase of the 100 mg kg^{-1} excretion curve has a slope which is not significantly different from the slopes of the monophasic curves recorded at lower dose levels. With respect to urinary excretion (Fig. 7) the curves are biphasic, possibly reflecting loss of two different metabolites, or the existence of two different physiological compartments. In this case, administration of a high dose of VCM depresses urinary excretion without altering the shape of the curve. This indicates that the fate of metabolised VCM, in contrast with the amount metabolised, is not altered by the level of exposure. This point is confirmed by the data given by Watanabe et al. (1976a) for the percentage of different metabolites in urine at different dose levels. These data are summarised below.

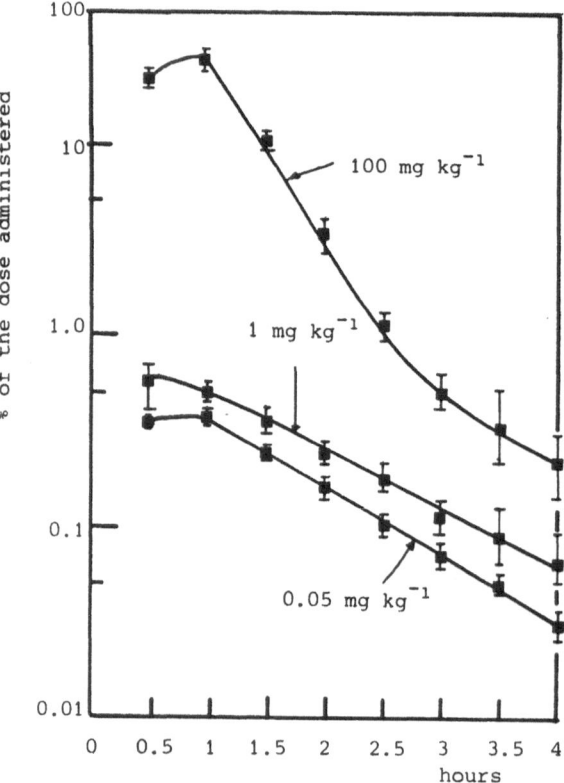

NOTE: From Watanabe et al. (1976a).
Each point represents the mean
± SE of the mean of five rats

FIGURE 6.   EXPIRED VINYL CHLORIDE EXPRESSED AS
PERCENTAGE OF THE DOSE ADMINISTERED

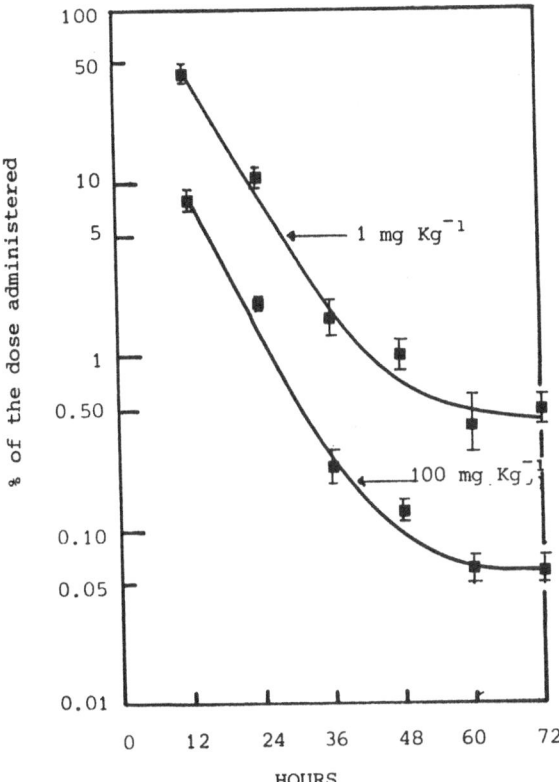

NOTE: From Watanabe et al. (1976a)
       Each point represents the mean
       ± SE of the mean for five rats

FIGURE 7. ^{14}C ACTIVITY EXCRETED IN THE URINE EXPRESSED
           AS PERCENTAGE OF THE DOSE ADMINISTERED

Dose (mg kg^{-1})	0.05	1.0	100
Number of animals	4	5	5

Percent in urine:

N-acetyl-S-(2-hydroxyethyl)-cysteine	30.4±2.0	36.2±3.9	29.1±2.0
Thiodiglycolic acid	25.6±1.9	23.7±1.1	25.4±0.9
Unidentified	38.6±2.9	34.5±4.6	36.6±2.0
Total recovery	94.6	94.4	91.1

Note: values are mean ± s.e.

The negligible effect of dose upon the fate of products of VCM metabolism is also reflected in the very similar distributions of the percentage of administered C-14 activity per gram of tissue in the bodies of rats at 72 h after oral dosing with [C-14]VCM (Watanabe et al., 1976a). These data are listed below.

Tissue	Dose (mg kg^{-1})		
	0.05	1.0	100
Liver	0.172±0.025	0.182±0.005	0.029±0.002
Skin	0.070±0.023	0.076±0.010	0.010±0.002
Carcass	0.027±0.007	0.046±0.002	0.007±0.001
Plasma	0.041±0.004	0.053±0.007	Not detected
Muscle	0.028±0.003	0.031±0.003	0.006±0.001
Lung	0.050±0.003	0.061±0.003	0.011±0.001
Fat	0.030±0.004	0.045±0.008	0.006±0.001

Note: values are mean ± s.e. (5 animals)

Withey (1976) studied retention of VCM in the blood of rats after intragastric, intravenous, or inhalation exposure. Following intragastric exposure, blood concentrations were very variable over the first two hours and Withey (1976) concluded that a complete pharmacokinetic analysis of absorption, distribution, metabolism and elimination for VCM administered by this route was not realistic. It should be noted that these remarks can only be taken to apply to VCM over a period ~2 h and should not be taken to apply with respect to VCM metabolites over longer periods.

Finally, it is noted that Green and Hathway (1978) reported that analyses of the livers of rats which had been exposed to 250 ppm of VCM in their drinking water for 2 y showed evidence of the presence of alkylating VCM metabolites bound to DNA in the form of etheno-deoxyadenosine and etheno-deoxycytidine.

9.4.2.3 Retention following inhalation and other non-gastric routes

The retention and metabolism of VCM following inhalation and other non-gastric routes has been studied by several groups. Green and Hathway (1975) gave the following data for excretion following intravenous and intraperitoneal injection of two different doses.

Dose (mg kg^{-1})	Time (h)	Excretion (% of dose) Intravenous			
		Exhaled air		Urine	Faeces
		VCM	CO$_2$		
0.25	0-24	99.0±0.8	0.1	0.5	0.1
	24-48	-	-	-	-
	48-72	-	-	-	-
	Total	99.0±0.8	0.1	0.5	0.1
450	0-24	-	-	-	-
	24-48	-	-	-	-
	48-72	-	-	-	-
	Total	-	-	-	-

Dose (mg kg^{-1})	Time (h)	Excretion (% of dose) Intraperitoneal			
		Exhaled air		Urine	Faeces
		VCM	CO$_2$		
0.25	0-24	43.2±4.6	10.3±2.2	41.5±4.8	1.6
	24-48	-	0.7	1.6	0.2
	48-72	-	-	-	-
	Total	43.2±4.6	11.0±1.2	43.1±5.7	1.8
450	0-24	96.2±4.1	0.7	2.5±0.9	0.1
	24-48	-	-	0.1	-
	48-72	-	-	-	-
	Total	96.2±4.1	0.7	2.6±0.9	0.1

The distinction between oral administration (Section 9.4.2.2) and intravenous administration is very marked and was attributed, by Green and Hathway (1975), to a highly efficient arterial-alveolar transfer which left a relatively low concentration of VCM available for biotransformation in the liver.

In a sequence of papers, Watanabe and his co-workers (Hefner et al., 1975a; Watanabe et al., 1976b; Watanabe et al., 1978) studied the fate of VCM, in rats following inhalation. Hefner et al. (1975a) used a closed inhalation apparatus and measured the decline in VCM levels due to metabolism of the VCM by rats contained within the apparatus. In the various studies conducted, VCM disappearance from the apparatus was always governed by first-order kinetics. Pretreatment with pyrazole was effective at blocking VCM metabolism at all levels of exposure, whereas ethanol was effective at low exposure levels (60 ppm VCM), but virtually ineffective at high levels (1000 ppm). SKF-525A, a microsomal oxidase inhibitor, had no effect at high exposures and a marginal effect only at low exposures, while pretreatment with 3-amino-1,2,4-triazole, an inhibitor of liver catalase activity, had only a limited effect at high exposure levels.

Hefner et al. (1975a) also reported that, following a 65 minute exposure to 49 ppm [C-14]VCM in this system, excretion was as listed below.

Percent of initially retained activity

	0-15 h	0-75 h
Urine	58.0	67.1
Faeces	2.7	3.8
Expired CO_2	9.8	14.0

Only 0.02% of the activity was expired as VCM. After 75 h, 1.6% of the activity remained in the liver, 3.6% in the skin, 0.2% in the kidneys and 7.6% in the remaining carcass.

On the basis of their results, Hefner et al. (1975a) considered that, in rats exposed to concentrations of VCM below 100 ppm, the VCM is predominantly metabolised via sequential oxidation to 2-chloroethanol, chloroacetaldehyde, and monochloroacetic acid by the alcohol dehydrogenase pathway. Above 220 ppm, this pathway was thought to be saturated and it was speculated that oxidation of the accumulating 2-chloroethanol might occur as follows.

$$ClCH_2\text{-}CH_2OH \underset{catalase}{\overset{H_2O_2}{\twoheadrightarrow}} ClHC_2\text{-}CH_2OOH \twoheadrightarrow ClCH_2\text{-}CHO$$

Direct epoxidation was also identified as a possible reaction.

Watanabe et al. (1976b) exposed rats to 10 or 1000 ppm of [C-14]VCM for 6 h and studied elimination of activity in expired air and urine in the period subsequent to exposure. Over the period 0.5 to 2.0 h post-exposure, loss in expired air was monophasic with half-lives of 20.4 and 22.4 min. at 10 and 1000 ppm respectively. Although these half-lives were not significantly different, the percentage of activity excreted in the expired air was almost an order of magnitude higher after the 1000 ppm exposure than it was after the 10 ppm exposure. Excretion of activity in urine was biphasic over the period of the study (Fig. 8) and the percentage of initial retained activity recovered in urine was very similar after exposure at the 10 and 1000 ppm levels. This is demonstrated by the percentage excretion listed below.

Percentage of initially retained C-14 activity

	10 ppm	1000 ppm
Expired as VCM	1.61±0.16	12.26±0.96
Expired as CO_2	12.09±0.43	12.30±0.63
Urine	67.97±1.71	56.29±1.96
Faeces	4.45±0.22	4.21±1.05
Carcass and tissues	13.84±1.16	14.48±0.52
Cage washings	0.15±0.08	0.23±0.09

Note: mean ± s.e. (4 animals)

The total µg equivalents of VCM recovered were 248 and 6642 per animal at exposures to 10 ppm and 1000 ppm respectively. For comparison, in a 6 h exposure a rat is estimated to inhale 36 l of air, corresponding to 1008 and 1.008×10^5 µg of VCM at the two exposure levels. Thus, the fractional

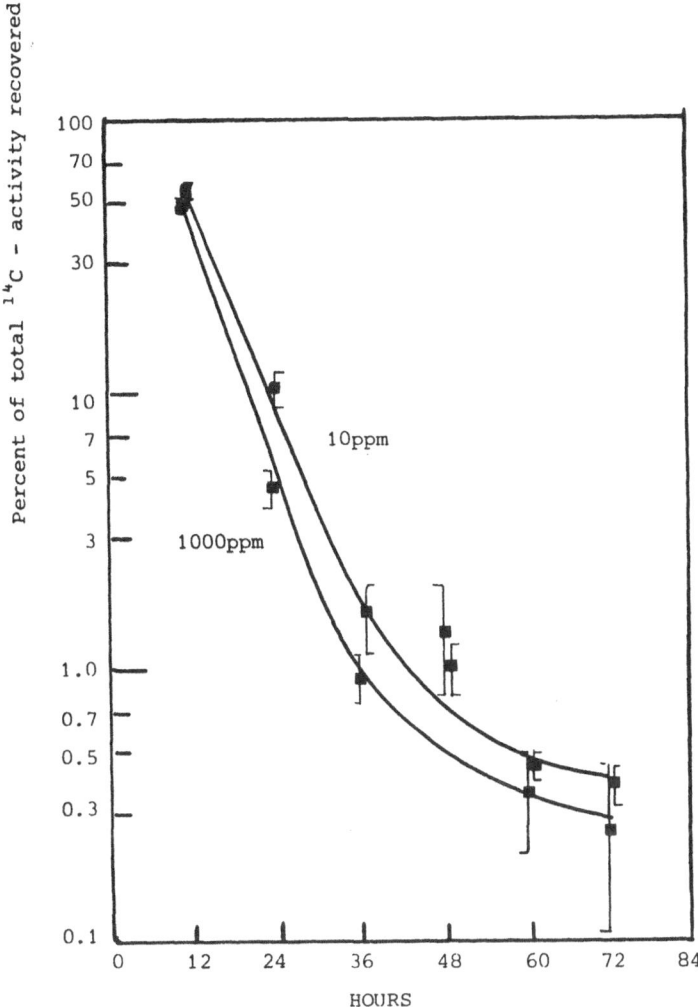

NOTE: From Watanabe et al. (1976b). Each point
represents mean ± SE for 4 animals.

FIGURE 8. EXCRETION OF C-14 IN URINE FOLLOWING EXPOSURE OF
RATS TO [C-14] VCM BY INHALATION

TABLE 2

EXCRETION AND RETENTION OF C-14 BY RATS FOLLOWING
SINGLE AND REPEATED EXPOSURES TO VCM[1]

	Single exposure[2]	Repeated exposure[3]
Expired as VCM	54.5±3.5	53.7±2.1
Expired as CO_2	8.0±1.4	9.6±1.6
Urine	27.1±2.1	25.7±1.4
Faeces	3.2±2.5	1.4±0.4
Carcass and tissues	7.3±2.5	9.7±1.6

Notes:

(1) From Watanabe et al. (1978). Results expressed as percentages of
the total activity retained at the end of a 6 h exposure to 5000 ppm
[C-14]VCM

(2) Mean ± s.e. (2 animals)

(3) Mean ± s.e. (3 animals)

TABLE 3

DISTRIBUTION OF C-14 IN RATS FOLLOWING SINGLE AND
REPEATED EXPOSURES TO VCM(1)

Tissue	Single exposure[2]	Repeated exposure[3]
Liver	0.119±0.022	0.157±0.028
Kidney	0.062±0.026	0.070±0.006
Fat	Not detected	Not detected
Skin	0.046±0.015	0.080±0.019
Carcass	0.030±0.014	0.039±0.011

Notes:

(1) From Watanabe et al. (1978). Results expressed as percentages
of the total activity retained at the end of a 6 h exposure to
5000 ppm [C-14]VCM

(2) Mean ± s.e. (3 animals)

(3) Mean ± s.e. (2 animals)

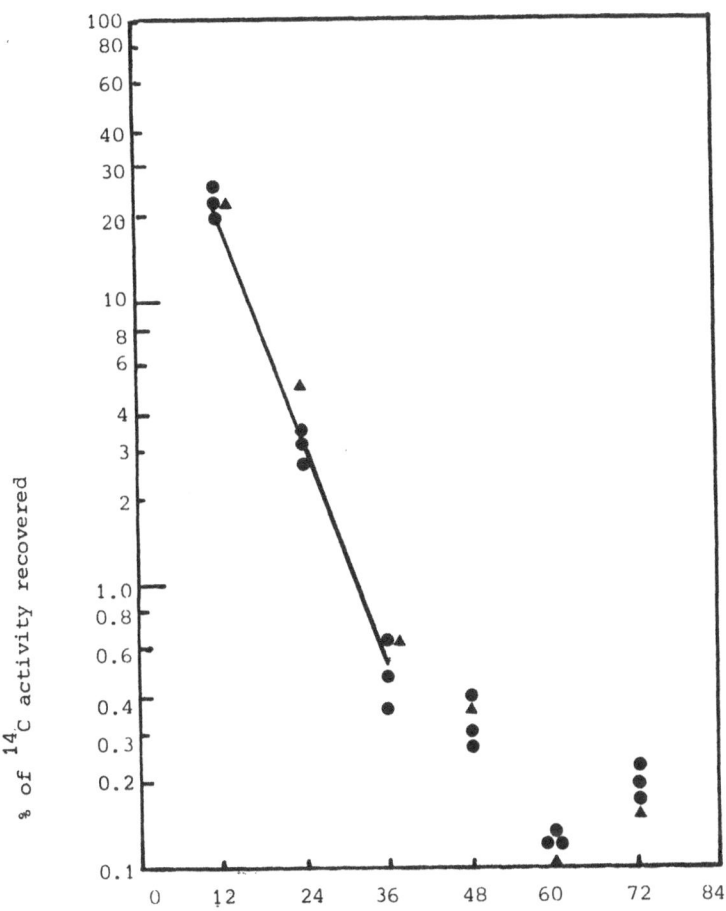

NOTES: From Watanabe et al. (1978)
▲ Repeated exposure
● Single exposure

FIGURE 9.   EXCRETION OF C-14 IN URINE FOLLOWING
             EXPOSURE OF RATS TO [C-14]VCM

retention at the end of a 6 h exposure is estimated to be 0.25 at 10 ppm, but only 0.066 at 1000 ppm. Taken together, these results indicate a saturation level for VCM exposure of about 270 ppm.

Watanabe et al. (1976b) also gave data for the tissue distribution of residual activity at 72 h after exposure. These data are listed below and indicate little effect of exposure level upon distribution.

Tissue	Percentage of initially retained activity per gram	
	10 ppm	1000 ppm
Liver	0.139±0.009	0.145±0.008
Skin	0.072±0.004	0.115±0.010
Carcass	0.048±0.004	0.049±0.004
Plasma	0.051±0.001	Not detected
Muscle	0.052±0.005	0.038±0.003
Lung	0.065±0.007	0.046±0.001
Fat	0.026±0.006	Not detected
Kidney	0.079±0.003	0.057±0.005

Note: mean ± s.e. (4 animals)

Similarly, as shown below, there was little effect of level of exposure upon the partition between different metabolites detected in urine.

Metabolite	Percentage of total urinary activity	
	10 ppm	1000 ppm
N-acetyl-S-(2-hydroxyethyl)-cysteine	40.6±3.9	39.0±2.4
Thiodiglycolic acid	25.9±3.6	17.6±2.1
Unidentified	30.4±2.2	39.4±1.2
Total recovery	96.9	96.0

Note: mean ± s.e. (4 animals)

More recently, Watanabe et al. (1978) compared the metabolism of [C-14]VCM in rats following a single 6 h exposure to 5000 ppm of VCM, or subsequent to repeated 6 h exposures (5 days per week for 7 weeks). Loss of activity via expiration of VCM was independent of mode of exposure, being monophasic over the period 0.5 to 3 h post-exposure and exhibiting a half-life of 30 minutes. Similarly, loss in urine exhibited an identical biphasic function in each case (Fig. 9). Distribution between the various routes of excretion and between the various tissues of the body was essentially identical (Tables 2 and 3) and very similar to results reported previously by this group.

Watanabe et al. (1978) also noted that aniline hydroxylase activities in liver were altered to the same extent in singly and repeatedly exposed animals and that hepatic macromolecular binding of [C-14]VCM metabolites was about 25% higher in repeated relative to single exposures.

On the basis of their various studies, Watanabe and co-workers (Gehring et al, 1978; 1979) proposed that the fractional metabolism of VCM in rats could be represented by a Michaelis-Menten formulation;

$$\upsilon = V_m S / (K_m + S)$$

where
υ (μg h^{-1}) is the rate of metabolism of VCM;

V_m (μg h^{-1}) is the maximum rate;

S (μg l^{-1}) is the concentration of VCM being inhaled; and

K_m (μg l^{-1}) is the Michaelis constant.

Best estimates of V_m and K_m were given as 1426±191 μg h^{-1} and 860±159 μg l^{-1} (307±57 ppm) respectively.

The metabolism of VCM in rats following inhalation has also been discussed by Bolt and co-workers (Bolt et al., 1976; Filser and Bolt, 1979). In closed system studies, Bolt et al. (1976) reported that ~40% of inspired VCM is absorbed by the lung. In the context of the experiments undertaken, this should be interpreted as absorbed and metabolised. Bolt et al. (1976) studied the inhibition of this metabolism by acute administration of various potential inhibitors, administered via intraperitoneal injection in DMSO, 30 minutes before commencement of exposure. Results from these studies are listed below.

Potential inhibitor		Percent inhibition
35 mg kg^{-1}	3-Bromophenyl-4(5)-imidazole	100
50 mg kg^{-1}	6-Nitro-1,2,3-benzothiadiazole	100
50 mg kg^{-1}	5,6-Dimethyl-1,2,3-benzothiadiazole	76
50 mg kg^{-1}	SKF 525A	76
50 mg kg^{-1}	Metyrapone	0
50 mg kg^{-1}	Pyrazole	66
100 mg kg^{-1}	Pyrazole	100

Studies were also conducted using agents known to induce drug metabolising enzymes in the endoplasmic reticulum of the liver. These agents were phenobarbital, 3-methylcholanthrene, rifampicin, ethanol, clotrimazol and DDT. Of these only clotrimazol and DDT caused substantial effects in respect of increasing metabolism.

Bolt et al. (1976) also gave data on the urinary excretion and tissue distribution of C-14 following a 5 h exposure of rats to 50 ppm of [C-14] VCM. The percentage urinary excretion of incorporated activity (mean ± s.e. for 3 animals) was 69.4±2.58, 1.74±0.48, 0.49±0.08 and 0.42±0.03 on days 1, 2, 3 and 4 after exposure respectively. Tissue distributions immediately and 48 h after the beginning of exposure showed high concentrations of C-14 activity in liver, spleen and kidney. These data, expressed as percent of initially incorporated activity per gram of tissue, are listed below.

Tissue	Percent of C-14 activity per gram	
	Immediately after exposure	48 h after beginning of exposure
Brain	0.171±0.008	0.038±0.004
Liver	1.86±0.30	0.32±0.02
Spleen	0.73±0.05	0.37±0.01
Kidney	2.13±0.43	0.21±0.03
Adipose tissue	0.22±0.06	0.044±0.004
Muscle	0.32±0.07	0.05±0.01

Note: mean ± s.e. (3 animals)

In a subsequent study, Filser and Bolt (1979) discussed the pharmacokinetics of VCM in rats in the context of other halogenated ethylenes. For VCM, distinction was made between a low concentration regime in which first-order kinetics operated and a high concentration regime, above saturation, where zero-order kinetics operated. For vinyl chloride, the air concentration corresponding to the saturation point, was determined to be 250 ppm.

Withey (1976) conducted a detailed study of the retention of VCM in blood following intravenous injection and inhalation exposure. The concentration data were well fitted by a biphasic curve:

$$C_1 = Ae^{-\alpha t} + Be^{-\beta t}$$

Withey (1976) interpreted this result in terms of a two compartment model such that

$$\frac{dQ_1}{dt} = -(k_{12} + k_e) Q_1 + k_{21} Q_2$$

and

$$\frac{dQ_2}{dt} = -k_{21} Q_2 + k_{12} Q_1$$

where Q_1 is the quantity of VCM in blood;
Q_2 is the quantity in other tissues;
K_e is the rate of loss via exhalation; and
k_{12}, k_{21} are exchange rates between the two compartments.

Values of fitted and derived parameters for various routes of exposure are listed below.

Rat weight (g)	Exposure(5 h) or dose	A	$\alpha(min.^{-1})$	B	$\beta(min.^{-1})$
			Fitted values		
368	1000 ppm	4.97	0.87	3.38	0.0454
324	1000 ppm	5.75	0.61	2.84	0.0486
355	3000 ppm	15.47	0.29	4.58	0.0224
351	3000 ppm	17.95	0.31	5.60	0.0193
414	7000 ppm	21.39	0.22	15.89	0.0240
314	7000 ppm	19.44	0.24	9.64	0.0240
428	2.867 mg*	31.40	0.0812	4.60	0.0168
358	2.815 mg*	24.10	0.0885	3.06	0.0143
434	2.943 mg+	18.70	0.0742	5.00	0.0180
312	2.630 mg+	8.20	0.0481	3.72	0.0168

Rat weight (g)	Exposure(5 h) or dose	k_{12}	k_{21}	k_e
		Derived values $(min.^{-1})$		
368	1000 ppm	0.3049	0.0737	0.5345
324	1000 ppm	0.1637	0.0699	0.4231
355	3000 ppm	0.0569	0.0284	0.2348
351	3000 ppm	0.0655	0.0249	0.2474
414	7000 ppm	0.0684	0.0383	0.1382
314	7000 ppm	0.0599	0.0341	0.1652
428	2.867 mg*	0.0185	0.0250	0.0545
358	2.815 mg*	0.0245	0.0227	0.0559
434	2.943 mg+	0.0176	0.0299	0.0448
312	2.630 mg+	0.0079	0.0266	0.0305

Note: * = Aqueous solution; + = oil solution

Examination of the inhalation data shows a trend to decreasing rate constants with increasing level of exposure. This is almost undoubtedly due to the failure of the model to include loss of VCM due to tissue metabolism. At higher levels of exposure, this pathway is reduced in significance because of saturation effects. With the reduction in importance of this route at high dose levels both α and β are reduced. It is noted that the lowest level of exposure used (1000 ppm) is four times the saturation level estimated for rats (see above).

Further data on rats derive from autoradiographic studies on frozen whole body sagittal sections (Duprat et al., 1977). These studies demonstrate that inhaled VCM is rapidly absorbed through the lungs and is strongly localised in the liver within 10 minutes of exposure.

In addition to the papers reviewed above, there have been several studies concerned with the macromolecular binding of VCM metabolites following inhalation (e.g. Bolt et al., 1976a). Osterman-Golkar et al. (1977) reported that, in mice, VCM is metabolically converted to a short-lived alkylating intermediate which introduces the 2-oxoethyl group onto nucleophilic sites in DNA and proteins. Consideration of the rate constants for proposed intermediates indicated that chloroethylene oxide, rather than chloracetaldehyde, is the main reactive metabolite. Laib and Bolt (1978) reported that, when rats were exposed to [C-14]VCM, radioactivity was incorporated into liver RNA in the physiological bases, 1,N^6-ethenoadenosine, and 3,N^4-ethenocytidine. Radioactive 3,N^4-ethenocytidine was also formed when polycytidylic acid was incubated

TABLE 4

IN VITRO EXPERIMENTS ON VCM METABOLISM

Reference	Comments
Kappus et al. (1975) Bolt et al. (1975)	VCM metabolites were bound to micro-somal proteins albumin and DNA, but not to Concanavalin A, which contains no cysteine. Addition of glutathione, or depression of cytochrome P-450, reduced macromolecular binding. Use of a xanthine oxidase test system demonstrated that the presence of O_2 radicals could potentiate covalent bonding.
Malaveille et al. (1975)	VCM caused mutation of Salmonella typhimurium in vitro. This response was potentiated by addition of micro-somal liver fractions, especially from phenobarbital pretreated animals.
Barbin et al. (1975)	VCM plus air was passed through a mouse liver microsomal system. The alkylating agents trapped were those that would be expected with chloroethylene oxide as an intermediate.
Salmon (1976)	Evidence of direct involvement of cytochrome P-450 in VCM metabolism.
Kappus et al. (1976)	Further evidence for involvement of the mixed function oxidase system in the metabolism of VCM with the resultant production of chloroethylene oxide.
Guengerich and Strickland (1977); Guengerich and Watanabe (1979)	Evidence that oxidation of VCM produces a metabolite which can destroy the heme of cytochrome P-450 and limit VCM metabolism. It was suggested that this metabolite differed from that reponsible for mutagenesis, since the latter must leave the site of its production.
Laib and Bolt (1977)	Binding as $1-N^6$-ethenoadenosine demonstrated for RNA in vitro.
Ivanetich et al. (1977)	Metabolism of VCM appears to be cata-lysed by more than one type of cyto-chrome P-450 and metabolites of VCM depress cytochrome P-450 activities.
Laib and Ottenwälder (1978)	VCM metabolites were found to be bound to adenosine, cytidine and DNA in rat liver microsomal suspensions.
Laib et al. (1979)	Formation of $1,N^6$-ethenoadenosine and $3,N^4$-ethenocytidine as a result of VCM metabolism in vitro.

TABLE 4 (Cont.)

Pessayre et al. (1979; 1979a)	Evidence to suggest that chloroethylene oxide is the VCM metabolite responsible for cytochrome P-450 destruction. The authors suggested that chloroethylene oxide not involved in this process, or transformed by the action of epoxide hydrolase, escapes to the cytosol where it is available for binding to glutathione. They also suggested that inducers affected both the production and degradation of VCM metabolites.
Sabadie et al. (1980)	Preparations derived from human liver specimens were shown to have very variable capacities for converting VCM into electrophiles mutagenic to S. typhimurium.
Laib et al. (1981)	On the basis of data presented here and previously, the authors suggested that attachment of VCM to adenosine or cytosine is limited to single stranded nucleic acid.

in vitro with rat liver microsomes, NADPH and [C-14]VCM. Subsequently, Bolt et al. (1980) reported that, in rats, irreversible binding of C-14 to proteins was proportional to the amount of [C-14]VCM metabolised rather than to the level of exposure. This point has also be made by Watanabe et al. (1978a) who additionally recorded the observation that pre-treatment with phenobarbital increased significantly the protein-bound to metabolised ratio in rat liver. Watanabe et al. (1978) also noted that the degree of protein binding was related to the degree of glutathione depression observed at different exposure concentrations. Binding of C-14 to the RNA and DNA of various mouse tissues, after intraperitoneal injection of [C-14]VCM has been studied by Bergman (1982) who gave data showing incorporation of radioactivity into all four bases, as well as $3,N^4$-ethenocytidine, $1,N^6$-ethenoadenosine and $1,N^6$-etheno-adenine.

Finally, with respect to inhalation, it is noted that Heger et al. (1982) have recently studied the relation between VCM exposure level and thiodiglycolic acid excretion in urine for 15 workers at a PVC processing plant and have found the two to be correlated (see also Muller et al., 1979). Results obtained so far are encouraging for developing a VCM exposure test based on thiodiglycolic acid excretion (Tarkowski et al., 1980), but it is noted that excretion is affected substantially by alcohol consumption and that the methods available may not be sufficiently sensitive to do more than identify that the threshold limit value has been exceeded (Draminski and Trojanowska, 1981).

9.4.3   Metabolism in vitro

There have been a substantial number of studies of VCM metabolism in vitro. These have mainly been related to identification, or investigation, of the metabolic pathways discussed in Section 9.4.1 and are not considered in detail herein. A brief summary of some of the relevant experiments is given in Table 4 and a short review has been given by Hopkins (1979b). The major point of relevance with respect to the development of pharmacokinetic models is the significance of the mixed function oxidase system and the interaction of VCM metabolites with cytochrome P-450 leading to the destruction of haem.

9.5   METABOLIC MODEL

As has been demonstrated, inhalation is likely to be the predominant route of exposure to VCM, both for the occupationally and the non-occupationally exposed (Section 9.2.4). For this reason, attention is concentrated on modelling the metabolism of VCM entering the body by this route.

In order to model the metabolism of inhaled VCM and its metabolites, the following points must be gaken into account.

-     Loss of VCM from the lungs is monophasic with a half-life of 20 to 30 minutes.
-     Loss of VCM metabolites in urine is biphasic with an initial phase exhibiting a half life ~2.7 h and a second phase of undefined half-life.

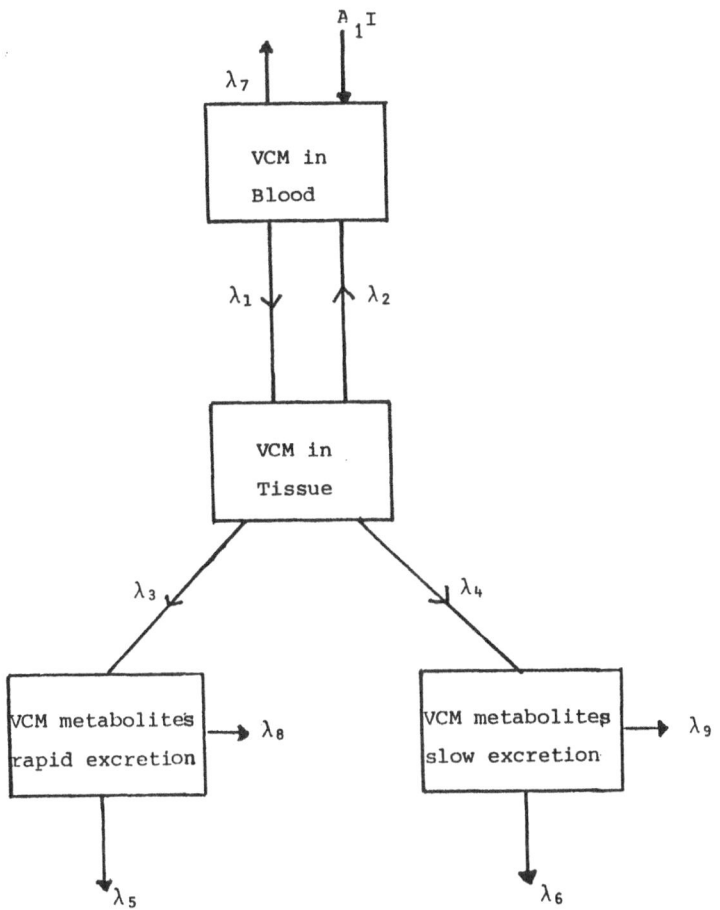

NOTES: I = Intake rate

A_1 = Fraction of inhaled VCM entering blood
λ_1, λ_2 = Blood: Tissue exchange rates
λ_3, λ_4 = Metabolic rates
λ_5, λ_6 = Excretion rates for identifiable metabolites
λ_7 = Unchanged VCM exhalation rate
λ_8, λ_9 = Rates of breakdown to non-specific metabolites

FIGURE 10.   MODEL FOR VCM METABOLISM IN MAN

- The fraction of VCM metabolised decreases as the level of exposure increases.

With regard to this last point, it is noted that, in rats, saturation does not occur until air concentrations of 250 to 300 ppm are reached. Thus, virtually all human exposures are likely to be in the non-saturated region where first-order kinetics should apply.

A model for VCM metabolism can have several applications. These include:

- interpretation of exhaled air measurements in terms of exposure;
- interpretation of urinary excretion measurements in terms of exposure;
- analysis of uptake and retention in target tissues with respect to understanding mechanisms of toxic action.

With regard to this last application, limited data on tissue distributions and the lack of understanding of relationships between nucleic acid alkylation and mutagenesis make it impossible, at present, to develop a relevant model. A conceptual model for the interpretation of exhaled air and urinary metabolite measurements is shown in Fig. 10. This model includes provision for loss to non-specific metabolites, which would include CO_2 lost by exhalation. It is emphasised that this model is for chemically identifiable metabolites of VCM and is not sufficiently complex to represent, in total, the metabolism of C-14 following inhalation of [C-14]VCM.

Taking the only well-defined specific metabolite of VCM to be thiodiglycolic acid and assuming that rat and human metabolism are closely similar, the following model parameters are estimated from the data given in Section 9.4.2.3.

Parameter	Value (h^{-1})	Basis
λ_1	18	Withey (1976)
λ_2	6	Adjusted so that ~33% of inhaled VCM is retained in a 6 h exposure.
λ_3	3	Withey (1976) and Watanabe (1976b) assuming that loss via exhalation is controlled by metabolic removed.
λ_4	0.3	Adjusted so that cumulative long-term excretion is 10% of cumulative short-terms excretion.
λ_5	0.03	} Watanabe et al. (1978), 75% loss in
λ_6	0.0038	} urine and 25% of that as thiodiglycolic } acid.
λ_7	50	Extrapolation from Withey (1976).
λ_8	0.13	} Watanabe et al. (1978). VCM meta-
λ_9	0.0162	} bolites other than thiodglycolic } acid in urine and including CO_2 } in breath.

9.6   REFERENCES

Anderson, H.A., Snyder, J., Lewinson, T., Woo, C., Lilis, R. and Selikoff, I.J., 1978. Levels of CEA among vinyl chloride and polyvinyl chloride exposed workers. Cancer, 42, (Suppl. 3), pp.1560-1567.

Bahlman, L.J., Alexander, V., Infante, P.F., Wagoner, J.K., Lane, J.M. and Bingham, E., 1979. Vinyl halides: carcinogenicity Vinyl bromide, vinyl chloride and vinylidene chloride. Am. Ind. Hyg. Assoc. J., 40, A30-A40.

Barbin, A., Brésil, H., Croisy, A., Jacquignon, P., Malaveille, C., Montesano, R. and Bartsch, H., 1975. Liver-microsome-mediated formation of alkylating agents from vinyl bromide and vinyl chloride. Biochem. Biophys. Res. Commun., 67, 596-603.

Bartsch, H. and Montesano, R., 1975. Mutagenic and carcinogenic effects of vinyl chloride. Mutat. Res., 32, 93-114.

Basler, A. and Röhrborn, G., 1980. Vinyl chloride: an example for evaluating mutagenic effects in mammals in vivo after exposure to inhalation. Arch. Toxicol., 45, 1-7.

Bergman, K., 1982. Reactions of vinyl chloride with RNA and DNA of various mouse tissues in vivo. Arch. Toxicol., 49, 117-129.

Berk, P.D., Martin, J.F., Young, R.S., Creech, J., Selikoff, I.J., Falk, H., Watanabe, P., Popper, H. and Thomas, L., 1976. Vinyl chloride-associated liver disease. Ann. Intern. Med., 84, 717-731.

Bolt, H.M. 1978. Metabolic activation of halogenated ethylenes. In: Remmer, H., Bolt, H.M., Bannasch, P. and Popper, H. (Eds.) Primary Liver Tumours. MTP Press, Lancaster, UK, pp.285-294.

Bolt, H.M., Kappus, H., Buchter, A. and Bolt, W., 1975. Metabolism of vinyl chloride. Lancet, 1, p.1425.

Bolt, H.M., Kappus, H., Buchter, A. and Bolt, W., 1976. Disposition of [1,2-^{14}C] vinyl chloride in the rat. Arch. Toxicol., 35, 153-162.

Bolt, H.M., Kappus, H., Kaufmann, R., Appel, K.E., Buchter, A. and Bolt, W., 1976a. Metabolism of ^{14}C-vinyl chloride in vitro and in vivo. INSERM Symp. Ser., 52, 151-164.

Bolt, H.M., Filsher, J.G., Laib, R.J., Ottenwälder, H., 1980. Binding kinetics of vinyl chloride and vinyl bromide at very low doses. Arch. Toxicol., (Suppl. 3), pp.129-142.

Bonse, G. and Henschler, D., 1976. Chemical reactivity, biotransformation, and toxicity of polchlorinated aliphatic compounds. CRC Crit. Rev. Toxicol., 4, 395-409.

Buffler, P.A., Wood, S., Eifler, C., Sucrez, L. and Kilian, D.J., 1979. Mortality experience of workers in a vinyl chloride monomer production plant. J. Occup. Med., 21, 195-203.

Connolly, R.B. and Jaeger R.J., 1979. Acute hepatoxicity of vinyl chloride and ethylene: modification by trichloropropene oxide, diethylmaleate and cysteine. Toxicol. Appl. Pharmacol., 50, 523-531.

Creech, J.L. and Johnson, M.N., 1974. Angiosarcoma of liver in the manu-facture of polyvinyl chloride. J. occup. Med., 16, 150-151.

Draminski, W. and Trojanowska, B., 1981. Chromatographic determination of thiodiglycolic acid - a metabolite of vinyl chloride. Arch. Toxicol., 48, 289-292.

Du, J.T., Sandoz, J.P., Tseng, M.T. and Tamburro, C.H., 1979. Biochemical alterations in livers of rats exposed to vinyl chloride. J. Toxicol. Environ. Health, 5, 1119-1132.

Duprat, P., Fabry, J.P., Gradiski, D. and Magadur, J.L., 1977. Metabolic approach to industrial poisoning: blood kinetics and distribution of ^{14}C-vinylchloride monomer. Acta Pharmacol. Toxicol., 41, (Suppl. 1), pp.142-143.

Feron, V.J. and Kroes, 1979. One year time sequence inhalation toxicity study of vinyl chloride in rats. II. Morphological changes in the respir-atory tract, ceruminous glands, brain, kidneys, heart and spleen. Toxic-ology, 13, 131-141.

Feron, V.J., Kruysse, A. and Til, H.P., 1979. One year time sequence inhalation toxicity study of vinyl chloride in rats. I. Growth, mortality, haematology, clinical chemistry and organ weights. Toxicology, 13, 25-29.

Feron, V.J., Spit, B.J., Immel, H.R. and Kroes, R., 1979a. One year time sequence inhalation toxicity study of vinyl chloride in rats. III. Morphological changes in the liver. Toxicology, 13, 143-154.

Filser, J.G. and Bolt, H.M., 1979. Pharmacokinetics of halogenated ethyl-enes in rats. Arch. Toxicol., 42, 123-136.

Fishbein, L., 1979. Potential halogenated industrial carcinogenic and mutagenic chemicals. 1. Halogenated unsaturated hydrocarbons. Sci. Tot. Environ., 11, 111-161.

Fleig, I. and Thiess, A.M., 1978. External chromosome studies undertaken on persons and animals with VC illness. Mutat. Res., 53, p.187.

Fox, A.J. and Collier, P.F., 1977. Mortality experience of workers exposed to vinyl chloride monomer in the manufacture of polyvinyl chloride in Great Britain. Br. J. Ind. Med., 34, 1-10.

Gehring, P.J., Watanabe, P.G. and Park, C.N., 1978. Resolution of dose-response toxicity data for chemicals requiring metabolic activation: example-vinyl chloride. Toxicol. Appl. Pharmacol., 44, 581-591.

Gehring, P.J., Watanabe, P.G. and Park, C.N., 1979. Risk of angiosarcoma in workers exposed to vinyl chloride as predicted from studies in rats. Toxicol. Appl. Pharmacol., 49, 15-21.

Gluszcz, M., 1981. Difficulties of an early diagnosis of liver damage in those exposed to vinyl chloride. Med. Pr., 32, 277-282.

Green, T. and Hathway, D.E., 1975. The biological fate in rats of vinyl chloride in relation to its oncogenicity. Chem.-Biol. Interact., 11, 545-562.

Green, T. and Hathway, D.E., 1977. The chemistry and biogenesis of the S-containing metabolites of vinyl chloride in rats. Chem.-Biol. Interact., 17, 137-150.

Green, T. and Hathway, D.E., 1978. Interactions of vinyl chloride with rat liver DNA in vivo. Chem.-Biol. Interact., 22, 211-224.

Griciute, L., 1978. The carcinogenicity of vinyl chloride. IARC Scientific Publications, 22, 3-11.

Guengerich, F.P. and Strickland, T.W., 1977. Metabolism of vinyl chloride: destruction of the heme of highly purified liver microsomal cytochrome P-450 by a metabolite. Molec. Pharmacol., 13, 993-1004.

Guengerich, F.P. and Watanabe, P.G., 1979. Metabolism of [^{14}C]- and [^{36}Cl]- labeled vinyl chloride in vivo and in vitro. Biochem. Pharmacol., 28, 589-596.

Haley, T.J., 1975. Vinyl chloride - how many unknown problems? J. Toxicol. Environ. Health, 1, 47-73.

Hefner, R.E. Jr., Watanabe, P.G. and Gehring, P.J., 1975. Percutaneous absorption of vinyl chloride. Toxicol. Appl. Pharmacol., 34, 529-532.

Hefner, R.E. Jr., Watanabe, P.G. and Gehring, P.J. 1975a. Preliminary studies on the fate of inhaled vinyl chloride monomer (VCM) in rats. Environ. Health Perspect., 11, 85-95.

Heger, M., Muller, G. and Norpoth, K., 1982. Investigations into the correlation between vinyl chloride (VCM)-uptake and excretion of its metabolites by 15 VCM-exposed workers. II. Measurements of the urinary excretion of the VCM-metabolite thiodiglycolic acid. Int. Arch. Occup. Environ. Health, 50, 187-196.

Hopkins, J., 1979. Vinyl chloride - part 1: metabolism. Food Cosmet. Toxicol., 17, 403-405.

Hopkins, J., 1979a. Vinyl chloride-part 2: mutagenicity. Food Cosmet. Toxicol., 17, 542-544.

Hopkins, J., 1979b. Vinyl chloride - part 3: macromolecular binding. Food Cosmet. Toxicol., 17, 681-683.

Infante, P., Wagoner, J.K. McMichael, A.J., Waxweiler, R.J. and Falk, H., 1976. Genetic risks of vinyl chloride. Lancet, 1, 734-735.

International Agency for Research on Cancer, 1979. Vinyl chloride, poly-vinyl chloride and vinyl chloride - vinyl acetate copolymers. IARC Monographs on the Evaluation of the Carcinogenic Risk of Chemicals to Humans, 19, 377-438.

International Agency for Research on Cancer, 1982. Vinyl Chloride. IARC Monographs on the Evaluation of the Carcinogenic Risk of Chemicals to Humans, 29, 260-262.

International Commission on Radiological Protection, 1975. Report of the Task Group on Reference Man. ICRP Publication 23, Pergamon Press, Oxford.

Ivanetich, K.M., Aronson, I. and Katz, I.D., 1977. The interaction of vinyl chloride with rat hepatic microsomal cytochrome P-450 in vitro. Biochem. Biophys. Res. Commun., 74, 1411-1418.

Jaeger, R.J., Reynolds, E.S., Conolly, R.B., Moslen, M.T., Szabo, S. and Murphy, S.D., 1974. Acute hepatic injury by vinyl chloride in rats pre-treated with phenobarbital. Nature (Lond.), 252, 724-726.

Jaeger, R.J., Murphy, S.D., Reynolds, E.S., Szabo, S. and Moslen, M.T., 1977. Chemical modification of acute hepatotoxicity of vinyl chloride monomer in rats. Toxicol. Appl. Pharmacol., 41, 597-607.

Kappus, H., Bolt, H.M., Buchter, A. and Bolt, W., 1975. Rat liver micro-somes catalyse covalent binding of ^{14}C-vinyl chloride to macromolecules. Nature (Lond.), 257, 134-135.

Kappus, H., Bolt, H.M., Buchter, A. and Bolt, W., 1976. Liver microsomal uptake of [^{14}C] vinyl chloride and transformation to protein alkylating metabolites in vitro. Toxicol. Appl. Pharmacol., 37, 461-471.

Laib, R.J. and Bolt, H.M., 1977. Alkylation of RNA by vinyl chloride metabolites in vitro and in vivo: formation of 1-N^6-etheno-adenosine. Toxicology, 8, 185-195.

Laib, R.J. and Bolt, H.M., 1978. Formation of 3,N^4-ethenocytidine moieties in RNA by vinyl chloride metabolites in vitro and in vivo. Arch. Toxicol., 39, 235-240.

Laib, R.J. and Ottenwälder, H., 1978. Alkylation of DNA and RNA by meta-bolites of vinyl chloride and vinyl bromide. Naunyn-Schmiedebergs Arch. Pharmacol. (Suppl.), 302, p.R21.

Laib, R.J., Stöchle G., Bolt, H.M. and Kunz W., 1979. Vinyl chloride and Trichlorethylene: comparison of alkylating effects of metabolites and induction of preneoplastic enzyme differences in rat liver. J. Cancer Res. Clin. Oncol., 94, 139-147.

Laib, R.J., Gwinner, L.M. and Bolt, H.M., 1981. DNA Alkylation by vinyl chloride metabolites: etheno derivatives of 7-alkylation of guanine? Chem.-Biol. Interact., 37, 219-231.

Lee, C.C., Bhandari, J.C., Winston, J.M., House, W.B., Dixon, R.L. and Woods, J.S., 1978. Carcinogenicity of vinyl chloride and vinylidene chloride. J. Toxicol. Environ. Health, 4, 15-30.

Lester, D., Greenberg, L.A. and Adams, W.R., 1963. Effects of single and repeated exposures of humans and rats to vinyl chloride. Amer. Ind. Hyg. Assoc. J., 24, 265-275.

Malaveille, C., Bartsch, H., Barbin, A., Camus, A.M., Montesano, R., Croisy, A. and Jacquignon, P., 1975. Mutagenicity of vinyl chloride, chlorethylene oxide, chloroacetaldehyde and chloroethanol. Biochem. Biophys. Res. Commun., 63, 363-370.

Monson, R.R., Peters, J.M. and Johnson, M.N., 1974. Proportional mortality among vinyl-chloride workers. Lancet, 2, 397-398.

Muller, G., Norpoth, K. and Wickramasinghe, P.W., 1979. An analytical method, using GC-MS, for the quantitative determination of urinary thiodiglycolic acid. Int. Arch. Occup. Environ. Health, 44, 185-191.

Nicholson, W.J., Hammond, E.C., Seidman, H. and Selikoff, I.J., 1975. Mortality experience of a cohort of vinyl chloride-polyvinyl chloride workers. Ann. N.Y. Acad. Sci., 246, 225-230.

Norpoth, K., Gottschalk, D., Gottschalk, I., Witting, U., Thomas, H., Eichner, D. and Schmidt, E.H., 1980. Influence of vinyl chloride monomer (VCM) and As_2O_3 on rat liver cell proliferation after partial hepatectomy. J. Cancer Res. Clin. Oncol., 97, 41-50.

Osterman-Golkar, S., Hultmark, D., Segerbäck, D., Calleman, C.J., Göthe, R., Ehrenberg, L. and Wachtmeister, C.A., 1977. Alkylation of DNA and proteins in mice exposed to vinyl chloride. Biochem. Biophys. Res. Commun., 76, 259-266.

Ott, M.G., Langner, R.R. and Holder, B.B., 1975. Vinyl chloride exposure in a controlled industrial environment. Arch. Environ. Health, 30, 333-339.

Pessayre, D., Wandscheer, J.C., Descatoire, V., Dolder, A. and Benhamou, J.-P., 1979. Effects of inducers on the in vivo covalent binding of a vinyl chloride metabolite to liver fractions. Biochem. Pharmacol., 28, 3667-3668.

Pessayre, D., Wandscheer, J.C., Descatoire, V., Artigou, J.Y. and Benhamou, J.P., 1979a. Formation and inactivation of a chemically reactive metabolite of vinyl chloride. Toxicol. Appl. Pharmacol., 49, 505-515.

Plugge, H. and Safe, S., 1977. Vinyl chloride metabolism. A review. Chemosphere, 6, 309-325.

Potter, H.R., 1976. Vinyl chloride - part 1. Fd. Cosmet. Toxicol., 14, 347-349.

Potter, H.R., 1976a. Vinyl chloride - part 2. Fd. Cosmet. Toxicol., 14, 498-501.

Reynolds, E.S., Moslen, M.T., Szabo, S., Jaeger, R.J., and Murphy, S.D., 1975. Hepatotoxicity of vinyl chloride and 1,1-dichloroethylene: role of mixed function oxidase system. Am. J. Pathol., 81, 219-231.

Reynolds, E.S., Moslen, M.T., Szabo, S. and Jaeger, R.J., 1975a. Vinyl chloride-induced deactivation of cytochrome P-450 and other components of the liver mixed function oxidase system: an in vivo study. Res. Commun. Chem. Pathol. Pharmacol., 12, 685-694.

Reynolds, E.S., Moslen, M.T., Szabo, S. and Jaeger, R., 1976a. Modulation of halothane and vinyl chloride induced acute injury to liver endoplasmic reticulum. Panminerva Med., 18, 367-374.

Sabadie, N., Malaveille, C., Camus, A.M. and Bartsch, H., 1980. Comparison of hydroxylation of benzo(a)pyrene with the metabolism of vinyl chloride, N-nitrosomorpholine, and N-nitroso-N-methylpiperazine to mutagens by human and rat liver microsomal fractions. Cancer Res., 40, 119-126.

Salmon, A.G., 1976. Cytochrome P-450 and the metabolism of vinyl chloride. Cancer Lett., 2, 109-114.

Suzuki, Y., 1980. Nonneoplastic effects of vinyl chloride in mouse lung. Environ. Res., 21, 235-253.

Tabershaw, I.R. and Gaffey, W.R., 1974. Mortality study of workers in the manufacture of vinyl chloride and its polymers. J. Occup. Med., 16, 509-518.

Tarkowski, S., Wiśniewska-Knpyl, J.M., Klimczak, J., Dramińiski, W. and Wróblewska, K., 1980. Urinary excretion of thiodiglycollic acid and hepatic content of free thiols in rats at different levels of exposure to vinyl chloride. J. Hyg. Epidemiol. Microbiol. Immunol., 24, 253-261.

Tatrai, E. and Ungváry, Gy., 1981. On the acute hepatotoxicity of inhaled vinyl chloride. Acta Morphol. Acad. Sci. Hung., 29, 221-226.

Thomas, L.B., Popper, H., Berk, P.D., Selikoff, I. and Falk, H., 1975. Vinyl chloride-induced liver disease. From idiopathic portal hypertension (Banti's syndrome) to angiosarcomas. New Engl. J. Med., 292, 17-22.

Van Esch, G.J. and Van Logten, M.J., 1975. Vinyl chloride. A report of a European assessment. Toxicology, 4, 1-4.

Viola, P.L., Bigotti, A. and Caputo, A., 1971. Oncogenic response of rat skin, lungs and bones to vinyl chloride. Cancer Res., 31, 516-522.

Watanabe, P.G., Hefner, R.E. Jr., and Gehring, P.J. 1976. Vinyl chloride induced depression of hepatic non-protein sulfhydryl content and effects on bromosulphalein (BSP) clearance in rats. Toxicology, 6, 1-8.

Watanabe, P.G., McGowan, G.R. and Gehring, P.J., 1976a. Fate of [^{14}C] vinyl chloride after single oral administration in rats. Toxicol. Appl. Pharmacol., 36, 339-352.

Watanabe, P.G., McGowan, G.R., Madrid, E.O. and Gehring, P.J., 1976b. Fate of [^{14}C]vinyl chloride following inhalation exposure in rats. Toxicol. Appl. Pharmacol., 37, 49-59.

Watanabe, P.G., Zempel, J.A. and Gehring, P.J. 1978. Comparison of the fate of vinyl chloride following single and repeated exposure in rats. Toxicol. Appl. Pharmacol., 44, 391-399.

Watanabe, P.G., Zempel, J.A., Pegg, D.G. and Gehring, P.J., 1978a. Hepatic macromolecular binding following exposure to vinyl chloride. Toxicol. Appl. Pharmacol., 44, 571-579.

Waxweiler, R.J., Stringer, W., Wagoner, J.K. and Jones, J., 1976. Neoplastic risk among workers exposed to vinyl chloride. Ann. N.Y. Acad. Sci., 271, 40-48.

Wiśniewska-Knypl, J.M., Klimczak, J. and Kolakowski, J., 1980. Monooxygenase activity and ultrastructural changes of liver in the course of chronic exposure of rats to vinyl chloride. Int. Arch. Occup. Environ. Health, 46, 241-249.

Withey, J.R., 1976. Pharmacodynamics and uptake of vinyl chloride monomer administered by various routes to rats. J. Toxicol. Environ. Health, 1, 381-394.

Appendix 10
Benzidine

CONTENTS

10.1   INTRODUCTION

Benzidine is an aromatic amine that does not occur naturally. It was first prepared in 1845 and has been used in the production of direct azo dyes since 1884 (Shriner et al. 1978; International Agency for Research on Cancer, 1982). Congeners of benzidine, in particular 3,3´-dichloro-benzidine, 3,3´-dimethylbenzidine and 3,3´-dimethoxybenzidine, are also widely used.

The physical and chemical properties of benzidine and its congeners have been summarised by Shriner et al. (1978). Benzidine is a colourless crystalline compound with a molecular weight of 184.23, a density of 1.25, a melting point of 115 to 128°C, depending on the speed of heating, and a boiling point of 400°C. It is soluble in alcohol and ether and is slightly soluble in water. 3,3´-dichlorobenzidine is also a colourless crystalline compound. It has a molecular weight of 253.1 and a melting point of 132 to 133°C; is soluble in ethanol, benzene and glacial acetic acid; is slightly soluble in dilute hydrochloric acid; and is almost insoluble in cold water. 3,3´-dimethylbenzidine is a white to reddish crystalline compound with a molecular weight of 212.28 and a melting point of 131 to 132°C. It is highly soluble in ethanol, ethyl ether and acetone; and is slightly soluble in water. 3,3´-dimethoxybenzidine is a colourless crystalline compound that turns violet on standing. It has a molecular weight of 244.3; melts at 137 to 138°C; is soluble in ethanol, ethyl ether, acetone, benzene and chloroform; and is poorly soluble in water.

Benzidine is both a primary aromatic amine and a diphenyl derivative. It undergoes chemical reactions which are characteristic for each class of compounds, as well as some which are peculiar to it alone. The benzidine derivatives mentioned above undergo similar chemical reactions to those displayed by benzidine, i.e. they can be acetylated, alkylated and diazotised. This last reaction is of commercial importance, as it is the first step in their use in the synthesis of azo dyes. The chemical structures of benzidine and its derivatives are shown in Fig. 1.

Benzidine and its salts are used principally in the manufacture of dyestuffs and at least 250 commercial dyes are based on these compound (Shriner et al. 1978). It also has uses in analytical chemistry, as a hardener for polyurethane and in various other, minor, applications. Benzidine congeners are used for similar purposes (Shriner et al. 1978; International Agency for Research on Cancer, 1982).

10.2   LEVELS OF EXPOSURE

Data on potential occupational and non-occupational exposure to benzidine and its congeners are very limited. At one time benzidine and its congeners were manufactured and used in open systems which permitted transfers to the atmosphere, the worker and the work site (Shriner et al., 1978). Some spot sample air levels in benzidine manufacturing plant have been given by Shriner et al. (1978) and the International Agency for Research on Cancer (1982), but the data are not sufficient for estimation of typical past or present levels of benzidine in air.

For non-occupational exposure, potential sources are river waters local to dye producing plants (International Agency for Research on Cancer, 1982; 1982a) and dyes or dyed products containing benzidine

BENZIDINE

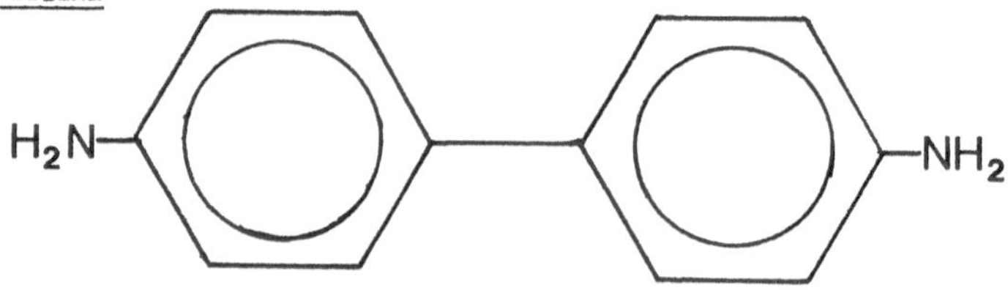

3,3' - DICHLOROBENZIDINE

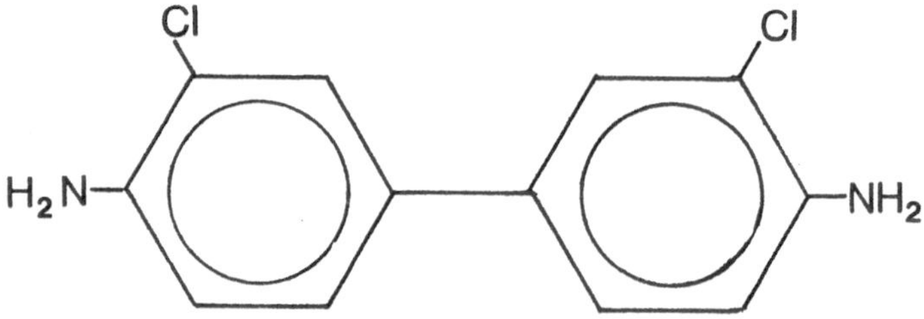

3,3' - DIMETHYLBENZIDINE

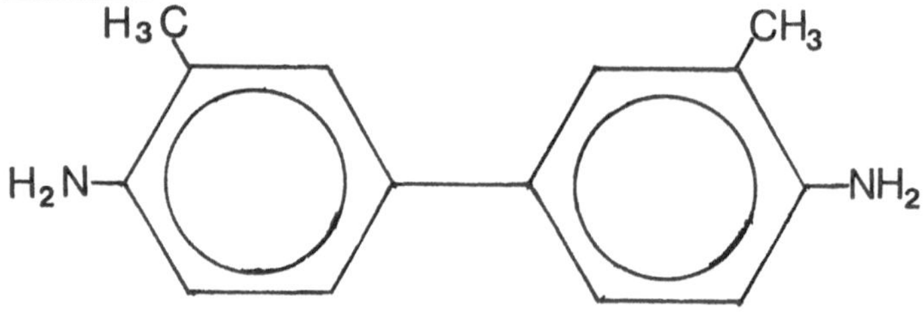

3,3' - DIMETHOXYLBENZIDINE

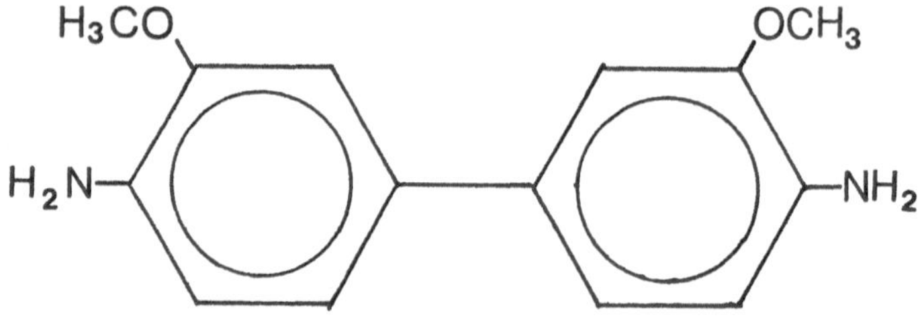

FIGURE 1. THE CHEMICAL STRUCTURE OF BENZIDINE AND ITS DERIVATIVES

(Boeniger et al., 1981). The data available are not sufficient to assess the number of individuals exposed, or the degree of exposure via these routes.

10.3   EFFECTS

The major effect of concern with respect to benzidine and its congeners is carcinogenesis, though other effects have been observed. Major reviews on human and animal carcinogenesis include those by Haley (1975) and the International Agency for Research on Cancer (1982; 1982a). With respect to the carcinogenic effect of benzidine on man, the International Agency for Research on Cancer (1982) summarised their conclusions as follows.

> "Occupational exposure to benzidine has been strongly
> associated with bladder cancer in numerous case reports
> from many countries. The association has also been
> observed in several epidemiological studies ..... There
> is sufficient evidence that benzidine is carcinogenic to
> man."

With respect to experiments on animals, the International Agency for Research on Cancer (1982) gave the following summary of the data available.

> "Benzidine and its dihydrochloride were tested in mice,
> rats and hamsters by oral administration, in mice and
> rats by subcutaneous administration and in rats by
> inhalation and intraperitoneally. Following its oral
> administration to mice .... it significantly increased
> the incidence of liver cell tumours (benign and malig-
> nant). In female rats it markedly increased the incidence
> of mammary tumours; and in male and female hamsters it
> increased the incidence of liver tumours following its
> oral administration. The subcutaneous administration of
> benzidine or its sulphate to rats produced a high inci-
> dence of Zymbal-gland tumours; colonic tumours were
> also reported .... The intraperitoneal administration
> of benzidine to rats resulted in a marked increase in
> the incidence of mammary and Zymbal-gland tumours. It
> was also tested in dogs by oral administration. ....
>
> The metabolites of benzidine, N,N´-diacetylbenzidine
> and N-hydroxy-N,N´-diacetylbenzidine, produced
> mammary and Zymbal-gland tumours in rats following
> their intraperitoneal injection."

With respect to 3,3´-dichlorobenzidine, the International Agency for Research on Cancer (1982a) noted data on the production of liver cell tumours in mice, hepatocellular carcinomas in dogs, mammary and Zymbal-gland tumours in rats, carcinomas of the urinary bladder in hamsters and dogs, and increased incidences of leukaemia in rats and mice. Data on man were limited to negative, but inconclusive, epidemiological studies. On the basis of these data, the International Agency for Research on Cancer (1982a) concluded that there is sufficient evidence that 3,3´-dichlorobenzidine is carcinogenic in mice, rats, hamsters and dogs, and that the epidemiological data are inadequate to evaluate its carcinogenicity to man.

With respect to cancer induction, two recent papers, not included in the above reviews, merit mention. Nelson et al. (1982) reported that liver tumours were induced in mice chronically exposed to benzidine dihydrochloride in drinking water. In this experiment, there were significant differences among the liver tumour survival distributions between different genetic crosses and between males and females. For man, Ohkawa et al. (1982) recorded 64 cases of uroepithelial cancer in Wakayama City, Japan, which could be associated with occupational exposure to benzidine or, in a few cases, β-napthylamine.

The difficulty of inducing bladder cancer in some species of animal, notably mice and rats, calls for comment, since it suggests that species distinctions in benzidine metabolism could influence the carcinogenic response (see Section 10.4). However, it is also noted that benzidine and its derivatives can cause tumours other than bladder cancers in animals. Similar tumours may occur in human populations, but, being less characteristic than bladder cancer, may be more difficult to recognise. It should also be noted that early reports associating benzidine exposure with bladder cancer in man often refer to mixed exposures to benzidine and the potent bladder carcinogen β-napthylamine (Haley, 1975).

With respect to other effects of benzidine it is noted that, under experimental conditions, it causes cirrhosis of the liver in rats, rabbits and dogs (Haley, 1975); can induce glomerulonephritis and nephrotic syndrome in experimental animals (Shriner et al., 1978); and has been associated with dermatitis, cystitis and haematouria in man (Shriner et al., 1978; Gimalt and Romaguera, 1981).

10.4   METABOLISM

The metabolism of benzidine has been reviewed by Shriner et al. (1978). Benzidine intake by exposed persons may be by inhalation or ingestion. However, for occupational exposure, transcutaneous absorption has been identified as the most significant route of exposure (Meigs et al., 1951; 1954). In this section, the metabolic pathways of benzidine and its congeners are reviewed. This is followed by an analysis of the pharmacokinetics of these substances.

10.4.1   Metabolic pathways

Benzidine and its congeners are wholly, or partly, transformed, in experimental animals, to a number of metabolites. These have been summarised by Shriner et al. (1978) and a list derived from that publication is given in Table 1. More recently, Tanaka (1981) has reported that, in rats, 3, 3´-dichlorobenzidine is metabolised to 3,3´-dichloro-N-acetylbenzidine and 3,3´-dichloro-N,N´-diacetylbenzidine.

The in vitro metabolism and macromolecular binding of benzidine and its derivatives have been summarised by the International Agency for Research on Cancer (1982). Benzidine is metabolised in vitro by liver

TABLE 1

METABOLITES FORMED BY BIOTRANSFORMATION OF BENZIDINE
AND ITS DERIVATIVES IN ANIMALS$^{(1)}$

Benzidine metabolites

Compound	Species
N-hydroxy acetylaminobenzidine	Human
Monoacetylbenzidine	Human, monkey, dog, mouse
Diacetylbenzidine	Human, dog, mouse
3-Hydroxybenzidine	Human, dog, rabbit, rat
3,3´-Dihydroxybenzidine	Human, rat
3-Hydroxybenzidine sulphate	Dog, rabbit
3-Hydroxybenzidine glucuronite	Dog, rabbit, mouse
3-Hydroxybenzidine hydrogen sulphate	Dog
4,4´-Diamino-3-diphenyl hydrogen sulphate	Dog, rat, mouse
4-Amino-4-hydroxybiphenyl	Dog
4´-Acetamido-4-aminodiphenyl	Guinea pig, rabbit, rat, mouse
4´-Acetamido-4-amino-3-diphenyl hydrogen sulphate	Guinea pig, rabbit, rat, mouse
4´-Amino-4-diphenylyl sulfamic acid	Guinea pig, rabbit, rat
N-Glucuronides	Guinea pig, rabbit, rat, mouse
4-Acetamido-4-diphenylyl sulfamic acid	Guinea pig, rabbit, rat
Monoacetylated 3-hydroxybenzidine glucuronide and/or ethereal sulphate	Mouse
N-Hydrogen sulphate and/or glucuronide	Mouse

3,3´-Dimethylbenzidine metabolites

Compound	Species
Diacetyl-o-tolidine	Human
5-Hydroxy-o-tolidine	Human
Monoacetyl-o-tolidine	Human
5-Ethereal sulphate of o-tolidine	Dog

Note:

Adapted from Shriner et al. (1978)

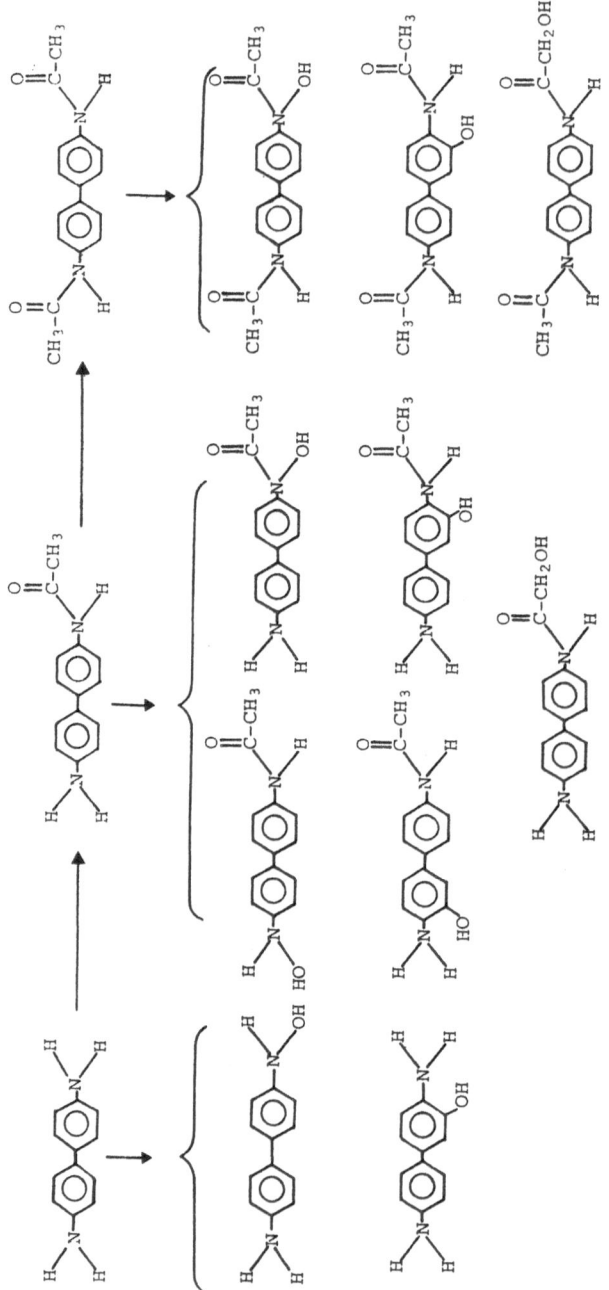

Note: From Morton et al. (1979)

FIGURE 2.   POTENTIAL ACETYLATED AND/OR MONOHYDROXYLATED METABOLITES OF BENZIDINE

cytosol from rats, mice, hamsters or guinea pigs to N-acetylbenzidine and N, N'-diacetylbenzidine. Hepatic microsomal preparations in vitro convert synthetic N,N'-diacetylbenzidine to N-hydroxy-N,N'-diacetylbenzidine and 3-hydroxy-N,N'-diacetylbenzidine by a NADPH-dependent reaction. Also, liver cytosol catalyses the binding of synthetic N-hydroxy-N-acetyl-N'-[1-^{14}C]-acetylbenzidine to tRNA (Morton et al., 1979). On the basis of these results, Morton et al. (1979) suggested the metabolic pathways shown in Fig. 2. In a second paper, Morton et al. (1980) demonstrated that liver cytosol from rats, mice and hamsters could catalyse the 3'-phosphoadenosine 5'-phosphosulphate-dependent metabolism of N-hydroxy-N, N'-diacetylbenzidine to a reactive electrophilic ester and suggested that this metabolite might be involved in the hepatocarcinogenicity of benzidine. More recently, Morton et al. (1981) have demonstrated that the two benzidine metabolites N,N'-diacetylbenzidine and N-hydroxy-N,N'-diacetylbenzidine are both potent inducers of mammary gland and Zymbal gland tumours in female CD rats.

Other data on the macromolecular binding of metabolites of benzidine have been given by Martin and Ekers (1980) and by Zenser et al. (1980). Martin and Ekers (1980) gave intraperitoneal injections of [H-3]benzidine to male rats and demonstrated binding of the radioactivity to hepatic RNA, DNA and protein. The degree of binding was maximal at 24 h after administration and the degree of binding followed the order RNA>DNA> protein at all times from 7 to 72 h after administration. The amount of radioactivity associated with hepatic DNA did not change between 1 and 28 days after administration. Chromatographic separation of acid hydrolised DNA demonstrated five different H-3 labelled products, but insufficient labelled material was obtained for further characterisation.

Zenser et al. (1980) used a renal inner medullary microsome preparation from rabbits to demonstrate the co-oxidative metabolism of benzidine to reactive metabolites which bound to DNA and tRNA. Co-oxidative metabolism of benzidine and subsequent binding was dependent upon specific fatty acid substrates and was blocked by inhibitors of prostaglandin endoperoxide synthetase. The authors suggested that it is metabolism in the renal medulla and excretion of metabolites into urine which makes benzidine a potent inducer of bladder cancer in man (see also Zenser et al., 1979). Zenser et al. (1980) also noted that glutathione and tRNA are competitors for binding to the metabolites formed from benzidine in the renal medulla.

Zenser and co-workers (Rapp et al. 1980) subsequently extended their work to demonstrate an identical pathway of metabolism in intact renal inner medullary slices. This study also demonstrated that inhibitors of the mixed function oxidase system had no effect on the renal medullary metabolism of benzidine and that fatty acids which are not substrates for prostaglandin endoperoxidase synthetase did not increase binding to medullary tissue. Binding was increased by arachidonic acid, but this arachidonic acid mediated binding could be prevented by inhibitors of prostaglandin endoperoxidase synthetase.

Other papers of interest with respect to benzidine biochemistry include the report by Cerniglia et al. (1982) that anaerobic bacterial suspensions isolated from faeces or intestinal contents, can metabolise benzidine and 3,3'-dimethylbenzidine based dyes to free amines. On this basis, Cerniglia et al. (1982) suggested that such bacteria may play a significant role in the aetiology of bladder cancers caused by such dyes.

In contrast, on the basis of in vitro experiments, Martin and Kennelly (1981) suggested that the mammalian liver may play only a minor or negligible role in the azo-reduction of dyes derived from benzidine or its congeners.

10.4.2   Transcutaneous absorption

Very few data are available concerning the transcutaneous absorption of benzidine. However, it is clear that this route can be a major source of uptake in occupationally exposed individuals. Thus, Meigs et al. (1951) reported that levels of quinonizable substances in the urine of men working in benzidine manufacture could not be accounted for by the levels of benzidine in air. Furthermore, for three individuals, the concentration of quinonizable substances in urine was directly proportional to the total content of aromatic amines in clothing. While the constant of proportionality is almost certain to have been determined by the type of clothing worn and local practices of industrial hygiene, it is nevertheless of interest to record that the constant of proportionality was ~0.005 mg of quinonizable substances per litre of urine for every mg of aromatic amines in clothing. This is indicative of skin absorption fractions in excess of 1%, very much higher than the value of 0.025% recorded in an experimental exposure of the skin of the forearm for 48 h (Meigs et al., 1951). Further studies (Meigs et al., 1954) showed enhanced excretion, presumably reflecting enhanced uptake, on hot humid days relative to cool dry days, but quantification of the degree of skin absorption cannot be given for these subjects.

10.4.3   Exposure by ingestion

There have been several studies on the metabolism of benzidine and its congeners following oral administration. Clayson et al. (1959) reported on various metabolites of benzidine in the urine of dogs and rabbits following oral exposure, but gave no quantitative data. However, Bradshaw and Clayson (1955) reported that continuous ether extraction of the urine of a dog fed benzidine at 500 mg d^{-1} for ten days enabled 400 mg of benzidine and 85 mg of 3-hydroxybenzidine to be isolated.

Ghetti (1960) reported on the elimination of total amines in the urine of a dog following oral dosing. The quantity eliminated corresponded to 12% of the administered dose and this elimination occurred during the first six days after exposure.

More recently, Hsu and Sikka (1982) studied the distribution and retention of U-^{14}C-labelled 3,3′-dichlorobenzidine in male rats following a 12 h period of fasting. The rats were given either a single dose of 6.4 or 40 mg kg^{-1}, or six daily doses of 6 mg kg^{-1}. Initial studies gave detailed tissue distributions (Table 2) which identified liver, kidney and lung as possible organs of accumulation. Further studies on the uptake and retention of C-14 label in these tissues, together with studies on 3,3′-dichlorobenzidine and C-14 derived from [C-14] 3,3′-dichlorobenzidine in blood plasma, gave the following multi-exponential uptake and retention functions following administration at the 40 mg kg^{-1} level.

TABLE 2

DISTRIBUTION OF RADIOACTIVITY IN SELECTED TISSUES OF RATS RECEIVING
A SINGLE ORAL DOSE (6.4 or 40 mg kg^{-1}) OF [^{14}C]
3,3´-DICHLOROBENZIDINE (DCB)

| | μg [^{14}C]DCB eq g^{-1} wet tissue | | | |
| Tissue | 24h | | 96h | |
	6.4 mg kg^{-1}	40 mg kg^{-1}	6.4 mg kg^{-1}	40 mg kg^{-1}
Heart	0.289±0.078	2.34±0.30	0.096±0.002	0.604±0.125
Lung	0.743±0.159	4.065±0.445	0.167±0.016	1.097±0.402
Pancreas	0.294±0.052	2.15±0.885	0.104±0.123	0.529±0.306
Spleen	0.309±0.059	3.355±0.940	0.174±0.020	0.891±0.096
Kidney	2.197±0.712	14.18±2.085	1.119±0.445	8.896±1.095
Testes	0.207±0.069	1.11±0.115	0.082±0.024	0.372±0.095
Liver	4.566±0.197	21.59±3.617	1.863±0.052	9.413±1.194
Stomach and contents	1.56±0.901	201.7±40.56	0.083±0.038	0.687±0.319
Small intestine and contents	10.90±3.509	41.89±11.23	0.129±0.011	1.701±0.473
Caecum and contents	19.07±5.497	114.5±48.46	0.216±0.053	3.080±0.426
Large instestine and contents	16.10±6.101	129.4±48.46	0.242±0.034	3.296±0.505
Muscle	0.123±0.022	1.335±0.148	0.050±0.013	0.375±0.505
Plasma	0.641±0.169	6.326±0.387	0.193±0.024	2.229±0.908
Erythrocytes	0.323±0.066	2.676±0.57	0.181±0.141	1.655±0.242

Note:

From Hsu and Sikka (1982). Mean ± s.d. for 3 animals

C-14 in plasma:

$$\dot{C} = 76.559e^{-0.412t} + 8.218e^{-0.021t} - 84.77e^{-0.437t}$$

3,3´-dichlorobenzidine in plasma:

$$C = 0.075e^{-0.124t} + 1.004e^{-0.051t} - 1.079e^{-0.326t}$$

C-14 in liver:

$$C = 184.10e^{-0.120t} + 20.649e^{-0.009t} - 204.749e^{-0.021t}$$

C-14 in kidney: .

$$C = 74.475e^{-0.097t} + 11.463e^{-0.005t} - 85.938e^{-0.128t}$$

C-14 in lung:

$$C = 99.753e^{-0.180t} + 5.447e^{-0.016t} - 105.200e^{-0.277t}$$

where C (µg or µg equivalents per ml plasma or per g tissue) is the
concentration in the tissue or fluid; and

t is the time in hours.

It is emphasised that these uptake and retention functions were derived
from limited and variable data, and should, therefore, be considered with
circumspection. Nevertheless, the following points are noted.

- The 3,3´-dichlorobenzidine was largely metabolised before it entered
  the blood plasma.
- Peak concentrations of metabolites in plasma and tissues were
  reached at 8 to 12 hours after exposure.
- The half-life of 3,3´-dichlorobenzidine metabolites in tissues was
  estimated at ~70 h.

Because these experiments extended over only 96 h, substantial
longer-term components of 3,3´-dichlorobenzidine metabolite retention in
tissues cannot be ruled out, and it is noted that Hsu and Sikka (1982)
reported that approximately half the C-14 in liver and kidney was
covalently bound to macromolecules at 72 h after exposure.

Hsu and Sikka (1982) also studied the distribution of C-14 in
tissues of the single and multiple exposure animals, and found very
little difference between the two groups. With respect to excretion they
reported that about 25% of C-14 from a single dose was excreted in the
urine and about 60% in the faeces over a 96 h period. Cannulation of the
bile duct was used to demonstrate that virtually all the faecal excretion
derived from the liver. High pressure liquid chromatographic analysis
demonstrated the same metabolites in urinary and bile extracts, but in
different proportions. The metabolites recovered in the urine were mostly
unconjugated compounds, whereas most of the metabolites in bile were
conjugates.

10.4.4   Exposure via other routes

There are a limited number of studies on the metabolism of benzidine and its congeners following exposure via routes other than those considered above. Baker and Deighton (1953) reported on the concentrations of free total diazotizable material in rat tissues 4 and 12 h after intraperitoneal injection of 100 mg kg^{-1} of benzidine. Results from this study are summarised below.

Tissue	Concentration (μg g^{-1})			
	Free		Total	
	4 h	12 h	4 h	12 h
Whole blood	16.2	1.0	35.0	17.5
Plasma	32.5	1.0	70.0	15.0
Blood cells	8.7	3.8	11.2	5.0
Liver	16.2	11.3	45.0	25.0
Spleen	21.2	6.3	46.2	17.5
Kidney	21.2	2.5	46.2	11.2
Stomach	275.8	20.0	310.0	80.0
Stomach contents	310.0	54.0	315.0	85.0
Small intestine	81.2	26.3	157.5	135.0
Small intestine contents	-	134.0	-	560.0
Caecum	2.5	13.8	21.2	75.0
Caecum contents	2.0	0.1	11.4	15.0
Colon	3.7	1.0	21.2	25.0
Urine	5.4	28.0	10.2	50.0
Miscellaneous	1.7	1.0	21.2	11.2
Carcass	81.2	8.8	82.5	36.2

Note:

'Miscellaneous' consisted of brain, pancreas, diaphragm, bladder, gonads, oesophagus, heart, thymus, lungs and adrenals; all analyses performed on pooled samples from four rats; small intestine contents were not analysed at 4 h.

Baker and Deighton (1953) also noted that by 12 h a portion of the injected amino groups were rendered non-diazotizable, since only 68% of the injected dose could be accounted for at that time, as compared with 93% at 4 h.

        Clayson et al. (1959) reported on the recovery of various metabolites of benzidine in the urine of mice, rats and guinea pigs following intraperitonal injection, but gave no quantitative data.

        Ghetti (1960) reported on the elimination of amines in the urine of dogs, following exposure to benzidine by inhalation, intratracheal instillation or subcutaneous injection. The percentages of the dose eliminated by these routes was 12, 4.2 and 24 for inhalation, intratracheal instillation and subcutaneous injection respectively. Similarly Bos et al. (1980) reported that, following intraperitoneal injection of [C-14]benzidine into the rat, 17% of the radioactivity was excreted in urine within 24h.

TABLE 3

DISTRIBUTION PATTERN 1 AND 4 h AFTER INTRAVENOUS ADMINISTRATION
OF 0.2 mg 3,3´-DICHLOROBENZIDINE-^{14}C AND BENZIDINE-^{14}C PER kg
BODY WEIGHT TO RATS AND DOGS. MEAN VALUES ($\bar{x}$) AND 95%
CONFIDENCE INTERVALS (wt_w) OR SINGLE VALUES (1)

	Benzidine						
	Rat				Dog		
	1 h		4 h		4 h		
	$\bar{x}$	wt_w	$\bar{x}$	wt_w	Dog 4	Dog 5	Dog 6
	Concentration in wet tissue ($\mu g\ g^{-1}$)						
Stomach	0.13	0.02	0.050	0.010	0.094	0.15	0.057
Small intestine	0.26	0.11	0.26	0.05	0.20	0.23	0.080
Large intestine	0.13	0.02	0.26	0.12	0.46	0.24	0.22
Kidney	0.27	0.03	0.13	0.03	0.24	0.32	0.21
Ureter	0.005 to 0.088		0.001 to 0.035		0.32	0.28	0.24
Urinary bladder	0.22	0.11	0.18(3)	0.08	2.2	2.3	3.3
Liver	0.81	0.22	0.53	0.11	0.79	0.78	0.56
Bile	-	-	-	-	30	19	7.9
Pancreas	0.13	0.02	0.044	0.011	0.036	0.053	0.043
Spleen	0.14	0.02	0.067	0.017	0.12	0.16	0.11
Adrenals	0.24(2)	0.05	0.086	0.024	0.081	0.096	0.080
Gonads (♂)	0.088	0.012	0.030	0.011	0.031	0.041	0.063
Lung	0.91	0.18	0.90	0.29	0.11	0.12	0.068
Heart	0.14	0.03	0.053	0.017	0.044	0.046	0.043
Skeletal muscle	0.093	0.019	0.030	0.006	0.030	0.026	0.054
Retroperitoneal fat	0.061	0.010	0.021	0.008	0.044	0.088	0.085
Subcutaneous fat	0.070	0.015	0.024	0.006	0.060	0.076	0.043
Brain	0.033	0.005	0.011	0.004	0.013	0.015	0.013
Mesenteric lymph nodes	0.10	0.03	0.036	0.013	0.061	0.068	0.053
Blood	0.16	0.06	0.066	0.027	0.076	0.10	0.058
Plasma	0.22	0.07	0.092	0.031	0.12	0.16	0.094
n	5		5		3		

TABLE 3 (Cont.)

	3,3´-Dichlorobenzidine						
	Rat				Dog		
	1 h		4 h		4 h		
	$\bar{x}$	wt_w	$\bar{x}$	wt_w	Dog 4	Dog 5	Dog 6
	Concentration in wet tissue ($\mu g\ g^{-1}$)						
Stomach	0.020	0.006	0.015	0.006	0.025	0.096	0.024
Small intestine	0.55	0.18	1.1	0.8	0.087	0.56	0.23
Large intestine	0.032	0.008	0.33	0.29	1.0	0.80	0.49
Kidney	0.096	0.024	0.078	0.011	0.078	0.046	0.041
Ureter	0.11	0.02	0.04	0.02	0.072	0.074	0.089
Urinary bladder	0.030	0.007	0.049	0.043	0.068	0.084	0.032
Liver	0.20	0.05	0.22	0.09	0.35	0.28	0.23
Bile	-	-	-	-	38	36	68
Pancreas	0.045	0.018	0.013	0.004	0.018	0.032	0.070
Spleen	0.024	0.005	0.012	0.002	0.013	0.022	0.044
Adrenals	0.24	0.13	0.086	0.037	0.050	0.032	0.045
Gonads (♂)	0.037	0.010	0.018(4)	0.003	0.018	0.020	0.017
Lung	0.41	0.16	0.28	0.10	0.073	0.044	0.057
Heart	0.032	0.010	0.014	0.004	0.017	0.015	0.021
Skeletal muscle	0.016	0.002	0.007	0.003	0.017	0.016	0.013
Retroperitoneal fat	0.12	0.05	0.018	0.012	0.093	0.056	0.18
Subcutaneous fat	0.12	0.04	0.017	0.008	0.092	0.044	0.089
Brain	0.014	0.005	0.005	0.003	-	0.013	0.012
Mesenteric lymph nodes	0.057	0.012	0.014	0.003	0.035	0.049	0.12
Blood	0.025	0.004	0.016	0.005	0.013	0.016	0.010
Plasma	0.041	0.007	0.028	0.008	0.026	0.031	0.019
n	5		5		3		

Notes:

(1)   From Kellner et al. (1973)
(2)   n = 4; 1 value = 0.49
(3)   n = 4; 1 value = 0.63
(4)   n = 4; 1 value = 0.055

TABLE 4

DISTRIBUTION PATTERN 7 AND 14 DAYS AFTER INTRAVENOUS ADMINISTRATION OF 0.2 mg 3,3'-DICHLOROBENZIDINE-[C-14] AND BENZIDINE[C-14] PER kg BODY WEIGHT TO RATS, DOGS AND MONKEYS. MEAN VALUES ($\bar{x}$) AND 95% CONFIDENCE INTERVAL (wt_W) OR SINGLE VALUES

Benzidine

	Rat 7 d		Rat 14 d		Dog 7 d		Dog 3	Monkey 7 d		Monkey 14 d
	$\bar{x}$	wt_W	$\bar{x}$	wt_W	Dog 1	Dog 2	Dog 3	M. 1	M. 2	M. 3

Concentration in wet tissue (μg g^{-1})

	$\bar{x}$	wt_W	$\bar{x}$	wt_W	Dog 1	Dog 2	Dog 3	M. 1	M. 2	M. 3
Kidney	0.009	<0.001	0.006	<0.001	0.012	0.013	0.020	0.007	0.008	0.004
Ureter	0.001	<0.001	0.002	<0.001	0.001	0.002	0.003	-	0.001	0.002
Urinary bladder	0.005	<0.001	0.006	<0.001	0.007	0.007	0.007	-	0.003	0.002
Liver	0.042	0.002	0.022	0.004	0.12	0.19	0.087	0.027	0.010	0.011
Bile	-	-	-	-	0.086	0.13	0.13	-	0.007	0.004
Spleen	0.005	<0.001	0.010	0.001	0.029	0.029	0.030	0.003	0.002	0.003
Adrenals	0.004	<0.001	0.003	<0.001	0.016	0.010	0.016	-	0.002	0.003
Gonads (♂)	<0.001	-	0.001	-	0.002	0.002	0.008	-	0.005♀	0.001
Lung	0.005	<0.001	0.005	<0.001	0.007	0.010	0.011	0.012	0.010	0.011

TABLE 4 (Cont.)

3,3'-Dichlorobenzidine

Concentration in wet tissue ($\mu g\ g^{-1}$)

	Rat 7 d $\bar{x}$	Rat 7 d wt_w	Rat 14 d $\bar{x}$	Rat 14 d wt_w	Dog 7 d Dog 1	Dog 7 d Dog 2	Dog 7 d Dog 3	Monkey 7 d M. 1	Monkey 14 d M. 2
Kidney	0.006	<0.001	0.002	0.001	0.014	0.010	0.007	0.018	0.009
Ureter	-	-	-	-	0.004	0.003	0.003	0.011	0.003
Urinary bladder	0.004	<0.001	0.002	<0.001	0.005	0.003	0.003	0.015	0.018
Liver	0.013	<0.001	0.004	<0.001	0.062	0.040	0.044	0.042	0.032
Bile	-	-	-	-	0.60	0.18	0.13	0.055	0.019
Spleen	0.004	<0.001	0.003	<0.001	0.004	0.005	0.004	0.012	0.006
Adrenals	0.015	0.003	0.006	<0.001	0.004	0.005	0.005	0.016	0.004
Gonads (♂)	0.002	<0.001	<0.001	-	0.002	0.002	0.002	0.006	0.001
Lung	0.004	<0.001	0.002	<0.001	0.036	0.023	0.031	0.012	0.013

Note:

From Kellner et al. (1973)

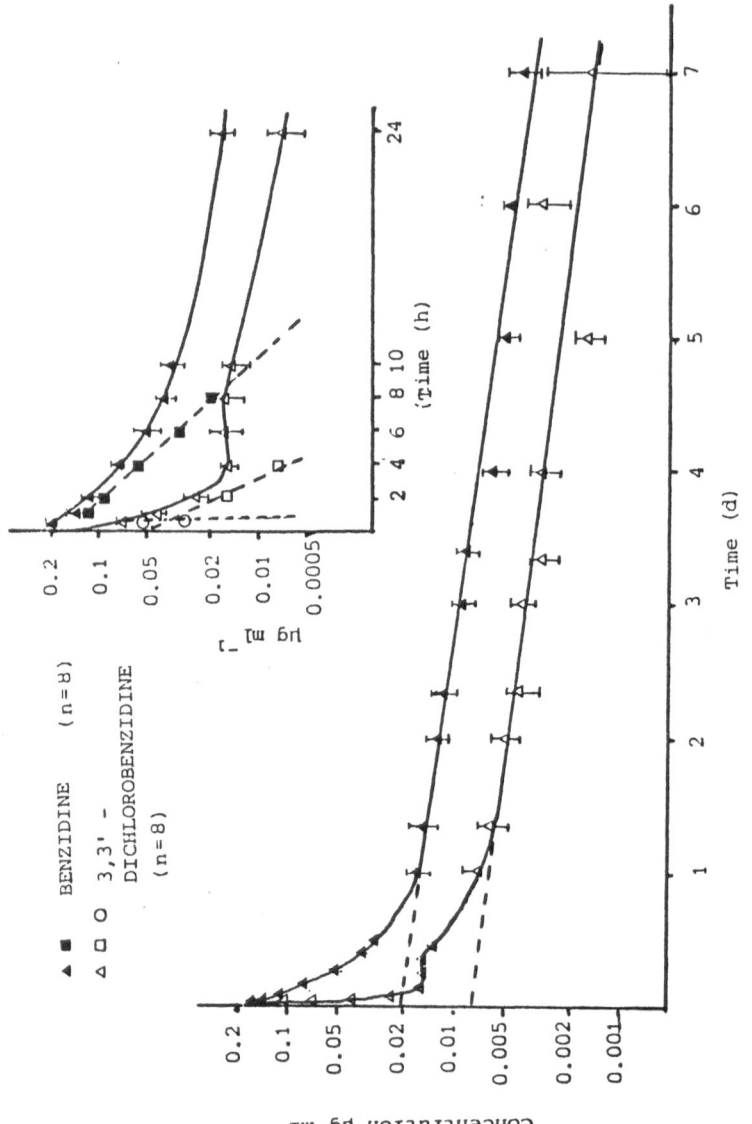

Note: from Kellner et al. (1973)

FIGURE 3   CONCENTRATION IN BLOOD AFTER INTRAVENOUS ADMINISTRATION OF 0.2 mg OF
C-14 LABELLED 3,3'-DICHLOROBENZIDINE OR BENZIDINE PER kg BODY WEIGHT TO RATS

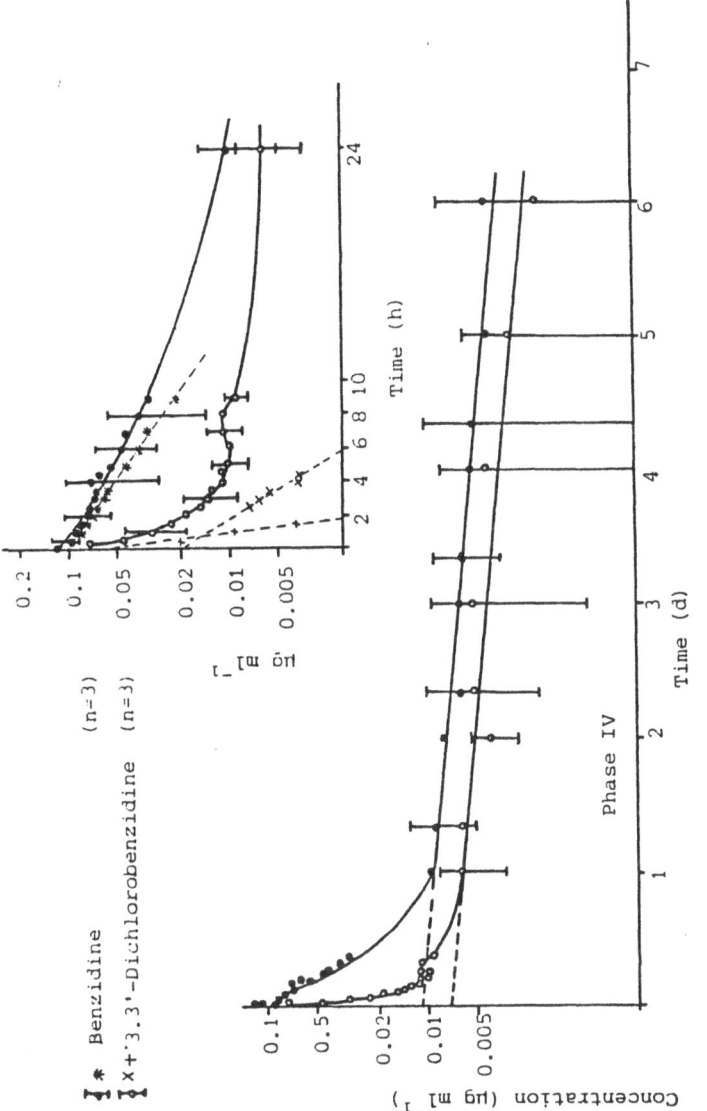

FIGURE 4.   CONCENTRATION IN BLOOD AFTER INTRAVENOUS ADMINISTRATION OF 0.2mg 3,3'-DICHLOROBENZIDINE-^{14}C AND BENZIDINE-^{14}C Kg^{-1} BODY WEIGHT TO DOGS.

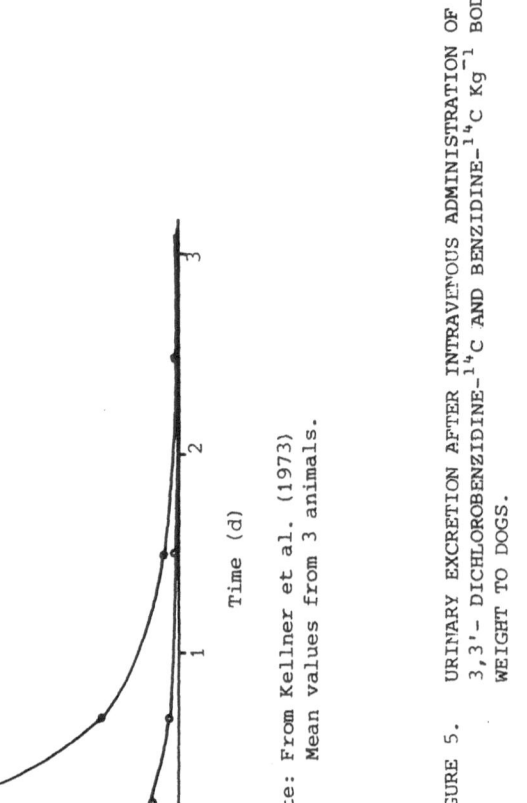

FIGURE 5.   URINARY EXCRETION AFTER INTRAVENOUS ADMINISTRATION OF 0.2mg 3,3'- DICHLOROBENZIDINE-^{14}C AND BENZIDINE-^{14}C Kg^{-1} BODY WEIGHT TO DOGS.

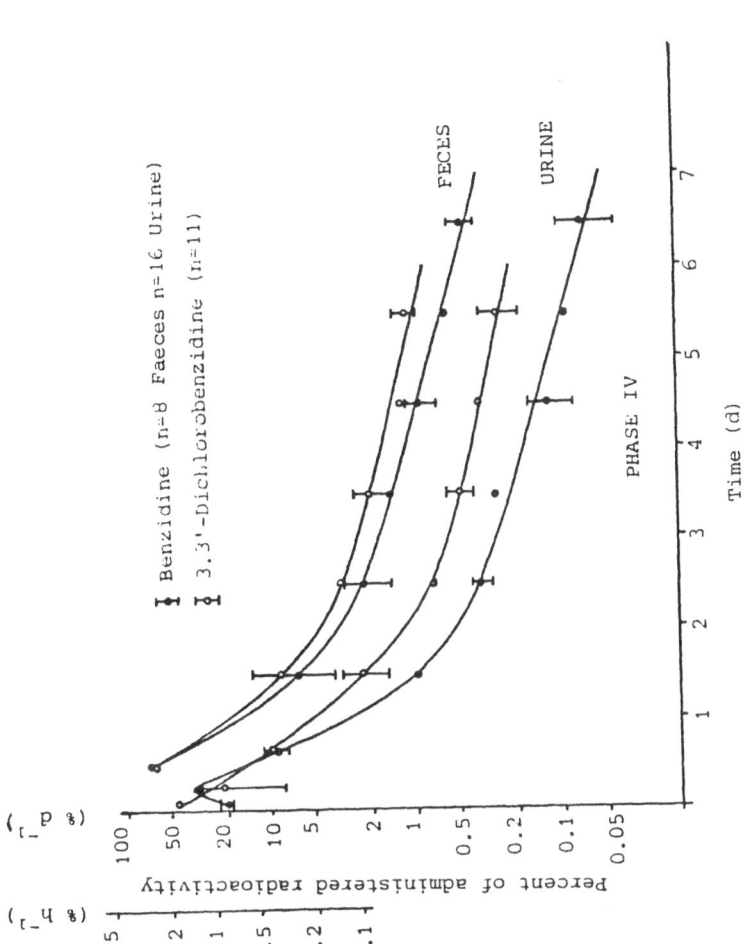

Note: from Kellner et al. (1973): mean values and 95% confidence limits.

FIGURE 6   EXCRETION WITH URINE AND FAECES AFTER INTRAVENOUS ADMINISTRATION OF
0.2 mg 3,3'-DICHLOROBENZIDINE-^{14}C AND BENZIDINE-^{14}C kg^{-1}

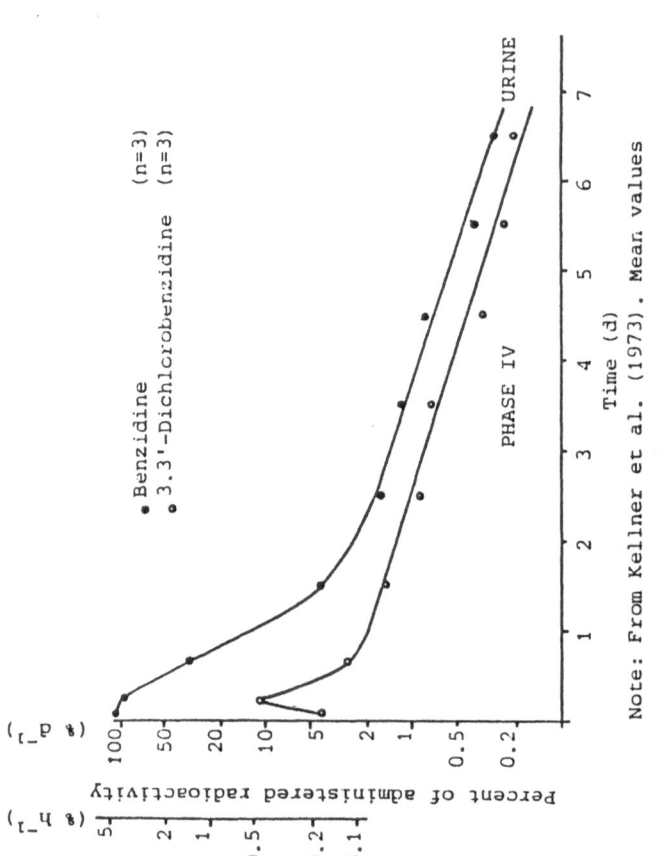

FIGURE 7.   EXCRETION IN URINE AFTER INTRAVENOUS ADMINISTRATION OF 0.2mg 3,3'-DICHLOROBENZIDINE-^{14}C AND BENZIDINE-^{14}C Kg^{-1} BODY WEIGHT TO DOGS.

Note: From Kellner et al. (1973). Mean values

Martin and Ekers (1980) reported that [H-3]benzidine injected intraperitoneally into male rats was bound to DNA and that significant amounts of radioactivity remained bound to DNA four weeks after injection. These authors also reported uptake and retention of H-3 for liver, kidney and lung. Two phases of loss were seen with half-lives of ~2 h and ≧24 h. In view of the potentially labile nature of H-3 bound to benzidine, the results of these studies are difficult to interpret.

Extensive studies on the metabolism of benzidine and 3,3´dichlorobenzidine in rats, dogs and monkeys were undertaken by Kellner et al. (1973). Time-dependent concentrations in blood for rats and dogs are shown in Figs. 3 and 4 respectively. The main distinction between the two compounds is a more rapid and larger early reduction in concentrations of the dichloro form, probably reflecting enhanced early excretion in the urine (Fig. 5). Both faecal and urinary excretion in rats, at 1 d or more after injection, exhibited similar biphasic curves for the two compounds (Fig. 6), with half-lives for the two components ~0.25 d and ~2 d. In the urine from dogs (Fig. 7) a similar early phase is exhibited for benzidine, but is much less apparent for 3,3´-dichlorobenzidine. The slower phase is seen for both compounds and again exhibits a half-life of about 2 d.

Kellner et al. (1973) also gave detailed data for the distribution of benzidine and 3,3´-dichlorobenzidine in various tissues. These data (Tables 3 and 4) indicate some accumulation of metabolites in liver, but are of limited relevance with respect to metabolic modelling.

10.5   CONSIDERATIONS IN MODELLING

The major potential route of exposure to benzidine and its congeners has been identified as transcutaneous. Unfortunately, the degree of systemic uptake by this route cannot be quantified, except that it can be in excess of 1% of the material applied to the skin. Furthermore, the time course of such uptake has not been studied.

With respect to metabolism, any model must rely almost completely on the studies of Kellner et al. (1973) and Hsu and Sikka (1982). While these papers give useful data at early times after exposure, i.e. in the first few days, the evidence suggests that metabolites of benzidine and its congeners are bound in tissues for many weeks. Furthermore, in vitro studies suggest substantial inter-species differences in benzidine metabolism, though this is not reflected in the work of Kellner et al. (1973).

On the basis of the data available, it is concluded that it is not currently possible to propose a metabolic model for benzidine that would be useful either in monitoring exposure or in interpreting dose-response data.

10.6   REFERENCES

Baker, R.K. and Deighton, J.G., 1953. The metabolism of benzidine in the rat. Cancer Res., 13, 529-531.

Boeniger, M.F., Stein, H.P., Choudhary, G. and Neumeister, C.E., 1981. Residual benzidine in imported and domestic benzidine dyes. Toxicol. Lett., 9, 415-420.

Bos, R.P., Brouns, R.M.E., Van Doorn, R., Theuws, J.L.G. and Henderson, P. Th., 1980. The appearance of mutagens in urine of rats after the administration of benzidine and some other aromatic amines. Toxicology, 16, 113-122.

Bradshaw, L. and Clayson, D.B., 1955. Metabolism of two aromatic amines in the dog. Nature (Lond.), 176, 974-975.

Cerniglia, C.E., Freeman, J.P., Franklin, W. and Pack, L.D., 1982. Metabolism of benzidine and benzidine-congener based dyes by human, monkey and rat intestinal bacteria. Biochem. Biophys. Res. Commun., 107, 1224-1229.

Clayson, D.B., Ward, E. and Ward, L., 1959. The fate of benzidine in various species. Acta unio int. cancrum, 15, 581-586.

Ghetti, G., 1960. Urinary excretion of several aromatic amines in workers employed in the production and use of benzidine, substituted benzidine and their salts. Med. Lav., 51, 102-114.

Gimalt, F. and Romaguera, C., 1981. Cutaneous sensitivity to benzidine. Derm. Beruf. Umwelt., 29, 95-97.

Haley, T.J., 1975. Benzidine revisited: a review of the literature and problems associated with the use of benzidine and its congeners. Clin. Toxicol., 8, 13-42.

Hsu, R.S. and Sikka, H.C., 1982. Disposition of 3,3´-dichlorobenzidine in the rat. Toxicol. Appl. Pharmacol., 64, 306-316.

International Agency for Research on Cancer, 1982. Benzidine and its sulphate, hydrochloride and dihydrochloride. IARC Monographs on Evaluation of the Carcinogenic Risk of Chemicals to Humans, 29, 149-183.

International Agency for Research on Cancer, 1982a. 3,3´-Dichlorobenzidine and its dihydrochloride. IARC Monographs on Evaluation of the Carcinogenic Risk of Chemicals to Humans, 29, 239-256.

Kellner, H.-M., Christ, O.E. and Lotzsch, K., 1973. Animal studies on the kinetics of benzidine and 3,3´-dichlorobenzidine. Arch. Toxicol., 31, 61-79.

Martin, C.N. and Ekers, S.F., 1980. Studies on the macromolecular binding of benzidine. Carcinogenesis, 1, 101-109.

Martin, C.N. and Kennelly, J.C., 1981. Rat liver microsomal azoreductase activity on four azo dyes derived from benzidine, 3,3´-dimethylbenzidine or 3,3´dimethyloxybenzidine. Carcinogenesis, 2, 307-312.

Meigs, J.W., Brown, R.M. and Sciarini, L.J., 1951. A study of exposure to benzidine and substituted benizidines in a chemical plant. A preliminary report. Arch. Ind. Hyg., 4, 533-540.

Meigs, J.W., Sciarini, L.J. and Van Sandt, W.A., 1954. Skin penetration by diamines of the benzidine group. Arch. Ind. Hyg., 9, 122-132, 1954.

Morton, K.C., King, C.M. and Baetcke, K.P., 1979. Metabolism of benzidine to N-hydroxy-N,N´-diacetylbenzidine and subsequent nucleic acid binding and mutagenicity. Cancer Res., 39, 3107-3113.

Morton, K.C., Beland, F.A., Evans, F.E., Fullerton, N.F. and Kadlubar, F.F., 1980. Metabolic activation of N-hydroxy-N,N´-diacetylbenzidine by hepatic sulfotransferase. Cancer Res., 40, 751-757.

Morton, K.C., Wang, C.Y., Garner, C.D. and Shirai, T., 1981. Carcinogenicity of benzidine, N,N´-diacetylbenzidine and N-hydroxy-N,N´diacetylbenzidine for female CD rats. Carcinogenesis, 2, 747-752.

Nelson, C.J., Baetcke, K.P., Frith, C.H., Kodell, R.L. and Schieferstein, G., 1982. The effect of sex, dose, time and cross on neoplasia in mice given benzidine dihydrochloride. Toxicol. Appl. Pharmacol., 64, 171-186.

Ohkawa, T., Fujinaga, T., Doi, J., Ebisuno, S., Takamatsu, M., Nakamura, J. and Kido, R., 1982. Clinical study on occupational uroepithelial cancer in Wakayama City. J. Urol., 128, 520-523.

Rapp, N.S., Zenser, T.V., Brown, W.W. and Davis, B.B., 1980. Metabolism of benzidine by a prostaglandin-mediated process in renal inner medullary slices. J. Pharmacol. Exp. Ther., 215, 401-406.

Shriner, C.R., Drury, J.S., Hammons, A.S., Towill, L.E., Lewis, E.B. and Opresko, D.M., 1978. Reviews on the Environmental Effects of Pollutants: II. Benzidine. EPA-600-1-78-024 (ORNL/EIS-86), US Environmental Protection Agency, Health Effects Research Laboratory, Cincinnati, OH.

Tanaka, K., 1981. Urinary metabolites of 3-3´ dichlorobenzidine and their mutagenicity. Sangyo Igaku, 23, 426-427.

Zenser, T.V., Mattammal, M.B., Ambrecht, H.J. and Davies, B.B., 1980. Benzidine binding to nucleic acids mediated by the peroxidative activity of prostaglandin endoperoxide synthetase. Cancer Res., 40, 2839-2845.

Zenser, T.V., Mattammal, M.B. and Davis, B.B., 1979. Co-oxidation of benzidine by renal medullary prostaglandin cyclooxygenase. J. Pharmacol. exp. Ther., 211, 460-464.

Appendix 11
Carbon Tetrachloride

CONTENTS

11.1   INTRODUCTION

Carbon tetrachloride, CCl_4, is usually encountered as a colourless liquid. It has a freezing point of -23°C and a boiling point of 76.7°C. Its molecular weight is 153.8, its density 1.585 and its vapour pressure at 20°C is 91.3 mm. CCl_4 is miscible with ethanol, diethyl ether, chloroform, benzene, solvent naptha and most fixed and volatile oils, but it is insoluble in water (International Agency for Research on Cancer, 1979).

CCl_4 decomposes to phosgene in the presence of limited quantities of water at 250°C. When dry it is non-reactive with iron and nickel, reacts slowly with copper and lead, but reacts strongly with aluminium and its alloys (International Agency for Research on Cancer, 1979).

Production of CCl_4 takes place on a large scale in many industrialised countries. In 1976, US production was more than 3.9×10^8 kg, while in Western Europe annual production is more than 3.2×10^8 kg. In 1977, Japan produced 5.15×10^7 kg of this compound (International Agency for Research on Cancer, 1979).

Carbon tetrachloride is mainly used as an intermediate in the production of fluorocarbons, with a major secondary use being its application as a solvent. Miscellaneous other applications relate to grain fumigation, pesticide production and petrol additive formulation (International Agency for Research on Cancer, 1979).

11.2   LEVELS OF EXPOSURE

11.2.1   Air

Concentrations of CCl_4 in air are typically given in terms of ppb, ppm, µg l^{-1} or mg m^{-3}. The relevant conversion factor is that 1 ppm is equal to 6.5 mg m^{-3}.

Permissible levels of carbon tetrachloride in the working environment vary from 20 mg m^{-3} in the USSR to 65 mg m^{-3} in the USA, Federal Republic of Germany and Sweden (International Agency for Research on Cancer, 1979). A concentration of 65 mg m^{-3}, in combination with a breathing rate of 20 l min.$^{-1}$ for an 8 h working day (International Commission on Radiological Protection, 1975), corresponds to a daily intake of 624 mg of CCl_4 by inhalation.

With respect to non-occupational exposure, it is noted that CCl_4 is formed in the troposphere by solar-induced photochemical reactions. Air samples at 42 locations in the US exhibited an average concentration of 1.4 µg m^{-3} and more than 86% of all measurements fell within the range 0.6 to 1.9 µg m^{-3} (International Agency for Research on Cancer, 1979). The International Agency for Research on Cancer (1979) also quoted data indicating variations in mean levels of CCl_4 in air varying from 0.4 to 10.3 µg m^{-3}, as well as the following data for concentrations at specified locations.

Location	Concentration ($\mu g\ m^{-3}$)
Rural	0.756
Rural	0.5-0.7
Japanese town	8.8
(concentrations correlated with positions of local chemical factories)	
Sites in Northern hemisphere	0.7
Sites in Southern hemisphere	0.434

Similar values have been listed by Fishbein (1979).

Overall, it seems that concentrations of 1 $\mu g\ m^{-3}$ are typical, except in the vicinity of factories producing or using CCl_4. In these locations, concentrations ~10 $\mu g\ m^{-3}$ may be anticipated.

At a breathing rate of 23 $m^3\ d^{-1}$ (International Commission on Radiological Protection, 1975), a concentration of 1 $\mu g\ m^{-3}$ corresponds to a daily intake of 23 μg by inhalation.

11.2.2   Water

CCl_4 has been found in rivers, lakes, raw-water, finished drinking water, effluent water from commercial manufacturing sources and sewage treatment plant effluent water (International Agency for Research on Cancer, 1979). Typical levels in various waters were summarised by Johns (1976) as follows.

	Range ($\mu g\ l^{-1}$)
Rainwater	0.01-1.0
Surface water	0.01-1.0
Potable water	0.01-1.0
Sea water	0.01-1.0

For comparison, Fishbein (1979) quoted a value of 2-3 ppb, i.e. 2-3 $\mu g\ l^{-1}$, derived from a survey of 80 US cities. However, CCl_4 was detected in only 12.5% of the finished waters and the maximum level recorded was 4 $\mu g\ l^{-1}$ (International Agency for Research on Cancer, 1979).

In view of the data reviewed above, it seems appropriate to assume that a typical concentration of CCl_4 in drinking water is ~1 $\mu g\ l^{-1}$, corresponding to a typical daily intake ~2 μg, considerably smaller than that by inhalation.

It is noted that accidental or deliberate ingestion of CCl_4 does occur, but this is not considered here.

11.2.3   Diet

The International Agency for Research on Cancer (1979) reported the following data for CCl_4 concentrations in a UK diet.

Component	Concentration ($\mu g\ kg^{-1}$)
Dairy produce	0.2-14
Meat	7-9
Oils and fats	0.7-18
Beverages	0.2-6
Fruits and vegetables	3-8

Johns (1976) listed the following concentration ranges as typical.

Item	Concentration ($\mu g\ kg^{-1}$)
Marine invertebrates	1-10
Fish	1-10
Water birds	1-100
Marine mammals	1-10
Fatty foods	1-10
Non-fatty foods	1

These data indicate that the average concentration of CCl_4 in dietary materials is likely to be ~5 $\mu g\ kg^{-1}$, corresponding to a daily dietary intake ~7 μg.

11.2.4   Other routes

It is noted that CCl_4 is used as a solvent and that transcutaneous absorption, or uptake through wounds and abrasions, may occur. This contribution to exposure cannot readily be quantified.

11.2.5   Summary

On the basis of data reviewed in this section, the following daily intakes of CCl_4 are estimated.

Medium	Intake (mg)	Comments
Air	<624	Occupational exposure, based on current limits
	0.023	Non-occupational: typical value
	0.23	Non-occupational: maximum value
Water	0.002	Non-occupational: typical value
Diet	~0.007	Non-occupational: typical value

These values indicate that inhalation is likely to be the main route of exposure to CCl_4, though ingestion in diet and water may be of significance in the non-occupationally exposed.

11.3   EFFECTS

The general toxic effects of CCl_4 have been summarised briefly by Hardie (1964) as follows

"Carbon tetrachloride is a strong metabolic poison; ingestion of 3-4 g liquid is known to be fatal after several days. It is less narcotic than chloroform and its use as an anaesthetic has been shown to be accompanied by much greater irritation of the subject than with chloroform. Toxic effects of carbon tetrachloride are evident upon contact of the liquid with the skin. When the substance was formerly used in shampoo mixtures, sufficient carbon tetrachloride was absorbed through the scalp to cause drowsiness and nausea. By removing the fats from the skin, carbon tetrachloride destroys the skin's resistance to physical irritation and infection; prolonged or repeated contact can cause a form of dermatitis.

Inhalation of high concentrations of carbon tetrachloride vapour can produce unconciousness in 1-2 min., and continued exposure can produce respiratory paralysis and even death. Sometimes upon exposure to a high concentration of the vapour fatal collapse occurs days later. Repeated exposure to concentrations of about 100 ppm has been known to have chronic toxic effects. ....

Chronic carbon tetrachloride poisoning is accompanied by nausea, vomiting, loss of appetite and colic, associated in nearly all cases with weakness, fatigue, headache, dizziness, and sometimes a burning sensation in the eyes. The appearance of jaundice is an important symptom, enabling an early diagnosis to be made."

A more detailed description of these various effects was given by Browning (1965).

The carcinogenic actions of CCl_4 were reviewed by the International Agency for Research on Cancer (1979). In mice and rats, CCl_4 produced both benign and malignant liver tumours, and there was an indication that such tumours were also induced in hamsters and trout. For man, no epidemiological studies were available, but three case reports were reviewed concerning the appearance of liver tumours, in association with cirrhosis, following exposure to CCl_4.

On the basis of the data available, the International Agency for Research on Cancer (1979) concluded as follows.

"There is sufficient evidence that carbon tetrachloride is carcinogenic in experimental animals. There are suggestive case reports of liver cancer in humans. In the absence of adequate data in humans, it is reasonable, for practical purposes, to regard carbon tetrachloride as if it presented a carcinogenic risk to humans."

In respect of other effects, CCl_4 has been reported to cause testicular degeneration in rats (Chatterjee, 1966), as well as some morphological and pulmonary surfactant changes in the lungs (Stewart et al., 1979). Damage to the placenta (Tsirel'nikov and Tsirel'nikova, 1976), delayed foetal development (Schwetz et al., 1974), and necrotic damage to the placenta and foetal liver (Von Roschlau and Rodenkirchen, 1969) have been reported in experimental studies on mice and rats.

Much of the experimental work on CCl_4 has been directed to its effects as a hepatotoxin, particularly with respect to the induction of characteristic fatty liver and necrosis. This subject has been discussed in several reviews by Recknagel and his co-workers (Recknagel and Ghosal, 1966; Recknagel, 1967; Recknagel and Glende, 1973; Recknagel et al., 1977) by Smuckler (1976), and by McCay and Poyer (1976).

Various theories for the induction of this liver injury were discussed by Recknagel (1967), who emphasised that the key feature is the metabolism of CCl_4 with the breaking of the carbon-chlorine bond followed by a metabolite induced lipoperoxidation reaction. Virtually all experimental work undertaken over the last 15 years has been related to the lipoperoxidation hypothesis, a brief summary of which is given below.

The lipoperoxidation hypothesis was reviewed and summarised by Recknagel et al. (1977). Release of the latent toxicological potential of CCl_4 requires cleavage of the CCl_3-Cl bond. This is carried out by the mixed function oxidase system present in the endoplasmic reticulum of hepatocytes and cells in some other tissues. The mechanism of cleavage appears to involve cytochrome P450. The CCl_3 radical produced by this cleavage attacks polyenoic fatty acids of phospholipids in the lipoprotein membrane in which cytochrome P450 is embedded and, as molecular oxygen enters the reaction, autocatalytic peroxidation of membrane lipids is initiated (Fig. 1). The process of peroxidative lipid decomposition underlies the unfolding of a spectrum of pathological changes which soon lead to fatty liver, loss of hepatic protein synthetic capability, imposition of subcellular structural deformities, loss of soluble liver enzymes into the plasma and eventual death of the cell. It should be noted that this hypothesis is specifically directed to explaining the processes underlying CCl_4 induced fatty liver and hepatic necrosis. It does not address itself to other processes which may be involved in the induction of hepatic neoplasia, e.g. covalent binding to DNA. Also, although there is agreement that free radical metabolites are the active molecular species (see Bini et al., 1975; Ingall et al., 1978), the relative contributions of lipid peroxidation and covalent binding in the aetiology of hepatic injury is still subject to controversy (Suarez et al., 1981).

Because the mixed function oxidase system is involved in the metabolism of CCl_4, it is not surprising that the hepatotoxity of this substance is affected by a wide range of inducers, or suppressors, of this system. A brief account of some experiments of interest is given below.

There have been several studies of the effects of CCl_4 on isolated rat hepatocytes. Thus, Stacey and Priestly (1978) reported that CCl_4 decreased membrane integrity, but that a wide range of chemicals reported to be hepatoprotective in other experimental models of CCl_4 toxicity had no effect in this system. In a second paper, Stacey and Priestly (1978a) reported that they could find no evidence of lipid peroxidation in isolated hepatocytes exposed to CCl_4. Casini and Farber (1981) reported that hepatocytes from phenobarbital pre-treated animals were more sensitive to CCl_4 induced cell killing than were cells from control

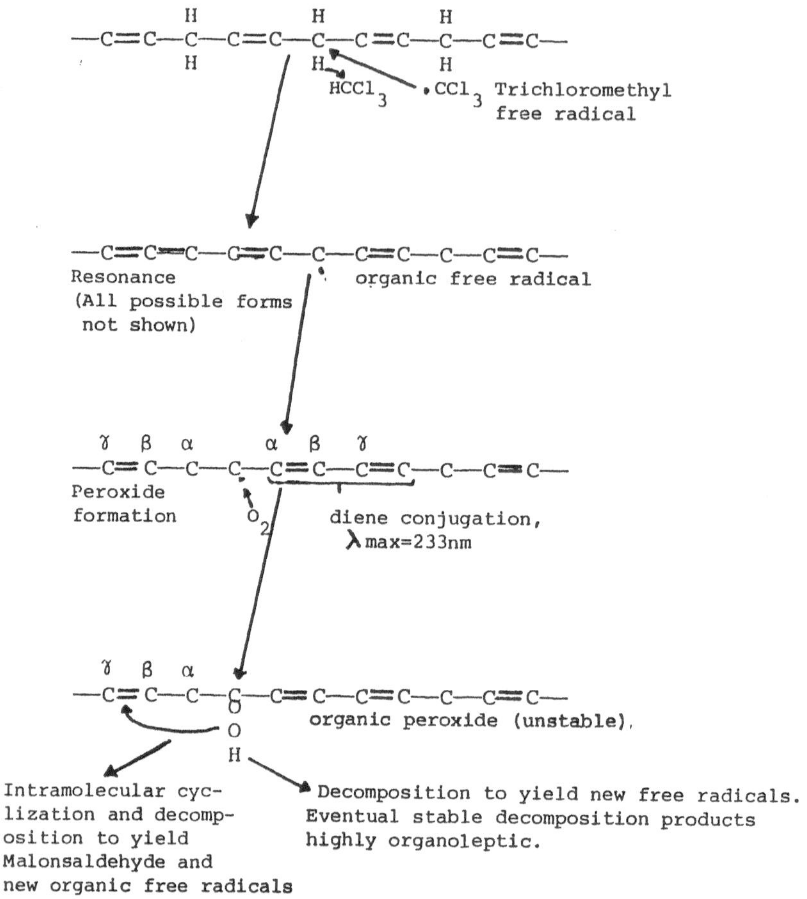

```
        H          H          H
—C≡C—C—C≡C—C—C≡C—C—C≡C—
        H          H          H
                   H      ·CCl₃  Trichloromethyl
                   HCCl₃         free radical
```

```
—C≡C≡C—C≡C—C—C≡C—C—C≡C—
Resonance              organic free radical
(All possible forms
 not shown)
```

```
  γ  β  α      α  β  γ
—C≡C—C—C—C≡C—C≡C—C—C≡C—
Peroxide
formation    O₂     diene conjugation,
                     λmax=233nm
```

```
  γ  β  α
—C≡C—C—C—C≡C—C≡C—C—C≡C—
          O
          O    organic peroxide (unstable),
          H
```

Intramolecular cyc-   Decomposition to yield new free radicals.
lization and decomp-   Eventual stable decomposition products
osition to yield   highly organoleptic.
Malonsaldehyde and
new organic free radicals

Note: From Recknagel et al. (1977).

FIGURE 1. AUTOCATALYTIC PEROXIDATION OF A POLYENOIC LONG-CHAIN
FATTY ACID INITIATED BY A TRICHLOROMETHYL FREE RADICAL.

TABLE 1

RECENT STUDIES ON THE INTERACTIONS OF CARBON TETRACHLORIDE
WITH OTHER SUBSTANCES IN INTACT ANIMALS

Reference	Comments
Matkovics et al. (1978)	Vitamin E was found to reduce, but not completely eliminate CCl_4 toxicity in rats.
Strubelt et al. (1978)	Chromic consumption of ethanol by rats was found to potentiate CCl_4 hepatotoxicity.
Curtis et al. (1979)	Pre-exposure to the photodegradation product of the chlorocarbon insecticide mirex was found to potentiate CCl_4 hepatotoxicity in rats.
Cagan and Klaassen (1979)	Rats as young as 4 days of age were demonstrated to be as susceptible as adults to CCl_4 induced hepatotoxicity, although they had a lower capacity to metabolise CCl_4.
Chang-Tsui and Ho (1980)	Acute or continuous administration of pentobarbital enhanced CCl_4-induced elevated levels of glutamate oxalacetate transaminase and glutamate pyruvate transaminase in mice.
Lowrey et al. (1981)	Pre-treatment with ethanol or isopropanol had no effect on the rate of decline or extent of depression of the liver microsomal calcium pump in CCl_4 treated rats. It was suggested that the mechanism of alcohol potentiation of CCl_4 induced hepatotoxicity probably resides in alteration of processes developing after the initial events of CCl_4 metabolism.
Saxena and Garg (1981)	Feeding of the liver tonic Liv-52 gave marked protection against CCl_4-induced lipid peroxidation in rats.
Suarez et al. (1981)	It was found that administration of diethylmaleate to fed and fasted rats produced a marked depletion of hepatic reduced glutathione and protected against CCl_4 hepatotoxicity in the fasted animals. The authors commented that the protective effect of diethylmaleate may be related to its ability to inhibit hepatic microsomal drug metabolism.

animals and that cell killing could be prevented by addition of SKF 525A to the culture medium. It was also noted that this protection was accompanied by evidence of decreased CCl_4 metabolism, as assessed by the extent of metabolite binding to total cellular lipids and proteins, and by the extent of formation of conjugated dienes accompanying the peroxidation of phospholipids isolated from total cell lipids.

Casini and Farber (1981) also found that the extent of CCl_4-induced cell death was determined by the Ca^{2+} concentration in the culture medium, while Stacey et al. (1982) found that lipid peroxidation occurred in hepatocytes exposed to CCl_4 in air, but did not occur when the cells were exposed to CCl_4 in a 95% O_2, 5% CO_2 mixture. In view of these results, extrapolation from studies on isolated hepatocytes to implications with respect to the intact liver requires considerable care.

There have been a wide variety of studies undertaken on the effects of various substances on the liver when administered in conjunction with CCl_4. Much of the earlier work was reviewed by Recknagel et al. (1977) in discussion of the lipid peroxidation hypothesis. Some more recent studies, summarised in Table 1, are all consistent with that hypothesis.

11.4   METABOLISM

There have been numerous experiments attempting to elucidate the mechanism of CCl_4 liver injury. Unfortunately, very few of these have any relevance to developing a pharmacokinetic model for CCl_4 metabolism. While it would be possible to discuss CCl_4 metabolism in the context of the lipid peroxidation hypothesis, or in terms of the degree of binding to various cellular constituents, this would be of limited relevance to the current review. Attention is, therefore, concentrated on the fragmentary data available concerning the gross features of CCl_4 metabolism.

11.4.1   Transcutaneous absorption

Stewart and Dodd (1964) reported on mean alveolar air concentrations of CCl_4 during and after immersion of one thumb in the solvent for thirty minutes. Clearance of CCl_4 was monophasic over the first 5 h after exposure with a half-life of ~2 h. On the basis of their data, Stewart and Dodd (1964) calculated that immersion of both hands for 30 minutes would be approximately equivalent to a thirty minute vapour exposure at 100 to 500 ppm. In comparison, topical application to both hands for thirty minutes was estimated to be equivalent to a vapour exposure of about 10 ppm for three hours. Interpretation of these data is difficult without comparable information on exposure by other routes.

11.4.2   Ingestion

There have been several studies on the retention of CCl_4 in the body following oral intakes. Fowler (1969) administered 1 ml kg^{-1} of CCl_4 by stomach tube to rabbits and reported the following distribution of CCl_4 and its metabolites.

Time (h)	Tissue	No. of rabbits	CCl_4 $(\mu g\ g^{-1})$	$CHCl_3$ $(\mu g\ g^{-1})$	$CCl_3.CCl_3$ $(ng\ g^{-1})$
6	Fat	5	787±289	4.7±0.5	4.1±1.2
	Liver	5	96±11	4.9±1.5	1.6±0.5
	Kidney	5	20±13	1.4±0.6	0.7±0.2
	Muscle	5	21±12	0.1±0.1	0.3±0.2
24	Fat	5	96±11	1.0±0.2	16.5±1.6
	Liver	5	7.7±1.3	1.0±0.4	4.2±1.8
	Kidney	5	6.9±3.9	0.4±0.2	2.2±1.1
	Muscle	5	1.3±0.6	0.1±0.1	0.5±0.2
44 (died)	Fat	1	23	1.4	10.0
	Liver	1	1.1	4.4	3.1
	Kidney	1	0.5	0.4	2.2
	Muscle	1	0.3	Trace	9.2
48	Fat	4	45±12	0.4±0.1	6.8±2.4
	Liver	4	3.8±0.1	0.8±0.2	1.0±0.3
	Kidney	4	0.5±0.3	0.2±0.0	Trace
	Muscle	4	0.5±0.3	0.1±0.1	Trace

Note: mean ± s.d.

Two additional, unidentified, metabolites were also recorded as being present.

In rats, Seawright and MacLean (1967) gave data on the expiration of $^{14}CCl_4$ and $^{14}CO_2$ after oral administration of $^{14}CCl_4$. About 70% of the dose was eliminated as $^{14}CCl_4$ in the first 24 h, while ~0.2 to 0.4% was exhaled as $^{14}CO_2$, with significantly less being exhaled in rats fed a protein-free diet, as compared with rats fed a stock diet. Concentrations of CCl_4 in blood and liver at 1 and 3 h after dosing are listed below.

Diet and treatment	Time (h)	CCl_4 in blood $(\mu g\ ml^{-1})$	CCl_4 in liver $(\mu g\ g^{-1}\ w.w.)$
Stock	1	26±11	296±168
	3	38±19	385±283
Protein-free	1	49±7	574±96
	3	49±13	575±178
Protein-free + DDT	1	39±12	455±159
	3	45±9	497±115

Note: mean ± s.d. (5 animals); administered dose 2.5 ml kg^{-1}

Similar results on loss in expired air, to 6 h post-exposure, were reported by Garner and MacLean (1969).

Reynolds (1967) recorded data on the levels of non-volatile radioactivity in liver following oral administration of C-14 or Cl-36 labelled CCl_4. These data, which are listed below, indicate that the amount of CCl_4 metabolised is determined by the amount administered.

Agent	Dose (µM)	Percentage of dose recovered as non-volatile activity in liver
$^{14}CCl_4$	50	0.53
	100	0.38
	3400	0.011
CCl_4^{36}	57	0.70
	330	0.44
$^{14}CCl_4$ (new born)	55	0.31

Rao and Recknagel (1969) reported that, following oral administration, only 0.0137% of C-14 administered as $^{14}CCl_4$ was incorporated into the lipids derived from the liver associated with 100 g body weight of rat. Incorporation peaked five minutes after intragastric administration indicating the rapid uptake of CCl_4 from the gastrointestinal tract.

In man, Stewart et al. (1963) reported on the loss of CCl_4 in expired air following ingestion of "one pint" of a solution composed of two parts CCl_4 and one part methanol. A multi-phasic loss curve was recorded, but, in view of the amount consumed and the therapeutic measures employed, this curve is difficult to interpret. However, it is notable that the long-term component of loss can be interpreted as exhibiting a half-life of ~50 h.

11.4.3   Inhalation

With respect to inhalation studies, reliance must be placed on the work of McCollister et al. (1951) and Stewart et al. (1961).

McCollister et al. (1951) studied the uptake of CCl_4 in monkeys exposed to 0.315 mg l^{-1}. The fractional absorption of CCl_4 was defined by:

$$A = (C_i - C_e)/C_i$$

where   A is the fractional absorption;

C$_i$ is the inhaled concentration; and

C$_e$ is the exhaled concentration.

Values of A for the three animals studied were 0.262, 0.367 and 0.283. Concentrations of C-14 in blood increased throughout the period of the experiment and an accumulation half-time cannot be derived from the data presented. However, decorporation over the 12 to 28 days post-exposure was biphasic, with components exhibiting half-lives of ~1 and 5 d respectively.

McCollister et al. (1951) also gave data on the tissue distribution of C-14 in a female monkey after exposure to 46 ppm of C-14 labelled CCl_4 for 300 minutes. These data are summarised below in terms of a distribution ratio, with blood taken as unity.

Tissue	Distribution ratio
Fat	7.94
Liver	3.03
Bone marrow	3.00
Blood	1.00
Brain	0.97
Kidney	0.74
Heart	0.45
Spleen	0.32
Muscle	0.19
Lung	0.13
Bone	0.13

Significant quantities of radioactivity were excreted in the urine and faeces of this animal, but only spot samples were taken and the results cannot readily be quantified.

In man, Stewart et al. (1961) exposed subjects to CCl_4 at ~10 ppm for 180 minutes or 49 ppm for 70 minutes. Subsequent to the exposure period, breath concentrations appeared to decline as a simple power function of time. Analysis of the data presented by Stewart et al.(1961) suggests a function of the form:

$$C_o t^{-\alpha}$$

where α is ~1 for the 49 ppm exposure and ~0.6 for the 10 ppm exposure.

11.5   CONSIDERATIONS IN DEVELOPMENT OF A METABOLIC MODEL

Data on the metabolism of CCl_4 are very limited. Significant transcutaneous absorption can occur, but human studies appear to be limited to immersion of one thumb for a thirty minute period. With regard to ingestion, investigations on man are limited to a single individual exposed to a very large volume of CCl_4 in combination with methanol, while experiments on rats were conducted for purposes other than the understanding of CCl_4 pharmacokinetics.

Inhalation, potentially the most significant route of exposure has been little better investigated and the data on monkeys and man are insufficient to generate a pharmacokinetic model applicable to exposure regimes other than those studied.

In terms of monitoring for exposure to CCl_4, analysis of the expired air seems a potentially useful method, particularly since components of loss of unchanged CCl_4 with half lives ~50 h may occur. If such a method were to be used, detailed experiments would have to be undertaken to characterise the uptake and loss of CCl_4 by humans at different levels.

11.6   REFERENCES

Bini, A., Vecchi, G., Virvoli, G., Vannini, V. and Cessi, C. 1975. Detection of early metabolites in rat liver after administration of CCl_4 and $CBrCl_3$. Pharmacol. Res. Commun., 7, 143-149.

Browning, E., 1965. Toxicity and Metabolism of Industrial Solvents. Elsevier, Amsterdam.

Cagen, S.Z. and Klaassen C.D., 1979. Hepatotoxicity of carbon tetrachloride in developing rats. Toxicol. Appl. Pharmacol., 50, 347-354.

Casini, A.F. and Farber, J.L., 1981. Dependence of the carbon-tetrachloride-induced death of hepatocytes on the extracellular calcium concentration. Am. J. Pathol., 105, 138-148.

Castro, J.A., Díaz-Gomez, M.I., de Ferreyra, E.C., de Castro, C.R., D'Acosta, N. and de Fenos, O.M., 1972. Carbon tetrachloride effect on rat liver and adrenals related to their mixed-function oxygenase content. Biochem. Biophy. Res. Commun., 47, 315-321.

Chang-Tsui, Y.-Y.H. and Ho, I.K., 1980. Enhancement of carbon tetrachloride elevated glutamate oxalacetate transaminase and glutamate pyruvate transaminase by acute and continuous pentobarbital administration in mice. Clin. Toxicol., 16, 41-50.

Chatterjee, A., 1966. Testicular degeneration in rats by carbon tetrachloride intoxication. Experientia, 22, 395-396.

Chen, W.-J., Chi, E.Y. and Smuckler, E.A., 1977. Carbon tetrachloride-induced changes in mixed function oxidases and microsomal cytochromes in rat lung. Lab. Invest., 36, 388-394.

Colby, H.D., Brogan, W.C. III and Miles, P.R., 1981. Carbon tetrachloride-induced changes in adrenal microsomal mixed-function oxidases and lipid peroxidation. Toxicology Appl. Pharmacol., 60, 492-499.

Curtis, L.R., Williams, W.L. and Mehendale, H.M., 1979. Biliary excretion dysfunction following exposure to photomirex and photomirex carbon tetrachloride combination. Toxicology, 13, 77-90.

Fishbein, L., 1979. Potential halogenated industrial carcinogenic and mutagenic chemicals II. Halogenated saturated hydrocarbons. Sci. Tot. Environ., 11, 163-195.

Fowler, J.S.L., 1969. Carbon tetrachloride metabolism in the rabbit. Br. J. Pharmacol., 37, 733-737.

Garner, R.C. and McLean, A.E.M., 1969. Increased susceptibility to carbon tetrachloride poisoning in the rat after pretreatment with oral phenobarbitone. Biochem. Pharmacol., 18, 645-650.

Hardie, D.W.F., 1964. Chlorocarbons and chlorohydrocarbons. Carbon Tetrachloride. In: Kirk, R.E. and Othmer, D.F. (Eds.) Encyclopedia of Chemical Technology, 2nd. edit., Vol. 5, John Wiley and Sons, New York, pp. 128-139.

Ingall, A., Lott, K.A.K. and Stater, T.F., 1978. Metabolic activation of carbon tetrachloride to a free-radical product: studies using a spin trap. Biochem. Soc. Trans., 6, 962-964.

International Agency for Research on Cancer, 1979. Carbon Tetrachloride. IARC Monographs on the Evaluation of the Carcinogenic Risk of Chemicals to Humans, 20, 371-399.

International Commission on Radiological Protection, 1975. Report of the Task Group on Reference Man. Pergamon Press, Oxford.

Johns, R., 1976. Air Pollution Assessment of Carbon Tetrachloride. PB 256 732, National Technical Information Service, Springfield, VA, USA.

Lowrey, K., Glende, E.A. Jr. and Recknagel, R.O., 1981. Failure of ethanol or isopropanol pretreatment to affect carbon-tetrachloride-induced inhibition of hepatic microsomal calcium pump activity. Drug Chem. Toxicol., 4, 263-273.

Matkovics, B., Novak, R., Szabo, L., Marik, M.Z. and Zsoldos, T., 1978. Effect of acute carbon tetrachloride intoxication on the lipid peroxidation and the enzymes of the peroxide metabolism of rat tissues. Gen. Pharmacol., 9, 329-332.

McCay, P.B. and Poyer, J.L., 1976. Enzyme-generated free radicals as initiators of lipid peroxidation in biological membranes. In: Martonosi, A. (Ed.). The Enzymes of Biological Membranes, Plenum Press, New York, pp.239-256.

McCollister, D.D., Beamer, W.H., Atchison, G.J. and Spencer, H.C., 1951. The absorption, distribution and elimination of radioactive carbon tetrachloride by monkeys upon exposure to low vapor concentrations. J. Pharmacol. Exp. Ther., 102, 112-124.

Rao, K.S. and Recknagel, R.O., 1969. Early incorporation of carbon-labelled carbon tetrachloride into rat liver particulate lipids and proteins. Exp. Mol. Pathol., 10, 219-228.

Recknagel, R.O., 1967. Carbon tetrachloride hepatotoxicity. Pharmacol. Rev., 19, 145-208.

Recknagel, R.O. and Ghoshal, A.K., 1966. Lipoperoxidation as a vector in carbon tetrachloride hepatotoxicity. Lab. Invest., 15, 132-148.

Recknagel, R.O. and Glende, E.A. Jr., 1973. Carbon tetrachloride hepatotoxicity: an example of lethal cleavage. CRC Critical Reviews in Toxicology, 2, 263-297.

Recknagel, R.O., Glende, E.A. Jr. and Hruszkewycz, A.M., 1977. Chemical mechanisms in carbon tetrachloride toxicity. In: Pryor, W.A. (Ed.). Free Radicals in Biology, Vol. III, Academic Press, New York, pp. 97-132.

Reynolds, E.S., 1967. Liver parenchymal cell injury. IV. Pattern of incorporation of carbon and chlorine from carbon tetrachloride into chemical constituents of liver in vivo. J. Pharmacol. Exp. Ther., 155, 117-126.

Saxena, A. and Garg, N.K., 1981. Effect of Liv-52 on membrane lipids in carbon tetrachloride induced hepatotoxicity in rats. Indian J. Exp. Biol., 19, 859-862.

Schwetz, B.A., Leong, B.K.J. and Gehring, P.J., 1974. Embryo- and foeto-toxicity of inhaled carbon tetrachloride, 1,1-dichloroethane and methyl ethyl ketone in rats. Toxicol. Appl. Pharmacol., 28, 452-464.

Seawright, A.A. and McLean, A.E.M., 1967. The effect of diet on carbon tetrachloride metabolism. Biochem. J., 105, 1055-1060.

Smuckler, E.A., 1976. Structural and functional changes in acute liver injury. Environ. Health Perspect., 15, 13-25.

Stacey, N. and Priestly, B.G., 1978. Dose-dependent toxicity of CCl_4 in isolated rat hepatocytes and the effects of hepatoprotective treatments. Toxicol. Appl. Pharmacol., 45, 29-39.

Stacey, N. and Priestly, B.G., 1978a. Lipid peroxidation in isolated rat hepatocytes: relationship to toxicity of CCl_4, ADP/Fe^{3+} and diethyl maleate. Toxicol. Appl. Pharmacol., 45, 41-48.

Stacey, N.H., Ottenwälder, H. and Kappus, H., 1982. CCl_4-induced lipid peroxidation in isolated rat hepatocytes with different oxygen concentrations. Toxicol. Appl. Pharmacol., 62, 421-427.

Stewart, R.D., Gay, H.H., Erley, D.S., Hake, C.L. and Peterson, J.E., 1961. Human exposure to carbon tetrachloride vapor. Relationship of expired air concentration to exposure and toxicity. J. occup. Med., 3, 586-590.

Stewart, R.D., Boettner, E.A., Southworth, R.R. and Cerny, J.C., 1963. Acute carbon tetrachloride intoxication. J. Am. Med. Assoc., 183, 994-997.

Stewart, R.D. and Dodd, H.C., 1964. Absorption of carbon tetrachloride, trichloroethylene, tetrachloroethylene, methylene chloride, and 1, 1, 1-trichloroethane through the human skin. Am. Ind. Hyg. Assoc. J., 25, 439-446.

Stewart, B.W., Le Mesurier, S.M. and Lykke, A.W.J., 1979. Correlation of biochemical and morphological changes induced by chemical injury to the lung. Chem.-Biol. Interact., 26, 321-338.

Strubelt, O., Obermeier, F., Siegers, C.-P. and Völpel, M., 1978. Increased carbon tetrachloride hepatotoxicity after low-level ethanol consumption. Toxicology, 10, 261-270.

Suarez, K.A., Griffin, K., Kopplin, R.P. and Bhonsle, P., 1981. Protective effect of diethylmaleate pretreatment on carbon tetrachloride hepatotoxicity. Toxicol. Appl. Pharmacol., 57, 318-324.

Tsirel'nikov, N.I. and Tsirel'nikova, T.G., 1976. Morphohistochemical study of the rat placenta after exposure to carbon tetrachloride at different stages of pregnancy. Byull. eksp. Biol. Med., 82, 1007-1009.

Von Roschlau, G. and Rodenkirchen, H., 1969. Histological examination of the diaplacental action of carbon tetrachloride and allyl alcohol in mice embryos. Exp. Path., 3, 255-263.

Appendix 12
Methyl Iodide

CONTENTS

12.1 INTRODUCTION

Methyl iodide, CH_3I, has a molecular weight of 141.95. It melts at -66.45°C and boils at 42.4°C. In the liquid state it is colourless with a pungent odour and exhibits a vapour pressure of 400 mm at 25°C. Methyl iodide is slightly soluble in water (0.014 g ml^{-1} at 20°C); soluble in acetone, benzene and carbon tetrachloride; and miscible with ethanol and ether. It reacts with many compounds as an alkylating agent and turns brown on exposure to light, due to decomposition and liberation of free iodine (International Agency for Research on Cancer, 1977).

Methyl iodide is used as a methylating agent in the preparation of pharmaceutical intermediates and in organic synthesis. It is also used in microscopy, and as a reagent in testing for pyridine. Additionally, methyl iodide has been investigated as a fumigant to control internal fungi of grain sorghum (International Agency for Research on Cancer, 1977).

Commercial production of methyl iodide has been reported as 10^6 to 10^7 kg in the Federal Republic of Germany, Spain and the UK and as 6×10^4 to 8×10^4 kg in Japan.

12.2 LEVELS OF EXPOSURE

Data on levels of methyl iodide in the environment are limited. The compound occurs in the sea as a natural product of marine algae, and the mean concentration in air over the Atlantic has been reported as 1.2×10^{-12} v/v. In contrast, a concentration of 8×10^{-11} v/v, has been detected in the air over New Brunswick, New Jersey (International Agency for Research on Cancer, 1977). It is noted that these cited values were incorrectly converted to µg l^{-1} in that publication.

No data on levels of occupational exposure appear to have been reported in the literature, but Threshold Limit Values, applicable in the US, have been quoted as 5 ppm for a time-weighted average and 10 ppm for short-term exposure (Fishbein, 1979). These values correspond to 28 and 56 µg l^{-1} respectively.

12.3 EFFECTS

Data on the effects of methyl iodide are limited. The International Agency for Research on Cancer (1977) reviewed studies on acute toxicity which showed that the LD_{50} in mice as a result of subcutaneous injection was 110 mg kg^{-1}. Oral doses of 50 mg kg^{-1} for 5 days per week over a month produced no effect, but 57 minutes exposure to 5 mg l^{-1} in air produced 50% mortality.

Two cases of human poisoning after industrial exposure to vapours of methyl iodide have been reported. The first showed symptoms of vertigo, diplopia, ataxia, delirium and serious mental disturbance. The second case was found to be drowsy, unable to walk and with slurred, incoherent, speech. Death occurred 7 to 8 days after exposure and autopsy revealed bronchopneumonia and congestion of all organs (International Agency for Research on Cancer, 1977).

Erythematous reactions to methyl iodide applied to human skin have also been reported (International Agency for Research on Cancer, 1977)

With respect to carcinogenesis, there appear to be no relevant human data. However, experiments on rats (Druckrey et al.,1970; Preussman, 1968) have shown that subcutaneous injection of methyl iodide can induce tumours at the site of injection. Also, experiments on mice (Poirier et al., 1975) indicated that intraperitoneal injection of methyl iodide may induce, or promote, pulmonary tumours.

The only other study of relevance to methyl iodide toxicity appears to be that of Ohmichi (1977) who reported that 57 mg kg⁻¹ of methyl iodide, injected subcutaneously into rabbits, could induce hyperglycaemia and hypertriglycaemia. Attention is directed to the large dosage used in this study.

12.4   METABOLISM

Only four papers relevant to the metabolism of methyl iodide have been identified.

Barnsley and Young (1965) subcutaneously injected methyl iodide in arachis oil into rats and analysed successive 24 h urine specimens for metabolic products. Such products were not identifiable by paper chromatography except in the first 24 h after injection. On the basis of their studies, Barnsley and Young (1965) proposed the metabolic pathways shown in Fig. 1, but did not quantify their significance relative to total methyl iodide metabolism, except in so far as that they noted that the amounts excreted did not appear to exceed 0.5% of the administered dose.

Johnson (1966) administered methyl iodide orally, or intravenously to female white rats. Results indicated that orally administered methyl iodide is rapidly converted to S-methylglutathione in the liver. In two experiments, 22 and 28% of oral doses of methyl iodide were accounted for in bile over the first 6 h after dosing, mainly in the form of S-methylglutathione, but also as S-methylcysteine. At a dose corresponding to the acute LD_{50}, less than 1% of orally administered methyl iodide was lost in the exhaled air in the 30 minutes after dosing.

From his data, Johnson (1966) calculated that 45 to 50% of a 50 to 70 mg dose of methyl iodide orally administered to a 200 g rat is accounted for by reactions with liver glutathione.

Morgan and Morgan (1967) and Morgan et al. (1967) studied the retention and metabolism of the iodide moiety of methyl iodide in human volunteers who inhaled [I-132]CH_3. In the first of these two papers, Morgan and Morgan (1967) defined retention, R, by:

$$R = (A_i - A_e)/A_i$$

where A_i was the activity inhaled; and

A_e the activity exhaled.

Retention in any one individual was extremely reproducible, as illustrated by the following sequence of results obtained over a two week interval.

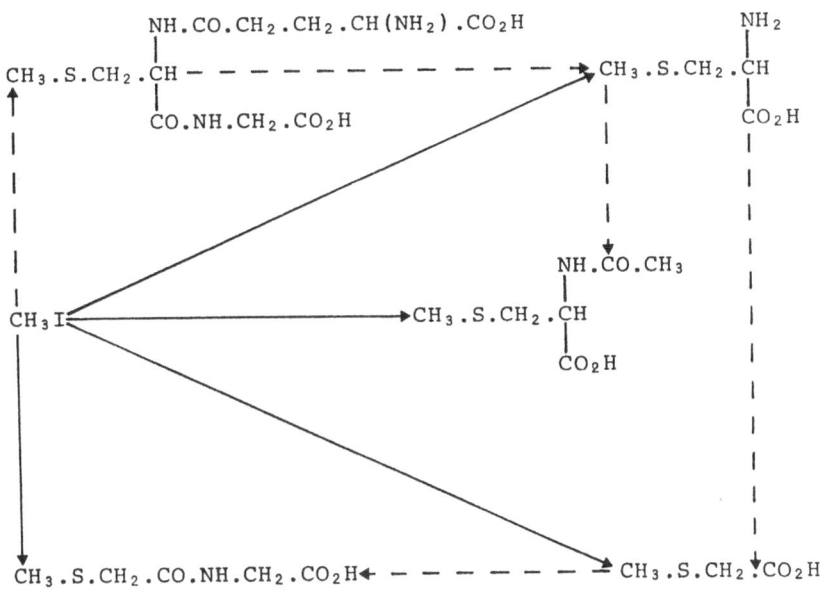

Note: From Barnsley and Young (1965)

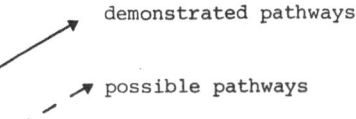 demonstrated pathways

possible pathways

FIGURE 1   PATHWAYS OF METHYL IODIDE METABOLISM

TABLE 1

MEASUREMENTS OF RESPIRATORY RATE; TIDAL, MINUTE AND TOTAL
VOLUMES; AND RESPIRATORY RETENTION OF METHYL IODIDE
IN EIGHTEEN HUMAN VOLUNTEERS[1]

Subject	Respiratory rate (breaths min.$^{-1}$)	Duration of breath (s)	Tidal volume (1)	Minute volume (1)	Vital capacity (1)	Retention (%)
A[2]	2.33	25.82	2.71	6.31	3.85	92
B	8.17	7.34	0.48	3.98	3.47	82
C	4.17	14.39	1.65	6.88	3.95	81
D	6.26	9.58	0.80	5.02	4.40	80
E	6.00	10.00	2.18	13.08	3.10	79
F	9.00	6.67	0.59	5.38	4.00	78
G	9.34	6.42	0.67	6.27	4.40	77
H	9.53	6.30	1.02	9.69	5.00	75
I	8.92	6.73	0.63	5.61	4.15	73
J	10.31	5.83	0.64	6.64	4.37	73
K	5.83	10.29	3.70	21.60	5.40	72
L	8.83	6.80	0.81	7.16	4.00	70
M	11.90	5.04	0.68	8.12	4.82	69
N	12.40	4.84	0.58	7.20	4.37	65
O	15.90	3.77	0.62	9.96	4.90	63
P	13.10	4.58	0.63	8.20	3.65	59
Q	14.30	4.20	1.06	15.18	4.70	54
R	19.50	3.08	0.37	7.20	3.08	53
Mean	9.8		1.10	8.5		72
Median	9.0		0.68	7.0		73
Normal range	10.1-13.1	5.9-4.6	0.58-0.90	5.8-10.3		

Notes:

(1)   From Morgan and Morgan (1967)
(2)   Only female subject

Tidal volume (l)	Minute volume (l)	R
1.16	11.57	0.738
0.94	9.38	0.762
0.92	9.23	0.735
1.00	9.97	0.756
0.94	9.43	0.759
0.91	9.11	0.755
$\bar{x}$ ± s.d. 0.98±0.09	9.78±0.84	0.751±0.012

Inter-subject variability was much larger (Table 1) and it was demonstrated that this variation was correlated highly with respiratory rate both on an inter- and on an intra-subject basis (Fig. 2).

Morgan and Morgan (1967) noted that their in vitro studies had shown that the reaction between methyl iodide and blood is extremely rapid at body temperatures, being complete within a matter of seconds. Correspondingly, in vivo there was no excretion of methyl iodide from the lungs at the end of the exposure period.

Morgan and Morgan (1967) also used their data to compute a half-time of clearance of methyl iodide from the lungs to the circulation. A value ~2 s was obtained.

Morgan et al. (1967) studied the metabolism of methyl iodide in human volunteers who inhaled [I-132]CH$_3$ in a single breath. In this study, the breath was held for 45 s following inspiration, ensuring that more than 99% of the methyl iodide was taken up into the body. For comparison, in a second experiment, one subject drank a solution of I-132 labelled sodium iodide. Comparison of the thyroid uptake and cumulative urinary excretion indicated no differences between the metabolism of I-132 in the two cases. Morgan et al. (1967) concluded that the similarity in thyroid uptake and urinary excretion rates, suggests that methyl iodide introduced by inhalation is broken down in vivo and that the organically bound iodine is converted to the iodide ion, which subsequently becomes involved in normal iodine metabolism. They noted that the absence of any apparent initial delay in thyroid uptake and urinary excretion following inhalation, suggest that this breakdown occurs very rapidly and commented that this conclusion was supported by the absence of organically bound iodine in the initial urine samples and demonstration, in vitro, of a factor in blood which produces a dramatic acceleration in the rate of hydrolysis of methyl iodide.

12.5 CONSIDERATIONS IN MODELLING AND THE DEVELOPMENT OF A MODEL RELEVANT TO MONITORING EXPOSURE

On the basis of data currently available, it is not possible to construct a detailed pharmacokinetic model for methyl iodide. If an individual is exposed to the vapour, ~75% of that inhaled will typically enter the circulation and be metabolised. Metabolism, which may occur in blood, liver and in other organs or tissues, involves the release of the iodide ion and further metabolism of the methyl group. In the liver, this further metabolism typically involves conjugation with glutathione. This conjugation and subsequent excretion of the conjugated products have not

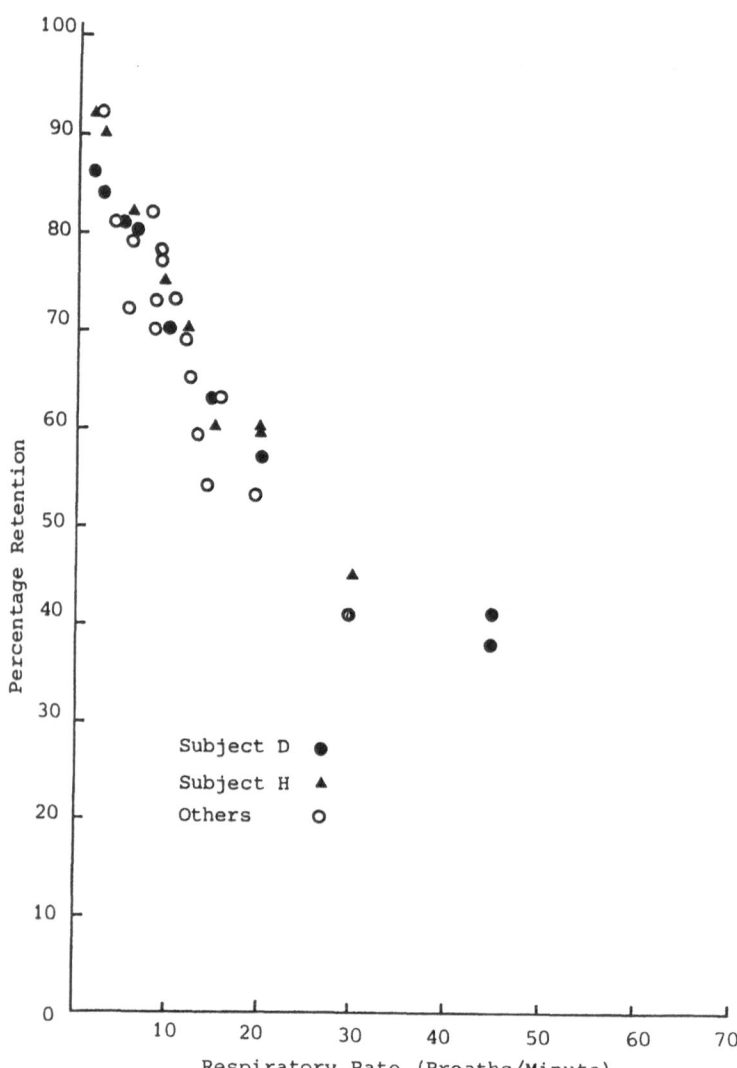

FIGURE 2   VARIATION OF PERCENTAGE RETENTION WITH
             RESPIRATORY RATE.

Note: From Morgan and Morgan (1967)

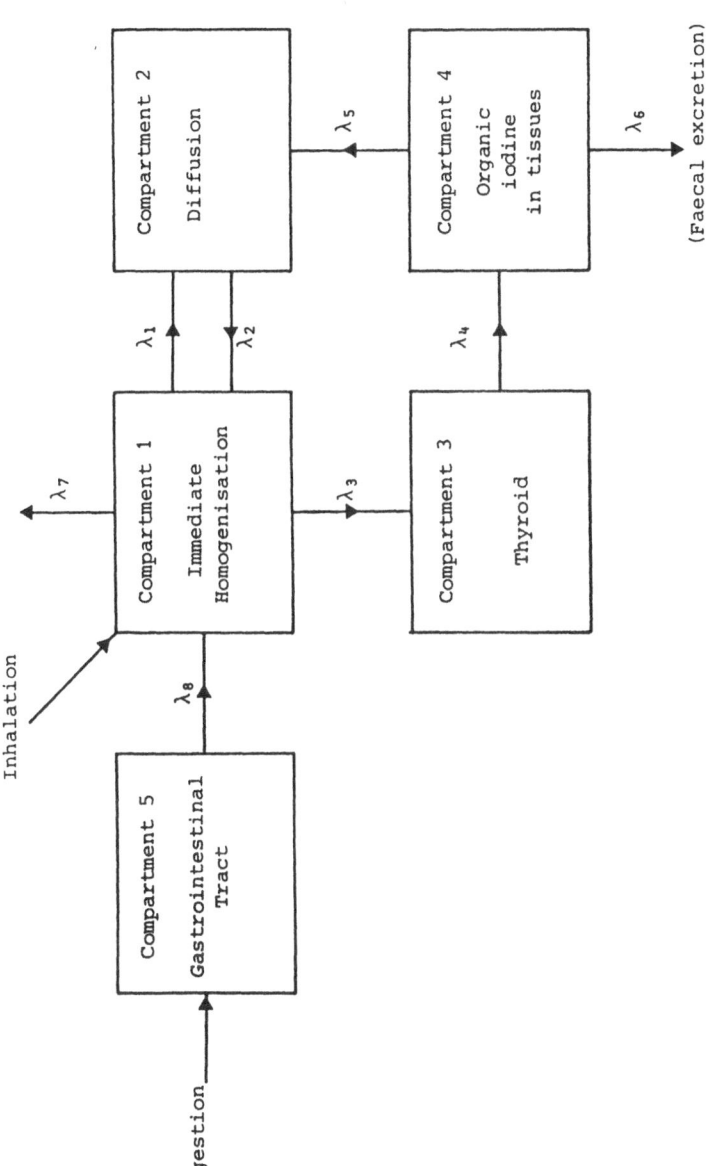

FIGURE 3   PROPOSED FIVE COMPARTMENT MODEL FOR THE METABOLISM OF IODINE.

Note: Adapted from Coughtrey et al. (1983)

been quantified in any detail. Furthermore, the products formed and excreted are unlikely to be specific to methyl iodide exposure.

With respect to the iodide released, an individual exposed to an atmosphere containing 5 ppm of methyl iodide would inhale ~2.7×10^5 µg of methyl iodide, corresponding to an uptake of 1.8×10^5 µg of iodine into the systemic circulation. This is very much more than the typical daily intake of iodine of 200 µg (International Commission on Radiological Protection, 1979) and suggests that exposure to methyl iodide could, in some circumstances, be monitored using a metabolic model for iodine. Such a model, which takes account of the effect of different levels of iodine intake on iodide metabolism, has been developed by Coughtrey et al. (1983). This model in illustrated in Fig. 3. For adult man, values of the various rate coefficients are as listed below.

Cofficient	Value (d^{-1})
λ_1	48
λ_2	18.7
λ_4	8.75×10^{-3}
λ_5	5.25×10^{-2}
λ_6	5.83×10^{-3}
λ_7	6.9

A value for λ_3 is estimated by consideration of the requirement to maintain homeostatic equilibrium. Thus,

$$\lambda_3 = \lambda_7(\lambda_5+\lambda_6)q_4/(I_{ING}+U_{INH}-\lambda_6 q_4)$$

where I_{ING} (mg d^{-1}) is the daily intake of iodine by ingestion;

U_{INH} (mg d^{-1}) is the daily uptake of iodine by inhalation; and

q_4 (mg) is the mass of organic iodine in tissues, which may be taken as 1.2 mg.

Thus, in this model, the thyroid effectively regulates its uptake of iodide and any excess is excreted in the urine.

It is noted that dietary iodine intakes can be very variable, depending on both locality and diet, and that this may need to be taken into account when using the above model for workplace monitoring.

12.6   REFERENCES

Barnsley, E.A. and Young, L., 1965. Biochemical studies of toxic agents. The metabolism of iodomethane. Biochem. J., 95, 77-81.

Coughtrey, P.J., Jackson, D. and Thorne, M.C., 1983. Radionuclide Distribution and Transport in Terrestrial and Aquatic Ecosystems. Vol. 3. A.A. Balkema, Rotterdam.

Druckrey, H., Kruse, H., Preussman, R., Ivankovic, S. and Landschütz, Ch., 1970. Cancerogene alkylierende Substanzen III. Alkyl-halogenide, -sulfate, -sulfonate und ringespannte Heterocyclen. Z. Krebsforsch., 74, 241-273.

Fishbein, L., 1979. Potential halogenated industrial carcinogenic and mutagenic chemicals II. Halogenated saturated hydrocarbons. Sci. Tot. Environ., 11, 163-195.

International Agency for Research on Cancer, 1977. Methyl iodide. IARC Monographs on the Evaluation of the Carcinogenic Risk of Chemicals to Humans, 15, 245-254.

International Commission on Radiological Protection, 1979. Limits for Intakes of Radionuclides by Workers. Part 1. Annals of the ICRP, 2, No. 3/4.

Johnson, M.K., 1966. Metabolism of iodomethane in the rat. Biochem. J., 98, 38-43.

Morgan, D.J. and Morgan, A., 1967. Studies on the retention and metabolism of inhaled methyl iodide-I. Retention of inhaled methyl iodide. Health Phys., 13, 1055-1065.

Morgan, A., Morgan, D.J., Evans, J.C. and Lister, B.A.J., 1967. Studies on the retention and metabolism of inhaled methyl iodide-II. Metabolism of methyl iodide. Health Phys., 13, 1067-1074.

Ohmichi, M., 1977. A comparative study of the effects of methyl iodide and cobalt chloride on the lipid metabolism in rabbits - with special reference to the cobalt alteration of coenzyme A, carnitine and their derivatives in rabbit liver. Nippon Eisegaku Zasshi, 32, 375-383.

Poirier, L.A., Stoner, G.D. and Shimkin, M.B., 1975. Bioassay of alkyl halides and nucleotide base analogs by pulmonary tumor response in strain A mice. Cancer Res., 35, 1411-1415.

Preussmann, R., 1968. Direct alkylating agents as carcinogens. Fd. Cosmet. Toxicol., 6, 576-577.